Neuroprognostication in Critical Care

Neuroprognostication in Critical Care

Edited by

David M. Greer
Boston University School of Medicine and Boston Medical Center

Neha S. Dangayach
Icahn School of Medicine at Mount Sinai and Mount Sinai Health System

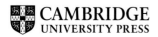

CAMBRIDGE
UNIVERSITY PRESS

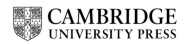

Shaftesbury Road, Cambridge CB2 8EA, United Kingdom

One Liberty Plaza, 20th Floor, New York, NY 10006, USA

477 Williamstown Road, Port Melbourne, VIC 3207, Australia

314–321, 3rd Floor, Plot 3, Splendor Forum, Jasola District Centre,
New Delhi – 110025, India

103 Penang Road, #05–06/07, Visioncrest Commercial, Singapore 238467

Cambridge University Press is part of Cambridge University Press & Assessment,
a department of the University of Cambridge.

We share the University's mission to contribute to society through the pursuit of
education, learning and research at the highest international levels of excellence.

www.cambridge.org
Information on this title: www.cambridge.org/9781108708272

DOI: 10.1017/9781108762489

First published 2024

A catalogue record for this publication is available from the British Library

Library of Congress Cataloging-in-Publication Data
Names: Greer, David M., 1966– editor. | Dangayach, Neha S., 1983– editor.
Title: Neuroprognostication in critical care / edited by David M. Greer, Neha S. Dangayach.
Description: Cambridge, United Kingdom ; New York : Cambridge University Press, 2024. |
Includes bibliographical references and index.
Identifiers: LCCN 2024006507 | ISBN 9781108708272 (paperback) | ISBN 9781108762489
(ebook)
Subjects: MESH: Critical Illness – therapy | Neurologic Examination | Decision Making,
Shared
Classification: LCC RC350.N49 | NLM WL 141 | DDC 616.8/0428–dc23/eng/20240214
LC record available at https://lccn.loc.gov/2024006507

ISBN 978-1-108-70827-2 Paperback
ISBN 978-1-108-76248-9 Cambridge Core

With gratitude to all of my residents, fellows and students over the many years, who have taught me far more than I could ever teach them; and to my wife, Stephanie, who has supported me through everything, everywhere.
David M. Greer

With the deepest love and respect for my parents, Subhash and Usha Dangayach who inspire me everyday with their positive thinking, an insatiable hunger for lifelong learning and a firm belief that nothing is impossible.
Neha S. Dangayach

Contents

Contributors

Alexander Allen
Department of Neurology, New York University School of Medicine, New York, NY, USA

Pria Anand
Department of Neurology, Boston Medical Center, Boston, MA, USA

Katharina Busl
Division of Neurocritical Care, Department of Neurology, University of Florida, Gainesville, FL, USA

Anna M. Cervantes-Arslanian,
Department of Neurology, Boston Medical Center, Boston, MA, USA

Tobias Cronberg
Lund University, Skåne University Hospital, Department of Clinical Sciences, Neurology, Lund, Sweden

Barry Czeisler
Department of Neurology, New York University School of Medicine, New York, NY, USA

Neha S. Dangayach
Department of Neurosurgery, Icahn School of Medicine at Mount Sinai, New York, NY, USA

Marie-Carmelle Elie-Turenne
Department of Emergency Medicine, University of Alabama at Birmingham School of Medicine, Birmingham, AL, USA

Brandon Foreman
Department of Neurology & Rehabilitation Medicine, University of Cincinnati, Cincinnati, OH, USA

Jonathan Gomez
Department of Neurology, Wake Forest School of Medicine, Winston Salem, NC, USA

Collin Herman
Department of Neurology, Wake Forest School of Medicine, Winston Salem, NC, USA

Shannon Hextrum
Department of Neurosurgery, Tulane University School of Medicine, New Orleans, LA, USA.

Zachary L. Hickman
Department of Neurosurgery, Icahn School of Medicine at Mount Sinai, New York, NY, USA
Department of Neurosurgery, NYC Health + Hospitals/Elmhurst, Queens, NY, USA

Salazar A. Jones
Department of Neurosurgery, Icahn School of Medicine at Mount Sinai, New York, NY, USA

Eyal Y. Kimchi
Department of Neurology, Massachusetts General Hospital, Boston, MA, USA

Matthew Kirschen
Department of Anesthesiology and Critical Care Medicine, Children's Hospital of Philadelphia, Perelman School of Medicine at the University of Pennsylvania, Philadelphia, PA, USA

Christopher L. Kramer
Department of Neurology, University of Chicago, Chicago, IL, USA

Natalie Kreitzer
Department of Emergency Medicine, University of Cincinnati, Cincinnati, OH, USA

Kerri L. LaRovere
Department of Neurology, Harvard Medical School and Boston Children's Hospital, Boston, MA, USA

Cappi Lay
Institute of Critical Care Medicine; Mount Sinai West, New York, NY, USA
Institute of Critical Care Medicine, Icahn School of Medicine at Mount Sinai, New York, NY, USA

Sarah Lelin
Institute of Critical Care Medicine, Mount Sinai Health System, New York, NY, USA

Ariane Lewis
Department of Neurology, NYU Langone Medical Center, New York, NY, USA

Aaron Sylvan Lord
Department of Neurology, NYU Langone Hospital – Brooklyn, Brooklyn, NY, USA
Department of Neurology and Neurosurgery, NYU Grossman School of Medicine, New York, NY, USA

Matthew B. Maas
Departments of Neurology and Anesthesiology, Northwestern University, Evanston, IL, USA

Carolina B. Maciel
Department of Neurology, University of Florida College of Medicine, Gainesville, FL, USA

Edward M. Manno
Ken and Ruth Davee Department of Neurology Northwestern University Feinberg School of Medicine
Chicago, IL, USA

Konstantinos Margetis
Department of Neurosurgery, Icahn School of Medicine at Mount Sinai, New York, NY, USA

Matthew Miller
Boston University School of Medicine, Boston, MA, USA

Sarah E. Nelson
Division of Neurosciences Critical Care, Departments of Anesthesiology and Critical Care Medicine, Neurology and Neurosurgery, The Johns Hopkins University School of Medicine, Baltimore, MD, USA

Charlene Ong
Department of Neurology, Boston University School of Medicine, Boston, MA, USA

Anuj D. Patel
Department of Neurology, MD Anderson Cancer Center, Houston, TX, USA

Pirouz Piran
Division of Neurosciences Critical Care, Departments of Anesthesiology and Critical Care Medicine, Neurology and Neurosurgery, The Johns Hopkins University School of Medicine, Baltimore, MD, USA

Michael A. Pizzi
Division of Neurocritical Care, Department of Neurology, University of Florida, Gainesville, FL, USA

Alejandro A. Rabinstein
Department of Neurology, Mayo Clinic, Rochester, MN, USA

Alexandra S. Reynolds
Department of Neurosurgery, Icahn School of Medicine at Mount Sinai, New York, NY, USA

Andrea O. Rossetti
Department of Clinical Neurosciences, University hospital (CHUV) and University of Lausanne, Switzerland

William Roth
Department of Neurology, University of Florida College of Medicine, Gainesville, FL, USA

Sophia L. Ryan
Department of Neurology, Icahn School of Medicine at Mount Sinai, New York, NY, USA

Rajbeer S. Sangha
Department of Neurology, University of Alabama, Birmingham, AL, USA

E. Alton Sartor
Department of Neurology, Boston University Chobanian & Avedisian School of Medicine, Boston, MA, USA

Aarti Sarwal
Department of Neurology, Wake Forest School of Medicine, Winston Salem, NC, USA

Thomas D. Schiano
Department of Medicine, Icahn School of Medicine at Mount Sinai, New York, NY, USA

Sanjeev Sivakumar
University of South Carolina School of Medicine-Greenville, Greenville, SC, USA

Jose I Suarez
Division of Neurosciences Critical Care, Departments of Anesthesiology and Critical Care Medicine, Neurology and Neurosurgery, The Johns Hopkins University School of Medicine, Baltimore, MD, USA

Kushak Suchdev
Boston University School of Medicine, Boston, MA, USA

Courtney Takahashi
Department of Neurology, Boston University Medical Center, Boston, MA, USA

Robert C. Tasker
Department of Neurology, Harvard Medical School and Boston Children's Hospital, Boston, MA, USA

Alexis Topjian
Department of Anesthesiology and Critical Care Medicine, Children's Hospital of Philadelphia, Perelman School of Medicine at the University of Pennsylvania, Philadelphia, PA, USA

Mark S. Wainwright
Department of Neurology, University of Washington School of Medicine, Seattle, WA, USA

Jeffrey Zimering
Department of Neurosurgery, Icahn School of Medicine at Mount Sinai, New York, NY, USA

Shared Decision Making

Neha S. Dangayach

Case Study 1.1 A 72-year-old woman with several risk factors for stroke including atrial fibrillation on coumadin, hypertension, and diabetes mellitus type II presented with sudden onset of left hemiparesis, left homonymous hemianopia, and right gaze preference with a National Institutes of Health Stroke Scale (NIHSS) of 15. Her head computed tomography (CT) did not show any acute signs of stroke or hemorrhage. Her CT angiogram showed a right middle cerebral artery (MCA) cut-off. Her International Normalized Ratio (INR) was 1.6 and she received intravenous thrombolysis. She was taken emergently for thrombectomy and despite a successful recanalization, her exam did not improve. Post-thrombetcomy head CT showed hemorrhagic transformation of her stroke. She was deemed to be at a high risk of developing malignant cerebral edema.

The Neurocritical Care, Neurosurgery, and Stroke team members discussed the options for managing her malignant cerebral edema and presented the evidence and consensus regarding hemicraniectomy to the family. The patient's husband and four adult children were present at this meeting. While her husband was regarded as the primary decision maker, it was well established during this meeting that all five family members would be participating in key management decisions and the patient's husband would be the one signing any consent forms. When the medical and surgical options for treatment of malignant cerebral edema were discussed with the family, the neurocritical care attending made it clear that the stroke could leave the patient debilitated with profound deficits, and while surgery would be a life-saving option it would not be a quality of life-preserving measure. She also acknowledged that while a lot had happened in the past few hours, it was imperative to give the family information

about these options and outcomes since the patient hadn't developed malignant edema yet but was likely to do so over the next few hours. Sharing the evidence and the consensus from the different teams was meant to help the family think about these options, and to allow them to weigh against the wishes and values of their loved one. She asked the family to think about what was the least possible quality of life that would make their loved one happy. After a couple of hours, the family shared that the patient would have wanted every possible chance to see her grandchildren even if she was bed bound. The patient was taken for a hemicraniectomy. She required a tracheostomy, a percutaneous gastrostomy (PEG) tube, and placement in a long-term acute care hospital (LTACH). All of these decisions upheld the principles of shared decision making (SDM) with the patient's family.

What Is Shared Decision Making?

Shared decision making (SDM) is a collaborative process that allows patients, or their surrogates, and clinicians to make healthcare decisions together, taking into account the best scientific evidence available, as well as the patient's values, goals, and preferences. This definition of SDM proposed by the Informed Medical Decisions Foundation [1] was endorsed by the American College of Critical Care Medicine (ACCM) and the American Thoracic Society (ATS) (Figure 1.1). Informed medical decision making may be used synonymously with SDM.[2] Critically ill patients may be too unstable or otherwise incapacitated (e.g., due to intubation, sedation), and may not be able to speak for themselves. In such situations, advance directives from the patient or conversations that they may have had with their families regarding

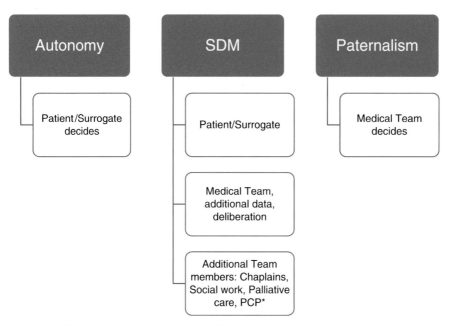

Figure 1.1 What medical decisions need to be made? What pros, cons, and uncertainties need to be weighed? Who makes medical decisions based on three different models? (Adapted from Xumei Cai et al., NCC 2015.[3].)

*PCP = Primary Care Physician

preferences for specific medical conditions or anticipated prognosis can help guide SDM. Families of such critically ill patients play a key role in medical decision making by sharing what they know about the patient's values, goals and wishes, while the medical team shares medical updates, information about prognosis and possible treatment options. Thus, with substituted judgment, medical teams are able to uphold the principles of patient-centered care and SDM in critical care, and particularly in neurocritical care.[3,4]

In this chapter, we discuss principles of SDM and how it can be applied in the neurocritical care setting, along with some strategies to overcome barriers.

Historical Perspective

Shared decision making was first introduced in 1982 by the President's Commission for the Study of Ethical Problems in Medicine and Biomedical and Behavioral Research.[5]

In 2010, federal healthcare reform in the United States included SDM. Since then, SDM has received increasing attention by healthcare providers and policy makers exploring opportunities to incorporate SDM into the standard of care. In October 2011, the National Academy for State Health Policy (NASHP) convened a meeting of state and federal officials, SDM experts, and consumer, provider, and purchaser representatives to discuss opportunities and challenges for implementation of SDM at the state level, and how these lessons from state experience could be applied to federal policies.[6] SDM has been included into federal rules for Accountable Care Organizations (ACOs). Countries like the United Kingdom have partnered with physician and patient champions to disseminate SDM decision aids to ensure successful implementation of SDM in health policy.[7]

Why Is SDM Important?

SDM helps improve clinical care and patient safety by encouraging the development and dissemination of the best possible evidence regarding risks and benefits of different management strategies in ways that patients can understand, and increases patient involvement in decision making. SDM interventions not only help in increasing active patient participation in informed decision making, but also help in setting realistic expectations, improving agreement between different stakeholders, and improving compliance with treatments as well as satisfaction with health outcomes.[8] SDM also has the potential to improve the health of populations and individual patients while helping reduce overall healthcare costs.[9] SDM along with decision aids have shown promising results for reducing unwarranted variations in care, as well as improving patient satisfaction.[6]

In an intensive care unit (ICU) setting, interventions such as feeding tube placement, tracheostomy, and initiation of renal replacement therapy tend to be important transitional aspects of a patient's care. While patients and families may not need to be involved in decision making about electrolyte replacement or antibiotic use, they almost always need to be involved in decision making about these important transitional aspects of care.[10] As new discoveries are made or practice changing evidence becomes available, SDM also helps in translating this new research into clinical practice.[11]

Models of SDM

Several models of SDM have been described that take patient preferences into account when more than one reasonable option is available. While these different models have not been studied specifically in the neurocritical care setting, they could all be reasonably adapted to facilitate SDM for neurocritical care. Examples of such models include Elwyn et al.'s model,[12] a three-step model to introduce choices with justification for each, describe options, and help patients explore preferences and make decisions. Another example is an expanded SDM model by Stacy et al. [13], which includes the family, surrogate decision makers, and interprofessional team members in SDM.

The process of SDM involves the following steps, regardless of the SDM model used:[5]

- Define and explain the problem.
- Define roles and desire for involvement.
- Present options.
- Discuss pros and cons.
- Share patient values and preferences.
- Discuss patient ability and self-efficacy.
- Offer knowledge and communication.
- Check and clarify understanding.
- Make or explicitly defer a decision.

- Arrange a follow-up.
- Come to a mutual agreement.

The Role of Family Meetings

Conducting family meetings with the above process in mind can help align the proposed options and outcomes with a patient's goals, values, and wishes. It is important to establish a partnership with surrogates early in the course of a critically ill patient's care.

The American College of Critical Care Medicine ((ACCM) recommends that family meetings with the multiprofessional ICU team should start within the first 24–48 hours of admission, and be scheduled at regular intervals and as needed.[14] Patients, surrogates, or family members can be invited to participate in rounds to build trust, improve understanding, and help establish rapport. This partnership can then be leveraged for making key medical decisions.[15] A proactive multidisciplinary approach can help prevent and reduce conflict. Protocolized family meetings at 72 hours are associated with higher satisfaction for families of critically ill patients. [16]

Identifying the Right Surrogate

While patients may have multiple family members who may wish to be involved in decision making, from a legal standpoint, different US states have provided guidance on what the hierarchy for surrogates should be for participation in decision making. Some states, such as New York and Massachusetts, allow for two-physician consent for life-saving procedures if no surrogates are identifiable despite reasonable attempts. In some situations, a state-appointed guardian may be needed. About 16% of critically ill patients may have neither decision-making capacity nor a surrogate.[28] Even when advance care planning (ACP) documentation is available, it needs to be put into the context of the acute neurological injury and anticipated prognosis.

Roles of Physicians in SDM

There are several aspects of critical care that will not benefit from patient or family input.

Therapies and practices sometimes provide no benefit or even cause disproportionate harm to certain populations of patients; thus, physicians should not offer interventions if they are convinced they would cause harm.

In situations where the prognosis is uncertain, that uncertainty should be shared clearly with surrogates. Prognosis in different patient-centered domains, such as physical, cognitive, and behavioral, should be emphasized whenever possible. Studies from different critical care settings show that preferences for participation in SDM vary depending on personal, familial, and cultural backgrounds. It is important to state the role and preference for what role surrogate decision makers may want to play. Surrogate decision makers may confuse their own interests or preferences with those of the patient. Surrogates should be asked to share any prior conversations regarding known wishes, and if no such conversations have occurred previously, they should be encouraged to make substituted judgments based on what they think the patient would say if they could speak for themselves. If that is not possible, the surrogates should work closely with the care team to help make decisions in the patient's best interests based on what they can best estimate would be what the patient would state if they were able (substituted judgment).

Role of Decision Aids in SDM

Decision aids are tools that help in sharing evidence-based information with patients and surrogates. Only a few decision aids have been studied in the neurocritical care setting. The International Patient Decision Aids Standards (IPDAS) Collaboration defines decision aids as tools that present treatment options in a balanced and evidence-based manner.[17]

It is also important to learn the different ways to communicate risk: (1) presenting absolute risk instead of relative risk; (2) highlighting incremental risk associated with treatment distinctly as compared to baseline risks; and (3) using pictographs to communicate risk and benefit if possible. Decision aids differ in important ways from other decision tools, should meet formal standards for framing the presentation of medical information to patients, and should be developed in line with the principles of SDM.[18]

Decision aids have been designed to achieve different goals, for example to improve knowledge about clinical issues and to discuss risks or benefits of different alternatives to treatments.[6]

Randomized controlled trials (RCTs) have shown that decision aids help improve the quality and efficiency of decision making and decrease conflict.[18–20]

Different formats for decision aids such videos [21] printed [22] and online materials have been [18] studied in RCTs. For ACP in patients with dementia, three RCTs [19,22,23] have shown that video-based decision aids improved understanding and increased patient satisfaction with their choices.

Literacy-adjusted decision aids for explaining ACP have been found to be more effective in helping patients complete a written advance directive. [5] Decisional conflict can be reduced with decision aids. A high-quality study by Hanson et al. found that a decision-making tool on feeding options in patients with advanced dementia in nursing homes led to significant decreases in decisional conflict.[22]

These trials on decision aids have not measured the impact on clinical outcomes.[18] While decision aids can improve knowledge, it is not clear that this translates into improved outcomes. Future research should focus on randomized controlled trials of decision aids and tools designed specifically for neurocritical care patients, and include outcomes beyond improvement in knowledge, such as whether care was consistent with preferences of the patient, as well as satisfaction with clinical care.[24,25]

Barriers to SDM in Critical Care

Shared decision making should be leveraged throughout the continuum of care for any critically ill patient, not just at key decision points. However, SDM can be challenging for various reasons, including the need to make time-sensitive decisions that may impact the ongoing life-saving measures, uncertainty about prognosis, and not knowing or misinterpreting the patient's *a priori* wishes given the sudden onset of an acute brain injury. Patients may have capacity for making one type of decision but may not be able to make other types of decisions depending on the timing of the injury and patient's clinical status. For example, a patient with a right MCA stroke may be able to understand that he has a stroke and is at risk of developing cerebral edema. This patient may be able to participate in decision making about a life-saving surgery such as hemicraniectomy. If this patient's clinical course is later complicated by new onset status epilepticus, they may no longer be able to participate in the decision making regarding the placement of a tracheostomy tube or feeding tube. The dynamic course of any acute brain injury may further complicate the ability to engage critically ill patients in SDM. Many critically ill patients are unable to make decisions for themselves due to fluctuating levels of consciousness, underlying neurological diseases, sedation, analgesia, toxic metabolic encephalopathy, and hemodynamic instability, among other reasons. SDM requires a substantial investment of time and effort from ICU teams, which may not always be possible in busy ICU settings.

Another area that may contribute to difficulties in decision making includes the perceived differences in prognosis between healthcare providers and families/surrogates. Education about SDM, upholding cultural and religious beliefs, is needed to ensure that healthcare providers understand the value system of patients better while guiding families in making appropriate decisions. Physician–surrogate discordance about prognosis can occur more than half the time in critically ill patients.[26] Such discordance is usually related to both misunderstandings by surrogates and differences in belief about the patient's prognosis.[27] Discordance in expected roles in SDM for surrogates can lead not only to miscommunication but also to anxiety and depression. However, clinicians rarely check for family understanding of the information, or elicit from the family members their preferred roles in decision making.[28]

There are several key issues in implementing SDM. There is a lack of dedicated training to understand and implement SDM in critically ill patients. Decisional conflict can arise from a lack of advance care planning, misinterpretation of patient's stated preferences, or misinterpretation of values and goals if these were not previously stated explicitly. Patients and surrogates may have different preferences for how much they want to be involved in the decision-making process. They may also differ in how much they rely on input from their care providers to make healthcare decisions. For example, older patients tend to rely more on physician guidance compared to younger patients; more educated patients prefer to be equal partners in making healthcare decisions compared to less educated patients.[18,29] Patients facing unfamiliar or uncertain situations may want to rely more on physicians or family members to help guide their preferences, both for participation in SDM as well as treatment decisions. Another issue may be a lack of availability of decision aids or validated decision tools in a language that the patient can understand. Patients and surrogates may experience difficulty in understanding numerical information and may prefer qualitative data.[5]

These barriers can be overcome with a multipronged approach. Engaging a multidisciplinary team in regular family meetings, establishing rapport with the surrogates early in the course of a critically ill patient, ideally within 24–48 hours of an ICU admission, clearly identifying and delineating roles in SDM, and, similarly, verbalizing the goals of treatment and expected prognosis, as well as acknowledging uncertainties can help overcome some of these barriers to SDM. Including education about SDM in medical school and training curricula can help physicians, nurses, and advanced practice providers (APPs) learn more about the key principles of SDM, how to apply those to their care settings, understand the gaps in literature, and become more familiar with regional health policies regarding SDM.

Participation in SDM may be limited by health literacy. Educated families may not participate as much as more educated families. The extent to which families want to participate in SDM is also variable. Approximately 15–30% of families preferred to play an active role in decision making for critically ill patients.[29,30] For others, SDM provides an opportunity to honor the patient by ensuring that the treatment plan is consistent with the patient's values, even if those values are different from those of the family members. In a study conducted in French ICUs, Pochard et al. reported that the strongest predictor of post-traumatic stress in surrogate decision makers was when they reported receiving inadequate information from the physician.[31] They also noted that active participation in decisions was associated with more post-traumatic stress symptoms.[31] This variability in preferences suggests that explicit discussion of roles in decision making may be a crucial step in the process of achieving appropriate family involvement in decisions.[32]

SDM in Neurocritical Care

Acknowledging Uncertainties in Neuroprognostication

Despite the progress in neurocritical care, there are still significant gaps in neuroprognostication for common neurocritical care diseases like subarachnoid hemorrhage (SAH), intracerebral hemorrhage (ICH), acute ischemic stroke, and traumatic brain injury ((TBI). This is further challenged by therapeutic nihilism in neurological emergencies, [33] where a nihilistic attitude could contribute to worse outcomes than what empiric evidence from retrospective or prospective cohorts may suggest. For instance, it is well known that in-hospital mortality after ICH is significantly influenced by the rate at which treating hospitals use do-not-resuscitate (DNR) orders, even after adjusting for case mix. This was thought to be not solely due to an individual patient's DNR order, but perhaps due to changes in the overall care once a patient was made DNR.[33] How we communicate the best evidence available for neuroprognostication while acknowledging the uncertainty in prognostication, in order to give patients a chance of meaningful recovery, is perhaps one of the most important aspects of SDM in neurocritical care. Quantifying what "recovery" means in different domains, including consciousness, physical functioning, cognitive and behavioral outcomes, as well as reintegration into life roles, such as the ability to return to work, can help all team members and surrogates better understand whether or not those outcomes might be in line with a patient's goals, values, and wishes.[34] Communicating prognosis while a patient is actively herniating or has impending herniation may become even more challenging when decisions about time-sensitive life-saving interventions need to be made without having certainty in what a patient's quality of life may be if they survive.

Surrogates often play an important role in medical decisions in neurocritical care for patients with severe acute brain injuries who cannot speak for themselves. It is important to determine patient preferences, understand goals, values, and wishes, and provide estimates of prognosis with the best possible evidence to guide decision making. Patient preferences can be determined by: (1) existing advance care documentation, (2) surrogate decision makers, (3) defining roles for surrogates and physicians, and (4) conducting effective and timely family meetings, based on studies of ICU families in crises.[3,35] The Control Preference Scale may help in understanding patient preferences regarding healthcare decision making. This scale includes questions regarding how patients prefer making final treatment decisions, whether they prefer making these decisions based on their doctor's opinion, whether they would like their doctor to share the decision-making responsibility, or whether their doctor would make the final decision after considering their opinion.[5]

How to Implement SDM in Neurocritical Care

Determining Capacity for Decision Making

Capacity for decision making can be determined by a qualified medical team member; the elements for assessing such capacity include but are not limited to determining how much the patient understands about their disease process, whether they understand the consequences of opting for or against a particular treatment recommendation, or whether they understand the uncertainties in prognostication. However, it must be kept in mind that this is not an absolute determination. Capacity for decision making can vary depending on a patient's clinical course or the type of decision. Patients may have the capacity for one type of decision but not for another (as described above in the section Barriers to SDM in Critical Care).[8] Using communication aids for nonverbal patients, such writing or communication boards [11] or computer interfaces,[13] can also help them participate more effectively in decision making.

Advanced Care Planning Documentation

Only a third of American adults have an advance care directive in place.[24] In a survey conducted by AARP (formerly the American Association of Retired Persons), while most people prefer to die at home, about 25% have not communicated their preferences to their families.[36] Studies have shown that prior documentation about advance care planning can help reduce stress for surrogates in medical decision making. There are several different types of advance care documents, such as Physician Orders for Life-Sustaining Therapies (POLST), Medical Orders for Life-Sustaining Therapies (MOLST), healthcare proxy forms, and written advance directives.

Key Issues with ACP Documents

These documents can sometimes have very little detail or may even lack any discussion about preferences [25] regarding specific treatments or procedures such as a PEG, tracheostomy tube, or renal replacement therapies, or the kind of quality of life a patient may consider acceptable.[27] Given the variabilities that exist in these documents, with the exception of POLST forms,[24] they are not legally binding.

Approach to SDM in Neurocritical Care

In a review about SDM in neurocritical care, the following approach was suggested:[3]

- Acknowledge uncertainty in prognosis.
- Agree on a time-limited trial of critical care to prevent premature withdrawal of life-sustaining therapy.
- If disagreement between surrogates and medical team members, offer a second opinion.
- Palliative care and ethics consultation may be beneficial in helping resolve conflict.

Family satisfaction with SDM in neurocritical care settings can be measured using the family satisfaction in the ICU (FS-ICU) questionnaire. In a study of 134 patients or surrogates completing this tool, researchers found that parents of patients in neurocritical care units have higher short-term satisfaction with SDM compared to other surrogates. In the ICU, about 20% surrogates or patients reported inconsistent caregiver–patient communication in the first 48 hours that made decision making difficult.[37]

SDM in Different Disease States in Neurocritical Care

SDM in TBI

In a qualitative study involving 20 adult TBI patients the authors found that participating in healthcare decision making helped patients regain their sense of autonomy.[38] While it is important

to maximize patients' participation in the decision-making process, this may not always be possible given the severity of the underlying TBI.

In a small qualitative study of SDM in severe TBI aiming to understand how surrogates decided to continue or withdraw life-sustaining therapy, 8/10 reported that they would make the same decision again. Surrogates used input from different sources to help guide treatment decisions, and described the need for support from a trauma advanced practice nurse or palliative care team. [39] In a recent study, Muehlschelgel et al. described a novel goals-of-care decision aid for surrogates of patients critically ill with TBI. This mixed methods study with qualitative interviews showed excellent usability, acceptability, and early feasibility in the neurocritical care environment. This methodology could potentially be used for developing other decision aids in neurology to promote SDM.[27] There is a lot of variability in predicting outcomes, and ongoing research can help harmonize how we prognosticate.[40] Although an unlimited endeavor for sustaining life seems unrealistic, treatment-limiting decisions should not deprive patients of a chance to achieve an outcome they would have considered acceptable.[41]

In severe TBI patients who develop life-threatening intractable intracranial hypertension, interventions with high morbidity such as surgical decompression or pharmacological coma have to be considered against a backdrop of uncertain outcomes, including prolonged states of disordered consciousness and severe disability. The clinical evidence available to guide shared decision making is limited in such situations.[34] There are no decision aids that could assist in rationally navigating available options, describing the nature and range of outcomes to surrogates, and incorporating patients' values into goals of care.[26]

SDM in Stroke (Including Ischemic and Hemorrhagic Stroke)

A commonly studied example of SDM in ischemic stroke care has been secondary stroke prevention in patients with atrial fibrillation.[42] Another area where several aspects of SDM have been studied is palliative care. Palliative care needs of serious or life-threatening stroke patients are enormous, including complex decision making, aligning treatment with goals, and symptom control. The care of stroke patients can become very compartmentalized, potentially leading to fragmentation as different key stake holders get involved during different phases of care and family-centered care are ultimately determined by the quality of interactions between patients, family members, and clinicians.

The following excerpt from the "Approaches to Overcome Challenges with Decision Making in Stroke: Recommendations from the American Heart Association (AHA) guideline statement on Palliative Care in Stroke" [43] provides some key recommendations for SDM in stroke patients

1. Providers should recognize that surrogate decision makers use many other sources of information in addition to the doctor's expertise in understanding their loved one's prognosis (Class I; Level of Evidence B).

2. Providers should recognize that making surrogate decisions has a lasting negative emotional impact on a sizeable minority of surrogates, who should be provided access to bereavement services (Class I; Level of Evidence B).

3. Providers should be knowledgeable and respectful of diverse cultural and religious preferences when establishing goals of care and refer to social workers and chaplains when appropriate (Class I; Level of Evidence B).

4. It might be useful for providers to practice self-awareness strategies (prognostic time out, self-reflection) of one's own biases and emotional state to minimize errors in prognostic estimates and goal setting recommendations (Class IIb; Level of Evidence B).

5. It might be reasonable for providers to recognize the existence of a possible self-fulfilling prophecy (i.e., a prediction that might directly or indirectly cause itself to become true) when prognosticating and making end-of-life decisions in patients with stroke (Class IIb; Level of Evidence B).

6. It might be reasonable for providers to be mindful of and to educate patients and surrogate decision makers about the possible cognitive biases (affective forecasting errors, focusing effects, and optimism bias) that might exist when discussing treatment options and establishing goals of care (Class IIb; Level of Evidence C).

7. Providers might consider the use of time-limited treatment trials with a well-defined outcome to better understand the prognosis or to allow additional time to optimize additional aspects of decision making (Class IIb; Level of Evidence C).

SDM in Spinal Cord Injuries and Neuromuscular Disorders

For patients who can speak for themselves or participate in decision making about life-sustaining therapies, such as patients with acute spinal cord injury or patients with neuromuscular emergencies such as myasthenic crisis or Guillain–Barré syndrome (GBS), they should be engaged early in the process for key decision points regarding tracheostomy and permanent feeding tube placement and transition of care.

SDM for Patients with Neurodegenerative Disorders

For patients with neurodegenerative disorders, multidisciplinary clinic teams typically follow these patients in outpatient settings as well, for example, a specialized clinic for patients with amyotrophic lateral sclerosis (ALS). Outpatient settings present important opportunities to discuss what an acceptable quality of life would be in the event of worsening or new deficits and what values should be kept in mind when instituting life-sustaining therapies in the event of critical illness. This will provide patients with the ability to participate in SDM prior to being in extremis. The burden of decision making in such situations will not be hindered by a lack of time or ability of the patient to engage key stakeholders, including family members, in the weeks or months preceding an inevitable deterioration. This will enable the team providing acute care to the patient to honor the patient's *a priori* stated values and wishes.

SDM in Cardiac Arrest

A pilot study conducted in two Canadian hospitals including patients and family members using a video-based SDM decision aid for cardiopulmonary resuscitation (CPR) found that a CPR decision video helped improve the knowledge about CPR for patients and family members. Such a video-based approach, along with discussions with the treating physician, may also help reduce decisional conflict and reduce the prevalence of medical orders for CPR in the Canadian hospital setting.[44]

For patients with preexisting disorders, chronic conditions, or underlying cancer, discussions about code status and their wishes regarding life-sustaining therapies in the event of cardiac arrest should be discussed prior to hospitalization in a controlled outpatient setting as much as possible. This allows the teams that know the patient best over a period of time to weigh appropriate treatment options and expected trajectories of recovery to guide patients and their families in the SDM process. When code status is not discussed in a timely fashion with the patient or their families in these situations, it may create unnecessary distress.

Education about SDM

Teaching trainees about SDM and how to conduct family meetings can help address gaps in how families are involved in this process on the frontlines. Advances in medicine help us now prolong life in ways not possible a few years ago, utilizing scoring systems to estimate prognosis in different domains. For example, while the Hunt and Hess score, first reported in literature in 1968 [45] and has stood the test of time for predicting mortality after SAH, it must be acknowledged that over the past two decades the outcomes for "poor grade" SAH patients have improved, with a third of these patients having good functional outcomes with aggressive care.[46,47] It is important to incorporate prognostic estimates from more recent studies while guiding families through SDM.

Conclusion

Shared decision making is a very important aspect of patient-centered care. More research is needed to improve our understanding of prognostication in neurocritical care and incorporate this improved understanding in the implementation of SDM. Similarly, studies that evaluate the effectiveness of different decision aids for neurocritical care patients can help incorporate the most effective decision aids for patients.

References

1. Informed Medical Decision Foundation. Healthwise. Available from: www.healthwise.org/specialpages/imdf.aspx

2. McNutt RA. Shared medical decision making: problems, process, progress. *JAMA.* 2004;**292**:2516–18.

3. Cai X, Robinson J, Muehlschlegel S, et al. Patient preferences and surrogate decision making in neuroscience intensive care units. *Neurocrit Care.* 2015;**23**(1):131–41.

4. Phillips J, Wendler D. Clarifying substituted judgement: the endorsed life approach. *J Med Ethics.* 2015;**41**(9):723–30.

5. Lin GA, Fagerlin A. Shared decision making state of the science. *Circ Cardiovasc Qual Outcomes.* 2014;**7**(2):328–34.

6. Shafir A, Rosenthal J. Shared decision making: advancing patient-centered care through state and federal implementation. National Academy for State Health Policy. *Open J Nurs.* 2012;**7**(7).

7. Légaré F, Witteman HO. Shared decision making: examining key elements and barriers to adoption into routine clinical practice. *Health Aff.* 2013;**32**(2):276–84.

8. Kon AA, Davidson JE, Morrison W, Danis M, White DB. Shared decision making in ICUs: an American College of Critical Care Medicine and American Thoracic Society policy statement. *Crit Care Med.* 2016;**44**(1):188–201.

9. Frosch DL, Moulton BW, Wexler RM, et al. Shared decision making in the United States: policy and implementation activity on multiple fronts. *Z Evid Fortbild Qual Gesundhwes.* 2011;**105**(4):305–12.

10. Turnbull AE, Sahetya SK, Needham DM. Aligning critical care interventions with patient goals: a modified Delphi study. *Heart Lung J Acute Crit Care.* 2016;**45**(6):517–24.

11. Shah ND, Mullan RJ, Breslin, M, et al. Translating comparative effectiveness into practice: the case of diabetes medications. *Med Care.* 2010;**48**(6 Suppl):S153–8.

12. Elwyn G, Frosch D, Thomson R, et al. Shared decision making: a model for clinical practice. *J Gen Intern Med.* 2012;**27**(10):1361–7.

13. Stacy D, Légaré F, Lewis K, et al. Decision aids for people facing health treatment or screening decisions. *Cochrane Database Syst Rev.* 2014;**1**:CD001431.

14. Davidson JE, Powers K, Hedayat KM, et al. Clinical practice guidelines for support of the family in the patient-centered intensive care unit: American College of Critical Care Medicine Task Force 2004–2005. *Crit Care Med.* 2007;**35**(2):605–22.

15. Davidson JE, Aslakson RA, Long AC, et al. Guidelines for family-centered care in the neonatal, pediatric, and adult ICU. *Crit Care Med.* 2017;**45**(1):103–28.

16. Piscitello GM, Parham WM, Huber MT, Siegler M, Parker WF. The timing of family meetings in the medical intensive care unit. *Am J Hosp Palliat Med.* 2019;**36**(12):1049–56.

17. Butler M, Ratner E, McCreedy E, Shippee N, Kane RL. Decision aids for advance care planning: an overview of the state of the science. Ann Inter Med. 2014;**161**(6):408–18.

18. Austin CA, Mohottige D, Sudore RL, Smith AK, Hanson LC. Tools to promote shared decision making in serious illness: a systematic review. JAMA Intern Med. 2015;**175**(7):1213–21.

19. Stirling C, Leggett S, Lloyd B, et al. Decision aids for respite service choices by carers of people with dementia: development and pilot RCT. *BMC Med Inform Decis Mak.* 2012;**12**(1):21.

20. Krones T, Budilivschi A, Karzig I, et al. Advance care planning for the severely ill in the hospital: a randomized trial. *BMJ Support Palliat Care.* 2019;**12**(e3):e411–e423.

21. Plaisance A, Witteman HO, LeBlanc A, et al. Development of a decision aid for cardiopulmonary resuscitation and invasive mechanical ventilation in the intensive care unit employing user-centered design and a wiki platform for rapid prototyping. *PLoS One.* 2018;**13**(2):e0191844.

22. Hanson LC, Carey TS, Caprio AJ, et al. Improving decision-making for feeding options in advanced dementia: a randomized, controlled trial. *J Am Geriatr Soc.* 2011;**59**(11):2009–16.

23. Volandes AE, Ferguson LA, Davis AD, et al. Assessing end-of-life preferences for advanced dementia in rural patients using an educational video: A randomized controlled trial. *J Palliat Med.* 2011;**14**(2):169–77.

24. Muehlschlegel S, Shutter L, Col N, Goldberg R. Decision aids and shared decision-making in neurocritical care: an unmet need in our neuroICUs. *Neurocrit Care.* 2015;**23**(1):127–30.

25. Muehlschlegel S, Hwang DY, Flahive J, et al. Goals-of-care decision aid for critically ill patients with TBI: development and feasibility testing. *Neurology.* 2020;**95**(2):e179–93.

26. White DB, Engelberg RA, Wenrich MD, Lo B, Curtis JR. Prognostication during physician-family discussions about limiting life support in intensive care units. *Crit Care Med.* 2007;**35**(2):442–8.

27. White DB, Ernecoff N, Buddadhumaruk P, et al. Prevalence of and factors related to discordance about prognosis between physicians and surrogate decision makers of critically ill patients. *JAMA.* 2016;**315**(19):2086–94.

28. White DB, Braddock CH, Bereknyei S, Curtis JR. Toward shared decision making at the end of life in intensive care units: opportunities for improvement. *Arch Intern Med.* 2007;**167**(5):461–7.

29. Levinson W, Kao A, Kuby A, Thisted RA. Not all patients want to participate in decision making: a national study of public preferences. J Gen Intern Med. 2005;**20**(6): 531–5.

30. Hauke D, Reiter-theil S, Hoster E, Hiddemann W, Winkler EC. The role of relatives in decisions concerning life-prolonging treatment in patients with end-stage malignant disorders: informants, advocates or surrogate decision-makers? *Ann Oncol.* 2011;**22**(12):2667–74.

31. Pochard F, Azoulay E, Chevret S, et al. Symptoms of anxiety and depression in family members of intensive care unit patients: ethical hypothesis regarding decision-making capacity. *Crit Care Med.* 2001;**29**(10):1893–7.

32. Hajizadeh N, Uhler L, Herman SW, Lester J. is shared decision making for end-of-life decisions associated with better outcomes as compared to other forms of decision making? A systematic literature review. *MDM Policy Pract.* 2016;**1**(1):238146831664223.

33. Hemphill JC, Newman J, Zhao S, Johnston SC. Hospital usage of early do-not-resuscitate orders and outcome after intracerebral hemorrhage. *Stroke.* 2004;**35**(5):1130–4.

34. Lazaridis C. Deciding under uncertainty: the case of refractory intracranial hypertension. *Front Neurol.* 2020;**11**:908.

35. Lazaridis C. End-of-life considerations and shared decision making in neurocritical care. *Contin Lifelong Learn Neurol.* 2018;**24**(6):1794–9.

36. Guengerich T. *Caregiving and End-of-Life Issues: A Survey of AARP Members in Florida.* Washington, DC: AARP; February 2009. Available from: https://assets.aarp.org/rgcenter/il/fl_eol_08 .pdf

37. Hwang D, Yagoda D, Perrey H, et al. Consistency of communication among intensive care unit staff as perceived by family members of patients surviving to discharge. *J Crit Care.* 2014;**29**(1):134–8.

38. Knox L, Douglas JM, Bigby C. "I've never been a yes person": decision-making participation and self-conceptualization after severe traumatic brain injury. *Disabil Rehabil.* 2017;**39**(22):2250–60.

39. Long B, Clark L, Cook P. Surrogate decision making for patients with severe traumatic brain injury. *J Trauma Nurs.* 2011;**18**(4):204–12

40. Lazaridis C. What does it mean to neuro-prognosticate? *AJOB Neurosci.* 2016;**7**:48–50.

41. Van Dijck JTJM, Bartels RHMA, Lavrijsen JCM, et al. The patient with severe traumatic brain

injury: clinical decision-making: the first 60 min and beyond. *Curr Opin Crit Care.* 2019 **25**:622–9.

42. Kunneman M, Branda ME, Hargraves IG, et al. Assessment of shared decision-making for stroke prevention in patients with atrial fibrillation: a randomized clinical trial. *JAMA Intern Med.* 2020;**180**(9):1215.

43. Holloway RG, Arnold RM, Creutzfeldt CJ, et al. Palliative and end-of-life care in stroke: a statement for healthcare professionals from the American Heart Association/American Stroke Association. *Stroke.* 2014;**45**(6):1887–916.

44. You JJ, Jayaraman D, Swinton M, Jiang X, Heyland DK. Supporting shared decision-making about cardiopulmonary resuscitation using a video-based decision-support intervention in a hospital setting: a multisite before–after pilot study. *CMAJ Open.* 2019;**7**(4):E630–7.

45. Hunt WE, Hess RM. Surgical risk as related to time of intervention in the repair of intracranial aneurysms. *J Neurosurg.* 1968;**28**(1):14–20.

46. de Oliveira Manoel AL, Goffi A, Marotta TR, et al. The critical care management of poor-grade subarachnoid haemorrhage. *Crit Care.* 2016;**20**:21.

47. Naval NS, Chang T, Caserta F, et al. Improved aneurysmal subarachnoid hemorrhage outcomes: a comparison of 2 decades at an academic center. *J Crit Care.* 2013;**28**(2):182–8.

Prognostication in Intracerebral Hemorrhage

Rajbeer S. Sangha and Matthew B. Maas

Background, Epidemiology, and Public Health Importance

Basic Overview of Intracerebral Hemorrhage

Intracerebral hemorrhage (ICH) refers to bleeding into brain parenchyma, with or without extension into the ventricles or convexity subarachnoid space. ICH that occurs in the absence of trauma, subacute infarction, tumor, or cerebrovascular malformations is called primary or spontaneous ICH. The management and prognosis of hemorrhagic brain tumors, large infarctions, severe traumatic brain injury, and ruptured vascular malformations are unique and determined by the structural injuries and pathologies underlying those conditions. For the remainder of this chapter, our use of the term ICH will refer to primary ICH unless otherwise stated. The mechanisms of injury in ICH may be considered in two categories: structural and biochemical. The extravasation of blood into the surrounding parenchyma leads to physical disruption and mechanical damage of the glial cells and neurons and, in severe cases, brain compression leading to herniation syndromes.[1] The second mechanism involves the breakdown of blood, release of inflammatory cytokines, and cerebral edema formation, all of which act to compound the original insult.[2]

Intracranial hemorrhages are generally categorized by etiology and location, which are frequently related. Deep hemorrhages occur in the basal ganglia, thalamus, internal capsule, cerebellum, or brainstem and are frequently attributable to rupture of a small perforating artery. Risk factors for deep hemorrhages include a chronic history of hypertension and advanced age. Lobar hemorrhages are defined as hemorrhages that occur at the periphery or in the cortical regions of the cerebrum. Spontaneous hemorrhages in these regions are most often secondary to coagulopathies or amyloid angiopathy. The accurate prediction of ICH outcomes is important for clinicians, as it requires making decisions regarding the allocation of scarce resources, discussing with family members at length the possible outcomes for their loved ones as well as a guide for design in clinical trials. For family members, prognostication of outcomes in ICH helps influence their decisions for long-term care and balancing previously expressed wishes of the patients themselves with their current and future clinical functional status. It has recently been estimated that at least 60 different prognostic tools have been published for post-ICH outcomes, yet nearly all converge upon a set of important clinical predictors and share a similar set of limitations.[3] This chapter will familiarize readers with those common prognostic data elements and the principles upon which prognostic assessments are based.

Intracerebral Hemorrhage Epidemiology

Intracerebral hemorrhage is a significant cause of morbidity and mortality worldwide, accounting for approximately 10–20% of all strokes.[4,5] Worldwide incidence is estimated at around 24.6 per 100,000 person-years (95% CI 19.7–30.7).[6] Significant variability across ethnicities has been noted in ICH, and in a systemic review the incidence rate per 100,000 person-years in Asians was 51.8, in Caucasians, 24.2, in Blacks, 22.9, and in Hispanics, 19.6.[6] The association of ICH and gender at this time has not yielded a definite trend, as a systematic review in 2009 indicated the incidence is higher in males and a 2010 meta-analysis found no significant difference between males and females.[6,7]

Major risk factors for spontaneous ICH include advancing age, hypertension, utilization of anticoagulant therapy, and presence of cerebral amyloid angiopathy (CAA). The incidence of ICH increases by almost double with each 10-year increase in age after the age of 35.[8,9] Hypertension is the most common cause of primary ICH, accounting for approximately 60–70% of all cases.[10] Cerebral amyloid angiopathy occurs due to the deposition of amyloid protein in the cerebral arteries, causing the blood vessels to leak more easily, and accounts for approximately 20% of ICH.[11]

Historical Approaches to Assessing Outcome for Intracerebral Hemorrhage

There is now a substantial literature on ICH outcomes. The two important attributes of all outcome studies are the time point at which outcome was ascertained and the outcome measure used. Most studies of ICH have used one of four assessment points: hospital discharge (including hospital survival), 30 days, 90 days, and long-term outcomes from 1 to 5 years. It may seem longer times to follow-up would be more rigorous and informative, but that isn't necessarily the case. Because of the severity of ICH, early death is common, and functional dependency requiring skilled nursing care often causes dislocation from the community and loss to follow-up over time, all of which impede ascertainment of outcomes over long time intervals. Moreover, several studies have shown that functional improvements after ICH happen mostly within the first 3 months, and that improvements between 3 and 12 months are often too slight to measure.[12,13] With respect to measurements, the ICH literature has used one of three approaches: mortality, global functional outcome scales, and domain-specific outcome scales. Outcome assessment methods will be discussed in a separate chapter, but it is important to note here that the modified Rankin Scale (mRS) is the predominant outcome instrument for ICH research.

Neuroprognostication in the Acute Setting

Clinical – Demographics

Clinical prognostic factors include demographic characteristics, medical comorbidities, and severity of initial neurological impairment. Demographics play a significant role in outcomes. One of the strongest predictors of outcomes is age, with increasing age correlating with worse outcomes

and mortality in multiple studies.[5,14,15] Outcomes also differ according to race and ethnicity. Caucasians were more likely to die and have a worse quality of life compared to Asians, and although there are substantial unadjusted difference between Caucasians and African Americans, most of the difference seems to be accounted for by other demographic, clinical, and socioeconomic factors.[16,17] While geographic variability around the world exists in terms of gender differences, multiple studies have demonstrated that females have a lower mortality rate in ICH than men.[18,19]

Clinical – Comorbidities

There are limited data describing the effect of comorbidities and outcomes following ICH. Several studies have shown that cancer is independently associated with poor outcomes, especially metastatic disease.[20,21] Patients with coagulopathies, including those with liver cancer, fare poorly.[22] ICH is more common among patients with end-stage renal disease, and among those patients, the risk for poor outcome is compounded by a prior history of stroke, diabetes, or malignancy.[23] A recent observational study evaluating a racially diverse population with detailed baseline assessments found that a variety of chronic comorbid diseases negatively influence potential functional recovery, including dementia, prior stroke, brain atrophy, diabetes, and cardiomyopathy.[24]

Clinical – Neurological Impairment

The severity of initial neurological impairment is commonly measured by the National Institutes of Health Stroke Scale (NIHSS) and the Glasgow Coma Scale (GCS). Although there is some collinearity between these measurements, the NIHSS provides a superior measurement of focal neurological deficit burden, whereas the GCS better characterizes impaired arousal. The GCS has been more commonly integrated into composite prognostic scales, as discussed later. In studies that compare individual prognostic factors or report the derivation of composite prognostic scores from individual factors, the GCS is consistently reported to be the most accurate individual prognostic factor, nearly as accurate as some multifactor composite risk prediction scores.[25–27]

Clinical – Medical Complications

Perihematomal Edema

Perihematomal edema (PHE) is the radiological manifestation of secondary injury, which includes a combination of cytotoxic edema the first few hours following injury followed by vasogenic edema that evolves during the subsequent 5 to 7 days. Thus far, the location of the ICH (lobar vs. basal ganglia) has not been demonstrated to be a predictor of PHE.[28,29] The data at this time point toward PHE playing an important role in outcomes in ICH. Early increase in PHE is associated with worse functional outcomes and death, and a greater rate of PHE expansion portends greater risk.[30–32] In a pooled analysis of patients from intensive blood pressure reduction in acute cerebral hemorrhage (INTERACT) trials, investigators found that absolute growth in PHE was an independent prognostic factor (adjusted OR 1.17; 95% CI 1.02–1.33 per 5 mL increase from baseline, $P = 0.025$).[33]

Respiratory Failure and Dysphagia

Approximately one-third of patients with ICH require mechanical ventilation, and need for early intubation and the presence of signs of brainstem dysfunction in intubated patients are indicators of higher mortality risk.[34] For patients who are mechanically ventilated, tracheostomy is an important procedure that is necessary to help with patients who require a prolonged weaning. In an analysis of 392 patients with supratentorial ICH, researchers found that 31% of mechanically ventilated patients required tracheostomy, or 9.9% of all patients. Factors that predisposed patients to tracheostomy included chronic obstructive pulmonary disease, hematoma volume, ganglionic location of the hematoma, and hydrocephalus.[35] The TRACH Score was developed to identify patients at risk for requiring tracheostomy.[36] The TRACH Score is calculated as follows: 3 + R – GCS/2, where GCS is the Glasgow Coma Scale score and R is the sum of points related to radiological characteristics, namely 2 points for thalamic location, 1.5 for hydrocephalus, and 3 for septum pellucidum shift. Scores range from –4.5 to 8. A score of –2 corresponds with approximately 20% likelihood of needing tracheostomy, a score of 0 at 60% likelihood, and 90% likelihood for a score of 2. Similarly, the GRAVo Score (GCS, Race, Age, ICH Volume) was developed to identify when patients are likely to require gastrostomy for management of persistent dysphagia.[37] It is calculated by assigning points as follows: GCS ≤ 12 (2 points), African American race (1), age > 50 (2) and ICH volume > 30 cm^3 (1), with scores ranging from 0 to 6. Score ranges of 0–1, 2–3, and 4–6 correspond to approximately 9%, 20%, and 63% likelihood of requiring gastrostomy, respectively. Both of these scores are similar to global severity scores for ICH.

Fever

Between 30 and 40% of ICH patients develop fever, most of whom do not have a clear infectious etiology and are presumed to have central fevers.[38,39] Risk factors for fever include larger hematoma, intraventricular hemorrhage (IVH), placement of an external ventricular drain (EVD) or surgical evacuation, positive microbial cultures and longer length of stay.[40] Depending on the location of the ICH, fever can have a variable incidence, with higher rates noted after lobar or basal ganglia ICH; the highest incidence occurs if the patient has IVH present.[41] A number of studies have looked at the prognostic significance of fever following ICH and have uniformly found an association between fever and poor outcomes, especially among those with likely central fever.[38,41,42] While studies have not demonstrated a clear benefit from temperature management intervention for ICH patients, guidelines recommend treating hyperthermia/fever for patients with ICH as "reasonable."[43] The presence of infection has been identified as an independent predictor of outcome in at least one study.[24] Disaggregating the influence of infection and fever is challenging in this population in which infection and central (noninfectious) fever are both common.

Hyperglycemia

Hyperglycemia is an independent predictor of 30-day and 3-month mortality.[44–46] Studies evaluating the role of aggressive glucose management in acute ischemic stroke and severe brain injury suggest that aggressive treatment is either not beneficial or can lead to worse outcomes, so the optimal way to address this potentially modifiable risk factor is uncertain.[47,48]

Imaging

Acutely, computed tomography (CT) is the most common and effective tool in the diagnosis and management of ICH. Head CT imaging gives valuable information and characteristics of an ICH, including hematoma volume, markers for possible hematoma growth, location, presence of perihematomal edema and cerebral shift, as well as factors that can affect prognosis including IVH and hydrocephalus.[49]

Hematoma Characteristics

The characteristics of the hematoma play a role in predicting prognosis. Both hematoma location and volume affect the mortality rate of ICH, with infratentorial ICH location being the highest predictor of 30-day mortality. This can be attributed to the limited space, rapid decompensation, and high risk of herniation for patients with a space-occupying lesion in the posterior fossa. Hematoma volume is the strongest predictor of 30-day mortality, and volume can be calculated from CT imaging by utilizing the ABC/2 method.[50] The ABC/2 method is a common approach to estimating hematoma volume that can be done without advanced imaging tools, wherein the product of the greatest hemorrhage diameter ("A"), the diameter perpendicular to A on the same axial slice ("B"), the number of CT slices with hemorrhage, and the slice thickness are divided by 2. For example, if a hematoma measures 3 cm in greatest axial diameter, a perpendicular measurement in widest section is 2 cm, the hematoma spans 6 axial slices that were acquired in 5 mm (0.5 cm) thickness, then the estimated hematoma volume is $(3*2*6*0.5)/2 = 9$ cm.[3] In the original derivation, slices with an area approximately 25–75% of the largest slice area were counted as a half slice and those with an area < 25% were not considered a hemorrhage slice, although many studies and clinical trials that use ABC/2 do not incorporate that adjustment.[50] Software programs have been developed and used to measure hematoma volumes with greater precision from source images.[51]

Comorbid Intraventricular and Subarachnoid Hemorrhage

Intraventricular hemorrhage can be primary (arising from a source within the intraventricular system or a lesion contiguous to the ventricles) or secondary, in which an ICH extends into the ventricular system, the latter accounting for approximately 70% of all cases. ICH patients with IVH

have lower initial GCS scores and larger ICH volumes, but taking those differences into consideration, the presence and extent of IVH is an independent risk factor for mortality and poor functional outcome.[52–54] Numerous interventions have been evaluated to mitigate the effects of blood in the ventricular system, most recently a trial of alteplase irrigation by ventricular drain, but have not achieved an impact on functional outcomes.[55] Blood can also dissect into the extra-axial space, most often in the case of lobar hemorrhages, causing subarachnoid hemorrhage. Subarachnoid extension of primary ICH is associated with greater burden of fever, more risk for early seizures, and worse functional outcomes.[56–58]

Hemorrhage Expansion by Hematoma Growth and Intraventricular Extension

Hemorrhage expansion occurs in the form of hematoma growth and delayed intraventricular hemorrhage. Given that larger parenchymal hematomas and intraventricular hemorrhage are associated with worse prognosis, it is not surprising that hematoma enlargement and delayed ventricular extension are deleterious. Hematoma growth occurs in up to 80% of patients with ICH and is associated with higher mortality and poor outcomes.[59] Patients with larger initial hematoma volumes, coagulopathy, liver disease, malignant hypertension at presentation, and diabetes appear to be at greatest risk.[60] When hematoma growth is defined based on its association with worsened outcomes, absolute growth ≥ 3 mL or relative growth ≥ 26% appear to be optimal thresholds, and hematoma growth at that magnitude occurs in around 30% of cases.[61] Intraventricular hemorrhage occurs when pressure in an expanding hematoma dissects through parenchyma into the ventricular system. Delayed intraventricular hemorrhage occurs in 10–20% of patients with ICH and no intraventricular blood at presentation and is independently associated with higher risk of death and worse functional outcomes.[62,63]

Angiographic Imaging Markers: The Spot, Swirl, and Blend Signs

Contrast enhancement within an acute primary parenchymal hematoma on CT angiography, called the spot sign, is a marker of extravasation and is associated with elevated risk of hematoma expansion and in-hospital mortality.[64,65] The spot sign has been associated with worse functional outcomes in retrospective studies, but the association could not be replicated in a large prospective cohort, and combining the spot sign with other prognostic information does not seem to improve prognostic accuracy.[66] The swirl sign was first described as regions of varying hypo- or isodensity within a region of hyperdensity in an active hematoma.[67] Further studies have called areas of variable density within the hematoma by names such as the "blend sign." Much of the research on these signs has focused on their predictive value for hematoma growth. In retrospective analyses, the swirl sign was an independent predictor of death and poor functional outcome.[68] In a meta-analysis, authors demonstrated that there were correlations between heterogeneity signs and poor outcomes (OR 3.60, 95% CI 1.98–6.54, $P < 0.001$) and mortality (OR 4.64, 95% CI 2.96–7.27, $P < 0.001$).[69] Other characteristics such a density heterogeneity of the ICH and hematoma shape (regular vs. irregular) have also been studied, and while they are predictive of ICH growth, they have yet to be validated for prognostication purposes.[70] Finally, chronic microvascular ischemic changes, also called leukoaraiosis, have been linked to poor outcomes in a variety of conditions, including worse outcomes in patients with ICH even after consideration of other prognostic risks.[71]

Scoring Systems and Other Approaches

ICH Score

The ICH Score was developed by Hemphill and colleagues by incorporating both clinical and radiographic variables as a method to stratify and predict 30-day mortality rates for patients with ICH.[53] The ICH Score is composed of three radiographic variables (hematoma volume, supratentorial versus infratentorial hemorrhage location, presence of intraventricular hemorrhage) as well as two clinical variables (GCS and age), as summarized in Table 2.1. The score's prognostic value has been validated by analyzing patients' functional outcomes at 30-day, 3 months, 6 months, and 12 months using the modified Rankin Scale; the prospective cohort showed the ICH score to be predictive across all time points, and these data could further be utilized

Table 2.1 ICH Score calculation and prognostic outcomes

Component	ICH Score points
Glasgow Coma Scale	
3–4	2
5–12	1
13–15	0
ICH volume (cm^3)	
≥ 30	1
< 30	0
Intraventricular hemorrhage	
Yes	1
No	0
Infratentorial origin of ICH	
Yes	1
No	0
Age (year)	
≥ 80	1
< 80	0
Total ICH Score	0–6

ICH Score	30-Day Mortality
0	0%
1	13%
2	26%
3	72%
4	97%
5	100%
6	100%

to help families plan for future care needs and end-of-life decisions.[13]

FUNC Score

Because the ICH Score was originally developed to characterize mortality risk, the FUNC Score was developed to prognosticate functional outcomes among survivors (Table 2.2).[72] The FUNC Score cohort had a more inclusive population that was felt to make it more widely generalizable as opposed to other prediction scores that were developed on patients. Further analysis by researchers have shown that the FUNC Score is able to accurately identify patients with a low chance of functional neurological recovery at discharge.[73] The ICH Score and FUNC Score are similar, and the ICH Score has subsequently been extensively validated for predicting functional outcomes.

17

Table 2.2 FUNC Score calculation

Component	FUNC Score points
ICH volume, cm^3	
< 30	4
30–60	2
> 60	0
Age, years	
< 70	2
70–79	1
≥ 80	0
ICH location	
Lobar	2
Deep	1
Infratentorial	0
GCS score	
≥ 9	2
≤ 8	0
Pre-ICH cognitive impairment	
No	1
Yes	0
Total FUNC Score	0–11

Other Scores

While numerous scores and prediction metrics are published on a yearly basis (e.g., 15,662 for all types of clinical diseases in 2005), only a small number of these scores and metrics undergo external validations and are sufficiently superior to enter clinical utilization and affect management or patient outcomes.[27,74] While multiple scores such as the ICH-FOS and Essen ICH have been published that report modestly superior accuracy when compared to the ICH Score, there has not been a shift toward their use by physicians.[75,76] Some scores have been created to address specific perceived deficiencies in the ICH Score. For example, the patients with early care limitations were excluded from the prognostic models for the max-ICH Score, but validation analysis showed that its accuracy was no greater for that population than the original ICH Score.[27,77] Numerous other scores have also been analyzed and compared to the ICH Score with minimal differences in their ability to predict outcomes.[27] A comparison of the four most commonly used prognostic scales for ICH (ICH Score, ICH-GS, modified ICH, and FUNC Score) again confirmed that there was no significant superiority between scores, and since the ICH Score is the most extensively validated and commonly used, there is no reason to adopt an alternative.[78]

Biomarkers

While there are a number of potential promising biomarkers that may help investigators with prognosticate outcomes following an ICH, there are limited data and research to support their use in clinical practice.[79] There is an association between tumor necrosis factor-α (TNF-α) levels following ICH and 3-month functional outcomes, but this is not a routinely available test in clinical practice. Changes in peripheral leukocyte counts have also been identified as a marker for the inflammatory process that occurs after ICH. In one study, researchers found that the increased leukocyte count measured between admission and the first 72 hours predicted worse discharge disposition and worse functional status at 3 months.[80] Other inflammatory markers with limited data include high-mobility group protein box-1 (HMGB-1), transmembrane protein CD34, C-reactive protein, serum interleukin (IL)-6, IL-10, IL-11, and intercellular adhesion molecule 1 (ICAM-1).[81–86]

Electrophysiology

While seizures are common after ICH, the data regarding early seizures affecting ICH outcomes are variable. Early seizure incidence following ICH in patients with continuous electroencephalogram (EEG) monitoring has been shown to be between 28 and 31%, and clinical seizures have been documented at rates between 5.5 and 24%. [87,88] In a prospective cohort of 562 patients, investigators reported no association between early seizures, mortality, or functional outcomes at 6 months.[89] Phenytoin, once widely used as a prophylaxis in acute ICH management, has been associated with worse outcomes, and prophylactic antiseizure medications are not recommended. [43,90,91] Limited data exist on EEG patterns and their ability to predict outcomes for patients. Claassen et al. found that periodic epileptiform discharges (PEDs) were independently associated with poor outcome.[88]

Other Approaches to Prognostication

Expert Opinion

A few of the formal clinical grading scales that have been mentioned above have been compared to the early clinical judgment of bedside clinicians in regard to their accuracy for estimating long-term mortality or functional outcome. The early subjective clinical judgment of physicians predicted outcomes more accurately than either the ICH Score or the FUNC Score.[92,93] Subjective factors such as psychosocial aspects of care that clinicians incorporate into their determination of ICH prognosis were topics that the investigators felt required further evaluation.[93,94]

Early Interval Reassessments

The Glasgow Coma Scale (GCS), introduced in 1974, has been utilized as a marker of level of consciousness in a person following brain injury. [95] Since then, it has been further utilized in a wide variety of assessments to aid in prognostication including in the ICH Score as discussed earlier in this chapter. However, early prognostication has been confounded by "self-fulfilling prophesies" by which physicians have limited aggressive care early due to severe initial symptoms, thus leading to worse outcomes.[96,97] Brief, serial neurological assessments, or "neurochecks," are commonly used in neurological intensive care units to monitor evolving symptoms and can be leveraged to trend the disease course.[98] Neurological fluctuations occur predominantly within the first 12 hours and stabilize within 5 days. Neurological status at day 5, measured for instance by the GCS, is an independent predictor of outcome for ICH, and utilization of the day 5 GCS can improve the accuracy of prognosticating outcomes for patients who have been stabilized after severe neurological injury (Figure 2.1). [99,100]

Effect of Therapeutic Interventions on Outcomes

While outcomes for patients with ICH have been improving in recent decades, there are few specific interventions that meaningfully alter the natural history of routine medical management. Given that some of these interventions were uncommon in the cohorts from which the major prognostic scores were developed, the effect of these

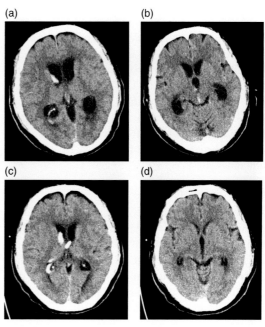

Figure 2.1 Imaging from a 62-year-old who presented to the emergency department with a small (1 cm^3) right thalamic ICH that had extended into the ventricles, causing hydrocephalus. Two slices of the baseline noncontrast head CT are shown in (a) and (b). The patient was comatose with initial GCS 7. The ICH Score was calculated to be 2, which corresponds to approximately 26% mortality and less than 20% chance of long-term functional independence (mRS ≤ 2). An external ventricular drain was inserted, and over the course of a few hours his GCS improved to 14 – alert with slight confusion and no motor deficits. Parts (c) and (d) show corresponding axial slices after ventriculostomy, with the ventricular catheter visible traversing the left foramen of Monroe. At 3-month reassessment, the patient was completely asymptomatic (mRS 0). The initial examination was severely impacted by a reversible complication that exaggerated the risk of poor outcome, whereas the neurological status reassessments over the first day clarified an expectation of good outcome.

interventions on outcomes should be considered when referencing those data.

Blood Pressure Control

As one of the primary risk factors in causing ICH, control of blood pressure (BP) has long been a target for physicians in ameliorating outcomes for patients presenting with spontaneous ICH. Sustained elevations in BP after the index event have been associated with increased ICH volume and worsened severity of the stroke.[101] Multiple studies have demonstrated an association with intensive BP reduction and attenuation of hematoma growth as well as limiting ICH progression, furthermore demonstrating improved 3-month function outcomes and mortality.[102–104] There have been two significant

randomized controlled trials that have been conducted to assess the effects of intensive BP reduction
in acute cerebral hemorrhage. Although there was
some evidence for a favorable trend in the
INTERACT2 study on a prespecified secondary analysis, INTERACT2 and ATACH-II were both negative with respect to their primary outcomes.
[105,106] More recently, a study that aggregated
individual-level data from these two trials showed
a modest beneficial effect of aggressive BP control on
outcomes.[107]

Surgical Decompression

Surgical intervention in ICH has been evaluated in
numerous trials that have now shown a positive
benefit in terms of patient outcomes including the
ISTICH and STICH II trials of open craniotomy
for hematoma evacuation and the MISTIE III trial
of minimally invasive surgery with thrombolysis
for hematoma evacuation.[108–110]

Reversal of Platelet Dysfunction

Antiplatelet agents have been associated with hematoma expansion and worse outcomes.[111–114]
Two approaches to normalizing platelet function
have been evaluated. The PATCH trial evaluated
platelet transfusion in patients with recent prior
antiplatelet medication use and found that transfusions were associated with increased mortality and
worse outcomes.[115] Desmopressin is used in
patients with congenital disorders such as von
Willebrand disease and is known to increase platelet
activity. Observational studies have reported
increased platelet activity and reduced hematoma
growth in acute ICH patients treated with desmopressin, but there is no clear evidence that patient
outcomes are influenced by that treatment.[116,117]

Neuroprognostication Over Time

Nearly all composite prognostic scores for ICH are
based on demographic information (e.g., age) and
variables that describe initial clinical severity.[27,78]
Most of the scoring systems developed for in-
hospital assessments have been developed for the
sake of predicting 3-month outcomes, or have been
developed for short-term outcomes but later validated for outcomes at 3 months or 1 year.[13,72]
As described in the prior section, adjusting prognostic estimates based on the trend of neurological
recovery over the first 5 days of the hospital course
improves prognostic accuracy, but beyond that there
are few data describing attempts to reevaluate

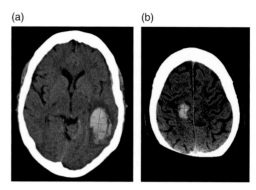

(a)   (b)

Figure 2.2 There is inherent uncertainty in estimating
prognosis that only time can resolve. Figure 2.2 shows axial slices
through the maximal hematoma cross section from initial
noncontrast head CTs from two cases of lobar ICH. These cases
illustrate how divergent outcomes can be from best predictions,
even when multiple reliable factors are considered together.
Part (a) shows a 30 cm³ left temporal ICH in an 82-year-old who
presented with GCS 14 and calculated ICH Score 2. Part (b)
shows a 4 cm³ right frontal ICH in a 72-year-old who presented
with GCS 14 and ICH Score 0. Despite equal neurological status
on admission and age and hematoma volume favoring the
patient with the right frontal hemorrhage, at 3 months that
patient was bed-bound and required continuous nursing care
(mRS 5), whereas the patient with the temporal lobe
hemorrhage had rehabilitated to minimal, nondisabling
symptoms (mRS 1) within the same time frame.

prognosis over time.[99] Functional outcomes
change minimally beyond 3 months, so the patient's
functional abilities at that timepoint are a reasonable
representation of the expected chronic disability.
[12,13] Cognition is clearly affected by ICH, but in
patterns that are fairly challenging to predict. The
development of early post-ICH dementia is associated with larger hemorrhages and lobar ICH location, but by 6 months there was no relationship
between dementia risk and any specific ICH characteristic.[118] Certain treatments may also influence cognitive outcomes, often in subtle ways.
Recent data have shown that the use of prophylactic
levetiracetam in the acute management of ICH is
associated with lower cognitive function as measured
from a patient-reported quality-of-life perspective
(Figure 2.2).[119]

Gaps in Current Knowledge and Future Research Directions

Biases and Confounding by Social Factors

Ethnic, religious, and racial group considerations
are important, as differences in these can drive
family decision making processes. Fraser et al.

found that Black patients were 76% less likely to withdraw life-sustaining therapy than White patients.[120] This was further seen in a recent prospective cohort where the investigators looked at whether race/ethnicity modified the implementation of comfort measures only (CMO) in patients with ICH. They found that Black patients were half as likely to be made CMO (OR 0.50, 5% CI 0.34–0.75; p = 0.01), and no statistically significant difference was observed in the Hispanic population.[121] Differences have also been noted between White patients of Hispanic ethnicity compared to non-Hispanic Whites.[122,123] Socioeconomic status may influence end-of-life care decisions separately from race and ethnicity, influencing decisions such as opting for long-term supportive care instead of palliative approaches.[17]

Biases and Confounding by Practitioner Perspectives

As previously described, there have been concerns that the early use of prognostic tools to direct care decisions leads to a self-fulfilling prophecy of a poor outcome.[97,124,125] One team of investigators attempted to develop an alternative prognostic scoring system to predict functional outcomes contingent on avoidance of early care limitations, and while the overall survival rates associated with avoiding early care limitations are higher, the specialized scoring algorithm does not perform more accurately than the usual ICH Score.[27,77] Avoidance of early care limitations was evaluated in a trial in which avoidance of do-not-resuscitate orders within the first 5 days of hospital care resulted a substantially lower mortality than predicted.[126]

Other Limitations

Generalizability

Most of the prognostic research on ICH outcomes comes from developed countries, but the incidence of ICH is higher in developing countries. While the underlying physiological principles illustrated by prognostic models are certainly relevant in all contexts (e.g., patients with larger hematoma volumes and worse GCS scores on admission are expected to have worse functional outcomes), the absolute rates of medication complications and poor outcomes differ in ways that are not well characterized.

Rehabilitation

The level of evidence to support specific rehabilitation interventions for post-stroke care is poor, and very few post-stroke rehabilitation data include a significant proportion of patients with intracerebral hemorrhage. More research is needed to establish evidence to support rehabilitation interventions and to determine the appropriate timing and duration of therapies.

Mobility Bias in Global Outcome Measures

Patients consistently report that cognition and other domains of independent function are important components of overall quality of life. Most prognostic data are evaluated based on their influence on global outcomes, often with the modified Rankin Scale, but the difference between good and poor outcomes on the mRS is overwhelmingly driven by mobility.[127] The mobility bias characteristics of global functional outcome scales has impeded the evaluation of clinical factors that are more likely to influence functions such as cognition rather than motor function. For example, delirium and exposure to antiseizure medications have been associated with worse cognitive outcomes, but not a change in global function as measured by the modified Rankin Scale.[119,128,129] The burden of cognitive and psychological symptoms is high after ICH, but consideration of cognitive and psychological outcomes requires sampling these outcomes in large cohorts of patients.[130] New web-based tools may help overcome the logistical burden of ascertaining outcomes across multiple discrete domains of function by using a patient-reported outcome paradigm.[127,131]

Conclusions

Intracerebral hemorrhage (ICH) develops unexpectedly and may severely incapacitate those affected, especially in the short term. There is a limited set of prognostic factors that strongly influence the likelihood of a favorable outcome, including the severity of neurological impairment, hematoma volume, and intraventricular hemorrhage extension at the time of initial presentation, along with age and premorbid disability. Early neurological changes occur in many patients, and those trends are informative as to the potential for recovery. Similarly, medical complications are common, can exacerbate morbidity, and can impede rehabilitation. Learning more about exposures that may influence outcomes more subtly overall or affect only particular symptoms and functional abilities will require broader use of domain-specific outcome measurements alongside common tools such as the modified Rankin Scale.

Various severity scoring systems exist and can provide an approximation of the range of potential likely outcomes, but the dynamics of the early hospital course, details about baseline functional status, and other unique factors are not incorporated and limit the specificity of those scores' prognostic accuracy. Expert perspectives are confirmed to be important for integrating all prognostic factors, adapting them to the local medical system and population, and educating families through decision-making steps, but even experts are vulnerable to cognitive biases that may be too pessimistic. Forthright conversations about prognosis are not to be avoided, but in many cases delayed for a few days to enable better clarity and then approached cautiously.

References

1. Hemphill JC. The intracerebral hemorrhage score: what it is and what it is not. *World Neurosurg.* 2019;**123**:157–8.

2. Keep RF, Hua Y, Xi G. Intracerebral haemorrhage: mechanisms of injury and therapeutic targets. *Lancet Neurol.* 2012;**11**:720–31.

3. Hemphill JC 3rd, Ziai W. The never-ending quest of intracerebral hemorrhage outcome prognostication. *JAMA Netw Open.* 2022;**5**: e221108.

4. Feigin VL, Lawes CM, Bennett DA, Barker-Collo SL, Parag V. Worldwide stroke incidence and early case fatality reported in 56 population-based studies: a systematic review. *Lancet Neurol.* 2009;**8**:355–69.

5. Sacco S, Marini C, Toni D, Olivieri L, Carolei A. Incidence and 10-year survival of intracerebral hemorrhage in a population-based registry. *Stroke.* 2009;**40**:394–9.

6. van Asch CJ, Luitse MJ, Rinkel GJ, et al. Incidence, case fatality, and functional outcome of intracerebral haemorrhage over time, according to age, sex, and ethnic origin: a systematic review and meta-analysis. *Lancet Neurol.* 2010;**9**:167–76.

7. Appelros P, Stegmayr B, Terent A. Sex differences in stroke epidemiology: a systematic review. *Stroke.* 2009;**40**:1082–90.

8. Broderick JP, Brott T, Tomsick T, Miller R, Huster G. Intracerebral hemorrhage more than twice as common as subarachnoid hemorrhage. *J Neurosurg.* 1993;**78**:188–91.

9. Stein M, Misselwitz B, Hamann GF, et al. Intracerebral hemorrhage in the very old: future demographic trends of an aging population. *Stroke.* 2012;**43**:1126–8.

10. McCormick WF, Rosenfield DB. Massive brain hemorrhage: a review of 144 cases and an examination of their causes. *Stroke.* 1973;**4**:946–54.

11. Manno EM. Update on intracerebral hemorrhage. *Continuum (Minneap Minn).* 2012;**18**:598–610.

12. Sreekrishnan A, Leasure AC, Shi FD, et al. Functional improvement among intracerebral hemorrhage (ICH) survivors up to 12 months post-injury. *Neurocrit Care.* 2017;**27**:326–33.

13. Hemphill JC 3rd, Farrant M, Neill TA Jr. Prospective validation of the ICH score for 12-month functional outcome. *Neurology.* 2009;**73**:1088–1094.

14. Radholm K, Arima H, Lindley RI, et al. Older age is a strong predictor for poor outcome in intracerebral haemorrhage: the INTERACT2 study. *Age Ageing.* 2015;**44**:422–7.

15. Gonzalez-Perez A, Gaist D, Wallander MA, McFeat G, Garcia-Rodriguez LA. Mortality after hemorrhagic stroke: data from general practice (The Health Improvement Network). *Neurology.* 2013;**81**:559–65.

16. Krishnan K, Beishon L, Berge E, et al. Relationship between race and outcome in Asian, Black, and Caucasian patients with spontaneous intracerebral hemorrhage: data from the Virtual International Stroke Trials Archive and Efficacy of Nitric Oxide in Stroke trial. *Int J Stroke.* 2018;**13**:362–73.

17. Garcia RM, Prabhakaran S, Richards CT, Naidech AM, Maas MB. Race, socioeconomic status, and gastrostomy after spontaneous intracerebral hemorrhage. *J Stroke Cerebrovasc Dis.* 2020;**29**:104567.

18. Vaartjes I, Reitsma JB, Berger-van Sijl M, Bots ML. Gender differences in mortality after hospital admission for stroke. *Cerebrovasc Dis.* 2009;**28**:564–71.

19. Zia E, Engstrom G, Svensson PJ, Norrving B, Pessah-Rasmussen H. Three-year survival and stroke recurrence rates in patients with primary intracerebral hemorrhage. *Stroke.* 2009;**40**: 3567–3573.

20. Gon Y, Todo K, Mochizuki H, Sakaguchi M. Cancer is an independent predictor of poor outcomes in

patients following intracerebral hemorrhage. *Eur J Neurol*. 2018;**25**:128–34.

21. Velander AJ, DeAngelis LM, Navi BB. Intracranial hemorrhage in patients with cancer. *Curr Atheroscler Rep*. 2012;**14**:373–81.

22. Lu Q, Chen L, Zeng J, et al. Clinical features of liver cancer with cerebral hemorrhage. *Med Sci Monit*. 2016;**22**:1716–23.

23. Lin CY, Chien CC, Chen HA, et al. The impact of comorbidity on survival after hemorrhagic stroke among dialysis patients: a nationwide population-based study. *BMC Nephrol*. 2014;**15**:186.

24. Woo D, Comeau ME, Venema SU, et al. Risk factors associated with mortality and neurologic disability after intracerebral hemorrhage in a racially and ethnically diverse cohort. *JAMA Netw Open*. 2022;**5**:e221103.

25. Parry-Jones AR, Abid KA, Di Napoli M, et al. Accuracy and clinical usefulness of intracerebral hemorrhage grading scores: a direct comparison in a UK population. *Stroke*. 2013;**44**:1840–5.

26. Ji R, Shen H, Pan Y, et al., Investigators CNSRC. A novel risk score to predict 1-year functional outcome after intracerebral hemorrhage and comparison with existing scores. *Crit Care*. 2013;**17**:R275.

27. Schmidt FA, Liotta EM, Prabhakaran S, Naidech AM, Maas MB. Assessment and comparison of the max-ICH score and ICH score by external validation. *Neurology*. 2018;**91**:e939–e946.

28. Gebel JM Jr, Jauch EC, Brott TG, et al. Natural history of perihematomal edema in patients with hyperacute spontaneous intracerebral hemorrhage. *Stroke*. 2002;**33**:2631–5.

29. McCarron MO, McCarron P, Alberts MJ. Location characteristics of early perihaematomal oedema. *J Neurol Neurosurg Psychiatry*. 2006;**77**:378–80.

30. Murthy SB, Moradiya Y, Dawson J, et al. Perihematomal edema and functional outcomes in intracerebral hemorrhage: influence of hematoma volume and location. *Stroke*. 2015;**46**:3088–92.

31. Wu TY, Sharma G, Strbian D, et al. Natural history of perihematomal edema and impact on outcome after intracerebral hemorrhage. *Stroke*. 2017;**48**:873–9.

32. Grunwald Z, Beslow LA, Urday S, et al. Perihematomal edema expansion rates and patient outcomes in deep and lobar intracerebral hemorrhage. *Neurocrit Care*. 2017;**26**:205–12.

33. Yang J, Arima H, Wu G, et al. Prognostic significance of perihematomal edema in acute intracerebral hemorrhage: pooled analysis from the intensive blood pressure reduction in acute cerebral hemorrhage trial studies. *Stroke*. 2015;**46**:1009–13.

34. Gujjar AR, Deibert E, Manno EM, Duff S, Diringer MN. Mechanical ventilation for ischemic stroke and intracerebral hemorrhage: indications, timing, and outcome. *Neurology*. 1998;**51**:447–51.

35. Huttner HB, Kohrmann M, Berger C, Georgiadis D, Schwab S. Predictive factors for tracheostomy in neurocritical care patients with spontaneous supratentorial hemorrhage. *Cerebrovasc Dis*. 2006;**21**:159–65.

36. Szeder V, Ortega-Gutierrez S, Ziai W, Torbey MT. The TRACH Score: clinical and radiological predictors of tracheostomy in supratentorial spontaneous intracerebral hemorrhage. *Neurocrit Care*. 2010;**13**:40–6.

37. Faigle R, Marsh EB, Llinas RH, Urrutia VC, Gottesman RF. Novel score predicting gastrostomy tube placement in intracerebral hemorrhage. *Stroke*. 2015;**46**:31–6.

38. Honig A, Michael S, Eliahou R, Leker RR. Central fever in patients with spontaneous intracerebral hemorrhage: predicting factors and impact on outcome. *BMC Neurol* 2015;**15**:6.

39. Georgilis K, Plomaritoglou A, Dafni U, Bassiakos Y, Vemmos K. Aetiology of fever in patients with acute stroke. *J Int Med*. 1999;**246**:203–9.

40. Gillow SJ, Ouyang B, Lee VH, John S. Factors associated with fever in intracerebral hemorrhage. *J Stroke Cerebrovasc Dis*. 2017;**26**:1204–8.

41. Schwarz S, Hafner K, Aschoff A, Schwab S. Incidence and prognostic significance of fever following intracerebral hemorrhage. *Neurology*. 2000;**54**:354–61.

42. Rincon F, Lyden P, Mayer SA. Relationship between temperature, hematoma growth, and functional outcome after intracerebral hemorrhage. *Neurocrit Care*. 2013;**18**:45–53.

43. Hemphill JC 3rd, Greenberg SM, Anderson CS, et al. Guidelines for the management of spontaneous intracerebral hemorrhage: a guideline for healthcare professionals from the American Heart Association/American Stroke Association. *Stroke*. 2015;**46**:2032–60.

44. Passero S, Ciacci G, Ulivelli M. The influence of diabetes and hyperglycemia on clinical course after intracerebral hemorrhage. *Neurology*. 2003;**61**:1351–6.

45. Lee SH, Kim BJ, Bae HJ, et al. Effects of glucose level on early and long-term mortality after intracerebral haemorrhage: the Acute Brain Bleeding Analysis Study. *Diabetologia*. 2010;**53**:429–34.

46. Kimura K, Iguchi Y, Inoue T, et al. Hyperglycemia independently increases the risk of early death in acute spontaneous intracerebral hemorrhage. *J Neurolog Sci.* 2007;**255**:90–4.

47. Oddo M, Schmidt JM, Carrera E, et al. Impact of tight glycemic control on cerebral glucose metabolism after severe brain injury: a microdialysis study. *Crit Care Med.* 2008;**36**:3233–8.

48. Johnston KC, Bruno A, Pauls Q, et al. Intensive vs standard treatment of hyperglycemia and functional outcome in patients with acute ischemic stroke: the SHINE Randomized Clinical Trial. *JAMA.* 2019;**322**:326–35.

49. Al-Mufti F, Thabet AM, Singh T, et al. Clinical and radiographic predictors of intracerebral hemorrhage outcome. *Interv Neurol.* 2018;**7**:118–36.

50. Kothari RU, Brott T, Broderick JP, et al. The ABCs of measuring intracerebral hemorrhage volumes. *Stroke.* 1996;**27**:1304–5.

51. Liotta EM, Prabhakaran S, Sangha RS, et al. Magnesium, hemostasis, and outcomes in patients with intracerebral hemorrhage. *Neurology.* 2017;**89**:813–19

52. Tuhrim S, Dambrosia JM, Price TR, et al. Intracerebral hemorrhage: external validation and extension of a model for prediction of 30-day survival. *Ann Neurol.* 1991;**29**:658–63.

53. Hemphill JC 3rd, Bonovich DC, Besmertis L, Manley GT, Johnston SC. The ICH score: a simple, reliable grading scale for intracerebral hemorrhage. *Stroke.* 2001;**32**:891–7.

54. Tuhrim S, Horowitz DR, Sacher M, Godbold JH. Volume of ventricular blood is an important determinant of outcome in supratentorial intracerebral hemorrhage. *Crit Care Med.* 1999;**27**:617–21.

55. Hanley DF, Lane K, McBee N, et al. Thrombolytic removal of intraventricular haemorrhage in treatment of severe stroke: results of the randomised, multicentre, multiregion, placebo-controlled CLEAR III trial. *Lancet.* 2017;**389**:603–11.

56. Guth JC, Gerard EE, Nemeth AJ, et al. Subarachnoid extension of hemorrhage is associated with early seizures in primary intracerebral hemorrhage. *J Stroke Cerebrovasc Dis.* 2014;**23**:2809–13.

57. Guth JC, Nemeth AJ, Rosenberg NF, et al. Subarachnoid extension of primary intracerebral hemorrhage is associated with fevers. *Neurocrit Care.* 2014;**20**:187–92.

58. Maas MB, Nemeth AJ, Rosenberg NF, et al. Subarachnoid extension of primary intracerebral

hemorrhage is associated with poor outcomes. *Stroke.* 2013;**44**:653–7.

59. Davis SM, Broderick J, Hennerici M, et al. Hematoma growth is a determinant of mortality and poor outcome after intracerebral hemorrhage. *Neurology.* 2006;**66**:1175–81.

60. Kazui S, Minematsu K, Yamamoto H, Sawada T, Yamaguchi T. Predisposing factors to enlargement of spontaneous intracerebral hematoma. *Stroke.* 1997;**28**:2370–5.

61. Dowlatshahi D, Demchuk AM, Flaherty ML, et al. Defining hematoma expansion in intracerebral hemorrhage: relationship with patient outcomes. *Neurology.* 2011;**76**:1238–44.

62. Maas MB, Nemeth AJ, Rosenberg NF, et al. Delayed intraventricular hemorrhage is common and worsens outcomes in intracerebral hemorrhage. *Neurology.* 2013;**80**:1295–9.

63. Moullaali TJ, Sato S, Wang X, et al. Prognostic significance of delayed intraventricular haemorrhage in the INTERACT studies. *J Neurol Neurosurg Psychiatry.* 2017;**88**:19–24.

64. Wada R, Aviv RI, Fox AJ, et al. CT angiography "spot sign" predicts hematoma expansion in acute intracerebral hemorrhage. *Stroke.* 2007;**38**:1257–62.

65. Delgado Almandoz JE, Yoo AJ, Stone MJ, et al. The spot sign score in primary intracerebral hemorrhage identifies patients at highest risk of in-hospital mortality and poor outcome among survivors. *Stroke.* 2010;**41**:54–60.

66. Rizos T, Dorner N, Jenetzky E, et al. Spot signs in intracerebral hemorrhage: useful for identifying patients at risk for hematoma enlargement? *Cerebrovasc Dis.* 2013;**35**:582–9.

67. Al-Nakshabandi NA. The swirl sign. *Radiology.* 2001;**218**:433.

68. Selariu E, Zia E, Brizzi M, Abul-Kasim K. Swirl sign in intracerebral haemorrhage: definition, prevalence, reliability and prognostic value. *BMC Neurol.* 2012;**12**:109.

69. Zhang D, Chen J, Xue Q, et al. Heterogeneity signs on noncontrast computed tomography predict hematoma expansion after intracerebral hemorrhage: a meta-analysis. *Biomed Res Int.* 2018; **2018**:6038193.

70. Barras CD, Tress BM, Christensen S, et al. Density and shape as CT predictors of intracerebral hemorrhage growth. *Stroke.* 2009;**40**:1325–31.

71. Caprio FZ, Maas MB, Rosenberg NF, et al. Leukoaraiosis on magnetic resonance imaging correlates with worse outcomes after spontaneous intracerebral hemorrhage. *Stroke.* 2013;**44**:642–6.

72. Rost NS, Smith EE, Chang Y, et al. Prediction of functional outcome in patients with primary

intracerebral hemorrhage: the FUNC score. *Stroke.* 2008;**39**:2304–9.

73. Garrett JS, Zarghouni M, Layton KF, Graybeal D, Daoud YA. Validation of clinical prediction scores in patients with primary intracerebral hemorrhage. *Neurocrit Care.* 2013;**19**:329–35.

74. Toll DB, Janssen KJ, Vergouwe Y, Moons KG. Validation, updating and impact of clinical prediction rules: a review. *J Clin Epidemiol.* 2008;**61**:1085–94.

75. Ji R, Shen H, Pan Y, et al. A novel risk score to predict 1-year functional outcome after intracerebral hemorrhage and comparison with existing scores. *Crit Care.* 2013;**17**:R275.

76. Weimar C, Benemann J, Diener HC. Development and validation of the Essen Intracerebral Haemorrhage Score. *J Neurol Neurosurg Psychiatry.* 2006;**77**:601–5.

77. Sembill JA, Gerner ST, Volbers B, et al. Severity assessment in maximally treated ICH patients: the max-ICH score. *Neurology.* 2017;**89**:423–31.

78. Gregorio T, Pipa S, Cavaleiro P, et al. Assessment and comparison of the four most extensively validated prognostic scales for intracerebral hemorrhage: systematic review with meta-analysis. *Neurocrit Care.* 2019;**30**:449–66.

79. Maas MB, Furie KL. Molecular biomarkers in stroke diagnosis and prognosis. *Biomark Med.* 2009;**3**:363–83.

80. Agnihotri S, Czap A, Staff I, Fortunato G, McCullough LD. Peripheral leukocyte counts and outcomes after intracerebral hemorrhage. *J Neuroinflammation.* 2011;**8**:160.

81. Silva Y, Leira R, Tejada J, et al. Molecular signatures of vascular injury are associated with early growth of intracerebral hemorrhage. *Stroke.* 2005;**36**:86–91.

82. Castillo J, Davalos A, Alvarez-Sabin J, et al. Molecular signatures of brain injury after intracerebral hemorrhage. *Neurology.* 2002;**58**:624–9.

83. Wang KW, Cho CL, Chen HJ, et al. Molecular biomarker of inflammatory response is associated with rebleeding in spontaneous intracerebral hemorrhage. *Eur Neurol.* 2011;**66**:322–7.

84. Fang HY, Ko WJ, Lin CY. Plasma interleukin 11 levels correlate with outcome of spontaneous intracerebral hemorrhage. *Surg Neurol.* 2005;**64**:511–17, discussion 517–518.

85. Di Napoli M, Godoy DA, Campi V, et al. C-reactive protein level measurement improves mortality prediction when added to the spontaneous intracerebral hemorrhage score. *Stroke.* 2011;**42**:1230–6.

86. Zhou Y, Xiong KL, Lin S, et al. Elevation of high-mobility group protein box-1 in serum correlates with severity of acute intracerebral hemorrhage. *Mediators Inflamm.* 2010;**2010**:142458.

87. Vespa PM, O'Phelan K, Shah M, et al. Acute seizures after intracerebral hemorrhage: a factor in progressive midline shift and outcome. *Neurology.* 2003;**60**:1441–6.

88. Claassen J, Jette N, Chum F, et al. Electrographic seizures and periodic discharges after intracerebral hemorrhage. *Neurology.* 2007;**69**:1356–65.

89. De Herdt V, Dumont F, Henon H, et al. Early seizures in intracerebral hemorrhage: incidence, associated factors, and outcome. *Neurology.* 2011;**77**:1794–1800.

90. Naidech AM, Garg RK, Liebling S, et al. Anticonvulsant use and outcomes after intracerebral hemorrhage. *Stroke.* 2009;**40**:3810–15.

91. Naidech AM, Beaumont J, Jahromi B, et al. Prabhakaran S, Kho A, Holl JL Evolving use of seizure medications after intracerebral hemorrhage: a multicenter study. *Neurology.* 2017;**88**:52–6.

92. Hwang DY, Dell CA, Sparks MJ, et al. Clinician judgment vs formal scales for predicting intracerebral hemorrhage outcomes. *Neurology.* 2016;**86**:126–33.

93. Hwang DY, Chu SY, Dell CA, et al. Factors considered by clinicians when prognosticating intracerebral hemorrhage outcomes. *Neurocrit Care.* 2017;**27**:316–25.

94. Chu SY, Hwang DY. Predicting outcome for intracerebral hemorrhage patients: current tools and their limitations. *Semin Neurol.* 2016;**36**:254–60.

95. Teasdale G, Jennett B. Assessment of coma and impaired consciousness. A practical scale. *Lancet.* 1974;**2**:81–4.

96. Hemphill JC 3rd, Newman J, Zhao S, Johnston SC. Hospital usage of early do-not-resuscitate orders and outcome after intracerebral hemorrhage. *Stroke.* 2004;**35**:1130–4.

97. Becker KJ, Baxter AB, Cohen WA, et al. Withdrawal of support in intracerebral hemorrhage may lead to self-fulfilling prophecies. *Neurology.* 2001;**56**:766–72.

98. Maas MB, Rosenberg NF, Kosteva AR, et al. Surveillance neuroimaging and neurologic examinations affect care for intracerebral hemorrhage. *Neurology.* 2013;**81**:107–12.

99. Maas MB, Francis BA, Sangha RS, et al. Refining prognosis for intracerebral hemorrhage by early reassessment. *Cerebrovasc Dis.* 2017;**43**:110–16.

100. Maas MB, Berman MD, Guth JC, et al. Neurochecks as a biomarker of the temporal profile and clinical impact of neurologic changes after intracerebral hemorrhage. *J Stroke Cerebrovasc Dis.* 2015;**24**:2026–31.

101. Dandapani BK, Suzuki S, Kelley RE, Reyes-Iglesias Y, Duncan RC. Relation between blood pressure and outcome in intracerebral hemorrhage. *Stroke.* 1995;**26**:21–4.

102. Sakamoto Y, Koga M, Yamagami H, et al. Systolic blood pressure after intravenous antihypertensive treatment and clinical outcomes in hyperacute intracerebral hemorrhage: the stroke acute management with urgent risk-factor assessment and improvement-intracerebral hemorrhage study. *Stroke.* 2013;**44**:1846–51.

103. Tsivgoulis G, Katsanos AH, Butcher KS, et al. Intensive blood pressure reduction in acute intracerebral hemorrhage: a meta-analysis. *Neurology.* 2014;**83**:1523–9.

104. Arima H, Anderson CS, Wang JG, et al. Lower treatment blood pressure is associated with greatest reduction in hematoma growth after acute intracerebral hemorrhage. *Hypertension.* 2010;**56**:852–8.

105. Anderson CS, Heeley E, Huang Y, et al. Rapid blood-pressure lowering in patients with acute intracerebral hemorrhage. *N Eng J Med.* 2013;**368**:2355–65.

106. Qureshi AI, Palesch YY, Barsan WG, et al. Intensive blood-pressure lowering in patients with acute cerebral hemorrhage. *N Eng J Med.* 2016;**375**:1033–43.

107. Moullaali TJ, Wang X, Martin RH, et al. Blood pressure control and clinical outcomes in acute intracerebral haemorrhage: a preplanned pooled analysis of individual participant data. *Lancet Neurol.* 2019;**18**:857–64.

108. Mendelow AD, Gregson BA, Fernandes HM, et al. Early surgery versus initial conservative treatment in patients with spontaneous supratentorial intracerebral haematomas in the International Surgical Trial in Intracerebral Haemorrhage (STICH): a randomised trial. *Lancet.* 2005;**365**:387–97.

109. Mendelow AD, Gregson BA, Rowan EN, et al. Early surgery versus initial conservative treatment in patients with spontaneous supratentorial lobar intracerebral haematomas (STICH II): a randomised trial. *Lancet.* 2013;**382**:397–408.

110. Hanley DF, Thompson RE, Rosenblum M, et al. Efficacy and safety of minimally invasive surgery with thrombolysis in intracerebral haemorrhage evacuation (MISTIE III): a randomised, controlled, open-label, blinded endpoint phase 3 trial. *Lancet* 2019;**393**:1021–32.

111. Yildiz OK, Arsava EM, Akpinar E, Topcuoglu MA. Previous antiplatelet use is associated with hematoma expansion in patients with spontaneous intracerebral hemorrhage. *J Stroke Cerebrovas Dis.* 2012;**21**:760–6.

112. Camps-Renom P, Alejaldre-Monforte A, Delgado-Mederos R, et al. Does prior antiplatelet therapy influence hematoma volume and hematoma growth following intracerebral hemorrhage? Results from a prospective study and a meta-analysis. *Eur J Neurol.* 2017;**24**:302–8.

113. Thompson BB, Béjot Y, Caso V, et al. Prior antiplatelet therapy and outcome following intracerebral hemorrhage: a systematic review. *Neurology.* 2010;**75**:1333–42.

114. Naidech AM, Jovanovic B, Liebling S, et al. Reduced platelet activity is associated with early clot growth and worse 3-month outcome after intracerebral hemorrhage. *Stroke.* 2009;**40**:2398–2401.

115. Baharoglu MI, Cordonnier C, Salman RA, et al. Platelet transfusion versus standard care after acute stroke due to spontaneous cerebral haemorrhage associated with antiplatelet therapy (PATCH): a randomised, open-label, phase 3 trial. *Lancet.* 2016;**387**:2605–13.

116. Naidech AM, Maas MB, Levasseur-Franklin KE, et al. Desmopressin improves platelet activity in acute intracerebral hemorrhage. *Stroke.* 2014;**45**:2451–3.

117. Feldman EA, Meola G, Zyck S, et al. Retrospective assessment of desmopressin effectiveness and safety in patients with antiplatelet-associated intracranial hemorrhage. *Crit Care Med.* 2019;**47**:1759–65.

118. Biffi A, Bailey D, Anderson CD, et al. Risk factors associated with early vs delayed dementia after intracerebral hemorrhage. *JAMA Neurol.* 2016;**73**:969–76.

119. Naidech AM, Beaumont J, Muldoon K, et al. Prophylactic Seizure medication and health-related quality of life after intracerebral hemorrhage. *Crit Care Med.* 2018;**46**:1480–15.

120. Fraser SM, Torres GL, Cai C, et al. Race is a predictor of withdrawal of life support in patients with intracerebral hemorrhage. *J Stroke Cerebrovasc Dis.* 2018;**27**:3108–14.

121. Ormseth CH, Falcone GJ, Jasak SD, et al. Minority patients are less likely to undergo withdrawal of care after spontaneous intracerebral hemorrhage. *Neurocrit Care.* 2018;**29**:419–25.

122. Zahuranec DB, Brown DL, Lisabeth LD, et al. Differences in intracerebral hemorrhage between Mexican Americans and non-Hispanic whites. *Neurology*. 2006;**66**:30–4.

123. Zahuranec DB, Brown DL, Lisabeth LD, et al. Ethnic differences in do-not-resuscitate orders after intracerebral hemorrhage. *Crit Care Med*. 2009;**37**:2807–11.

124. Zahuranec DB, Brown DL, Lisabeth LD, et al. Early care limitations independently predict mortality after intracerebral hemorrhage. *Neurology*. 2007;**68**:1651–7.

125. Zahuranec DB, Morgenstern LB, Sánchez BN, et al. Do-not-resuscitate orders and predictive models after intracerebral hemorrhage. *Neurology*. 2010;**75**:626–33.

126. Morgenstern LB, Zahuranec DB, Sánchez BN, et al. Full medical support for intracerebral hemorrhage. *Neurology*. 2015;**84**:1739–44.

127. Naidech AM, Beaumont JL, Berman M, et al. Dichotomous "good outcome" indicates mobility more than cognitive or social quality of life. *Crit Care Med*. 2015;**43**:1654–9.

128. Naidech AM, Beaumont JL, Rosenberg NF, et al. Intracerebral hemorrhage and delirium symptoms. Length of stay, function, and quality of life in a 114-patient cohort. *Am J Respir Crit Care Med*. 2013;**188**:1331–7.

129. Rosenthal LJ, Francis BA, Beaumont JL, et al. Agitation, delirium, and cognitive outcomes in intracerebral hemorrhage. *Psychosomatics*. 2017;**58**:19–27.

130. Francis BA, Beaumont J, Maas MB, et al. Depressive symptom prevalence after intracerebral hemorrhage: a multi-center study. *J Patient Rep Outcomes*. 2018;**2**:55.

131. Naidech AM, Beaumont JL, Berman M, et al. Web-based assessment of outcomes after subarachnoid and intracerebral hemorrhage: a new patient centered option for outcomes assessment. *Neurocrit Care*. 2015;**23**:22–7.

Prognostication in Acute Ischemic Stroke

Alexander Allen and Barry M. Czeisler

Background

Stroke represents one of the most prominent causes of disability and mortality worldwide and poses significant costs to healthcare services. As many as 24.9 million people living worldwide have suffered an ischemic stroke, and projections suggest that by 2030, an additional 3.4 million adults older than 18 years in the United States will have had a stroke.[1] Stroke can be deadly, with mortality rates at 1 year post-stroke (both ischemic and hemorrhagic) running from 8 to 36%, with the higher mortality rates occurring in the elderly. [1] But more than this, stroke leads to disability in a large number of patients. Approximately half of stroke survivors remain disabled, with 20% requiring care at a facility.[2] These sobering data highlight the economic and medical importance of understanding stroke mechanisms, stroke management, and stroke prognosis.

Despite the potential catastrophic outcomes of stroke, not all patients suffer significant morbidity, and some patients even show considerable improvement over time. Outcomes from stroke range from full recovery, through varying degrees of disability, to death. Efforts to predict stroke outcome not only provide expectations for patients, physicians, and families, but understanding a patient's prognosis may also inform decisions about acute management.[3] Consequently, researchers are working to better understand what clinical, biochemical, radiographic, and electrophysiological factors may predict a patient's outcome after ischemic stroke. Great effort has been invested to this end, and many prognostic measures and scales have been proposed. However, due to the clinical heterogeneity of ischemic stroke as well as the various constellations of comorbidities and complications unique to each stroke patient, an ideal prognostic measure or scale remains elusive.

The immense number of prognostic variables and scales poses a challenge to the understanding of stroke prognostication. Moreover, debate continues concerning the validity and applicability of such information. Finally, at the most elementary level, debate exists about whether an adequate measure of outcome has been established. For all these reasons, it is important not to lose the forest for the trees. We will attempt to organize and simplify the extensive data to provide a sense of how the various variables and scales convey prognostic information at different time points.

Defining Prognostication, Outcomes, and Common Neurological Scales

Neurological prognosis after stroke is often expressed in terms of a functional scale at a certain period in time (Table 3.1). Understanding the significance of such findings requires knowing what functional scale has been used and what values of that functional scale represent favorable or unfavorable outcomes.

Modified Rankin Scale (mRS)

The mRS is an ordinal scale from 0 to 6 that assesses the degree of disability after stroke, ranging from no symptoms to death.[4] Commonly, mRS of 0–2 (functional independence) is felt to represent a good or favorable outcome, whereas mRS of 3–6 represents a poor or unfavorable outcome. However, mRS 3 (ability to ambulate but lack of independence in activities of daily living) can be considered either favorable or unfavorable depending on the study, and can therefore affect the dichotomized cutoff utilized. In some studies, the mRS alone at a period of time such as 30 days has been proposed to serve as a reliable proxy for long-term functional outcomes,[5] but more often, the mRS is used as a measure of outcome potentially predicted by another variable. Whereas the

Table 3.1 Common neurological scales involved in prognostication

Scale	Component	Significance
Modified Rankin Scale (mRS)	0	No symptoms
	1	No significant disability despite symptoms. Able to carry out all usual duties and activities
	2	Slight disability. Unable to carry out all previous activities but able to look after own affairs without assistance
	3	Moderate disability. Requires some help but able to walk without assistance
	4	Moderate severe disability. Unable to walk and attend to bodily needs without assistance
	5	Severe disability. Bedridden, incontinent, and requiring constant nursing care and attention
	6	Dead
Barthel Index for Activities of Daily Living	Feeding	Independent (+10)
		Requires help (+5)
	Bathing	Independent (+5)
	Grooming	Independent (+5)
	Dressing	Independent (+10)
		Requires help (+5)
	Bowel control	Continent (+10)
		Occasional accident (+5)
	Bladder control	Continent (+10)
		Occasional accident (+5)
	Toilet use	Independent (+10)
		Requires help (+5)
	Transfers (bed to chair and back)	Independent (+15)
		Needs minor help (+10)
		Needs major help (1–2 people) but can sit (+5)
	Mobility on level surfaces	Independent, with any aid, > 50 yards (+15)
		Walks with help of one person > 50 yards (+10)
		Wheelchair independent > 50 yards (+5)
	Stairs	Independent (+10)
		Needs assistance (+5)
Cerebral Performance Category (CPC)	1	Good cerebral performance: Conscious, alert, able to work, mild neurological or psychological deficit
	2	Moderate cerebral disability: Conscious, sufficient function for independent activities of daily living, able to work in a sheltered environment
	3	Severe cerebral disability: Conscious, dependent on others for daily support because of impaired brain function, ranging from ambulatory to severe dementia or paralysis
	4	Coma or vegetative state: Any degree of coma or vegetative state without the presence of all brain death criteria
	5	Brain death
Extended Glasgow Outcome Scale (GOS-E)	1: Dead	
	2: Vegetative state	No obvious cortical function

29

Table 3.1 (cont.)

Scale	Component	Significance
	3: Lower severe disability	Able to follow commands but needs help with all activities and unable to live alone
	4: Upper severe disability	Able to follow commands, needs help with most activities, unable to live alone
	5: Lower moderate disability	Able to live independently, requires some assistance, unable to return to work or school
	6: Upper moderate disability	Able to live independently, requires little assistance, unable to return to work or school
	7: Lower good recovery	Able to return to work or school with mild difficulty
	8: Upper good recovery	Able to return to normal activities
Functional Independence Measure (FIM)	Eating Grooming Bathing Dressing (upper body) Dressing (lower body) Toileting Bladder control Bowel control Bed, chair, wheelchair transfers Toilet transfers Tub and shower transfers Walking/wheelchair Locomotion Stair locomotion Comprehension Expression Social interaction Problem solving Memory	A numeric score is assigned to each category: 1: Total assistance or not testable 2: Maximal assistance (≥ 25% independent) 3: Moderate assistance (≥ 50% independent) 4: Minimal assistance (≥ 75% independent) 5: Supervision 6: Modified independence (device) 7: Complete independence
	Level of consciousness	0: Alert 1: Not alert, but arousable with minimal stimulation 2: Not alert, requires repeated stimulation to attend 3: Coma
	Level of consciousness questions	0: Patient able to state month and own age 1: Patient answers one of the two correctly 2: Patient answers both incorrectly
	Level of consciousness commands	0: Patient blinks eyes and opens/closes a fist 1: Patient performs one of the two tasks 2: Patient performs neither task
	Horizontal extraocular movement	0: Normal 1: Partial gaze palsy but can be overcome 2: Partial gaze palsy but can be overcome with oculocephalic reflex 3: Forced gaze palsy that cannot be overcome
National Institutes of Health Stroke Scale (NIHSS)	Visual fields	0: No visual loss 1: Partial hemianopia 2: Complete hemianopia 3: Patient is bilaterally blind 3: Bilateral hemianopia
	Facial palsy	0: Normal symmetry 1: Minor paralysis (flat nasolabial fold, asymmetric smile) 2: Partial paralysis of lower face 3: Unilateral upper and lower face paralysis 3: Bilateral complete face paralysis
	Left upper extremity drift	0: No drift for 10 seconds 1: Drift but does not hit bed

Table 3.1 (cont.)

Scale	Component	Significance
		2: Drifts and hits bed
		3: Some effort against gravity
		4: No effort against gravity
		5: No movement
		0: Amputation or joint fusion
	Right upper extremity drift	0: No drift for 10 seconds
		1: Drift but does not hit bed
		2: Drifts and hits bed
		3: Some effort against gravity
		4: No effort against gravity
		5: No movement
		0: Amputation or joint fusion
	Left lower extremity drift	0: No drift for 5 seconds
		1: Drifts but does not hit bed
		2: Drifts and hits bed
		3: Some effort against gravity
		4: No effort against gravity
		5: No movement
		0: Amputation/joint fusion
	Right lower extremity drift	0: No drift for 5 seconds
		1: Drifts but does not hit bed
		2: Drifts and hits bed
		3: Some effort against gravity
		4: No effort against gravity
		5: No movement
		0: Amputation/joint fusion
	Limb ataxia	0: No ataxia
		1: Ataxia in 1 limb
		2: Ataxia in 2 limbs
		0: Does not understand test
		0: Paralyzed
		0: Amputation/joint fusion
	Sensation	0: No sensory loss
		1: Mild/moderate loss, less sharp/more dull, can sense being touched
		2: Complete loss and cannot sense being touched
		2: No response or quadriplegic
		2: Coma/unresponsive
	Language/aphasia	0: No aphasia
		1: Mild/moderate aphasia with some obvious changes but no significant limitations
		2: Severe aphasia with fragmented expression, inference needed, and inability to identify materials
		3: Mute/global aphasia with no usable speech or comprehension
		3: Coma/unresponsive
	Dysarthria	0: Normal
		1: Mild/moderate but can be understood
		2: Severe, with unintelligible slurring
		3: Mute/anarthric
		0: Intubated/unable to test
	Extinction/inattention	0: No abnormality
		1: Visual, tactile, auditory, spatial, or personal inattention
		1: Extinction to bilateral simultaneous stimulation
		2: Profound hemi-attention
		2: Extinction to > 1 modality

dichotomous approach outlined above attempts to split the mRS into favorable and unfavorable groups of numbers, an mRS ordinal (shift) analysis has been proposed as a means by which to assess all changes in mRS across the range of its values. The ordinal analysis approach has gained traction for use in clinical trials because it does not require as large a sample size and may lower the risk of overvaluing a beneficial transition at one of the distributions while disregarding harm at the other end.[6]

Barthel Index for Activities of Daily Living

The Barthel Index quantifies a patient's capabilities in various activities of daily living, including feeding, bathing, grooming, dressing, bowel and bladder habits, toilet use, transfers, mobility, and use of stairs. The index aims to establish the degree of independence from help provided by people and does not penalize the use of aids if needed. It ranges from 0 to 100, with 100 being independent in all activities.[7]

Cerebral Performance Category (CPC)

The CPC serves as an assessment of outcome after severe brain damage such as cardiac arrest. This scale ranges from 1 through 5, with a lower score indicating good cerebral performance with an alert conscious state with only mild neurological or psychological deficit and a higher score indicating varying degrees of cerebral disability up to brain death.[8]

Glasgow Outcome Scale (GOS) and Extended Glasgow Outcome Scale (GOS-E)

The GOS serves as a global scale for functional outcome that separates patients into one of five categories, ranging from 1 (dead) to 5 (good recovery). The GOS emphasizes ability to follow commands, to live independently, and to return to normal activities.[9,10] An extended, more detailed version of this scale has been created to provide a more accurate assessment, ranging from 1 (dead) to 8 (upper good recovery).

Functional Independence Measure (FIM)

The FIM is an 18-item assessment that evaluates feeding, grooming, bathing, upper and lower body dressing, and toileting to assess a patient's level of disability and to follow changes in a patient's functional status over time. Each item is scored from 1 (requiring total assistance) to 7 (totally independent).[11]

National Institutes of Health Stroke Scale (NIHSS)

The NIHSS serves as an ordinal scale ranging from 0–42 and consists of 11 items to measure neurological dysfunction across domains including language, coordination, strength, sensation, and neglect. Higher numbers indicate greater stroke severity. One should note that the NIHSS places greater emphasis on deficits associated with dominant hemisphere function compared to nondominant hemisphere or posterior circulation function, and consequently nondominant hemisphere stroke may receive a lower NIHSS scores compared to an infarct of comparable size affecting the dominant hemisphere. While the NIHSS alone was not devised for prognostic purposes, it is often used in conjunction with other clinical information in prognostic scoring systems.[4] Changes in the NIHSS are often used to define neurological changes, such as early neurological deterioration (any of ≥ 2 point increase in the NIHSS; ≥ 1 point increase in level of consciousness or motor item of the NIHSS; or any new neurological deficit within the first 3 days of admission)[12] or early neurological improvement (various definitions ranging from NIHSS improvement ≥ 4 points form baseline; an NIHSS 0, 1, or improvement ≥ 8; an NIHSS ≤ 3 or improvement ≥ 10; an NIHSS improvement by 20%; or a NIHSS score of 0 or 1).[13]

Prognostication by Outcomes

In terms of mortality and overall functional outcome, a daunting number of scales has been devised to address the prognosis of a variety of ischemic stroke scenarios. Many scales have aimed to incorporate easily attainable clinical information to assist with long-term prognostication for guiding expectations and potentially influencing management decisions. However, the clinical heterogeneity of stroke has made it challenging to devise a one-size-fits-all score. These features, as well as flaws in study designs in development of these scales, have limited applicability of the various scales and scores and the accuracy of their conclusions. Nevertheless, many of these are the best tools we have to assist with prognostication for our patients. Table 3.2 provides a summary of scores used to prognosticate mortality and functional outcome.

Mortality

Studies evaluating mortality in stroke have identified age, sex, vascular comorbidities, level of consciousness on presentation, the overall NIHSS, stroke subtype, and modified Rankin Scale as variables potentially influencing mortality at different time points. The presence of hemorrhagic conversion has also been associated with increased mortality.[14] Of the variety of biomarkers evaluated, hyperglycemia and acute kidney injury have been suggested to increase the risk of mortality.[15–18] These various features have been incorporated into the various scales as outlined below.

Early Mortality (In-Hospital to 1 Month)

Scores

Ischemic Stroke Risk Score (iScore): The iScore uses age, sex, stroke subtype, preadmission dependence for care, glucose level at the time of admission, and presence of comorbidities including atrial fibrillation, history of heart failure, history of myocardial infarction, active tobacco use, active cancer, and current use of dialysis. It has also been proposed to predict favorable 3-month outcomes after receiving tissue plasminogen activator (tPA) and to predict risk of intracerebral hemorrhage after receiving tPA. The score was evaluated in patients from Korea, Canada, and China and has been externally validated across 15 studies. An online calculator exists to calculate the score and provide both the score and its interpretation (www.sorcan.ca/iscore/). Criticisms of the score are that the validation cohort was partially derived from the derivation cohort, that the score requires substantial baseline information, and that generalizability of the scale is uncertain. [3,19–27]

JAGUAR score: The JAGUAR score uses Japan Coma Scale score, age, initial glucose level, time of hospital arrival from symptom onset, presence of atrial fibrillation, and pre-stroke mRS to predict chance of severe disability or death at 1 month in patients with ischemic stroke who cannot undergo endovascular intervention. The score has not been externally validated.[28]

NIHSS: In patients who undergo mechanical thrombectomy, a 24-hour NIHSS ≥ 14 may be associated with higher mortality at 1 month.[29]

PLAN score: The PLAN score uses pre-admission history of dependence on others for care, history of congestive heart failure, history of atrial fibrillation, active cancer, level of consciousness, age, and the presence of focal neurological deficits to predict severe disability at discharge, 30-day mortality, and 1-year mortality in patients who have and have not received tPA. The score was evaluated in patients from Canada and China and was externally validated in two studies. One criticism of the score is that the derivation cohort excluded patients receiving tPA and that the validation cohort included patients who received tPA.[3,22,25–27,30–32]

SOAR score: SOAR score uses age, presence of intracerebral hemorrhage, stroke type, and mRS to predict inpatient and 7-day mortality. The score was evaluated in patients from the United Kingdom and has not been externally validated. Criticisms of the score are that sex is not included in the final model despite there being significant associations in both univariate and multivariate analyses, and that excluding patients based on missing data may have increased bias.[3,25]

Clinical Factors

Seizures occurring during hospital admission for stroke have been associated with higher in-hospital mortality, more severe strokes, and higher rates of admission to the intensive care unit (ICU).[33] The presence of global aphasia may be associated with higher short-term risk of death.[34] Additionally, acute kidney injury (greater than 0.3 mg/dL increase in creatinine or 50% increase above baseline creatinine) occurring while in the hospital has been associated with a higher in-hospital mortality, and the rates of mortality may increase relative to the severity of renal dysfunction.[16,17] While it is unclear whether acute kidney injury has a causal relationship to ischemic stroke mortality, the presence of renal dysfunction in this context could contribute to homeostatic changes that may worsen stroke prognosis independent of other risk factors.

Biomarkers

Studies suggest that elevated troponin or elevated uric acid are associated with in-hospital mortality. [35,36] A higher neutrophil-to-lymphocyte ratio may be also associated with greater in-hospital mortality.[37,38] However, most biomarker studies

Table 3.2 Selection of scales predicting mortality and functional outcome

Scale	Populations	Stroke type	Outcome	Variables	Values	Points
				Age	< 61 years	+3
					61–70 years	+2
					71–80 years	+1
					> 80 years	+0
					90–100	+9
					80–89	+8
					70–79	+7
					60–69	+6
				Bispectral index	50–59	+5
					40–49	+4
					30–39	+3
					20–29	+2
					10–19	+1
ABMB	China	Ischemic stroke with impaired consciousness	Recovery of consciousness		0–9	+0
					Localize to pain	+3
					Flexing upper extremity to pain	+2
				Motor response	Extend upper extremity to pain	+1
					No response to pain	+0
					Pupil and corneal reflexes present	+4
				Brainstem response	One pupil wide and fixed	+3

Score	Population	Cohorts	Outcome	Parameter	Value	Points
					Pupil or corneal reflexes absent	+2
					Pupil and corneal reflexes absent	+1
					Absent pupil, corneal, and cough reflex	+0

A score > 13 at days 3–5 is associated with recovery of consciousness.

Score	Population	Cohorts	Outcome	Parameter	Value	Points
ASTRAL	Ischemic stroke	Switzerland China European cohorts	mRS at 3 months Mortality at 5 years	Initial glucose	< 3.7 or > 7.3 mmol/L	+1
				Age	Years	+1 per every 5 years
				Visual field deficit	Present	+2
				Level of consciousness	Decreased	+3
				Symptom onset to treatment time	> 3 hours	+2

Predictive of poor outcome (mRS 3–6) if ≥ 31. Higher mortality at 5 years for scores 35–59.

Score	Population	Cohorts	Outcome	Parameter	Value	Points
CONUT	Stroke patients	Japan	mRS at 3 months	Serum albumin	3.00–3.49 g/dL	+2
					2.50–2.99	+4
					< 2.50	+6
				Total lymphocyte count	≥ 1,600 lymphocytes/mm³	+3
				Total cholesterol	140–179 mg/dL	+1
						+2

Table 3.2 (cont.)

Scale	Populations	Stroke type	Outcome	Variables	Values	Points
					100–139 mg/dL	
					< 100 mg/dL	+3

A score ≥ 5 at admission is associated with poor outcome (mRS 3–6).

Scale	Populations	Stroke type	Outcome	Variables	Values	Points
				Hyperdense vessels or early ischemic changes on computed tomography (CT)	Present	+1 for each if present
				Pre-stroke mRS	> 1	+1
DRAGON	Finland Denmark Spain Australia	Anterior and posterior circulation strokes in patients receiving thrombolysis	mRS at 3 months	Age	65–79	+1
					> 79	+2
				Initial glucose	> 8 mmol/L	+1
				Symptom onset to treatment time	> 90 min	+1
				NIHSS	0–4	+0
					5–9	+1
					10–15	+2
					> 15	+3

Favorable outcome (mRS 0–2) is associated with DRAGON score ≤ 3.
Unfavorable outcome (mRS 5–6) is associated with DRAGON score 8–10.

Scale	Populations	Stroke type	Outcome	Variables	Values	Points
FSV	Canada Scotland	Ischemic and hemorrhagic stroke	mRS at 6 months	Lifts both arms	Present	+2
				Walks unassisted	Present	+1
				Age	< 80 years	+1
				Verbal GCS	Normal	+1

Favorable outcome (mRS 0–2) if ≥ 4.

				Pre-stroke mRS	0–5	Subtract the mRS
HIAT	United States	Ischemic stroke patients receiving intra-arterial treatment	Poor discharge outcome or in-hospital mortality	Age	> 75 years	+1
				NIHSS	> 18	+1
				Admission glucose level	> 150 mg/dL	+1

A score of 3 is associated with high chance of poor outcome (mRS 4–6).

					0–5	
iSCORE for 1-year outcome	Korea Canada China	Ischemic stroke Separately evaluated in patients who received tissue plasminogen activator (tPA)	Death at 30 days Death at 1 year Disability at 30 days Discharge to facility/institution mRS at 3 months after tPA Intracerebral hemorrhage after tPA	Age	Years	+1 for every year
				Sex	Male	+5
				Canadian Neurologic Scale (CNS)	0	+70
					≤ 4	+40
					5–7	+25
					> 8	0
				Stroke type	Lacunar	0
					Nonlacunar	+15
					Undetermined	+20
				History of atrial fibrillation	Present	+5
				History of congestive heart failure	Present	+10
				History of myocardial infarction	Present	+5
				Current smoking	Present	+5
				Cancer	Present	+15
				Dialysis	Yes	+40
				Pre-stroke dependence	Present	+20
				Initial glucose	≥ 7.5 mmol/L	+10

Table 3.2 (cont.)

Scale	Populations	Stroke type	Outcome	Variables	Values	Points
	Online calculator available at www.sorcan.ca/iscore Higher scores suggest higher risk of unfavorable outcomes (mRS > 2). Cutoff < 200 may be associated with favorable 3-month outcomes after tPA (mRS 0–2). Cutoff ≥ 200 may be associated with no significant improvement after tPA as well as increased risk of hemorrhage.					
				Japan Coma Scale	1-digit	+2
					2-digit	+4
					3-digit	+5
				Age	> 75 years	+1
				Initial glucose level	> 140 mg/dL	+1
JAGUAR	Japan	Ischemic stroke and unable to receive endovascular intervention	Severe disability or death at 1 month	Time of arrival from symptom onset	> 4.5 hours	+1
				Atrial fibrillation	Present	+1
				Pre-arrival mRS	> 2	+1
	A score ≥ 6 may be associated with high chance of severe disability (mRS 5–6) or death at 1 month.					
				Pre-stroke dependence	Present	+1.5
				Cancer	Present	+1.5
				History of congestive heart failure	Present	+1.0
PLAN	Canada China	Ischemic stroke, patients who did and did not receive tPA	Death at 1 month Death at 1 year mRS at discharge	History of atrial fibrillation	Present	+1.0
				Level of consciousness	Reduced	+5.0
				Age	Decades	+1.0 per decade
				Arm weakness	Significant	+2.0

A higher score portends a worse outcome.
A score ≥ 18 may be associated with 65% chance of severe disability (mRS 5–6), 50% mortality at 30 days, and 74% chance of mortality at 1 year.

				Leg weakness	Significant	+2.0
				Neglect or aphasia	Present	+1.0 for either or both
RNI	China	Anterior circulation large-vessel occlusion	mRS at 3 months	24-hour NIHSS	(Baseline NIHSS − 24-hour NIHSS)/Baseline NIHSS × 100%	Percent
				7-day NIHSS	([Baseline NIHSS] − [7-day NIHSS])/(Baseline NIHSS) × 100%	Percent

Favorable outcome (mRS 0–2) if ≥ 28% for 24-hour NIHSS.
Favorable outcome (mRS 0–2) if ≥ 42% for 7-day NIHSS.

				Intracranial stenosis	Present	+1
				Cortical nonlacunar-appearing acute infarcts	One infarct present	+1
					> 1 infarct	+2
SIGNAL2	Singapore	Mild ischemic stroke (post-stroke mRS ≤ 2)	Post-stroke cognitive impairment at 6 month and 1 year	Global cortical atrophy (GCA) score	GCA 1	+1
					GCA ≥ 2	+2
				Years of education	< 6 years	+2
				Age	50–64 years	+2
					≥ 65 years	+4
				Chronic lacunar infarcts	≥ 2	+2

Table 3.2 (cont.)

Scale	Populations	Stroke type	Outcome	Variables	Values	Points
			mRS at 3 months	Leukoaraiosis (Fazekas score)	Fazekas 2	+1
					Fazekas 3	+2

A score ≥ 7 may be associated with higher risk of cognitive impairment.

Scale	Populations	Stroke type	Outcome	Variables	Values	Points
SNARL		Ischemic stroke with endovascular intervention		Symptomatic hemorrhage	No	+2
				NIHSS	> 20	+0
					10–20	+1
					< 10	+3
				Age	> 80 years	+0
					60–79 years	+1
					< 60 years	+2
				Reperfusion	TICI ≥ 2b	+3
				Occlusion location	M2 or distal	+1

Low chance of favorable outcome (mRS < 3) if ≤ 3.
High chance of favorable outcome (mRS < 3) if ≥ 7.

Scale	Populations	Stroke type	Outcome	Variables	Values	Points
SOAR	United Kingdom	Stroke	Death at 7 days Death in hospital	Age	≤ 65 years	+0
					66–85 years	+1
					> 85 years	+2
				Stroke type	Hemorrhagic	+1
				Stroke subtype	Lacunar	+0
					Partial anterior circulation	+0
					Posterior circulation	+1
					Total anterior circulation	+2
				Pre-stroke mRS	≤ 2	+0
					3–4	+1
					5	+2

Poor outcome (inpatient and 7-day mortality) if ≥ 3.

				Factor	Value	Points
				Intracranial hemorrhage	Present	+1
				Age	65–84 years	+1
					> 85 years	+2
TACS	United Kingdom	Total anterior circulation stroke	In-hospital mortality	Pre-stroke mRS	4–5	+1
				No clear left or right lateralization of stroke	No clear lateralization	+1
				Congestive heart failure	Present	+1

A score ≥ 2 may portend a > 50% chance of mortality.

				Factor	Value	Points
				Age	≤ 59	0
					60–79	+1
					≥ 80	+2
THRIVE	International	Ischemic stroke patients who receive tPA, have thrombectomy, or have neither done	mRS at 3 months Death at 3 months	NIHSS	≤ 10	0
					11—20	+2
					≥ 80	+4
				Diabetes	Present	+1
				History of hypertension	Present	+1
				History of atrial fibrillation	Present	+1

Greater chance of poor outcome (mRS > 2) if ≥ 3.

Table 3.3 Biomarker predictors of unfavorable outcome at 3 months

Serum biomarker	Association	References
Brain-derived neurotrophic factor (BDNF)	Lower levels associated with poor outcome	[68] [302] [303] [304] [305] [306]
D-dimer	Elevated levels associated with poor outcome	[307]
Fatty acid-binding protein 4	Elevated levels associated with poor outcome	[308]
Glutamate	Elevated levels associated with poor outcome	[68] [309] [310] [311]
Heart fatty acid binding protein (H-FABP)	Elevated levels associated with poor outcome	[2] [312]
Lipids	Lower total cholesterol, triglycerides, and high-density lipoprotein (HDL) associated with poor outcomes. This association may be more prominent in males than females	[313] [314] [315] [316] [317]
Lipoprotein(a)	Elevated levels associated with poor outcome in patients with diabetes	[318]
Monocyte chemoattractant protein–1 (MCP–1)	Elevated levels associated with poor outcome in patients with NIHSS > 12	[319]
N-terminal prohormone of brain natriuretic peptide (NT-proBNP)	Elevated levels associated with poor outcome	[120]
Omega–3 polyunsaturated fatty acids	Lower levels associated with poor outcome	[320]
Platelet count-to-volume ratio	Elevated levels associated with poor outcome	[321]
Platelet distribution width	Lower levels associated with poor outcome	[322] [323]
Platelet-to-lymphocyte ratio	Elevated levels associated with poor outcome	[324] [325] [324]
Platelet-to-neutrophil ratio	Lower levels associated with poor outcome	[326]
Platelet volume	Elevated levels associated with poor outcome (but data is inconsistent)	[327] [328] [329] [330] [331] [332] [323] [333] [334]
Stress hyperglycemia ratio (glucose/HbA1c)	Elevated levels associated with poor functional outcome after mechanical thrombectomy for anterior circulation proximal occlusion	[335] [336] [337] [338]
Tau	Elevated levels associated with poor outcome	[68] [339]
T3 (free)	Lower levels associated with poor outcome	[340] [341] [342] [343] [344] [345] [346] [347]
Thyroid autoantibodies	Elevated levels associated with poor outcome	[348]
Toll-like receptors 2 and 4	Elevated levels associated with poor outcome	[349]
Troponin	Elevated levels associated with poor outcome	[70] [71] [72] [73] [35] [74] [68] [69]
Uric acid	Elevated levels associated with poor outcome	[36] [350] [351] [352]
Urine albumin	Elevated levels associated with poor outcome	[353] [354] [355]
Vitamin D	Low levels associated with poor outcome	[356] [357] [358] [359] [359] [360] [361].

Table 3.3 (cont.)

Serum biomarker	Association	References
White blood cell count (WBC) count and differential	Elevated WBCs associated with poor outcome Elevated neutrophils associated with poor outcome Elevated monocytes associated with poor outcome Lower lymphocytes associated with poor outcome	[362] [363] [364] [365] [366] [367] [368] [369] [370] [371] [372] [373] [374] [375] [376] [377] [378] [379] [380] [381] [382] [383] [384] [385] [386]

Table 3.4 Biomarker predictors of favorable outcome at 3 months

Serum biomarker	Association	References
Insulin-like growth factor (IGF–1)	Elevated levels associated with favorable outcome	[387]
Mannose-binding lectin	Low levels associated with favorable outcome	[388] [389] [390]
Lipids	Higher triglyceride-to-HDL ratio has been associated with favorable outcome	[391]

have been studied for longer-term functional outcome, as discussed further below.

Late Mortality (3 Months and Beyond)

Scores

CHADS2: The CHADS2 score helps assess the risk of stroke in patients with nonvalvular atrial fibrillation and considers a patient's history of congestive heart failure, history of hypertension, age, history of diabetes mellitus, and any history of cerebral ischemia. Variations on this score have been studied, and the CHADS2-Vasc score has been employed more commonly to this end and considers additional variables such as history of previous myocardial infarction, presence of peripheral artery disease or aortic plaque, younger age ranges, and sex. From a stroke prognosis perspective, in patients with nonvalvular atrial fibrillation, higher CHADS2 scores in admission may be associated with poor outcomes and higher mortality at 2 years.[39]

Ischemic Stroke Risk Score (iScore): See details above for early mortality.

PLAN score: See details above for early mortality.

Stroke Prognosis Instrument (SPI): The SPI score uses age, diabetes, acute severe hypertension, neurovascular event type, and history of coronary artery disease (CAD) to predict risk of stroke or death within 2 years of transient ischemic attack (TIA) or minor stroke. The score was evaluated in patients from Canada and was externally validated across four different cohorts. Criticisms of the score were that excluding patients with missing data and previous strokes may have increased bias.[3,40]

Totaled Health Risk in Vascular Events (THRIVE) score: The THRIVE score uses age, NIHSS, hypertension, diabetes, and atrial fibrillation to predict 3-month mRS and 3-month mortality in patients who receive tPA, undergo thrombectomy, or have neither intervention. It was originally developed to support identifying patients who may benefit from thrombectomy. It has been examined in over 16 external validation studies. However, criticisms of the score are that its final sample size is unclear, that it is unclear how missing data were handled, that the initial set of candidate predictors was limited, it was unclear how cutoffs were determined, and that it may have insufficient predictive performance to merit its use clinically. [3,41–54]

Clinical Factor

Acute kidney injury has also been associated with higher 3-month mortality.[18,55]

Functional Outcome

Extensive efforts have focused on attempting to identify determinants of functional outcome at various time points after ischemic stroke. Close attention has been given to the 3-month period following ischemic stroke, though functional outcomes at hospital discharge and months beyond have also been considered. A variety of clinical factors have been considered, including age, pre-stroke mRS, time to presentation, time to intra-arterial intervention in cases of large vessel occlusion, presence of various focal neurological deficits, components of the GCS, NIHSS, and change in NIHSS, history of cardiac comorbidities such as congestive heart failure, the motor exam, brainstem reflexes, and years of education. Radiographically, the presence of hemorrhage, reperfusion status following endovascular intervention, the location of a large vessel occlusion, the presence of intracranial stenoses, the presence of cortical atrophy, and the extent of white matter disease have been suggested to convey prognostic information. Even basic laboratory information such as the glucose level, serum albumin, total lymphocyte count, and total cholesterol levels have been factored into algorithms to prognosticate functional outcomes. Scores predictive of functional outcome, unfavorable and favorable, are outlined in Tables 3.3 and 3.4.

Early Functional Outcome (In-Hospital to 1 Month)
Scores

Houston Intra-Arterial Therapy (HIAT) score: The HIAT score uses age, NIHSS, and admission glucose level to predict the chance of poor outcome at discharge or in-hospital mortality in stroke patients undergoing intra-arterial intervention. The score was evaluated in patients from the United States and has not been externally validated.[56,57]

Ischemic Stroke Risk Score (iScore): See details above in section on early mortality.

JAGUAR score: See details above in section on early mortality.

PLAN Score. See details above in section on early mortality.

Total Anterior Circulation Stroke (TACS) score: The TACS score uses presence of hemorrhage, age, pre-stroke mRS, history of congestive heart failure, and presence of exam findings that suggest a lateralization of the stroke to predict mortality in patients with a total anterior circulation stroke, defined as homonymous hemianopia, other cortical signs, and unilateral weakness affecting at least two of the face, upper extremity, and lower extremity. The score was evaluated in the United Kingdom and has not been externally validated.[58]

Imaging

Infarct volume: Final infarct volumes less than 10 cm^3 may strongly predict return to home in nonagenarian patients.[59] Higher infarct volumes at 3 days have been found to correlate with worsened functional outcomes at 30 days. [60]

Collateral circulation: In patients with large vessel occlusions, poor pial collaterals seen on vascular imaging have been associated with larger infarct volumes and poor functional outcomes at discharge.[61–63] Conversely, favorable collaterals may be associated with good discharge outcomes in patients who undergo thrombectomy at times greater than 6 hours after the last known well time.[64]

Leukoariosis: Severe leukoaraiosis is associated with larger cortical infarct volumes and poor functional outcomes at 30 days.[65,66]

Biomarkers

Acute phase reactants, cardiac markers, and metabolic markers may have a role in helping to predict discharge outcomes. Elevated fibrinogen Y, an isoform of fibrinogen, may be associated with unfavorable outcome at discharge.[67] Elevated troponin levels also are associated with poor outcomes at hospital discharge and at 3 months, which may relate to cardiac complications occurring in patients with ischemic stroke or may reflect preexisting ischemic heart disease, congestive heart failure, comorbid atrial fibrillation, or active cancer. [35,68–74] Post-stroke hyperglycemia is associated with neurological deterioration, larger infarct size, poor functional recovery, and increased mortality rates, and elevated fasting plasma glucose levels in non-diabetic patients with acute ischemic stroke may be associated with poor outcomes at discharge.[75–86] Elevated ferritin levels have also been associated with worsened outcome at discharge.[87] Elevated BUN-to-creatinine ratio may also be associated with poor outcome at discharge and at 30 days. [88,89]

Late Functional Outcome (90 Days and Beyond)
Scores

ABMB score: The ABMB score uses age, bispectral index, motor response, and brainstem reflexes to predict recovery of consciousness in patients with impaired consciousness following a large stroke. The score was evaluated in patients from China and has not been externally validated. [90]

Acute Stroke Registry and Analysis of Lausanne (ASTRAL) score: The ASTRAL score is an integer-based point system that uses age, NIHSS, time to presentation, presence of a visual field defect, initial glucose level, and level of consciousness to predict an unfavorable outcome at 90 days. The score was evaluated in Chinese and European cohorts and externally validated across seven studies. Criticisms of the score include bias related to participant selection due to excluding patients with pre-stroke dependence and patients with any missing any data, unclear consideration of treatment effects, and unclear blinding during scale development. [3,15,22,43,91–95]

CHADS2-related scores: The CHADS2 score aids physicians in risk assessment of patients with atrial fibrillation to identify patients at higher risk for stroke, and assigns points based on the presence of CHF, hypertension, age, diabetes, and prior stroke or TIA. The CHADS2-Vasc score expands on the original score in terms of its age ranges, use of sex, and use of peripheral vascular comorbidities. However, this score has also been used as a potential prognostic marker after ischemic stroke. In patients who received tPA, a higher CHADS2 score may be associated with unfavorable 3-month outcomes in patients who received tPA,[96] or in patients with coronary artery disease without atrial fibrillation.[97]

CONUT score: The prevalence of malnutrition in ischemic stroke may range from 8–34% and may be an independent risk factor for morbidity and mortality.[98] Malnourishment on admission may be associated with higher rates of pneumonia, other infections, gastrointestinal hemorrhage, and bedsores. The CONUT score uses serum albumin, total lymphocyte count, and total cholesterol level to predict poor outcomes at 3 months in patients with stroke. It has not been externally validated.[98]

DRAGON: The DRAGON score incorporates the presence of a hyperdense vessel sign and early signs of ischemia on computed tomography (CT), pre-stroke mRS, age, initial glucose level, onset to treatment time, and admission NIHSS to predict favorable and unfavorable 3-month outcomes in patients with anterior and posterior circulation strokes receiving thrombolysis. The score was evaluated in patients from Finland, Denmark, Spain, and Australia and has been externally validated across 10 studies. Criticisms of the score include it being unclear whether any blinding

method was applied for assigning mRS scores, no clear description of the multivariable method for selecting final predictors, and potential for misinterpretation of early infarct and hyperdense vessel signs. [3,24,91,92,99–104]

Five Simple Variables (FSV): The FSV score considers age, pre-stroke mRS, motor function of the upper extremities, and verbal responses of the Glasgow Coma Scale to predict favorable 6-month outcomes. The score was evaluated in patients from Canada and Scotland and has been externally validated in one study. Criticisms of the score include that the sample size may have been insufficient for the number of tested candidate predictors, that participants with missing data were excluded from analysis, and that blinding was unclear.[3,31,32,93]

NIHSS: The NIHSS can be used to measure baseline dysfunction and to track early neurological changes after ischemic stroke. Baseline function prior to the ischemic stroke also has an impact on outcome. In one study, baseline NIHSS ≤ 6 was associated with favorable 3-month outcomes by the Barthel Index and Glasgow Outcome Scale, whereas a score ≥ 16 was associated with a higher chance of death or severe disability.[105] Early changes in the neurological exam, represented by changes in the NIHSS score from admission to later points during the admission, may convey prognostic information. [13,106,111] Early neurological improvement (reduction in NIHSS by 10 or more points or absolute score of 4 or less at 2 hours) or continuous neurological improvement (reduction in NIHSS by 8 or more between 2 and 24 hours or absolute score of 4 within 24 hours) have been associated with favorable 3-month outcomes independent of the presence of thrombolysis or endovascular intervention. In patients who receive tPA, early neurological improvement or continuous neurological improvement may be associated with favorable 3-month outcomes.[112] A 24-hour post-tPA NIHSS ≤ 11 has been associated with favorable 3-month outcomes.[113] Conversely, early neurological deterioration has been associated with poor 3-month outcomes. Post-thrombolysis NIHSS ≥ 15 or ≥ 20 may be associated with unfavorable 3-month outcome.[113,114] Early neurological stability – that is, minimal change in the NIHSS over time – may also be associated with poor 3-month functional outcomes in patients with initial NIHSS score > 4.[115] While cutoffs may vary across different studies, in general a higher baseline NIHSS generally portends a poor functional prognosis, and as time passes, the threshold at which the NIHSS will predict an unfavorable outcome decreases.[116]

Relative Neurological Improvement (RNI) score: The RNI score uses changes in the baseline NIHSS score at 24 hours and 7 days to predict favorable 3-month mRS in patients with anterior circulation large-vessel occlusion stroke. The score was evaluated in patients from China and has not been externally validated.[117]

SIGNAL2 score: The SIGNAL2 score uses presence of intracranial stenosis, presence of cortical nonlacunar-appearing acute infarcts, global cortical atrophy score, number of years of education, age, presence of chronic lacunar infarcts, and leukoaraiosis score to predict risk of post-stroke cognitive impairment at 6 months and 1 year in patients with mild ischemic stroke. The score was studied in patients from Singapore and has not been externally validated.[118]

SNARL score: The SNARL score uses the presence of intracranial hemorrhage, NIHSS, age, endovascular reperfusion status, and occlusion location to predict favorable mRS at 3 months in patients who undergo endovascular intervention for large vessel occlusion. Criticisms of the score are that interpretation of imaging findings may be subject to high interobserver variability.[3,119]

Totaled Health Risk in Vascular Events (THRIVE) score: See above at 90-day mortality.

Clinical Factors

Data suggest that female sex may be an independent risk factor for unfavorable function outcome after ischemic stroke.[120] Efforts to understand the molecular basis of this observation suggest that females may have a higher inflammatory response and sex-related differences in lipid profiles, though the etiology of this association remains uncertain. Short-term weight loss after stroke may occur in up to a quarter of patients, and it may be associated with unfavorable outcomes at 3 months and may reflect malnutrition and the need for proper nutrition following stroke.[121]

Some specific neurological deficits can affect ultimate neurological prognosis. Post-stroke aphasia represents an early marker of unfavorable outcome in ischemic stroke. This may relate to challenges imposed by a receptive aphasia in which patients may have difficulty participating in rehabilitation and in turn diminish its potential gains. Similarly, the lasting effects from an expressive aphasia may present functional challenges that amount to an inability to live independently. Accordingly, the presence of aphasia at 24 hours after onset, even in patients who received thrombolysis, is associated with poor outcome.[122] Unilateral spatial neglect after nondominant hemispheric infarction can also impact outcome. The incidence of unilateral spatial neglect varies widely and may occur in 18–82% of right hemisphere strokes.[123] It often leads to loss of autonomy in that a patient may not eat food on the left side of the plate, may collide with objects in the left side of space, may skip the initial part of sentences when reading, may not dress the left side of the body, and may have marked difficulty moving the left side of the body even in the absence of motor dysfunction. Functionally, neglect and other right hemisphere deficits such as anosognosia may interfere with a patient's ability to participate in rehabilitation which may significantly compromise the recovery process [124] and ultimately lead to worsened outcomes at 90 days.[123]

Post-stroke depression is also associated with prognosis, as it may interfere with cognitive and physical recovery and may also impact participation in acute rehabilitation. Persistent depression at 3 months and 12 months has been associated with unfavorable functional outcomes, and the persistence of anxiety and depression in young patients after stroke may even be associated with poor functional outcomes up to a decade following the stroke.[125] Resolution of depression within a year may in turn be associated with favorable outcomes.[126]

Imaging

Extensive data suggest an independent prognostic role for multiple radiographic factors for 3-month outcomes. Baseline imaging findings, infarct location, infarct volume, presence or absence of hemorrhagic transformation, degree of collateral circulation, and recanalization/reperfusion status all have prognostic implications.

Baseline imaging findings: Radiographically, a variety of measures suggest a role for white matter disease in post-stroke cognitive impairment. A higher burden of small vessel disease (white matter hyperintensities, lacunar infarcts, cerebral microhemorrhages, enlarged perivascular spaces) may correlate with poor performance on cognitive testing and measures of functional independence after stroke.[127–130] In patients who receive thrombolysis, severe leukoaraiosis on the baseline CT may be associated with poor 3-month outcomes and may be associated with a higher risk of symptomatic intracerebral hemorrhage.[131–137] In patients who undergo mechanical thrombectomy, severe leukoaraiosis may be associated with futile recanalization and poor 3-month outcomes.[138–141] Otherwise, in younger patients with ischemic stroke – mean age around 40 years – moderate or severe leukoaraiosis may be associated with unfavorable 3-month outcomes and higher rates of death after 2 years. [142,143] Severe leukoaraiosis is also associated with poor functional outcome at 1 year.[144] The degree of periventricular hyperintensities has also been associated with poor motor outcomes following stroke as well as poor cognitive outcomes and poor recovery from neglect.[127–129,145,146]

Infarct location: In terms of location, left hemisphere strokes involving the uncinate fasciculus, precuneus, and angular gyrus may be associated with poor 90-day outcomes, and right hemisphere strokes involving the parietal lobe and putamen may be associated with poor 90-day outcomes (mRS).[147] A basilar or vertebral artery occlusion has been associated with poor 3-month outcomes in patients with posterior circulation strokes.[148] Specific involvement of the corticospinal tracts may also portend worsened outcomes, since weakness contributes so much to disability and weight heavily into scales such as the mRS. According, abnormal descending corticospinal tract diffusion-weighted imaging (DWI) hyperintensities and early apparent diffusion coefficient (ADC) dropout in the descending corticospinal tracts is associated with poor NIHSS motor outcomes at 3 months. [4,149] Ischemic stroke involving primary motor cortex on brain magnetic resonance imaging (MRI) is similarly associated with less favorable outcomes (mRS) at 3 months.[150] Additional involvement of the somatosensory cortex and intraparietal sulcus may preferentially be associated with worse motor recovery and functional outcomes.[4,151] Poor verbal and visual memory (immediate and delayed recall and recognition) may be associated with left hemisphere strokes, subcortical strokes, and large infarct volume. [152] Lower scores on standardized cognitive tests such as the Montreal Cognitive Assessment (MoCA) may be associated with strokes involving the left inferior frontal gyrus, left superior temporal gyrus, hippocampus, parahippocampal gyrus, left middle temporal gyrus, and the left thalamus.[153] Right hemisphere strokes may affect attention and prosody as well as visual–spatial memory and geographic orientation.[154]

Infarct volume: Infarct volume has also been felt to carry prognostic significance and has been the focus of considerable review. Volumes ≥ 10 mL at 1 week after admission may be associated with a Barthel Index < 95 at 6 months, and in malignant middle cerebral artery (MCA) strokes, infarcts ≥ 300 mL may be associated with poor functional outcomes at 6 months regardless of whether the patient undergoes decompressive hemicraniectomy to relieve edema.[155] Final infarct volumes of ≥ 133 mL at 48 hours after the stroke was shown to be highly specific for unfavorable 3-month outcomes.[156] A DWI infarct volume > 70 mL in conjunction with an NIHSS > 20 may be associated with poor 3-month outcomes.[157] Seven days post-stroke DWI volumes ≤ 3.4 mL may be associated with complete independence at 3 months in patients who receive thrombolysis, whereas volumes ≥ 90 mL may be associated with unfavorable 3-month outcomes and volumes ≥ 115 mL may be associated with death at 90 days. In patients receiving thrombolysis, an infarct volume of < 16 mL may be associated with favorable 3-month outcomes.[158] In patients undergoing mechanical thrombectomy, higher pretreatment infarct volume may increase the number needed to treat to achieve functional independence in thrombectomy of proximal intracranial occlusion, with the number needed to treat increasing to 10 for an infarct volume of 80 mL and 15 for a volume of 135 mL.[159] Change in infarct volume over time also is important. Infarct growth of 14–16 mL from admission to day 7 may be associated with poor 3-month outcomes.[160,161] When comparing DWI 2 hours after thrombolysis and 24 hours after thrombolysis, every 1 mL increase in infarct volume may portend a 10% decrease in the odds of early neurological improvement, whereas for every 1 mL decrease in stroke volume, there may be a 10% increase in the odds of early neurological improvement.[162] After endovascular therapy, a growth in infarct size of ≥ 12 mL compared with baseline is associated with poor 3-month outcomes.[163]

Hemorrhagic transformation: Hemorrhagic transformation type 2 and parenchymal hemorrhage type 2 have been associated with poor 3-month outcomes.[14]

Collateral circulation: An incomplete circle of Willis is, expectedly, associated with poor 3-month outcomes following noncardioembolic strokes.[164] Patients with favorable collaterals may have better 3- to 6-month outcomes and lower rates of intracerebral hemorrhage after receiving IV thrombolysis.[165–167] Patients with distal hyperintense vessels seen on fluid-attenuated inversion recovery (FLAIR) may have lower NIHSS scores, smaller infarct volumes, and favorable 3-month outcomes, as these vessels may represent leptomeningeal collaterals,[168] although not universally so.[169] An opercular index score has been proposed to describe collateral robustness and predict outcome inpatients undergoing thrombectomy of M1, M2, or distal internal carotid artery (ICA) occlusions and is calculated from the number of opacified M3 opercular branches on the unaffected side divided by the number on the stroke side, with a ratio ≥ 2 associated with poor 3-month outcomes.[170] On catheter angiography, an incomplete large vessel occlusion found prior to intra-arterial therapy is associated with a threefold higher chance of 3-month favorable outcome compared to complete large vessel occlusions.[171] In contrast, microcirculatory obstructions, defined as contrast stasis and absence of capillary blush in sites distal to large vessel occlusions, is associated with poor 3-month outcomes.[172]

Reperfusion and recanalization: Serial imaging of cerebral CT angiography (CTA) and CT perfusion (CTP) at days 0 and 1 after ischemic stroke suggest that radiographic reperfusion on day 1 may be associated with favorable 3-month outcomes, whereas radiographic recanalization may not be associated with favorable outcomes.[173] A decrease in the intensity of a FLAIR hyperintense middle cerebral artery vessel 1 hour following thrombolysis may be associated with favorable 3-month outcomes. [174] In patients who have received alteplase, poor collateral recruitment on CT angiography within 24 hours of receiving alteplase may be associated with poor 3-month outcomes and higher mortality.[175] After thrombectomy, reduced flow signal of the ipsilateral recanalized MCA on transcranial doppler is associated with poor 3-month outcomes.[176] In terms of reperfusion, Thrombolysis in Cerebral Infarction (TICI) scores of 2b or higher are associated with favorable 3-month outcomes.[177] A higher number of device passes during intra-arterial therapy is associated with poor functional outcomes in large vessel occlusion, with the rate of recanalization dropping by nearly 40% for every pass and the likelihood of a favorable 3-month outcome dropping based on the number of passes (58% for more than one pass, 50% for more than two, 48% for more than three, 38% for more than four, and 25% for five or more).[178]

Biomarkers

Numerous biomarkers have been evaluated with respect to 3-month functional outcomes. However, the applicability of biomarkers as independent predictors of prognosis has been limited by a variety of technical considerations and relate to problems with identifying an ideal biological sample (blood, urine, cerebrospinal fluid [CSF]), differing assays used for single biomarkers, variations in the accepted reference ranges of various biomarkers, and limited predictive values. [2,68,179,180] Coupled with the clinical heterogeneity of stroke as well as the fact that many studies evaluating various biomarkers have had small sample sizes and were performed opportunistically rather than through carefully prespecified designs, the generalizability of potentially useful biomarkers has been limited.[68] With these considerations in mind, multiple observations have been made about various prospective biomarkers, which are summarized in Tables 3.3 and 3.4.

Potential biomarkers explored in 6-month prognosis include brain natriuretic peptide (BNP) and creatinine. In patients with atrial fibrillation, elevated BNP is associated with higher rates of in-hospital mortality, recurrent stroke, and poor functional outcome at 6 months.[181–184] Otherwise, the presence of an elevated creatinine is associated with poor 6-month outcomes and may be associated with risk of recurrent stroke. [55,185–189]

Electrophysiology

Both quantitative and qualitative electroencephalogram (EEG) have been used to guide prognostication. Measures of brain activity (delta/alpha ratio) and functional connectivity (magnitude squared coherence and weighted phase lag index, which represent ways to compare connectivity between electrodes quantitatively) may differ between the ipsilesional and contralesional hemisphere after ischemic stroke and may be associated with poor 3-month outcomes in this context.[190] Status epilepticus occurring within 3 months of stroke may be associated with poor functional outcomes due to impairment of neuroplasticity potentially related to the seizure activity as well as the antiepileptics used to treat the seizures. Status epilepticus lasting longer than 12 hours may be most strongly associated with poor outcomes.[191]

Neurophysiological measures such as EEG and motor evoked potentials have been evaluated with respect to 6-month prognosis. The pairwise derived brain symmetry index, a measure to evaluate global asymmetry along homologous channel pairs, may help estimate hemisphere damage in patients with ischemic stroke and thereby predict poor 6-month outcomes relative to the degree of asymmetry present.[192–194] Recordable motor evoked potentials immediately following the stroke as well as an improvement in central conduction time after 2 weeks may both be associated with higher functional outcomes at 2 weeks and at 6 months.[195–197]

Specific Outcomes

In large part due to their implications for stroke prognosis, close attention has been given to certain clinical scenarios that may complicate ischemic stroke. Such situations include hemorrhagic transformation of ischemic infarcts, early neurological deterioration, recurrent stroke, post-stroke seizures, post-stroke pneumonia, and post-stroke depression. Additionally, the prognosis for language recovery after ischemic stroke–related aphasia can be important in these patients.

Hemorrhagic Transformation of Ischemic Infarcts

As noted above, the presence of advanced hemorrhagic transformation carries a poor prognosis for good functional outcomes.

Clinical Factors

Higher NIHSS scores, presence of various cardiovascular comorbidities, use of antithrombotics, higher blood pressure, and functional status before the stroke have all been proposed as clinical determinants potentially associated with hemorrhagic transformation of an infarct.

Imaging

Radiographically, a lower CT ASPECTS value as well as the presence of a hyperdense MCA sign have also been found to contribute to a higher risk of hemorrhagic transformation of infarcts in the scales below. CT perfusion data have suggested a potential independent risk of hemorrhagic conversion in patients with particular perfusion imaging values, specifically a relative cerebral blood flow < 0.48 and Tmax > 14 seconds with volumes of > 5 mL.[198,199] The presence of cerebral microhemorrhages may be associated with greater rates of hemorrhagic transformation in patients who receive tPA.[200]

Biomarkers

Elevated hemoglobin A1c and elevated matrix metalloproteinase–9 (MMP-9, an enzyme released from astrocytes and microglia involved in inflammatory responses) may be associated with higher rates of symptomatic intracranial hemorrhage following thrombolysis.[2,68,179,201–206]

Scores (see Table 3.5)

Hemorrhagic Transformation (HT) score: The HT score uses CT ASPECTS, NIHSS, the presence of a hyperdense MCA sign, and presence of atrial fibrillation on admission electrocardiogram (EKG) to predict higher risk of hemorrhagic transformation in patients with acute MCA territory stroke. The score has not been externally validated.[207]

Symptomatic Intracranial Hemorrhage (sICH) score: The sICH score uses the presence of valvular heart disease, use of aspirin, systolic blood pressure prior to thrombolysis, NIHSS, platelet count, and need for IV antihypertensive medications during thrombolysis to predict the risk of symptomatic intracerebral hemorrhage in patients with ischemic stroke who receive tPA. The score was evaluated in patients from Thailand [24] and has been externally validated in one study.[208]

TURN score: The TURN score uses pre-stroke mRS and baseline NIHSS to predict symptomatic intracerebral hemorrhage after receiving tPA. The score was evaluated in patients from the United States and has not been externally validated. [209–211]

Early Neurological Deterioration

Clinical Factors

Higher NIHSS score and histories of diabetes and myocardial infarction may be associated with neurological deterioration.[212] Seizures can also be associated with deterioration.[33]

Imaging

Radiographically, lenticulostriate infarctions associated with branch atheromatous disease (infarcts > 15 mm or more in diameter and spanning > 3 axial sections) may be associated with higher rates of infarct enlargement and neurological deterioration.[213] Moreover, an increase in infarct volume of > 11 mL seen on ADC 3–5 days after a stroke may be associated with cerebral edema and neurological deterioration.[161] Severe leukoaraiosis is also associated with recurrent stroke.[214–216]

Table 3.5 Scores predictive of hemorrhagic transformation

Scale	Populations	Stroke type	Outcome	Variables	Values	Points
Hemorrhagic transformation (HT)	Russia	Ischemic middle cerebral artery (MCA) territory stroke	Hemorrhagic transformation	ASPECTS	0–2	+3
					3–4	+2
					5–6	+1
					7–10	+0
				NIHSS	> 23	+3
					18–23	+2
					12–17	+1
					0–11	+0
				Hyperdense MCA vessel sign	Present	+1
				Atrial fibrillation on electrocardiogram (EKG)	Present	+1

A score ≥ 2 suggests higher risk of hemorrhagic transformation.

Scale	Populations	Stroke type	Outcome	Variables	Values	Points
sICH	Thailand	Ischemic stroke patients receiving tPA	Symptomatic intracranial hemorrhage	Valvular heart disease	Present	+2
				Use of aspirin	Present	+1.5
				Systolic blood pressure > 140 prior to thrombolysis	Present	+1.0
				NIHSS	10–20 or ≥ 20	+2.0
				Platelet count	< 250,000	+1.0
				IV antihypertensives required during thrombolysis	Present	+1.0

A score ≥ 8 may be associated with > 50% risk of symptomatic hemorrhage.

Scale	Populations	Stroke type	Outcome	Variables	Values	Points
TURN	United States	Ischemic stroke patients receiving tPA	Symptomatic intracranial hemorrhage	Pre-stroke mRS	mRS number	mRS * 0.27
					Initial NIHSS	NIHSS * 0.10
					TURN value	TURN = −4.65 + (mRS * 0.27) + (NIHSS * 0.10)
					TURN predictor	TURN predictor = $e^{(TURN)} * (1+e^{(TURN)})$%

A TURN predictor ≥ 3.5% may be associated with higher risk of symptomatic ICH.

Table 3.6 Score predictive of neurological deterioration

Scale	Populations	Stroke type	Outcome	Variables	Values	Points
WORSEN	Japan China	Ischemic stroke or TIA	Early neurological deterioration	HbA1c	> 7.4%	+1
				Prior myocardial infarction	Present	+2
				Radiological findings	Internal carotid artery (ICA) occlusion	+3
					Middle carotid artery (MCA) M1 occlusion	+2
					Striatocapsular infarction	+1
					Pontine infarction	+1
				Infarct diameter	15–30 mm	+1
				Low-density lipoprotein (LDL) cholesterol	> 140 mg/dL	+1
				Initial NIHSS	> 8	+2

WORSEN score > 3 is associated with early neurological deterioration.

Biomarkers

Biomarkers are of less utility here, but serum hypoalbuminemia may predict in-hospital deterioration.[217,218]

Score (See Table 3.6)

WORSEN score The WORSEN score uses history of diabetes, history of myocardial infarction, presence of ICA occlusion, presence of MCA M1 occlusion, presence of striatocapsular infarction, presence of pontine infarction, the size of the infarct, low-density lipoprotein (LDL) level, and NIHSS score to predict neurological deterioration within 1 week of admission in patients with ischemic stroke who do not receive tPA or undergo endovascular intervention.[212] The score was evaluated in patients from Japan and was externally validated in one study.[219]

Recurrent Stroke

Clinical Factors

Clinical features potentially associated with recurrent stroke include age, presence of vascular comorbidities, smoking history, and prior TIA or stroke. [220]

Imaging

Brain imaging: The presence of intracranial atherosclerotic disease, whether the primary mechanism of the stroke or found incidentally, carries a higher risk of recurrent stroke. [221,222] The risk of recurrent stroke may further increase in patients with intracranial atherosclerosis across two or more large intracranial arteries.[221]. Even in strokes felt to result from a cardioembolic mechanism, the presence of intracranial atherosclerosis may be associated with a higher risk of stroke recurrence or death at 18 months.[223] A perfusion mismatch (Tmax > 6 seconds involving > 15 mL of tissue) in strokes due to intracranial atherosclerosis may be associated with a higher risk of recurrent stroke.[224] In patients with TIA or nondisabling ischemic stroke, a low mean flow velocity and a high pulsatility index on transcranial doppler ultrasound may be independently associated with a higher risk of recurrent stroke or vascular events over 2 years. [225] Additionally, the presence of a carotid plaque (but not necessarily the intima-media thickness) may be associated with risk of recurrent vascular events within 10 years.[226]

Cardiac imaging: In patients with cardi-oembolic strokes from atrial fibrillation, a lower left atrial appendage wall velocity on transthoracic echocardiography 1 week after the stroke may be associated with cerebrovas-cular death or recurrent ischemic stroke.[227] Also, patients with lower left atrial remodel-ing index may be associated with higher risk of recurrent cerebrovascular events.[228] Furthermore, left atrial enlargement, espe-cially severe enlargement, may be associated with higher 90-day risk of recurrent stroke and systemic embolization.[229]

Biomarkers

Elevated hemoglobin A1c, low serum albumin, and a history of chronic kidney disease may be associated with poor functional outcomes as well as recurrent stroke.[55,185–189,230–246]

Scores (See Table 3.7)

Small Vessel Disease (SVD) score: The SVD score uses presence of lacunar infarcts, presence of microhemorrhages, number of perivascular spaces in the basal ganglia, and presence of peri-ventricular and deep white matter T2/FLAIR hyperintensities to predict the chance of recurrent stroke in patients with stroke. The score has not been externally validated.[247]

Essen Stroke Risk Score (ESRS): The ESRS uses age, presence of arterial hypertension, presence of diabetes, history of myocardial infarction, presence of other cardiovascular disease, presence of periph-eral artery disease, smoking history within the last 5 years, and history of a prior TIA or ischemic stroke before the presenting event to predict risk of recur-rent stroke over 1 year in patients with ischemic stroke or TIA. The was evaluated in patients from Germany and has been externally validated.[220]

Stroke Prognosis Instrument (SPI): See mor-tality at 2 years above.

Post-Stroke Epilepsy

Clinical Factors

Higher NIHSS, mechanism and location of stroke, and occurrence of seizures shortly after the stroke may increase the risk of post-stroke epilepsy.[248]

Imaging

Cortical infarct location and/or involvement of the MCA territory can increase the risk of post-stroke epilepsy.[248]

Score (See Table 3.8)

SeLECT score. The SeLECT score uses NIHSS, presence of a large-artery atherosclerotic mechan-ism, early seizures (within 7 days) after stroke, pre-sence of cortical involvement of the stroke, and involvement of the MCA territory to predict increased risk of late seizures (after 7 days) follow-ing ischemic stroke. The score was evaluated in patients from Switzerland, Austria, and Germany. The score was developed under the premise that the injury resulting from a stroke may increase the risk of seizures in life, but given that early post-stroke seizures alone are not sufficient to establish the diagnosis of epilepsy since they may have been provoked from the stroke, the score works to iden-tify patients who may go on to develop post-stroke epilepsy. This score has been externally validated in three additional cohorts.[248]

Post-Stroke Pneumonia

Post-stroke pneumonia has been associated with a poor prognosis in multiple studies (see section below) and has been associated with higher mor-bidity, mortality, length of hospital stay, and over-all medical costs.[249–254] It is defined as pneumonia occurring within 7 days of admission for stroke and may complicate as many as 14% of strokes.[255,256] It has been felt to carry the high-est attributable rise in mortality (10–31%) of all medical complications following stroke.[257]

Clinical Factors

Higher age, higher baseline disability, presence of atrial fibrillation, male sex, presence of dysphagia, and higher NIHSS scores have all been shown to predict post-stroke pneumonia.[249,251,258] Possible determinants of morbidity and mortality in stroke-associated pneumonia include older age, higher pre-stroke disability, history of dementia, higher NIHSS scores, presence of dysphagia, sex, history of lung cancer, hyperglycemia, and ele-vated C-reactive protein levels.[255]

Imaging

Severe leukoaraiosis has also been associated with higher rates of pulmonary infections following ischemic stroke.[259]

Biomarkers

Elevated admission glucose is associated with post-stroke pneumonia.[252]

Table 3.7 Scores predictive of recurrent stroke

Scale	Populations	Stroke type	Outcome	Variables	Values	Points
ESRS	Germany	Ischemic stroke or TIA	Stroke recurrence	Age	≥ 65–75 years	+1
					≥ 75 years	+2
				Arterial hypertension	Present	+1
				Diabetes mellitus	Present	+1
				History of myocardial infarction	Present	+1
				Other cardiovascular disease	Present	+1
				Peripheral artery disease	Present	+1
				Smoking history within the last 5 years	Present	+1
				Previous TIA or ischemic stroke	Present	+1

A score > 2 is associated with higher risk of recurrent stroke over 1 year.

Scale	Populations	Stroke type	Outcome	Variables	Values	Points
SPI	United States Canada	TIA or minor stroke	Stroke at 2 years	Age	> 65	+3
				Diabetes mellitus	Present	+3
				Acute severe hypertension	Present	+2
				Type of event	TIA	+0
					Stroke	+2
				History of coronary heart disease	Present	+1

Low risk (0–2)
Medium risk (3–6)
High risk (7–11)

Scale	Populations	Stroke type	Outcome	Variables	Values	Points
SVD	China	Ischemic stroke	Recurrent stroke	Lacunar infarcts	Present	+1
				Microhemorrhages	Present	+1
				Basal ganglia perivascular spaces	> 10 present	+1
				Severe periventricular or moderate/severe deep white matter magnetic resonance imaging (MRI) hyperintensities	Present	+1

A score of 3 is associated with 16% chance of recurrent stroke.
A score of 4 is associated with a 25% chance of recurrent stroke.

Table 3.8 Scores predictive of post-stroke epilepsy

Scale	Populations	Stroke type	Outcome	Variables	Values	Points
				Stroke severity	NIHSS 0–3	0
					NIHSS 4–10	+1
					NIHSS ≥11	+2
A2DS2	Switzerland Austria Germany Italy	Ischemic stroke	Post-stroke epilepsy	Large artery atherosclerosis	Present	+1
				Early seizure (≤ 7 days)	Present	+3
				Cortical involvement of infarct	Present	+2
				MCA territory of infarct	Present	+1

Risk of post-stroke epilepsy at 5 years
0–3 = 1–6%
4–5 = 11–18%
5–6 = 18–29%
7–8 = 45–65%
9 = 83%

Scores (See Table 3.9)

A2DS2 score: The A2DS2 score, named for its variables, uses age, presence of atrial fibrillation, sex, presence of dysphagia, and NIHSS to predict risk of developing pneumonia in patients with ischemic stroke. A higher score estimates a greater risk for pneumonia. The score was evaluated in patients from China and has been externally validated in two studies.[249,258]

ISAN score: The ISAN score, also named for its variables, uses sex, age, pre-stroke mRS, and NIHSS to predict risk of developing pneumonia in patients with ischemic stroke. The score divides patients into low, medium, high, and highest risk classes. The score was evaluated in European and Asian populations. The score has been externally validated in two studies. [249,251]

Acute Ischemic Stroke-Associated Pneumonia Score (AIS-APS): The AIS-APS uses age, medical history, pre-stroke mRS, presence of dysphagia, infarct type, and admission glucose to predict risk of developing pneumonia in an acute cerebrovascular event. The score divides patients into very low, low, intermediate, high, and very high risk categories. The score was evaluated in patients from China and has been externally validated in one study.[249.252]

Fiberoptic Endoscopic Dysphagia Severity Scale (FEDSS): The FEDSS uses the degree of dysphagia on a fiberoptic endoscopic exam to predict the risk of poor 3-month functional outcome in patients with dysphagia following first-ever acute ischemic or hemorrhagic stroke. While not directly related to pneumonia, aspiration in the setting of dysphagia may increase the risk for stroke-related pneumonia. The score was evaluated in German patients and has not been externally validated.[254]

Post-Stroke Depression
Clinical Factors

Clinical features found to increase the risk of post-stroke depression include higher NIHSS score on presentation, younger age, female sex, and history of premorbid psychiatric disorders.[260–262]

Imaging

Leukoaraiosis,[263] presence of lobar microhemorrhages,[264] and moderate to severe enlargement of perivascular spaces [265] are associated with post-stroke depression. Left-sided lenticulocapsular locations as well as frontal lobe and basal ganglia locations are also associated with higher rates of post-stroke depression.[266,267]

Table 3.9 Scores predictive of post-stroke pneumonia

Scale	Populations	Stroke type	Outcome	Variables	Values	Points
A2DS2	China	Ischemic stroke	Risk of pneumonia	Age	> 75 years	+1
				Atrial fibrillation	Present	+1
				Male sex	Present	+1
				Dysphagia	Present	+2
				NIHSS	5–15	+3
					≥ 16	+5
About 0.3% chance with score of 0 About 39.4% with score of 10						
AIS-APS	China	Cerebrovascular event	Risk of pneumonia	Age	60–69	+2
					70–79	+5
					≥ 80	+7
				Atrial fibrillation	Present	+1
				Congestive heart failure	Present	+3
				Chronic obstructive pulmonary disease	Present	+3
				Current smoking	Present	+1
				Pre-stroke mRS	> 3	+2
				Admission NIHSS	5–9	+2
					10–14	+5
					≥ 15	+8
				Admission GCS	3–8	+3
				Dysphagia	Present	+3
				Infarct type	Total anterior circulation infarct	+2
					Posterior circulation infarct	+2
				Admission glucose	> 11.1 mmol/L	+2
Very low risk 0–6 Low risk 7–13 Intermediate risk 14–20 High risk 21–27 Very high risk 28–35						
FEDSS	Germany	First-ever ischemic or hemorrhagic stroke	mRS at 3 months	Degree of dysphagia on fiberoptic endoscopic exam	Soft solid food with no penetration or aspiration and/or only mild/moderate residue in valleculae or pyriforms	+1

Table 3.9 (cont.)

Scale	Populations	Stroke type	Outcome	Variables	Values	Points
					Soft solid food penetration/ aspiration and/ or massive residues in valleculae or pyriforms	+2
					Liquid penetration with protective reflex	+3
					Liquid penetration/ aspiration with insufficient protective reflex	+4
					Puree penetration with protective reflex	+4
					Penetration/ aspiration with insufficient or no protective reflex	+5
					Penetration/ aspiration of saliva	+6
Poor outcome if > 4						
				Age	60–69	+3
					70–79	+4
					80–89	+6
					≥ 90	+8
ISAN	China	Ischemic stroke	Risk of pneumonia	Pre-stroke mRS	2–5	+2
				NIHSS	5–15	+4
					16–20	+8
					≥ 21	+10

Low risk 0–5
Medium risk 6–10
High risk 11–14
Highest risk > 15

Biomarkers

Elevated serum leptin levels and elevated insulin-like growth factor (IGF-1) levels may be associated with post-stroke depression.[268,269]

Language Recovery after Stroke

The extent of language recovery varies largely on the degree of cortical involvement of the language centers.[4] As an example, the severity of auditory comprehension deficits appears to correlate strongly with the extent of injury to the posterior superior temporal gyrus, and patients with damage to less than half of the gyrus may have better overall comprehension after 6 months. Lesions of the dominant superior temporal gyrus may be more likely to cause a persistent global aphasia compared to involvement of the inferior frontal gyrus or pre/post central gyri, and sparing of the superior temporal gyrus may be associated with recovery of aphasia. Patients with aphasia in the setting of subcortical strokes may have less severe aphasia compared to cortical infarcts, and this observation has been in line with data suggesting that the initial severity of the aphasia may carry a poor prognosis due to disruption of the ability of neuronal speech networks to reorganize following a stroke.[4,270] Otherwise, perfusion imaging has suggested potential markers for language prognosis. Normal or near-normal hyperemic relative cerebral blood flow in the subinsular ribbon or angular gyrus regions may be associated with improvement of language function by discharge in strokes not resulting from a proximal large vessel occlusion.[271] Diffusion–perfusion mismatch on MR perfusion imaging may be associated with early recovery of language, with mismatches > 20% potentially being associated with total language improvement within 1 week.[272]

Gaps in Knowledge and Ongoing Research

Given the considerable heterogeneity of ischemic stroke, a single measure of prognosis remains elusive. The numerous potential mechanisms of stroke, the myriad underlying combinations of preexisting comorbidities as well as potential complications and acute courses following stroke, the relatively limited sample sizes of patients available to study, and variations in study designs have left us with numerous questions about how best to utilize the information from these various measures. Further complicating the situation, access to various biochemical assays and imaging techniques may not be available in less advanced healthcare settings. However, given the established challenges with clinical prognostication based on expert experience alone, there remains an ongoing need for adequate prognostication tools.

Ongoing studies aim to identify a potential prognostic role for genetic biomarkers, gastrointestinal biomes, advanced imaging techniques, and serological biomarkers.

Genetic biomarkers. Micro-ribonucleic acid (miRNA) represents small noncoding RNAs that play a role in post-transcriptional gene regulation and may have a role in hypertension, atherosclerosis, atrial fibrillation, diabetes, and dyslipidemia. [273] Some miRNAs isolated from peripheral blood may be associated with the occurrence and development of post-stroke depression.[274] Some miRNA antagonists may reduce focal cerebral damage. Systematic reviews of multiple studies with several hundred cases and controls have implicated 22 miRNAs as potential prognostic markers, but significant heterogeneity in study design limit the generalizability of conclusions based on this data so far.[275,276] Concerning other genetic markers, a variant of the GTP cyclohydrolase gene, if present, may be associated with future vascular events and death 5 years after initial ischemic stroke.[277]. A single nucleotide polymorphism variant of the p53 tumor suppressor protein may be associated with early neurological deterioration.[278] Higher concentrations of matrix metalloproteinase 9 messanger RNA (mRNA) may be associated with poor outcome and death within 6 months.[279] Increased peripheral expression of the gene *MCEMP1* may be associated with higher functional disability and mortality at 1 month.[280] A *VEGF* polymorphism (+936CIT) may be associated with poor outcome at 90 days after ischemic stroke.[281] Elevated levels of platelet stromal interaction molecule (STIM1) and orai1 calcium influx channels may be associated with poor outcomes and poor functional recovery at 3 months.[282] Elevated high-mobility group-box protein (HMGB1) levels may be associated with larger infarct volumes and predict poor 1-year outcomes.[283] Lower levels of plasma epoxyeicosatrienoic acid may be associated with early neurological deterioration in minor ischemic stroke, and polymorphisms of the *EPHX2* gene may be associated with lower levels of these acids.[284] A polymorphism of the resistin gene promoter may be associated with stroke severity and in-hospital mortality.[285] A polymorphism of the alpha-2-antiplasmin gene may be associated with better prognosis in cryptogenic strokes.[286] In patients with minor stroke or TIA taking aspirin and clopidogrel who have reduced renal functional, those patients with a CYP2C19 loss of function allele may be associated with higher risk of new stroke. Single nucleotide polymorphisms of the *CRP* gene may be associated with poor 3-month outcome of first-time large artery atherosclerotic strokes.[287] Elevated levels of tumor necrosis factor-α-induced protein 8-like 2 (TIPE2) mRNA in peripheral blood, in combination with the NIHSS score, may be associated with higher 3-month mortality.[288] Increased levels of an miRNA-125b-5p may be associated with an unfavorable outcome at 3 months.[289] Finally, a variant of *CYP3A4* (related with statin pharmacokinetics and risk of cardiovascular disease) has been associated with poor ischemic stroke outcomes at 1 year.[290]

Gastrointestinal microbiome. Emerging data have started to explore how the gastrointestinal system may affect the pathogenesis of various neurological diseases. Patients with acute stroke have been found potentially to have changes in their gut microbiomes, with higher numbers of opportunistic pathogens and lower numbers of beneficial flora.[291] Efforts to understand the significance of these findings have been limited given how microbes vary from one person to another and given how microbiomes may vary relative to clinical comorbidities, diet, and lifestyle. However, the utility of gut microbiomes has been demonstrated in helping to characterize disease diagnosis, activity, and treatment efficacy in inflammatory bowel disease. It has also been used in cirrhosis to help predict 90-day hospitalization rates. A stroke dysbiosis index (SDI) has been devised based on sequencing the 16S ribosome RNA genes from fecal samples in patients with acute ischemic stroke and healthy controls, and a higher index has been proposed to relate to more severe brain injury and higher chances of unfavorable outcomes. Higher levels of Enterobacteriaceae and lower levels of Clostridiaceae and Lachnospira from stool samples may relate to an elevated inflammatory response after infection or stroke, which may in turn relate to severe brain injury and poor stroke outcome.

Advanced imaging. The utility of advanced MRI and CT techniques remains under investigation. Functional MRI is under investigation to determine whether it may play a role in predicting motor outcomes after stroke.[292] Fractional anisotropy using MRI diffusion tensor imaging has been used in multiple different studies to evaluate white matter integrity to identify a possible role in predicting motor and cognitive outcomes.[293–299] Additionally, a role for axial diffusivity on diffusion tensor imaging remains under investigation.[300] Otherwise, amide proton transfer–weighted imaging MRI has been used to generate images based on amide protons which helps to evaluate protein content and pH, has a role for evaluating central nervous system (CNS) neoplasms as well as other CNS diseases, and may have a role in ascertaining the severity of stroke.[301]

Conclusion

The extensive body of data exploring variables involved in stroke prognosis reflects decades of efforts to understand better how a patient will progress after an ischemic stroke. The many prognostic measures created have attempted to unify this information and represent a small step in the direction of reconciling the complexities inherent to each patient with the heterogeneity of various stroke mechanisms. The pursuit of such information will prove invaluable for informing expectations about recovery and optimizing the use of acute treatment options as we understand the significance of variables available in the acute phases of stroke. Though much remains to be done, ongoing research continues to push forward in exciting directions to demystify the complexities of stroke prognostication.

References

1. Benjamin EJ, Virani SS, Callaway CW, et al. Heart disease and stroke statistics-2018 update: a report from the American Heart Association. *Circulation.* 2018;137(12):e67–492.

2. Makris K, Haliassos A, Chondrogianni M, Tsivgoulis G. Blood biomarkers in ischemic stroke: potential role and challenges in clinical practice and research. *Crit Rev Clin Lab Sci.* 2018;55(5):294–328.

3. Drozdowska BA, Singh S, Quinn TJ. Thinking about the future: a review of prognostic scales used in acute stroke. *Front Neurol.* 2019;10:274.

4. Etherton MR, Rost NS, Wu O. Infarct topography and functional outcomes. *J Cereb Blood Flow Metab.* 2018;38(9):1517–32.

5. Rost NS, Bottle A, Lee J-M, et al. Stroke severity is a crucial predictor of outcome: an international prospective validation study. *J Am Heart Assoc.* 2016;5(1):e002433.

6. Ganesh A, Luengo-Fernandez R, Wharton RM, Rothwell PM, Oxford Vascular Study. Ordinal vs dichotomous analyses of modified Rankin Scale, 5-year outcome, and cost of stroke. *Neurology.* 2018;91(21):e1951–60.

7. Quinn TJ, Langhorne P, Stott DJ. Barthel Index for stroke trials: development, properties, and application. *Stroke.* 2011;42(4):1146–51.

8. Ajam K, Gold LS, Beck SS, et al. Reliability of the Cerebral Performance Category to classify neurological status among survivors of ventricular fibrillation arrest: a cohort study. *Scand J Trauma Resusc Emerg Med.* 2011;**19**:38.

9. Teasdale GM, Pettigrew LE, Wilson JT, Murray G, Jennett B. Analyzing outcome of treatment of severe head injury: a review and update on advancing the use of the Glasgow Outcome Scale. *J Neurotrauma.* 1998;**15**(8):587–97.

10. Jennett B, Bond M. Assessment of outcome after severe brain damage. *Lancet.* 1975;**1**(7905):480–4.

11. Linacre JM, Heinemann AW, Wright BD, Granger CV, Hamilton BB. The structure and stability of the Functional Independence Measure. *Arch Phys Med Rehabil.* 1994;**75**(2):127–32.

12. Lee S-J, Lee D-G. Distribution of atherosclerotic stenosis determining early neurologic deterioration in acute ischemic stroke. *PLoS One.* 2017;**12**(9):e0185314.

13. Kharitonova T, Mikulik R, Roine RO, et al. Association of early National Institutes of Health Stroke Scale improvement with vessel recanalization and functional outcome after intravenous thrombolysis in ischemic stroke. *Stroke.* 2011;**42**(6):1638–43.

14. van Kranendonk KR, Treurniet KM, Boers AMM, et al. Hemorrhagic transformation is associated with poor functional outcome in patients with acute ischemic stroke due to a large vessel occlusion. *J Neurointerv Surg.* 2019;**11**(5):464–8.

15. Ntaios G, Faouzi M, Ferrari J, et al. An integer-based score to predict functional outcome in acute ischemic stroke: the ASTRAL score. *Neurology.* 2012;**78**(24):1916–22.

16. Khatri M, Himmelfarb J, Adams D, et al. Acute kidney injury is associated with increased hospital mortality after stroke. *J Stroke Cerebrovasc Dis.* 2014;**23**(1):25–30.

17. Gadalean F, Simu M, Parv F, et al. The impact of acute kidney injury on in-hospital mortality in acute ischemic stroke patients undergoing intravenous thrombolysis. *PLoS One.* 2017;**12**(10): e0185589.

18. Shi J, Liu Y, Liu Y, et al. Dynamic changes in the estimated glomerular filtration rate predict all-cause mortality after intravenous thrombolysis in stroke patients. *Neurotox Res.* 2019;**35**(2):441–50.

19. Saposnik G, Kapral MK, Liu Y, et al. IScore: a risk score to predict death early after hospitalization for an acute ischemic stroke. *Circulation.* 2011;**123**(7):739–49.

20. Saposnik G, Reeves MJ, Johnston SC, Bath PMW, Ovbiagele B, VISTA Collaboration. Predicting clinical outcomes after thrombolysis using the iScore: results from the Virtual International Stroke Trials Archive. *Stroke.* 2013;**44**(10):2755–9.

21. Sung S-F, Chen Y-W, Hung L-C, Lin H-J. Revised iScore to predict outcomes after acute ischemic stroke. *J Stroke Cerebrovasc Dis.* 2014;**23**(6):1634–9.

22. Wang W-Y, Sang W-W, Jin D, et al. The prognostic value of the iScore, the PLAN Score, and the ASTRAL Score in acute ischemic stroke. *J Stroke Cerebrovasc Dis.* 2017;**26**(6):1233–8.

23. Bushnell C. Another score to predict ischemic stroke mortality? *Circulation.* 2011;**123**(7):712–13.

24. Van Hooff R-J, Nieboer K, De Smedt A, et al. Validation assessment of risk tools to predict outcome after thrombolytic therapy for acute ischemic stroke. *Clin Neurol Neurosurg.* 2014;**125**:189–93.

25. Mattishent K, Kwok CS, Mahtani A, et al. Prognostic indices for early mortality in ischaemic stroke – meta-analysis. *Acta Neurol Scand.* 2016;**133**(1):41–8.

26. Xu J, Tao Y, Xie X, et al. A comparison of mortality prognostic scores in ischemic stroke patients. *J Stroke Cerebrovasc Dis,* 2016;**25**(2):241–7.

27. Chu X, Yang Y, Zhang F, Ye R, Chu W. Validation of iScore and PLAN Score for death in thrombectomy in acute stroke due to anterior circulation large artery occlusion. *J Stroke Cerebrovasc Dis.* 2018;**27**(11):3261–5.

28. Widhi Nugroho A, Arima H, Takashima N, et al. The JAGUAR score predicts 1-month disability/ death in ischemic stroke patient ineligible for recanalization therapy. *J Stroke Cerebrovasc Dis.* 2018;**27**(10):2579–86.

29. Chen C-J, Chuang T-Y, Hansen L, et al. Predictors of 30-day mortality after endovascular mechanical thrombectomy for acute ischemic stroke. *J Clin Neurosci.* 2018;**57**:38–42.

30. O'Donnell MJ, Fang J, D'Uva C, et al. The PLAN score: a bedside prediction rule for death and severe disability following acute ischemic stroke. *Arch Intern Med.* 2012;**172**(20):1548–56.

31. Reid JM, Dai D, Delmonte S, et al. Simple prediction scores predict good and devastating outcomes after stroke more accurately than physicians. *Age Ageing.* 2017;**46**(3):421–6.

32. Ayis SA, Coker B, Rudd AG, Dennis MS, Wolfe CDA. Predicting independent survival after stroke: a European study for the development and validation of standardised stroke scales and prediction models of outcome. *J Neurol Neurosurg Psychiatry.* 2013;**84**(3):288–96.

33. Huang C-W, Saposnik G, Fang J, Steven DA, Burneo JG. Influence of seizures on stroke

outcomes: a large multicenter study. *Neurology*. 2014;**82**(9):768–76.

34. Oliveira FF de, Damasceno BP. Global aphasia as a predictor of mortality in the acute phase of a first stroke. *Arq Neuropsiquiatr*. 2011;**69**(2B):277–82.

35. Fan Y, Jiang M, Gong D, Man C, Chen Y. Cardiac troponin for predicting all-cause mortality in patients with acute ischemic stroke: a meta-analysis. *Biosci Rep [Internet]*. 2018;**38**(2).

36. Karagiannis A, Mikhailidis DP, Tziomalos K, et al. Serum uric acid as an independent predictor of early death after acute stroke. *Circ J*. 2007;**71** (7):1120–7.

37. Celikbilek A, Ismailogullari S, Zararsiz G. Neutrophil to lymphocyte ratio predicts poor prognosis in ischemic cerebrovascular disease. *J Clin Lab Anal*. 2014;**28**(1):27–31.

38. Fang Y-N, Tong M-S, Sung P-H, et al. Higher neutrophil counts and neutrophil-to-lymphocyte ratio predict prognostic outcomes in patients after non-atrial fibrillation-caused ischemic stroke. *Biomed J*. 2017;**40**(3):154–62.

39. Tokunaga K, Yamagami H, Koga M, et al. Associations between pre-admission risk scores and two-year clinical outcomes in ischemic stroke or transient ischemic attack patients with non-valvular atrial fibrillation. *Cerebrovasc Dis*. 2018;**45**(3–4):170–9.

40. Kernan WN, Viscoli CM, Brass LM, et al. The stroke prognosis instrument II (SPI-II): a clinical prediction instrument for patients with transient ischemia and nondisabling ischemic stroke. *Stroke*. 2000;**31**(2):456–62.

41. Kamel H, Patel N, Rao VA, et al. The totaled health risks in vascular events (THRIVE) score predicts ischemic stroke outcomes independent of thrombolytic therapy in the NINDS tPA trial. *J Stroke Cerebrovasc Dis*. 2013;**22**(7):1111–16.

42. You S, Han Q, Xiao G, et al. [The role of THRIVE score in prediction of outcomes of acute ischemic stroke patients with atrial fibrillation]. *Zhonghua Nei Ke Za Zhi*. 2014;**53**(7):532–6.

43. Kuster GW, Dutra LA, Brasil IP, et al. Performance of four ischemic stroke prognostic scores in a Brazilian population. *Arq Neuropsiquiatr*. 2016;**74**(2):133–7.

44. Raza SA, Rangaraju S. A review of pre-intervention prognostic scores for early prognostication and patient selection in endovascular management of large vessel occlusion stroke. *Interv Neurol*. 2018;**7** (3-4):171–81.

45. Flint AC, Faigeles BS, Cullen SP, et al. THRIVE score predicts ischemic stroke outcomes and thrombolytic hemorrhage risk in VISTA. *Stroke*. 2013;**44**(12):3365–9.

46. Flint AC, Kamel H, Rao VA, Cullen SP, Faigeles BS, Smith WS. Validation of the Totaled Health Risks In Vascular Events (THRIVE) score for outcome prediction in endovascular stroke treatment. *Int J Stroke*. 2014;**9**(1):32–9.

47. Flint AC, Gupta R, Smith WS, et al. The THRIVE score predicts symptomatic intracerebral hemorrhage after intravenous tPA administration in SITS-MOST. *Int J Stroke*. 2014;**9**(6):705–10.

48. Chen W, Liu G, Fang J, et al. external validation of the totaled health risks in vascular events score to predict functional outcome and mortality in patients entered into the China National Stroke Registry. *J Stroke Cerebrovasc Dis*. 2016;**25** (10):2331–7.

49. Boehme AK, Rawal PV, Lyerly MJ, et al. Investigating the utility of previously developed prediction scores in acute ischemic stroke patients in the stroke belt. *J Stroke Cerebrovasc Dis*. 2014;**23** (8):2001–6.

50. Fjetland L, Roy S, Kurz KD, et al. Neurointerventional treatment in acute stroke. Whom to treat? (Endovascular treatment for acute stroke: utility of THRIVE score and HIAT score for patient selection). *Cardiovasc Intervent Radiol*. 2013;**36**(5):1241–6.

51. Ishkanian AA, McCullough-Hicks ME, Appelboom G, et al. Improving patient selection for endovascular treatment of acute cerebral ischemia: a review of the literature and an external validation of the Houston IAT and THRIVE predictive scoring systems. *Neurosurg Focus*. 2011;**30**(6):E7.

52. Kastrup A, Brunner F, Hildebrandt H, et al. THRIVE score predicts clinical and radiological outcome after endovascular therapy or thrombolysis in patients with anterior circulation stroke in everyday clinical practice. *Eur J Neurol*. 2017;**24**(8):1032–9.

53. Kurre W, Aguilar-Pérez M, Niehaus L, et al. Predictors of outcome after mechanical thrombectomy for anterior circulation large vessel occlusion in patients aged ≥80 years. *Cerebrovasc Dis*. 2013;**36**(5–6):430–6.

54. Lei C, Wu B, Liu M, et al. Totaled health risks in vascular events score predicts clinical outcomes in patients with cardioembolic and other subtypes of ischemic stroke. *Stroke*. 2014;**45**(6):1689–94.

55. Laible M, Möhlenbruch MA, Pfaff J, et al. Influence of renal function on treatment results after stroke thrombectomy. *Cerebrovasc Dis*. 2017;**44**(5–6):351–8.

56. Hallevi H, Barreto AD, Liebeskind DS, et al. Identifying patients at high risk for poor outcome after intra-arterial therapy for acute ischemic stroke. *Stroke*. 2009;**40**(5):1780–5.

57. Liggins JTP, Yoo AJ, Mishra NK, et al. A score based on age and DWI volume predicts poor outcome following endovascular treatment for acute ischemic stroke. Int J *Stroke*. 2015;**10** (5):705–9.

58. Wood AD, Gollop ND, Bettencourt-Silva JH, et al. A 6-point TACS score predicts in-hospital mortality following total anterior circulation stroke. *J Clin Neurol*. 2016;**12**(4):407–13.

59. Tonetti DA, Gross BA, Desai SM, et al. Final infarct volume of <10 cm^3 is a strong predictor of return to home in nonagenarians undergoing mechanical thrombectomy. *World Neurosurg*. 2018;**119**:e941–6.

60. Vogt G, Laage R, Shuaib A, Schneider A, VISTA Collaboration. Initial lesion volume is an independent predictor of clinical stroke outcome at day 90: an analysis of the Virtual International Stroke Trials Archive (VISTA) database. *Stroke*. 2012;**43**(5):1266–72.

61. Christoforidis GA, Mohammad Y, Kehagias D, Avutu B, Slivka AP. Angiographic assessment of pial collaterals as a prognostic indicator following intra-arterial thrombolysis for acute ischemic stroke. *AJNR Am J Neuroradiol*. 2005;**26**(7) :1789–97.

62. Liu X-T, Wang W, Wang L-J, et al. [Correlation of collateral circulation and prognosis in patients with acute cerebral infarction]. Zhonghua Yi Xue Za Zhi. 2011;**91**(11):766–8.

63. Galego O, Jesus-Ribeiro J, Baptista M, et al. Collateral pial circulation relates to the degree of brain edema on CT 24 hours after ischemic stroke. *Neuroradiol J*. 2018;**31**(5):456–63.

64. Sharma R, Llinas RH, Urrutia V, Marsh EB. Collaterals predict outcome regardless of time last known normal. *J Stroke Cerebrovasc Dis*. 2018;**27** (4):971–7.

65. Liou L-M, Chen C-F, Guo Y-C, et al. Cerebral white matter hyperintensities predict functional stroke outcome. *Cerebrovasc Dis*. 2010;**29**(1):22–7.

66. Henninger N, Khan MA, Zhang J, Moonis M, Goddeau RP Jr. Leukoaraiosis predicts cortical infarct volume after distal middle cerebral artery occlusion. *Stroke*. 2014;**45**(3):689–95.

67. van den Herik EG, Cheung EYL, de Lau LML, et al. γ′/total fibrinogen ratio is associated with short-term outcome in ischaemic stroke. *Thromb Haemost*. 2011;**105**(3):430–4.

68. Whiteley W, Chong WL, Sengupta A, Sandercock P. Blood markers for the prognosis of ischemic stroke: a systematic review. *Stroke*. 2009;**40**(5):e380–9.

69. Ahn S-H, Lee J-S, Kim Y-H, et al. Prognostic significance of troponin elevation for long-term mortality after ischemic stroke. *J Stroke Cerebrovasc Dis*. 2017;**19**(3):312–22.

70. Scheitz JF, Mochmann H-C, Erdur H, et al. Prognostic relevance of cardiac troponin T levels and their dynamic changes measured with a high-sensitivity assay in acute ischaemic stroke: analyses from the TRELAS cohort. *Int J Cardiol*. 2014;**177**(3):886–93.

71. Beaulieu-Boire I, Leblanc N, Berger L, Boulanger J-M. Troponin elevation predicts atrial fibrillation in patients with stroke or transient ischemic attack. *J Stroke Cerebrovasc Dis*. 2013;**22** (7):978–83.

72. Furtner M, Ploner T, Hammerer-Lercher A, Pechlaner R, Mair J. The high-sensitivity cardiac troponin T assay is superior to its previous assay generation for prediction of 90-day clinical outcome in ischemic stroke. *Clin Chem Lab Med*. 2012;**50**(11):2027–9.

73. Csecsei P, Pusch G, Ezer E, et al. Relationship between cardiac troponin and thrombo-inflammatory molecules in prediction of outcome after acute ischemic stroke. *J Stroke Cerebrovasc Dis*. 2018;**27**(4):951–6.

74. He L, Wang J, Dong W. The clinical prognostic significance of hs-cTnT elevation in patients with acute ischemic stroke. *BMC Neurol*. 2018;**18** (1):118.

75. Xing L, Liu S, Tian Y, et al. C-R relationship between fasting plasma glucose and unfavorable outcomes in patients of ischemic stroke without diabetes. *J Stroke Cerebrovasc Dis*. 2019;**28** (5):1400–8.

76. Osei E, Fonville S, Zandbergen AAM, et al. Impaired fasting glucose is associated with unfavorable outcome in ischemic stroke patients treated with intravenous alteplase. *J Neurol*. 2018;**265**(6):1426–31.

77. Wang F, Jiang B, Kanesan L, Zhao Y, Yan B. Higher admission fasting plasma glucose levels are associated with a poorer short-term neurologic outcome in acute ischemic stroke patients with good collateral circulation. *Acta Diabetol*. 2018;**55** (7):703–14.

78. Zhou J, Wu J, Zhang J, et al. Association of stroke clinical outcomes with coexistence of hyperglycemia and biomarkers of inflammation. *J Stroke Cerebrovasc Dis*. 2015;**24**(6):1250–5.

79. Cao W, Ling Y, Wu F, et al. Higher fasting glucose next day after intravenous thrombolysis is independently associated with poor outcome in acute ischemic stroke. *J Stroke Cerebrovasc Dis.* 2015;**24**(1):100–3.

80. Ntaios G, Egli M, Faouzi M, Michel P. J-shaped association between serum glucose and functional outcome in acute ischemic stroke. *Stroke.* 2010;**41**(10):2366–70.

81. Kostulas N, Markaki I, Cansu H, Masterman T, Kostulas V. Hyperglycaemia in acute ischaemic stroke is associated with an increased 5-year mortality. *Age Ageing.* 2009;**38**(5):590–4.

82. Fuentes B, Castillo J, San José B, et al. The prognostic value of capillary glucose levels in acute stroke: the GLycemia in Acute Stroke (GLIAS) study. *Stroke.* 2009;**40**(2):562–8.

83. Stead LG, Gilmore RM, Bellolio MF, et al. Hyperglycemia as an independent predictor of worse outcome in non-diabetic patients presenting with acute ischemic stroke. *Neurocrit Care.* 2009;**10**(2):181–6.

84. Baird TA, Parsons MW, Phan T, et al. Persistent poststroke hyperglycemia is independently associated with infarct expansion and worse clinical outcome. *Stroke.* 2003;**34**(9):2208–14.

85. Bruno A, Levine SR, Frankel MR, et al. Admission glucose level and clinical outcomes in the NINDS rt-PA Stroke Trial. *Neurology.* 2002;**59**(5):669–74.

86. Nardi K, Milia P, Eusebi P, et al. Predictive value of admission blood glucose level on short-term mortality in acute cerebral ischemia. *J Diabetes Complications.* 2012;**26**(2):70–6.

87. Garg R, Aravind S, Kaur S, et al. Role of serum ferritin as a prognostic marker in acute ischemic stroke: a preliminary observation. *Ann Afr Med.* 2020;**19**(2):95–102.

88. Schrock JW, Glasenapp M, Drogell K. Elevated blood urea nitrogen/creatinine ratio is associated with poor outcome in patients with ischemic stroke. *Clin Neurol Neurosurg.* 2012;**114**(7):881–4.

89. Cortés-Vicente E, Guisado-Alonso D, Delgado-Mederos R, et al. Frequency, risk factors, and prognosis of dehydration in acute stroke. *Front Neurol.* 2019;**10**:305.

90. Hu Y, Wang C, Yan X, Fu H, Wang K. Prediction of conscious awareness recovery after severe acute ischemic stroke. *J Neurol Sci.* 2017;**383**:128–34.

91. Ntaios G, Gioulekas F, Papavasileiou V, Strbian D, Michel P. ASTRAL, DRAGON and SEDAN scores predict stroke outcome more accurately than physicians. *Eur J Neurol.* 2016;**23**(11):1651–7.

92. Asuzu D, Nystrom K, Amin H, et al. Comparison of 8 scores for predicting symptomatic intracerebral hemorrhage after IV thrombolysis. *Neurocrit Care.* 2015;**22**(2):229–33.

93. Cooray C, Mazya M, Bottai M, et al. External validation of the ASTRAL and DRAGON scores for prediction of functional outcome in stroke. *Stroke.* 2016;**47**(6):1493–9.

94. Liu G, Ntaios G, Zheng H, et al. External validation of the ASTRAL score to predict 3- and 12-month functional outcome in the China National Stroke Registry. *Stroke.* 2013;**44**(5):1443–5.

95. Papavasileiou V, Milionis H, Michel P, et al. ASTRAL score predicts 5-year dependence and mortality in acute ischemic stroke. *Stroke.* 2013;**44**(6):1616–20.

96. Koga M, Kimura K, Shibazaki K, et al. CHADS2 score is associated with 3-month clinical outcomes after intravenous rt-PA therapy in stroke patients with atrial fibrillation: SAMURAI rt-PA Registry. *J Neurol Sci.* 2011;**306**(1–2):49–53.

97. Hoshino T, Ishizuka K, Shimizu S, Uchiyama S. CHADS2 score predicts functional outcome of stroke in patients with a history of coronary artery disease. *J Neurol Sci.* 2013;**331**(1–2):57–60.

98. Naito H, Nezu T, Hosomi N, et al. Controlling nutritional status score for predicting 3-mo functional outcome in acute ischemic stroke. *Nutrition.* 2018;**55–56**:1–6.

99. Zhang X, Liao X, Wang C, et al. Validation of the DRAGON Score in a Chinese population to predict functional outcome of intravenous thrombolysis-treated stroke patients. *J Stroke Cerebrovasc Dis.* 2015;**24**(8):1755–60.

100. Giralt-Steinhauer E, Rodríguez-Campello A, Cuadrado-Godia E, et al. External validation of the DRAGON score in an elderly Spanish population: prediction of stroke prognosis after IV thrombolysis. *Cerebrovasc Dis.* 2013;**36**(2):110–4.

101. Ovesen C, Christensen A, Nielsen JK, Christensen H. External validation of the ability of the DRAGON score to predict outcome after thrombolysis treatment. *J Clin Neurosci.* 2013;**20**(11):1635–6.

102. Strbian D, Seiffge DJ, Breuer L, et al. Validation of the DRAGON score in 12 stroke centers in anterior and posterior circulation. *Stroke.* 2013;**44**(10):2718–21.

103. Baek JH, Kim K, Lee Y-B, et al. Predicting stroke outcome using clinical- versus imaging-based scoring system. *J Stroke Cerebrovasc Dis.* 2015;**24**(3):642–8.

104. Wang A, Pednekar N, Lehrer R, et al. DRAGON score predicts functional outcomes in acute

ischemic stroke patients receiving both intravenous tissue plasminogen activator and endovascular therapy. *Surg Neurol Int.* 2017;**8**:149.

105. Adams HP Jr, Davis PH, Leira EC, et al. Baseline NIH Stroke Scale score strongly predicts outcome after stroke: a report of the Trial of Org 10172 in Acute Stroke Treatment (TOAST). *Neurology.* 1999;**53**(1):126–31.

106. Jia X-Y, Huang M, Zou Y-F, et al. Predictors of poor outcomes in first-event ischemic stroke as assessed by magnetic resonance imaging. *Clin Invest Med.* 2016;**39**(3):E95–104.

107. Soize S, Fabre G, Gawlitza M, et al. Can early neurological improvement after mechanical thrombectomy be used as a surrogate for final stroke outcome? *J Neurointerv Surg.* 2019;**11**(5):450–4.

108. Song Y-M, Lee GH, Kim JI. Timing of neurological improvement after acute ischemic stroke and functional outcome. *Eur Neurol.* 2015;**73**(3-4):164–70.

109. Heitsch L, Ibanez L, Carrera C, et al. Early neurological change after ischemic stroke is associated with 90-day outcome. *Stroke.* 2021;**52**(1):132–41.

110. Sajobi TT, Menon BK, Wang M, et al. Early trajectory of stroke severity predicts long-term functional outcomes in ischemic stroke subjects: results from the ESCAPE Trial (Endovascular Treatment for Small Core and Anterior Circulation Proximal Occlusion with Emphasis on Minimizing CT to Recanalization Times). *Stroke.* 2017;**48**(1):105–10.

111. Kim D-H, Nah H-W, Park H-S, et al. Factors associated with early dramatic recovery following successful recanalization of occluded artery by endovascular treatment in anterior circulation stroke. *J Clin Neurosci.* 2017;**46**:171–5.

112. Yeo LLL, Paliwal P, Teoh HL, et al. Early and continuous neurologic improvements after intravenous thrombolysis are strong predictors of favorable long-term outcomes in acute ischemic stroke. *J Stroke Cerebrovasc Dis.* 2013;**22**(8):e590–6.

113. Rangaraju S, Frankel M, Jovin TG. Prognostic value of the 24-hour neurological examination in anterior circulation ischemic stroke: a post hoc analysis of two randomized controlled stroke trials. *Interv Neurol.* 2016;**4**(3–4):120–9.

114. Johnston KC, Wagner DP. Relationship between 3-month National Institutes of Health Stroke Scale score and dependence in ischemic stroke patients. *Neuroepidemiology.* 2006;**27**(2):96–100.

115. Irvine HJ, Battey TW, Ostwaldt A-C, et al. Early neurological stability predicts adverse outcome after acute ischemic stroke. *Int J Stroke.* 2016;**11**(8):882–9.

116. Wu Z, Zeng M, Li C, et al. Time-dependence of NIHSS in predicting functional outcome of patients with acute ischemic stroke treated with intravenous thrombolysis. *Postgrad Med J.* 2019;**95**(1122):181–6.

117. Pu J, Wang H, Tu M, et al. Combination of 24-hour and 7-day relative neurological improvement strongly predicts 90-day functional outcome of endovascular stroke therapy. *J Stroke Cerebrovasc Dis.* 2018;**27**(5):1217–25.

118. Kandiah N, Chander RJ, Lin X, et al. Cognitive impairment after mild stroke: development and validation of the SIGNAL2 Risk Score. *J Alzheimers Dis.* 2016;**49**(4):1169–77.

119. Prabhakaran S, Jovin TG, Tayal AH, et al. Posttreatment variables improve outcome prediction after intra-arterial therapy for acute ischemic stroke. *Cerebrovasc Dis.* 2014;**37**(5):356–63.

120. Rodríguez-Castro E, Rodríguez-Yáñez M, Arias S, et al. Influence of sex on stroke prognosis: a demographic, clinical, and molecular analysis. *Front Neurol.* 2019;**10**:388.

121. Kim Y, Kim CK, Jung S, et al. Prognostic importance of weight change on short-term functional outcome in acute ischemic stroke. *Int J Stroke.* 2015;**10**(Suppl A100):62–8.

122. Kremer C, Perren F, Kappelin J, Selariu E, Abul-Kasim K. Prognosis of aphasia in stroke patients early after iv thrombolysis. *Clin Neurol Neurosurg.* 2013;**115**(3):289–92.

123. Luvizutto GJ, Moliga AF, Rizzatti GRS, et al. Unilateral spatial neglect in the acute phase of ischemic stroke can predict long-term disability and functional capacity. *Clinics.* 2018;**73**:e131.

124. Spaccavento S, Cellamare F, Falcone R, Loverre A, Nardulli R. Effect of subtypes of neglect on functional outcome in stroke patients. *Ann Phys Rehabil Med.* 2017;**60**(6):376–81.

125. Maaijwee NAMM, Tendolkar I, Rutten-Jacobs LCA, et al. Long-term depressive symptoms and anxiety after transient ischaemic attack or ischaemic stroke in young adults. *Eur J Neurol.* 2016;**23**(8):1262–8.

126. El Husseini N, Goldstein LB, Peterson ED, et al. Depression status is associated with functional decline over 1-year following acute stroke. *J Stroke Cerebrovasc Dis.* 2017;**26**(7):1393–9.

127. Molad J, Kliper E, Korczyn AD, et al. Only white matter hyperintensities predicts post-stroke

cognitive performances among cerebral small vessel disease markers: results from the TABASCO Study. *J Alzheimers Dis.* 2017;**56**(4):1293–9.

128. Li J, Zhao Y, Mao J. Association between the extent of white matter damage and early cognitive impairment following acute ischemic stroke. *Exp Ther Med.* 2017;**13**(3):909–12.

129. Khan M, Heiser H, Bernicchi N, et al. Leukoaraiosis predicts short-term cognitive but not motor recovery in ischemic stroke patients during rehabilitation. *J Stroke Cerebrovasc Dis.* 2019;**28**(6):1597–603.

130. Sillanpää N, Pienimäki J-P, Protto S, et al. Chronic infarcts predict poor clinical outcome in mechanical thrombectomy of sexagenarian and older patients. *J Stroke Cerebrovasc Dis.* 2018;**27**(7):1789–95.

131. Arba F, Palumbo V, Boulanger J-M, et al. Leukoaraiosis and lacunes are associated with poor clinical outcomes in ischemic stroke patients treated with intravenous thrombolysis. *Int J Stroke.* 2016;**11**(1):62–7.

132. Kongbunkiat K, Wilson D, Kasemsap N, et al. Leukoaraiosis, intracerebral hemorrhage, and functional outcome after acute stroke thrombolysis. *Neurology.* 2017;**88**(7):638–45.

133. Fierini F, Poggesi A, Pantoni L. Leukoaraiosis as an outcome predictor in the acute and subacute phases of stroke. *Expert Rev Neurother.* 2017;**17**(10):963–75.

134. Chen Y, Yan S, Xu M, et al. More extensive white matter hyperintensity is linked with higher risk of remote intracerebral hemorrhage after intravenous thrombolysis. *Eur J Neurol.* 2018;**25**(2):380–e15.

135. Liu Y, Zhang M, Chen Y, et al. The degree of leukoaraiosis predicts clinical outcomes and prognosis in patients with middle cerebral artery occlusion after intravenous thrombolysis. *Brain Res.* 2018;**1681**:28–33.

136. Yang C-M, Hung C-L, Su H-C, et al. Leukoaraiosis and risk of intracranial hemorrhage and outcome after stroke thrombolysis. *PLoS One.* 2018;**13**(5):e0196505.

137. Liu X, Li T, Diao S, et al. The global burden of cerebral small vessel disease related to neurological deficit severity and clinical outcomes of acute ischemic stroke after IV rt-PA treatment. *Neurol Sci.* 2019;**40**(6):1157–66.

138. Zhang J, Puri AS, Khan MA, Goddeau RP Jr, Henninger N. Leukoaraiosis predicts a poor 90-day outcome after endovascular stroke therapy. *AJNR Am J Neuroradiol.* 2014;**35**(11):2070–5.

139. Gilberti N, Gamba M, Premi E, et al. Leukoaraiosis is a predictor of futile recanalization in acute ischemic stroke. *J Neurol.* 2017;**264**(3):448–52.

140. Guo Y, Zi W, Wan Y, et al. Leukoaraiosis severity and outcomes after mechanical thrombectomy with stent-retriever devices in acute ischemic stroke. *J Neurointerv Surg.* 2019;**11**(2):137–40.

141. Liu Y, Gong P, Sun H, et al. Leukoaraiosis is associated with poor outcomes after successful recanalization for large vessel occlusion stroke. *Neurol Sci.* 2019;**40**(3):585–91.

142. Jeong SH, Ahn SS, Baik M, et al. Impact of white matter hyperintensities on the prognosis of cryptogenic stroke patients. *PLoS One.* 2018;**13**(4):e0196014.

143. Putaala J, Haapaniemi E, Kurkinen M, et al. Silent brain infarcts, leukoaraiosis, and long-term prognosis in young ischemic stroke patients. *Neurology.* 2011;**76**(20):1742–9.

144. Leonards CO, Ipsen N, Malzahn U, et al. White matter lesion severity in mild acute ischemic stroke patients and functional outcome after 1 year. *Stroke.* 2012;**43**(11):3046–51.

145. Senda J, Ito K, Kotake T, et al. Association of leukoaraiosis with convalescent rehabilitation outcome in patients with ischemic stroke. *Stroke.* 2016;**47**(1):160–6.

146. Kamakura CK, Ueno Y, Sakai Y, et al. White matter lesions and cognitive impairment may be related to recovery from unilateral spatial neglect after stroke. *J Neurol Sci.* 2017;**379**:241–6.

147. Yassi N, Churilov L, Campbell BCV, et al. The association between lesion location and functional outcome after ischemic stroke. *Int J Stroke.* 2015;**10**(8):1270–6.

148. Sylaja PN, Puetz V, Dzialowski I, et al. Prognostic value of CT angiography in patients with suspected vertebrobasilar ischemia. *J Neuroimaging.* 2008;**18**(1):46–9.

149. DeVetten G, Coutts SB, Hill MD, et al. Acute corticospinal tract Wallerian degeneration is associated with stroke outcome. *Stroke.* 2010;**41**(4):751–6.

150. Kaya D, Dincer A, Arman F, et al. Ischemic involvement of the primary motor cortex is a prognostic factor in acute stroke. *Int J Stroke.* 2015;**10**(8):1277–83.

151. Shelton FN, Reding MJ. Effect of lesion location on upper limb motor recovery after stroke. *Stroke.* 2001;**32**(1):107–12.

152. Schouten EA, Schiemanck SK, Brand N, Post MWM. Long-term deficits in episodic memory after ischemic stroke: evaluation and prediction of verbal and visual memory performance based on lesion characteristics. *J Stroke Cerebrovasc Dis.* 2009;**18**(2):128–38.

153. Munsch F, Sagnier S, Asselineau J, et al. Stroke location is an independent predictor of cognitive outcome. *Stroke.* 2016;**47**(1):66–73.

154. Shatzman S, Mahajan S, Sundararajan S. Often overlooked but critical: poststroke cognitive impairment in right hemispheric ischemic stroke. *Stroke.* 2016;**47**(9):e221–3.

155. Freyschlag CF, Boehme C, Bauer M, et al. The volume of ischemic brain predicts poor outcome in patients with surgically treated malignant stroke. *World Neurosurg.* 2019;**123**:e515–19.

156. Boers AMM, Jansen IGH, Beenen LFM, et al. Association of follow-up infarct volume with functional outcome in acute ischemic stroke: a pooled analysis of seven randomized trials. *J Neurointerv Surg.* 2018;**10**(12):1137–42.

157. Schaefer PW, Pulli B, Copen WA, et al. Combining MRI with NIHSS thresholds to predict outcome in acute ischemic stroke: value for patient selection. *AJNR Am J Neuroradiol.* 2015;36(2):259–64.

158. Kruetzelmann A, Köhrmann M, Sobesky J, et al. Pretreatment diffusion-weighted imaging lesion volume predicts favorable outcome after intravenous thrombolysis with tissue-type plasminogen activator in acute ischemic stroke. *Stroke.* 2011;**42**(5):1251–4.

159. Xie Y, Oppenheim C, Guillemin F, et al. Pretreatment lesional volume impacts clinical outcome and thrombectomy efficacy. *Ann Neurol.* 2018;**83**(1):178–85.

160. Cho K-H, Kwon SU, Lee DH, et al. Early infarct growth predicts long-term clinical outcome after thrombolysis. *J Neurol Sci.* 2012;**316**(1–2):99–103.

161. Battey TWK, Karki M, Singhal AB, et al. Brain edema predicts outcome after nonlacunar ischemic stroke. *Stroke.* 2014;**45**(12):3643–8.

162. Simpkins AN, Dias C, Norato G, Kim E, Leigh R, NIH Natural History of Stroke Investigators. Early change in stroke size performs best in predicting response to therapy. *Cerebrovasc Dis.* 2017;**44**(3–4):141–9.

163. Deng W, Teng J, Liebeskind D, Miao W, Du R. Predictors of infarct growth measured by apparent diffusion coefficient quantification in patients with acute ischemic stroke. *World Neurosurg.* 2019;**123**:e797–802.

164. Zhou H, Sun J, Ji X, et al. Correlation between the integrity of the circle of Willis and the severity of initial noncardiac cerebral infarction and clinical prognosis. *Medicine (Baltimore).* 2016;**95**(10): e2892.

165. Leng X, Lan L, Liu L, Leung TW, Wong KS. Good collateral circulation predicts favorable outcomes in intravenous thrombolysis: a systematic review and meta-analysis. *Eur J Neurol.* 2016;**23** (12):1738–49.

166. Madelung CF, Ovesen C, Trampedach C, et al. Leptomeningeal collateral status predicts outcome after middle cerebral artery occlusion. *Acta Neurol Scand.* 2018;**137**(1):125–32.

167. Wufuer A, Wubuli A, Mijiti P, et al. Impact of collateral circulation status on favorable outcomes in thrombolysis treatment: a systematic review and meta-analysis. *Exp Ther Med.* 2018;**15**(1):707–18.

168. Huang X, Liu W, Zhu W, et al. Distal hyperintense vessels on FLAIR: a prognostic indicator of acute ischemic stroke. *Eur Neurol.* 2012;**68**(4):214–20.

169. Dong X, Nao J. Fluid-attenuated inversion recovery vascular hyperintensities in anterior circulation acute ischemic stroke: associations with cortical brain infarct volume and 90-day prognosis. *Neurol Sci.* 2019;**40**(8):1675–82.

170. Copelan A, Chehab M, Brinjikji W, et al. Opercular Index Score: a CT angiography-based predictor of capillary robustness and neurological outcomes in the endovascular management of acute ischemic stroke. *J Neurointerv Surg.* 2017;**9**(12):1179–86.

171. Maus V, You S, Kalkan A, et al. Incomplete large vessel occlusions in mechanical thrombectomy: an independent predictor of favorable outcome in ischemic stroke. *Cerebrovasc Dis.* 2017;**44** (3–4):113–21.

172. Arsava EM, Arat A, Topcuoglu MA, et al. Angiographic microcirculatory obstructions distal to occlusion signify poor outcome after endovascular treatment for acute ischemic stroke. *Transl Stroke Res.* 2018;**9**(1):44–50.

173. Carbone F, Busto G, Padroni M, et al. Radiologic cerebral reperfusion at 24 h predicts good clinical outcome. *Transl Stroke Res.* 2019;**10**(2):178–88.

174. Sakuta K, Saji N, Aoki J, et al. Decrease of hyperintense vessels on fluid-attenuated inversion recovery predicts good outcome in t-PA patients. *Cerebrovasc Dis.* 2016;**41** (3–4):211–8.

175. Yeo LLL, Paliwal P, Low AF, et al. How temporal evolution of intracranial collaterals in acute

stroke affects clinical outcomes. *Neurology.* 2016;**86**(5):434–41.

176. Kneihsl M, Niederkorn K, Deutschmann H, et al. Abnormal blood flow on transcranial duplex sonography predicts poor outcome after stroke thrombectomy. *Stroke.* 2018;**49**(11):2780–2.

177. Dekker L, Geraedts VJ, Hund H, et al. Importance of reperfusion status after intra-arterial thrombectomy for prediction of outcome in anterior circulation large vessel stroke. *Interv Neurol.* 2018;**7**(3–4):137–47.

178. García-Tornel Á, Requena M, Rubiera M, et al. When to stop. *Stroke.* 2019;**50**(7):1781–8.

179. Branco JP, Costa JS, Sargento-Freitas J, et al. [Neuroimaging and blood biomarkers in functional prognosis after stroke]. *Acta Med Port.* 2016;**29**(11):749–54.

180. Katan M, Elkind MSV. Inflammatory and neuroendocrine biomarkers of prognosis after ischemic stroke. *Expert Rev Neurother.* 2011;**11** (2):225–39.

181. Shibazaki K, Kimura K, Iguchi Y, et al. Plasma brain natriuretic peptide predicts death during hospitalization in acute ischaemic stroke and transient ischaemic attack patients with atrial fibrillation. *Eur J Neurol.* 2011;**18**(1):165–9.

182. Rost NS, Biffi A, Cloonan L, et al. Brain natriuretic peptide predicts functional outcome in ischemic stroke. *Stroke.* 2012;**43**(2):441–5.

183. Shibazaki K, Kimura K, Aoki J, et al. Brain natriuretic peptide level on admission predicts recurrent stroke after discharge in stroke survivors with atrial fibrillation. *Clin Neurol Neurosurg.* 2014;**127**:25–9.

184. Menon B, Ramalingam K, Conjeevaram J, Munisusmitha K. Role of brain natriuretic peptide as a novel prognostic biomarker in acute ischemic stroke. *Ann Indian Acad Neurol.* 2016;**19**(4):462–6.

185. Jang SY, Sohn MK, Lee J, et al. Chronic kidney disease and functional outcomes 6 months after ischemic stroke: a prospective multicenter study. *Neuroepidemiology.* 2016;**46**(1):24–30.

186. Jeon JW, Jeong HS, Choi DE, et al. Prognostic relationships between microbleed, lacunar infarction, white matter lesion, and renal dysfunction in acute ischemic stroke survivors. *J Stroke Cerebrovasc Dis.* 2017;**26**(2):385–92.

187. Synhaeve NE, van Alebeek ME, Arntz RM, et al. Kidney dysfunction increases mortality and incident events after young stroke: the FUTURE study. *Cerebrovasc Dis.* 2016;**42**(3–4):224–31.

188. Wang I-K, Liu C-H, Yen T-H, et al. Renal function is associated with 1-month and 1-year mortality in patients with ischemic stroke. *Atherosclerosis.* 2018;**269**:288–93.

189. Widhi Nugroho A, Arima H, Miyazawa I, et al. The association between glomerular filtration rate estimated on admission and acute stroke outcome: the Shiga Stroke Registry. *J Atheroscler Thromb.* 2018;**25**(7):570–9.

190. Van Kaam RC, van Putten MJAM, Vermeer SE, Hofmeijer J. Contralesional brain activity in acute ischemic stroke. *Cerebrovasc Dis.* 2018;**45** (1–2):85–92.

191. Santamarina E, Abraira L, Toledo M, et al. Prognosis of post-stroke status epilepticus: effects of time difference between the two events. *Seizure.* 2018;**60**:172–7.

192. Sheorajpanday RVA, Nagels G, Weeren AJTM, van Putten MJAM, De Deyn PP. Quantitative EEG in ischemic stroke: correlation with functional status after 6 months. *Clin Neurophysiol.* 2011;**122**(5):874–83.

193. Xin X, Gao Y, Zhang H, Cao K, Shi Y. Correlation of continuous electroencephalogram with clinical assessment scores in acute stroke patients. *Neurosci Bull.* 2012;**28**(5):611–7.

194. Zappasodi F, Olejarczyk E, Marzetti L, et al. Fractal dimension of EEG activity senses neuronal impairment in acute stroke. *PLoS One.* 2014;**9**(6):e100199.

195. Vang C, Dunbabin D, Kilpatrick D. Correlation between functional and electrophysiological recovery in acute ischemic stroke. *Stroke.* 1999;**30** (10):2126–30.

196. Hendricks HT, Pasman JW, van Limbeek J, Zwarts MJ. Motor evoked potentials in predicting recovery from upper extremity paralysis after acute stroke. *Cerebrovasc Dis.* 2003;**16**(3):265–71.

197. Nascimbeni A, Gaffuri A, Granella L, Colli M, Imazio P. Prognostic value of motor evoked potentials in stroke motor outcome. *Eura Medicophys.* 2005;**41**(2):125–30.

198. Souza LCS, Payabvash S, Wang Y, et al. Admission CT perfusion is an independent predictor of hemorrhagic transformation in acute stroke with similar accuracy to DWI. *Cerebrovasc Dis.* 2012;**33**(1):8–15.

199. Yassi N, Parsons MW, Christensen S, et al. Prediction of poststroke hemorrhagic transformation using computed tomography perfusion. *Stroke.* 2013;**44**(11):3039–43.

200. Nagaraja N, Tasneem N, Shaban A, et al. Cerebral microbleeds are an independent predictor of hemorrhagic transformation following intravenous alteplase administration in acute

ischemic stroke. *J Stroke Cerebrovasc Dis.* 2018;**27**(5):1403–11.

201. Simats A, García-Berrocoso T, Montaner J. Neuroinflammatory biomarkers: from stroke diagnosis and prognosis to therapy. *Biochim Biophys Acta.* 2016;**1862**(3):411–24.

202. Worthmann H, Tryc AB, Goldbecker A, et al. The temporal profile of inflammatory markers and mediators in blood after acute ischemic stroke differs depending on stroke outcome. *Cerebrovasc Dis.* 2010;**30**(1):85–92.

203. Ramos-Fernandez M, Bellolio MF, Stead LG. Matrix metalloproteinase-9 as a marker for acute ischemic stroke: a systematic review. *J Stroke Cerebrovasc Dis.* 2011;**20**(1):47–54.

204. Gori AM, Giusti B, Piccardi B, et al. Inflammatory and metalloproteinases profiles predict three-month poor outcomes in ischemic stroke treated with thrombolysis. *J Cereb Blood Flow Metab.* 2017;**37**(9):3253–61.

205. Zhong C, Yang J, Xu T, et al. Serum matrix metalloproteinase-9 levels and prognosis of acute ischemic stroke. *Neurology.* 2017;**89**(8):805–12.

206. Liu S-Y, Cao W-F, Wu L-F, et al. Effect of glycated hemoglobin index and mean arterial pressure on acute ischemic stroke prognosis after intravenous thrombolysis with recombinant tissue plasminogen activator. *Medicine.* 2018;**97**(49):e13216.

207. Kalinin MN, Khasanova DR, Ibatullin MM. The hemorrhagic transformation index score: a prediction tool in middle cerebral artery ischemic stroke. *BMC Neurol.* 2017;**17**(1):177.

208. van Asch Charlotte JJ, Velthuis Birgitta K, Greving Jacoba P, et al. External validation of the secondary intracerebral hemorrhage score in the Netherlands. *Stroke.* 2013;**44**(10):2904–6.

209. Asuzu D, Nyström K, Amin H, et al. TURN: a simple predictor of symptomatic intracerebral hemorrhage after iv thrombolysis. *Neurocrit Care.* 2015;**23**(2):166–71.

210. Asuzu D, Nyström K, Amin H, et al. Validation of TURN, a simple predictor of symptomatic intracerebral hemorrhage after IV thrombolysis. *Clin Neurol Neurosurg.* 2016;**146**:71–5.

211. Asuzu D, Nyström K, Schindler J, et al. TURN score predicts 90-day outcome in acute ischemic stroke patients after IV thrombolysis. *Neurocrit Care.* 2015;**23**(2):172–8.

212. Miyamoto N, Tanaka R, Ueno Y, et al. Analysis of the usefulness of the WORSEN score for predicting the deterioration of acute ischemic stroke. *J Stroke Cerebrovasc Dis.* 2017;**26**(12):2834–9.

213. Nakase T, Yamamoto Y, Takagi M, Japan Branch Atheromatous Disease Registry Collaborators. The impact of diagnosing branch atheromatous disease for predicting prognosis. *J Stroke Cerebrovasc Dis.* 2015;**24**(10):2423–8.

214. Melkas S, Sibolt G, Oksala NKJ, et al. Extensive white matter changes predict stroke recurrence up to 5 years after a first-ever ischemic stroke. *Cerebrovasc Dis.* 2012;**34**(3):191–8.

215. Andersen SD, Larsen TB, Gorst-Rasmussen A, et al. White matter hyperintensities improve ischemic stroke recurrence prediction. *Cerebrovasc Dis.* 2017;**43**(1–2):17–24.

216. Nam K-W, Kwon H-M, Lim J-S, Han M-K, Lee Y-S. Clinical relevance of abnormal neuroimaging findings and long-term risk of stroke recurrence. *Eur J Neurol.* 2017;**24**(11):1348–54.

217. Vahedi A, Lotfinia I, Sad RB, Halimi M, Baybordi H. Relationship between admission hypoalbuminemia and inhospital mortality in acute stroke. *Pak J Biol Sci.* 2011;**14**(2):118–22.

218. Lin L-C, Lee T-H, Chang C-H, et al. Predictors of clinical deterioration during hospitalization following acute ischemic stroke. *Eur Neurol.* 2012;**67**(3):186–92.

219. Xu Y, Chen Y, Chen R, et al. External validation of the WORSEN score for prediction the deterioration of acute ischemic stroke in a Chinese population. *Front Neurol.* 2020;**11**:482.

220. Liu Y, Wang Y, Li WA, Yan A, Wang Y. Validation of the Essen Stroke Risk Score in different subtypes of ischemic stroke. *Neurol Res.* 2017;**39**(6):504–8.

221. Kim B-S, Chung P-W, Park K-Y, et al. Burden of intracranial atherosclerosis is associated with long-term vascular outcome in patients with ischemic stroke. *Stroke.* 2017;**48**(10):2819–26.

222. Lee S-J, Lee D-G, Lim D-S, Hong S. Impact of intracranial atherosclerotic stenosis on the prognosis in acute ischemic stroke patients with cardioembolic source. *Eur Neurol.* 2015;**73**(5–6):271–7.

223. Tian L, Yue X, Xi G, et al. Multiple intracranial arterial stenosis influences the long-term prognosis of symptomatic middle cerebral artery occlusion. *BMC Neurol.* 2015;**15**:68.

224. Sacchetti DC, Cutting SM, McTaggart RA, et al. Perfusion imaging and recurrent cerebrovascular events in intracranial atherosclerotic disease or carotid occlusion. *Int J Stroke.* 2018;**13**(6):592–9.

225. Wijnhoud AD, Koudstaal PJ, Dippel DWJ. The prognostic value of pulsatility index, flow velocity, and their ratio, measured with TCD ultrasound, in

patients with a recent TIA or ischemic stroke. *Acta Neurol Scand*. 2011;**124**(4):238–44.

226. Yoon HJ, Kim KH, Park H, et al. Carotid plaque rather than intima-media thickness as a predictor of recurrent vascular events in patients with acute ischemic stroke. *Cardiovasc Ultrasound*. 2017;**15**(1):19.

227. Tamura H, Watanabe T, Nishiyama S, et al. Prognostic value of low left atrial appendage wall velocity in patients with ischemic stroke and atrial fibrillation. *J Am Soc Echocardiogr*. 2012;**25**(5):576–83.

228. Hashimoto N, Watanabe T, Tamura H, et al. Left atrial remodeling index is a feasible predictor of poor prognosis in patients with acute ischemic stroke. *Heart Vessels*. 2019;**34**(12):1936–43.

229. Paciaroni M, Agnelli G, Falocci N, et al. Prognostic value of trans-thoracic echocardiography in patients with acute stroke and atrial fibrillation: findings from the RAF study. *J Neurol*. 2016;**263**(2):231–7.

230. Harima K, Honda S, Mikami K, et al. Collagen-induced platelet aggregates, diabetes, and aspirin therapy predict clinical outcomes in acute ischemic stroke. *J Stroke Cerebrovasc Dis*. 2019;**28**(8):2302–10.

231. Akhtar N, Kamran S, Singh R, et al. The impact of diabetes on outcomes after acute ischemic stroke: a prospective observational study. *J Stroke Cerebrovasc Dis*. 2019;**28**(3):619–26.

232. Wang H, Cheng Y, Chen S, et al. Impact of elevated hemoglobin A1c levels on functional outcome in patients with acute ischemic stroke. *J Stroke Cerebrovasc Dis*. 2019;**28**(2):470–6.

233. Gofir A, Mulyono B, Sutarni S. Hyperglycemia as a prognosis predictor of length of stay and functional outcomes in patients with acute ischemic stroke. *Int J Neurosci*. 2017;**127**(10):923–9.

234. Dong X-L, Guan F, Xu S-J, et al. Influence of blood glucose level on the prognosis of patients with diabetes mellitus complicated with ischemic stroke. *J Res Med Sci*. 2018;**23**:10.

235. McCall SJ, Alanazi TA, Clark AB, et al. Hyperglycaemia and the SOAR stroke score in predicting mortality. *Diab Vasc Dis Res*. 2018;**15**(2):114–21.

236. Zhu Z, Yang J, Zhong C, et al. Abnormal glucose regulation, hypoglycemic treatment during hospitalization and prognosis of acute ischemic stroke. *J Neurol Sci*. 2017;**379**:177–82.

237. Shafa MA, Ebrahimi H, Iranmanesh F, Sasaie M. Prognostic value of hemoglobin A1c in nondiabetic and diabetic patients with acute ischemic stroke. *Iran J Neuro.l* 2016;**15**(4):209–13.

238. Luitse MJ, Velthuis BK, Kappelle LJ, van der Graaf Y, Biessels GJ, DUST Study Group. Chronic hyperglycemia is related to poor functional outcome after acute ischemic stroke. *Int J Stroke*. 2017;**12**(2):180–6.

239. Jing J, Pan Y, Zhao X, et al. Prognosis of ischemic stroke with newly diagnosed diabetes mellitus according to hemoglobin A1c criteria in Chinese population. *Stroke*. 2016;**47**(8):2038–44.

240. Lattanzi S, Bartolini M, Provinciali L, Silvestrini M. Glycosylated hemoglobin and functional outcome after acute ischemic stroke. *J Stroke Cerebrovasc Dis*. 2016;**25**(7):1786–91.

241. Wu S, Wang C, Jia Q, et al. HbA1c is associated with increased all-cause mortality in the first year after acute ischemic stroke. *Neurol Res*. 2014;**36**(5):444–52.

242. Wu S, Shi Y, Wang C, et al. Glycated hemoglobin independently predicts stroke recurrence within one year after acute first-ever non-cardioembolic strokes onset in a Chinese cohort study. *PLoS One*. 2013;**8**(11):e80690.

243. Tanaka R, Ueno Y, Miyamoto N, et al. Impact of diabetes and prediabetes on the short-term prognosis in patients with acute ischemic stroke. *J Neurol Sci*. 2013;**332**(1–2):45–50.

244. Kamouchi M, Matsuki T, Hata J, et al. Prestroke glycemic control is associated with the functional outcome in acute ischemic stroke: the Fukuoka Stroke Registry. *Stroke*. 2011;**42**(10):2788–94.

245. Kaarisalo MM, Räihä I, Sivenius J, et al. Diabetes worsens the outcome of acute ischemic stroke. *Diabetes Res Clin Pract*. 2005;**69**(3):293–8.

246. Zhang Q, Lei Y-X, Wang Q, et al. Serum albumin level is associated with the recurrence of acute ischemic stroke. *Am J Emerg Med*. 2016;**34**(9):1812–16.

247. Lau KK, Li L, Schulz U, et al. Total small vessel disease score and risk of recurrent stroke: Validation in 2 large cohorts. *Neurology*. 2017;**88**(24):2260–7.

248. Galovic M, Döhler N, Erdélyi-Canavese B, et al. Prediction of late seizures after ischaemic stroke with a novel prognostic model (the SeLECT score): a multivariable prediction model development and validation study. *Lancet Neurol*. 2018;**17**(2):143–52.

249. Zapata-Arriaza E, Moniche F, Blanca P-G, et al. External validation of the ISAN, A2DS2, and AIS-APS scores for predicting stroke-associated pneumonia. *J Stroke Cerebrovasc Dis*. 2018;**27**(3):673–6.

250. Ramírez-Moreno JM, Martínez-Acevedo M, Cordova R, et al. External validation of the A2SD2 and ISAN scales for predicting infectious respiratory complications of ischaemic stroke. *Neurologia.* 2019;**34**(1):14–21.

251. Zhang R, Ji R, Pan Y, et al. External validation of the prestroke independence, sex, age, National Institutes of Health Stroke Scale score for predicting pneumonia after stroke using data from the China National Stroke Registry. *J Stroke Cerebrovasc Dis.* 2017;**26**(5):938–43.

252. Ji R, Shen H, Pan Y, et al. Novel risk score to predict pneumonia after acute ischemic stroke. *Stroke.* 2013;**44**(5):1303–9.

253. Hoffmann S, Malzahn U, Harms H, et al. Development of a clinical score (A2DS2) to predict pneumonia in acute ischemic stroke. *Stroke.* 2012;**43**(10):2617–23.

254. Warnecke T, Ritter MA, Kroger B, et al. Fiberoptic endoscopic dysphagia severity scale predicts outcome after acute stroke. *Cerebrovasc Dis.* 2009;**28**(3):283–9.

255. Tinker RJ, Smith CJ, Heal C, et al. Predictors of mortality and disability in stroke-associated pneumonia. *Acta Neurol Belg.* 2019;**121**:379–85.

256. Hotter B, Hoffmann S, Ulm L, et al. external validation of five scores to predict stroke-associated pneumonia and the role of selected blood biomarkers. *Stroke.* 2021;**52**(1):325–30.

257. Kishore AK, Vail A, Chamorro A, et al. How is pneumonia diagnosed in clinical stroke research? A systematic review and meta-analysis. *Stroke.* 2015;**46**(5):1202–9.

258. Li Y, Song B, Fang H, et al. External validation of the A2DS2 score to predict stroke-associated pneumonia in a Chinese population: a prospective cohort study. *PLoS One.* 2014;**9**(10): e109665.

259. Duan Y, Chen F, Lin L, Wei W, Huang Y. Leukoaraiosis rather than lacunes predict poor outcome and chest infection in acute ischemic stroke patients. *Int J Clin Exp Med.* 2015;**8**(10):19304–10.

260. Huff W, Steckel R, Sitzer M. [Poststroke depression: risk factors and effects on the course of the stroke]. *Nervenarzt.* 2003;**74**(2):104–14.

261. Głodzik-Sobańska L, Słowik A, Borratyńska A, Szczudlik A. [Depressive symptoms following ischemic stroke]. *Neurol Neurochir Pol.* 2003;**37**(1):17–25.

262. Zhang T, Wang C, Liu L, et al. A prospective cohort study of the incidence and determinants of post-stroke depression among the mainland Chinese patients. *Neurol Res.* 2010;**32**(4):347–52.

263. Arsava EM, Bayrlee A, Vangel M, et al. Severity of leukoaraiosis determines clinical phenotype after brain infarction. *Neurology.* 2011;**77**(1):55–61.

264. Tang WK, Chen Y, Liang H, et al. Cerebral microbleeds as a predictor of 1-year outcome of poststroke depression. *Stroke,* 2014;**45**(1):77–81.

265. Liang Y, Chan YL, Deng M, et al. Enlarged perivascular spaces in the centrum semiovale are associated with poststroke depression: A 3-month prospective study. *J Affect Disord.* 2018;**228**:166–72.

266. Wichowicz HM, Gąsecki D, Landowski J, et al. Clinical utility of chosen factors in predicting post-stroke depression: a one year follow-up. *Psychiatr Pol.* 2015;**49**(4):683–96.

267. Nishiyama Y, Komaba Y, Ueda M, et al. Early depressive symptoms after ischemic stroke are associated with a left lenticulocapsular area lesion. *J Stroke Cerebrovasc Dis.* 2010;**19**(3):184–9.

268. Jiménez I, Sobrino T, Rodríguez-Yáñez M, et al. High serum levels of leptin are associated with post-stroke depression. *Psychol Med.* 2009;**39**(7):1201–9.

269. Zhang W, Wang W, Kuang L. The relation between insulin-like growth factor 1 levels and risk of depression in ischemic stroke. *Int J Geriatr Psychiatry.* 2018;**33**(2):e228–33.

270. Alferova VV, Shklovskij VM, Ivanova EG, et al. [The prognosis for post-stroke aphasia]. *Zh Nevrol Psikhiatr Im S S Korsakova.* 2018;**118**(4):20–9.

271. Payabvash S, Kamalian S, Fung S, et al. Predicting language improvement in acute stroke patients presenting with aphasia: a multivariate logistic model using location-weighted atlas-based analysis of admission CT perfusion scans. *AJNR Am J Neuroradiol.* 2010;**31**(9):1661–8.

272. Reineck LA, Agarwal S, Hillis AE. "Diffusion-clinical mismatch" is associated with potential for early recovery of aphasia. *Neurology.* 2005;**64**(5):828–33.

273. Koutsis G, Siasos G, Spengos K. The emerging role of microRNA in stroke. *Curr Top Med Chem.* 2013;**13**(13):1573–88.

274. Yan H, Fang M, Liu X-Y. Role of microRNAs in stroke and poststroke depression. *Sci World J.* 2013;**2013**:459692.

275. Jin F, Xing J. Circulating pro-angiogenic and anti-angiogenic microRNA expressions in patients with acute ischemic stroke and their

association with disease severity. *Neurol Sci.* 2017;**38**(11):2015–23.

276. Dewdney B, Trollope A, Moxon J, et al. Circulating microRNAs as biomarkers for acute ischemic stroke: a systematic review. *J Stroke Cerebrovasc Dis.* 2018;**27**(3): 522–30.

277. Tang L, Zhang L, Ding H, Tu W, Yan J. GTP cyclohydrolase 1 gene 3'-UTR C+243T variant predicts worsening outcome in patients with first-onset ischemic stroke. *J Huazhong Univ Sci Technolog Med Sci.* 2010;**30**(6):694–8.

278. Gomez-Sanchez JC, Delgado-Esteban M, Rodriguez-Hernandez I, et al. The human Tp53 Arg72Pro polymorphism explains different functional prognosis in stroke. *J Exp Med.* 2011;**208**(3):429–37.

279. Graham CA, Chan RWY, Chan DYS, et al. Matrix metalloproteinase 9 mRNA: an early prognostic marker for patients with acute stroke. *Clin Biochem.* 2012;**45**(4-5):352–5.

280. Raman K, O'Donnell MJ, Czlonkowska A, et al. Peripheral blood *MCEMP1* gene expression as a biomarker for stroke prognosis. *Stroke.* 2016;**47**(3):652–8.

281. Zhao J, Bai Y, Jin L, et al. A functional variant in the 3'-UTR of VEGF predicts the 90-day outcome of ischemic stroke in Chinese patients. *PLoS One.* 2017;**12**(2):e0172709.

282. Dong M, Zheng N, Ren LJ, Zhou H, Liu J. Increased expression of STIM1/Orai1 in platelets of stroke patients predictive of poor outcomes. *Eur J Neurol.* 2017;**24**(7):912–19.

283. Tsukagawa T, Katsumata R, Fujita M, et al. Elevated serum high-mobility group box-1 protein level is associated with poor functional outcome in ischemic stroke. *J Stroke Cerebrovasc Dis.* 2017;**26**(10):2404–11.

284. Yi X, Lin J, Li J, Zhou Q, Han Z. Epoxyeicosatrienoic acids are mediated by EPHX2 variants and may be a predictor of early neurological deterioration in acute minor ischemic stroke. *J Atheroscler Thromb.* 2017;**24**(12):1258–66.

285. Bouziana SD, Tziomalos K, Goulas A, et al. Major adipokines and the -420C>G resistin gene polymorphism as predictors of acute ischemic stroke severity and in-hospital outcome. *J Stroke Cerebrovasc Dis.* 2018;**27**(4):963–70.

286. Wzorek J, Karpiński M, Wypasek E, et al. Alpha-2-antiplasmin Arg407Lys polymorphism and cryptogenic ischemic cerebrovascular events: association with neurological deficit. *Neurol Neurochir Pol.* 2018;**52**(3):352–8.

287. Ye Z, Zhang H, Sun L, et al. GWAS-supported CRP gene polymorphisms and functional outcome of large artery atherosclerotic stroke in Han Chinese. *Neuromol Med.* 2018;**20**(2):225–32.

288. Zhang Y-Y, Huang N-N, Fan Y-C, et al. Peripheral tumor necrosis factor-a-induced protein 8-like 2 mRNA level for predicting 3-month mortality of patients with acute ischemic stroke. *J Neurol.* 2018;**265**(11):2573–86.

289. He X-W, Shi Y-H, Zhao R, et al. Plasma levels of miR-125b-5p and miR-206 in acute ischemic stroke patients after recanalization treatment: a prospective observational study. *J Stroke Cerebrovasc Dis.* 2019;**28**(6):1654–61.

290. Li S, Shi C-H, Liu X-J, et al. Association of CYP3A4*1G and CYP3A5*3 with the 1-year outcome of acute ischemic stroke in the Han Chinese population. *J Stroke Cerebrovasc Dis.* 2019;**28**(7):1860–5.

291. Xia G-H, You C, Gao X-X, et al. Stroke Dysbiosis Index (SDI) in gut microbiome are associated with brain injury and prognosis of stroke. *Front Neurol.* 2019;**10**:397.

292. Du J, Yang F, Zhang Z, et al. Early functional MRI activation predicts motor outcome after ischemic stroke: a longitudinal, multimodal study. *Brain Imaging Behav.* 2018;**12**(6):1804–13.

293. Koyama T, Marumoto K, Miyake H, Domen K. Relationship between diffusion tensor fractional anisotropy and motor outcome in patients with hemiparesis after corona radiata infarct. *J Stroke Cerebrovasc Dis.* 2013;**22**(8):1355–60.

294. Bigourdan A, Munsch F, Coupé P, et al. Early fiber number ratio is a surrogate of corticospinal tract integrity and predicts motor recovery after stroke. *Stroke.* 2016;**47**(4):1053–9.

295. Maximova MY, Popova TA, Konovalov RN. [Prognosis of motor function recovery in ischemic stroke using diffusion tensor MRI]. *Zh Nevrol Psikhiatr Im S S Korsakova.* 2016;**116**(8 Pt 2):57–64.

296. Schaapsmeerders P, Tuladhar AM, Arntz RM, et al. Remote lower white matter integrity increases the risk of long-term cognitive impairment after ischemic stroke in young adults. *Stroke.* 2016;**47**(10):2517–25.

297. Etherton MR, Wu O, Cougo P, et al. Integrity of normal-appearing white matter and functional outcomes after acute ischemic stroke. *Neurology.* 2017;**88**(18):1701–8.

298. Nakashima A, Moriuchi T, Mitsunaga W, et al. Prediction of prognosis of upper-extremity function following stroke-related paralysis using

brain imaging. *J Phys Therapy Sci.* 2017;**29**
(8):1438–43.

299. Koyama T, Koumo M, Uchiyama Y, Domen K. Utility of fractional anisotropy in cerebral peduncle for stroke outcome prediction: comparison of hemorrhagic and ischemic strokes. *J Stroke Cerebrovasc Dis.* 2018;**27**(4):878–85.

300. Moulton E, Valabregue R, Lehéricy S, Samson Y, Rosso C. Multivariate prediction of functional outcome using lesion topography characterized by acute diffusion tensor imaging. *Neuroimage Clin.* 2019;**23**:101821.

301. Lin G, Zhuang C, Shen Z, et al. APT weighted MRI as an effective imaging protocol to predict clinical outcome after acute ischemic stroke. *Front Neurol.* 2018;**9**:901.

302. Rodier M, Quirié A, Prigent-Tessier A, et al. Relevance of post-stroke circulating BDNF levels as a prognostic biomarker of stroke outcome. impact of rt-PA treatment. *PLoS One.* 2015;**10**(10):e0140668.

303. Lasek-Bal A, Jędrzejowska-Szypułka H, Różycka J, et al. Low concentration of BDNF in the acute phase of ischemic stroke as a factor in poor prognosis in terms of functional status of patients. *Med Sci Monit.* 2015;**21**:3900–5.

304. Rezaei S, Asgari Mobarake K, Saberi A, Keshavarz P, Leili EK. Brain-derived neurotrophic factor (BDNF) Val66Met polymorphism and post-stroke dementia: a hospital-based study from northern Iran. *Neurol Sci.* 2016;**37**(6):935–42.

305. Wang J, Gao L, Yang Y-L, et al. low serum levels of brain-derived neurotrophic factor were associated with poor short-term functional outcome and mortality in acute ischemic stroke. *Mol Neurobiol.* 2017;**54**(9):7335–42.

306. Xu H-B, Xu Y-H, He Y, et al. Decreased serum brain-derived neurotrophic factor may indicate the development of poststroke depression in patients with acute ischemic stroke: a meta-analysis. *J Stroke Cerebrovasc Dis.* 2018;**27**(3):709–15.

307. Hsu P-J, Chen C-H, Yeh S-J, et al. High plasma D-dimer indicates unfavorable outcome of acute ischemic stroke patients receiving intravenous thrombolysis. *Cerebrovasc Dis.* 2016;**42**(1-2):117–21.

308. Li S, Bi P, Zhao W, et al. Prognostic utility of fatty acid-binding protein 4 in patients with type 2 diabetes and acute ischemic stroke. *Neurotox Res.* 2018;**33**(2):309–15.

309. Cheng S-Y, Zhao Y-D, Li J, et al. Plasma levels of glutamate during stroke is associated with

development of post-stroke depression. *Psychoneuroendocrinology.* 2014;**47**:126–35.

310. Meng X-E, Li N, Guo D-Z, et al. High plasma glutamate levels are associated with poor functional outcome in acute ischemic stroke. *Cell Mol Neurobiol.* 2015;**35**(2):159–65.

311. Geng L-Y, Qian F-Y, Qian J-F, Zhang Z-J. The combination of plasma glutamate and physical impairment after acute stroke as a potential indicator for the early-onset post-stroke depression. *J Psychosom Res.* 2017;**96**:35–41.

312. Tu W-J, Zeng X-W, Deng A, et al. Circulating FABP4 (fatty acid-binding protein 4) is a novel prognostic biomarker in patients with acute ischemic stroke. *Stroke.* 2017;**48**(6):1531–8.

313. Li W, Liu M, Wu B, et al. Serum lipid levels and 3-month prognosis in Chinese patients with acute stroke. *Adv Ther.* 2008;**25**(4):329–41.

314. Lai Y-T, Hsieh C-L, Lee H-P, Pan S-L. Are higher total serum cholesterol levels associated with better long-term motor function after ischemic stroke? *Nutr Neurosci.* 2012;**15**(6):239–43.

315. Tziomalos K, Giampatzis V, Bouziana SD, et al. Prognostic significance of major lipids in patients with acute ischemic stroke. *Metab Brain Dis.* 2017;**32**(2):395–400.

316. Deng Q-W, Wang H, Sun C-Z, et al. Triglyceride to high-density lipoprotein cholesterol ratio predicts worse outcomes after acute ischaemic stroke. *Eur J Neurol.* 2017;**24**(2):283–91.

317. Cuadrado-Godia E, Jiménez-Conde J, Ois A, et al. Sex differences in the prognostic value of the lipid profile after the first ischemic stroke. *J Neurol.* 2009;**256**(6):989–95.

318. Wang H, Zhao J, Gui Y, et al. Elevated lipoprotein (A) and risk of poor functional outcome in Chinese patients with ischemic stroke and type 2 diabetes. *Neurotox Res.* 2018;**33**(4):868–75.

319. Bonifačić D, Toplak A, Benjak I, et al. Monocytes and monocyte chemoattractant protein 1 (MCP-1) as early predictors of disease outcome in patients with cerebral ischemic stroke. *Wien Klin Wochenschr.* 2016;**128**(1-2):20–7.

320. Song T-J, Cho H-J, Chang Y, et al. low plasma proportion of omega 3-polyunsaturated fatty acids predicts poor outcome in acute non-cardiogenic ischemic stroke patients. *J Stroke Cerebrovasc Dis.* 2015;**17**(2):168–76.

321. Quan W, Chen Z, Yang X, et al. Mean platelet volume/platelet count ratio as a predictor of 90-day outcome in large artery atherosclerosis stroke patients. *Int J Neurosci.* 2017;**127**(11):1019–27.

322. Gao F, Chen C, Lyu J, et al. Association between platelet distribution width and poor outcome of acute ischemic stroke after intravenous thrombolysis. *Neuropsychiatr Dis Treat.* 2018;**14**:2233–9.

323. Xie D, Xiang W, Weng Y, et al. Platelet volume indices for the prognosis of acute ischemic stroke patients with intravenous thrombolysis. *Int J Neurosci.* 2019;**129**(4):344–9.

324. Altintas O, Altintas MO, Tasal A, Kucukdagli OT, Asil T. The relationship of platelet-to-lymphocyte ratio with clinical outcome and final infarct core in acute ischemic stroke patients who have undergone endovascular therapy. *Neurol Res.* 2016;**38**(9):759–65.

325. Chen Z, Huang Y, Li S, et al. Platelet-to-white blood cell ratio: a prognostic predictor for 90-day outcomes in ischemic stroke patients with intravenous thrombolysis. *J Stroke Cerebrovasc Dis.* 2016;**25**(10):2430–8.

326. Jin P, Li X, Chen J, et al. Platelet-to-neutrophil ratio is a prognostic marker for 90-days outcome in acute ischemic stroke. *J Clin Neurosci.* 2019;**63**:110–5.

327. Pikija S, Cvetko D, Hajduk M, Trkulja V. Higher mean platelet volume determined shortly after the symptom onset in acute ischemic stroke patients is associated with a larger infarct volume on CT brain scans and with worse clinical outcome. *Clin Neurol Neurosurg.* 2009;**111**(7):568–73.

328. Mayda-Domaç F, Misirli H, Yilmaz M. Prognostic role of mean platelet volume and platelet count in ischemic and hemorrhagic stroke. *J Stroke Cerebrovasc Dis.* 2010;**19**(1):66–72.

329. Arévalo-Lorido JC, Carretero-Gómez J, Álvarez-Oliva A, et al. Mean platelet volume in acute phase of ischemic stroke, as predictor of mortality and functional outcome after 1 year. *J Stroke Cerebrovasc Dis.* 2013;**22**(4):297–303.

330. Peng F, Zheng W, Li F, et al. Elevated mean platelet volume is associated with poor outcome after mechanical thrombectomy. *J Neurointerv Surg.* 2018;**10**(1):25–8.

331. Oji S, Tomohisa D, Hara W, et al. Mean platelet volume is associated with early neurological deterioration in patients with branch atheromatous disease: involvement of platelet activation. *J Stroke Cerebrovasc Dis.* 2018;**27**(6):1624–31.

332. İnanç Y, Giray S, İnanç Y. Mean platelet volume, C-reactive protein, and prognosis in patients with acute ischemic stroke following intravenous thrombolytic treatment. *Med Sci Monit.* 2018;**24**:3782–8.

333. Staszewski J, Pogoda A, Data K, et al. The mean platelet volume on admission predicts unfavorable stroke outcomes in patients treated with IV thrombolysis. *Clin Interv Aging.* 2019;**14**:493–503.

334. Du J, Wang Q, He B, et al. Association of mean platelet volume and platelet count with the development and prognosis of ischemic and hemorrhagic stroke. *Int J Lab Hematol.* 2016;**38**(3):233–9.

335. Chen X, Liu Z, Miao J, et al. High stress hyperglycemia ratio predicts poor outcome after mechanical thrombectomy for ischemic stroke. *J Stroke Cerebrovasc Dis.* 2019;**28**(6):1668–73.

336. Marulaiah SK, Reddy MP, Basavegowda M, Ramaswamy P, Adarsh LS. Admission hyperglycemia an independent predictor of outcome in acute ischemic stroke: A longitudinal study from a tertiary care hospital in South India. *Niger J Clin Pract.* 2017;**20**(5):573–80.

337. Jing J, Pan Y, Zhao X, et al. Insulin resistance and prognosis of nondiabetic patients with ischemic stroke: the ACROSS-China study (Abnormal Glucose Regulation in Patients With Acute Stroke Across China). *Stroke.* 2017;**48**(4):887–93.

338. Pan Y, Jing J, Chen W, et al. Post-glucose load measures of insulin resistance and prognosis of nondiabetic patients with ischemic stroke. *J Am Heart Assoc.* 2017;**6**(1).

339. Bielewicz J, Kurzepa J, Czekajska-Chehab E, Stelmasiak Z, Bartosik-Psujek H. Does serum Tau protein predict the outcome of patients with ischemic stroke? *J Mol Neurosci.* 2011;**43**(3):241–5.

340. Wang Y, Zhou S, Bao J, Pan S, Zhang X. Low T3 levels as a predictor marker predict the prognosis of patients with acute ischemic stroke. *Int J Neurosci.* 2017;**127**(7):559–66.

341. Suda S, Muraga K, Kanamaru T, et al. Low free triiodothyronine predicts poor functional outcome after acute ischemic stroke. *J Neurol Sci.* 2016;**368**:89–93.

342. Dhital R, Poudel DR, Tachamo N, et al. Ischemic stroke and impact of thyroid profile at presentation: a systematic review and meta-analysis of observational studies. *J Stroke Cerebrovasc Dis.* 2017;**26**(12):2926–34.

343. Suda S, Aoki J, Shimoyama T, et al. Low free triiodothyronine at admission predicts poststroke infection. *J Stroke Cerebrovasc Dis.* 2018;**27**(2):397–403.

344. Jiang X, Xing H, Wu J, et al. Prognostic value of thyroid hormones in acute ischemic stroke – a meta analysis. *Sci Rep*. 2017;7(1):16256.

345. Suda S, Shimoyama T, Nagai K, et al. Low free triiodothyronine predicts 3-month poor outcome after acute stroke. *J Stroke Cerebrovasc Dis*. 2018;27(10):2804–9.

346. Feng X, Zhou X, Yu F, et al. Low-normal free triiodothyronine and high leukocyte levels in relation to stroke severity and poor outcome in acute ischemic stroke with intracranial atherosclerotic stenosis. *Int J Neurosci*. 2019;129 (7):635–41.

347. Li L-Q, Xu X-Y, Li W-Y, Hu X-Y, Lv W. The prognostic value of total T3 after acute cerebral infarction is age-dependent: a retrospective study on 768 patients. *BMC Neurol*. 2019;19(1):54.

348. Cho H-J, Kim S-S, Sung S-M, Jung D-S. Impact of thyroid autoantibodies on functional outcome in patients with acute ischemic stroke. *J Stroke Cerebrovasc Dis*. 2014;23(7):1915–20.

349. Brea D, Blanco M, Sobrino T, Ramos-Cabrer P, Castillo J. [The levels of expression of toll-like receptors 2 and 4 in neutrophils are associated with the prognosis of ischaemic stroke patients]. *Rev Neurol*. 2011;52(1):12–9.

350. Seet RCS, Kasiman K, Gruber J, et al. Is uric acid protective or deleterious in acute ischemic stroke? A prospective cohort study. *Atherosclerosis*. 2010;209(1):215–19.

351. Kurzepa J, Bielewicz J, Stelmasiak Z, Bartosik-Psujek H. Serum bilirubin and uric acid levels as the bad prognostic factors in the ischemic stroke. *Int J Neurosci*. 2009;119(12):2243–9.

352. Wang P, Li X, He C, et al. Hyperuricemia and prognosis of acute ischemic stroke in diabetic patients. *Neurol Res*. 2019;41(3):250–6.

353. Cuadrado-Godia E, Ois A, Garcia-Ramallo E, et al. Biomarkers to predict clinical progression in small vessel disease strokes: prognostic role of albuminuria and oxidized LDL cholesterol. *Atherosclerosis*. 2011;219(1):368–72.

354. Das S, Yadav U, Ghosh KC, et al. A clinical study of ischaemic strokes with micro-albuminuria for risk stratification, short-term predictive value and outcome. *J Indian Med Assoc*. 2012;110 (12):908–10, 919.

355. Li F, Chen Q-X, Peng B, et al. Microalbuminuria in patients with acute ischemic stroke. *Neurol Res*. 2019;41(6):498–503.

356. Turetsky A, Goddeau RP Jr, Henninger N. Low serum vitamin D is independently associated with larger lesion volumes after ischemic stroke. *J Stroke Cerebrovasc Dis*. 2015;24(7):1555–63.

357. Park K-Y, Chung P-W, Kim YB, et al. Serum vitamin D status as a predictor of prognosis in patients with acute ischemic stroke. *Cerebrovasc Dis*. 2015;40(1–2):73–80.

358. Daumas A, Daubail B, Legris N, et al. Association between admission serum 25-hydroxyvitamin D levels and functional outcome of thrombolyzed stroke patients. *J Stroke Cerebrovasc Dis*. 2016;25 (4):907–13.

359. Xu T, Zhong C, Xu T, et al. Serum 25-hydroxyvitamin D deficiency predicts long-term poor prognosis among ischemic stroke patients without hyperglycaemia. *Clin Chim Acta*. 2017;471:81–5.

360. Wei Z-N, Kuang J-G. Vitamin D deficiency in relation to the poor functional outcomes in nondiabetic patients with ischemic stroke. *Biosci Rep*. 2018;38(2):BSR20171609.

361. Alfieri DF, Lehmann MF, Oliveira SR, et al. Vitamin D deficiency is associated with acute ischemic stroke, C-reactive protein, and short-term outcome. *Metab Brain*. Dis 2017;32 (2):493–502.

362. Grau AJ, Boddy AW, Dukovic DA, et al. Leukocyte count as an independent predictor of recurrent ischemic events. *Stroke*. 2004;35 (5):1147–52.

363. Elkind MSV, Cheng J, Rundek T, Boden-Albala B, Sacco RL. Leukocyte count predicts outcome after ischemic stroke: the Northern Manhattan Stroke Study. *J Stroke Cerebrovasc Dis*. 2004;13 (5):220–7.

364. Nardi K, Milia P, Eusebi P, et al. Admission leukocytosis in acute cerebral ischemia: influence on early outcome. *J Stroke Cerebrovasc Dis*. 2012;21(8):819–24.

365. Nikanfar M, Shaafi S, Hashemilar M, Oskouii DS, Goldust M. Evaluating role of leukocytosis and high sedimentation rate as prognostic factors in acute ischemic cerebral strokes. *Pak J Biol Sci*. 2012;15(8):386–90.

366. Kumar AD, Boehme AK, Siegler JE, et al. Leukocytosis in patients with neurologic deterioration after acute ischemic stroke is associated with poor outcomes. *J Stroke Cerebrovasc Dis*. 2013;22(7):e111–7.

367. Ye J-K, Zhang J-T, Kong Y, et al. [Relationship between white blood cell count, neutrophils ratio and erythrocyte sedimentation rate and short clinical outcomes among patients with acute ischemic stroke at hospital admission]. *Zhonghua Liu Xing Bing Xue Za Zhi*. 2012;33(9):956–60.

368. Kim J, Song T-J, Park JH, et al. Different prognostic value of white blood cell subtypes in

73

patients with acute cerebral infarction. *Atherosclerosis.* 2012;**222**(2):464–7.

369. Wu J, Zhang J, Xu T, et al. [Neutrophil ratio/blood glucose and poor short outcome among patients with acute ischemic stroke]. *Zhonghua Liu Xing Bing Xue Za Zhi.* 2014;**35**(7):861–4.

370. Heikinheimo T, Putaala J, Haapaniemi E, Kaste M, Tatlisumak T. Leucocyte count in young adults with first-ever ischaemic stroke: associated factors and association on prognosis. *Int J Stroke.* 2015;**10**(2):245–50.

371. Furlan JC, Vergouwen MDI, Fang J, Silver FL. White blood cell count is an independent predictor of outcomes after acute ischaemic stroke. *Eur J Neurol.* 2014;**21**(2):215–22.

372. Qu X, Shi J, Cao Y, Zhang M, Xu J. Prognostic value of white blood cell counts and c-reactive protein in acute ischemic stroke patients after intravenous thrombolysis. *Curr Neurovasc Res.* 2018;**15**(1):10–17.

373. Zheng X, Zeng N, Wang A, et al. Prognostic value of white blood cell in acute ischemic stroke patients. *Curr Neurovasc Res.* 2018;**15**(2):151–7.

374. Malhotra K, Goyal N, Chang JJ, et al. Differential leukocyte counts on admission predict outcomes in patients with acute ischaemic stroke treated with intravenous thrombolysis. *Eur J Neurol.* 2018;**25**(12):1417–24.

375. Chen J, Zhang Z, Chen L, et al. Correlation of changes in leukocytes levels 24 hours after intravenous thrombolysis with prognosis in patients with acute ischemic stroke. *J Stroke Cerebrovasc Dis.* 2018;**27**(10):2857–62.

376. Shi J, Peng H, You S, et al. Increase in neutrophils after recombinant tissue plasminogen activator thrombolysis predicts poor functional outcome of ischaemic stroke: a longitudinal study. *Eur J Neurol.* 2018;**25**(4):687.

377. Xue J, Huang W, Chen X, et al. Neutrophil-to-lymphocyte ratio is a prognostic marker in acute ischemic stroke. *J Stroke Cerebrovasc Dis.* 2017;**26**(3):650–7.

378. Qun S, Tang Y, Sun J, et al. Neutrophil-to-lymphocyte ratio predicts 3-month outcome of acute ischemic stroke. *Neurotox Res.* 2017;**31**(3):444–52.

379. Zhang J, Ren Q, Song Y, et al. Prognostic role of neutrophil-lymphocyte ratio in patients with acute ischemic stroke. *Medicine.* 2017;**96**(45):e8624.

380. Duan Z, Wang H, Wang Z, et al. Neutrophil-lymphocyte ratio predicts functional and safety outcomes after endovascular treatment for acute ischemic stroke. *Cerebrovasc Dis.* 2018;**45**(5–6):221–7.

381. Pektezel MY, Yilmaz E, Arsava EM, Topcuoglu MA. Neutrophil-to-lymphocyte ratio and response to intravenous thrombolysis in patients with acute ischemic stroke. *J Stroke Cerebrovasc Dis.* 2019;**28**(7):1853–9.

382. Maestrini I, Strbian D, Gautier S, et al. Higher neutrophil counts before thrombolysis for cerebral ischemia predict worse outcomes. *Neurology.* 2015;**85**(16):1408–16.

383. Pikija S, Sztriha LK, Killer-Oberpfalzer M, et al. Neutrophil to lymphocyte ratio predicts intracranial hemorrhage after endovascular thrombectomy in acute ischemic stroke. *J Neuroinflammation.* 2018;**15**(1):319.

384. Inanc Y, Inanc Y. The effects of neutrophil to lymphocyte and platelet to lymphocyte ratios on prognosis in patients undergoing mechanical thrombectomy for acute ischemic stroke. *Ann Ital Chir.* 2018;**89**:367–73.

385. Liberale L, Montecucco F, Bonaventura A, et al. Monocyte count at onset predicts poststroke outcomes during a 90-day follow-up. *Eur J Clin Invest.* 2017;**47**(10):702–10.

386. Ren H, Liu X, Wang L, Gao Y. Lymphocyte-to-monocyte ratio: a novel predictor of the prognosis of acute ischemic stroke. *J Stroke Cerebrovasc Dis.* 2017;**26**(11):2595–602.

387. De Smedt A, Brouns R, Uyttenboogaart M, et al. Insulin-like growth factor I serum levels influence ischemic stroke outcome. *Stroke.* 2011;**42**(8):2180–5.

388. Osthoff M, Katan M, Fluri F, et al. Mannose-binding lectin deficiency is associated with smaller infarction size and favorable outcome in ischemic stroke patients. *PLoS One.* 2011;**6**(6):e21338.

389. Zhang Z-G, Wang C, Wang J, et al. Prognostic value of mannose-binding lectin: 90-day outcome in patients with acute ischemic stroke. *Mol Neurobiol.* 2015;**51**(1):230–9.

390. Song F-Y, Wu M-H, Zhu L-H, et al. Elevated serum mannose-binding lectin levels are associated with poor outcome after acute ischemic stroke in patients with type 2 diabetes. *Mol Neurobiol.* 2015;**52**(3):1330–40.

391. Deng Q-W, Li S, Wang H, et al. The short-term prognostic value of the triglyceride-to-high-density lipoprotein cholesterol ratio in acute ischemic stroke. *Aging Dis.* 2018;**9**(3):498–506.

Prognostication in Subarachnoid Hemorrhage

Pirouz Piran, Sarah E. Nelson, and Jose I. Suarez

Introduction

Nontraumatic aneurysmal subarachnoid hemorrhage (aSAH) accounts for 5% of all strokes and carries an exceptionally high disease-specific burden: half of patients with aSAH are younger than 55 years, one-third die within the initial days to weeks after ictus, and most survivors have long-term disability or cognitive impairment.[1] For those who survive, there are both short- and long-term consequences that can significantly reduce quality of life. In addition, aSAH can lead to loss of many years of productive life in survivors. Modifiable risk factors for aSAH include hypertension, smoking, and excessive alcohol intake.[2] The global decrease in aSAH incidence has paralleled a decrease in mean blood pressure and smoking prevalence.[3]

Brain injury after aSAH can be divided into early and delayed stages, which include both systemic and cerebral factors.[4] Early brain injury (EBI) is a direct consequence of aneurysmal rupture.[5] EBI is composed of transient global ischemia, mechanical injury to the brain, blood–brain barrier breakdown, and cerebral edema that occurs within the first 72 hours after symptom onset. Other early complications include rebleeding, elevated intracranial pressure (ICP) and hydrocephalus, seizures, and cardiac and pulmonary dysfunction. Later complications include global and delayed cerebral ischemia (DCI), hyponatremia, fever, and endocrine abnormalities. Appropriate management of these complications plays a pivotal role in the prognosis of these patients.

While the case fatality rate of aSAH has improved, the overall mortality rate remains high (up to 45% in some studies).[6] This is mainly related to the fact that most randomized controlled trials (RCT) on aSAH to date have failed to show significant improvement in outcomes.

Out of the 50 or more RCTs, only two studies showed promising results in regard to improvement of prognosis:

1. British Aneurysm Nimodipine Trial (BRANT)[7] to determine the efficacy of oral nimodipine on reducing cerebral infarction and poor outcome, and
2. International Subarachnoid Aneurysm Trial (ISAT),[8] which compared the safety and efficacy of endovascular coiling with microsurgical clipping in patients who are eligible for either treatment, found better survival free of disability at 1 year in the patients who underwent coiling.

Another factor that has been difficult to tease out is that of prognostication in aSAH. Many practitioners are reluctant to discuss a patient's potential outcome when there is significant prognostic uncertainty. Reliable prognostication tools can help patients and families decide on appropriate treatments and develop realistic expectations. Patients and their families require prognostication to emotionally, financially, and socially prepare for death or disability.[9] Historically, there has been much interest in prognostication of patients with aSAH. Many grading systems have been developed not only to predict outcome but also to give clinicians the ability to compare and study aSAH patients with different clinical conditions at various stages of this disease. In this chapter, we will describe the proposed grading systems to measure severity of aSAH and prognosis.

Grading

Admission neurological status after aSAH reflects the severity of EBI and is a larger predictor of death or severe disability than any other factor or complications that occur as a consequence of aneurysm rupture.[10,11] While admission neurological status can be a great predictor of poor outcome, prognostication based only on clinical and diagnostic criteria that are present on admission can result in withholding treatment in up to 30% of patients who subsequently experience favorable outcomes.[12]

The main grading scales for assessment of EBI and of outcome in patients with aSAH are the clinical World Federation of Neurosurgical Societies (WFNS) grading scale and Hunt and Hess scale.[13] The WFNS grading system uses Glasgow Coma Scale (GCS) and the presence of neurological deficits to grade the severity of aSAH. Similarly, the Hunt and Hess score system classifies aSAH patients based on clinical condition. Both scales range from a score of 1 to 5. Both are used as predictors of prognosis/outcome, with higher grades correlating to lower survival rate. Table 4.1 compares the WFNS and Hunt and Hess scores.

The Hunt and Hess scoring system was developed in 1968, mainly to help neurosurgeons decide on the surgical risk and the appropriate time of operating after aSAH onset. The authors of this scale thought that the most important aspects of aSAH were (1) the intensity of meningeal inflammatory reaction, (2) the severity of neurological deficit, and (3) the level of arousal. Later, the scale

Table 4.1 Comparison between the Hunt and Hess and the WFNS scales

Grade	Hunt and Hess	WFNS
1	Asymptomatic or minimal headache and slight nuchal rigidity	GCS 15, no motor deficit
2	Moderate-severe headache, nuchal rigidity, cranial nerve palsy	GCS 13 to 14, no motor deficit
3	Drowsiness, confusion, or mild focal deficit,	GCS 13 to 14 with motor deficit
4	Stupor, moderate-to-severe hemiparesis, possibly early decerebrate rigidity and vegetative disturbances	GCS 7 to 12, with or without motor deficit
5	Deep coma, decerebrate rigidity, moribund appearance	GCS 3 to 6, with or without motor deficit

Abbreviations: GCS: Glasgow Coma Scale; WFNS: World Federation of Neurosurgical Societies.

was modified to adjust for the presence of (a) systemic disease (such as hypertension and diabetes) and (b) cerebral vasospasm on angiography. If either systematic disease or cerebral vasospasm were present, the grade would be advanced by one point. While the Hunt and Hess scale may have better predictive capabilities than WFNS, it has been criticized as being subjective since it relies on vague terminologies, such as mild and moderate headache, which translate into significant interrater variability. Even the authors in their original paper admitted that their classification system is arbitrary and that the margins between categories may be ill defined. The inter-observer variability for the Hunt and Hess scale is moderate (kappa 0.41 to 0.48). In addition, Hunt and Hess grades 1 and 2 are very similar in terms of prognostication, since as long as the level of consciousness is normal, headache and/ or stiff neck have no significant effect on outcome.

The GCS measures neurological function in three domains: eye opening, verbal response, and motor response. The GCS has been used to predict aSAH outcome in different studies. The main limitation of this score is that the outcome is not significantly different among patients with a verbal score of 5 regardless of the score on other domains. In the same fashion, outcome appears to be similar between patients with GCS 13 and 14.[14] These findings led to the creation of new scales that would report each domain of the GCS separately.

In 1988, an expert opinion committee developed the WFNS scale. The main difference between the WFNS and Hunt and Hess scales is that the WFNS is more objective and avoids the vague subjective terminology present in the Hunt and Hess scale. As mentioned above, the WFNS scale is composed of the GCS plus neurological deficits as an additional fourth axis. However, prognostication data regarding the WFNS scale are conflicting, and some studies have shown that there is no meaningful difference in outcome between WFNS grades 2 and 3 or between grades 3 and 4.

Timing of aSAH grading has been the subject of debate as well. In addition, acute hydrocephalus and the presence of an intracerebral hematoma can affect initial grading. Some experts now recommend assigning grades after completing the initial neurological resuscitation via cerebrospinal fluid (CSF) drainage and/or craniotomy. Giraldo et al. [15] demonstrated that the WFNS grade after neurological resuscitation was a better predictor of outcome than the WFNS grade on admission.

Not all grading scales focus on the clinical outcome. The radiological Fisher score [16] and the more recent modified Fischer score,[17] both of which evaluate the amount of subarachnoid blood (Table 4.2) and presence of intraventricular blood, serve as indicators to predict vasospasm risk and development of delayed cerebral ischemia (DCI) from vasospasm, respectively (Figures 4.1 and 4.2).

Physiological derangements also are common in the acute phase of aSAH and have been used for grading and predicting outcome. For example, the systemic inflammatory response syndrome (SIRS) and Acute Physiology and Chronic Health

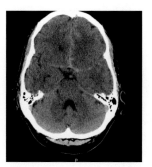

Figure 4.2 Patient with modified Fisher grade-I aSAH.

Table 4.2 Comparison between the Fisher and modified Fisher scales

Grade	Fisher scale	Modified Fisher scale
0		No SAH or IVH
1	No blood detected	Focal or diffuse, thin SAH, no IVH
2	Diffuse or thin layer of blood less than 1 mm thick (interhemispheric, insular, or ambient cisterns)	Focal or diffuse, thick SAH, no IVH
3	Localized clots and/or layers of blood greater than 1 mm thick in the vertical plane	Focal or diffuse, thin SAH, no IVH
4	Intracerebral or intraventricular clots with diffuse or absent blood in basal cisterns	Focal or diffuse, thick SAH with IVH

Abbreviations: IVH: intraventricular hemorrhage; SAH: subarachnoid hemorrhage.

Evaluation (APACHE) II scores have been shown to correlate with aSAH outcome.[18],19] Claassen et al. [20] showed that hypoxemia (arterio-alveolar gradient > 125 mmHg), metabolic acidosis (serum bicarbonate < 20 mmol/L), hyperglycemia (glucose > 180 mg/dL), and cardiovascular instability (MAP < 70 or > 130 mmHg) within 24 hours of admission were independently associated with death or severe disability at 3 months. The same study also showed that in-hospital re-bleeding, aneurysm size of > 10 mm, intraventricular hemorrhage (IVH), level of consciousness at onset, Hunt and Hess grade, and age were independent predictors of poor outcome at 3 months. The authors designed the SAH Physiologic Derangement Score (SAH-PDS) based on the important independent contributors to poor outcome in their study. The predictive value of the SAH-PDS was equivalent to that of admission GCS. This important study also showed that the physiological subcomponent of the APACHE-II score was associated with the outcome of death and severe disability but did not independently predict this outcome, which was similar to the findings in other studies. In addition, development of physiological complications such as hyperglycemia, decreased renal function, and fever are associated with poor outcomes; therefore, addressing these physiological derangements are recommended to improve the outcome of these patients.

Scores such as Hunt and Hess and WFNS focus mainly on the clinical condition of aSAH patients at the time of presentation. This approach has potential drawbacks, since relying purely on clinical condition using a grading system does not take into account comorbid factors, such as the patient's age, the location and size of the aneurysm, and the density of the hemorrhage. However, these comorbid factors do have an impact on the outcome of aSAH patients. For example, Ogilvy

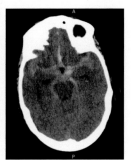

Figure 4.1 Patient with modified Fisher grade-IV aSAH.

77

and Carter [21] showed that factors other than clinical condition are strongly associated with outcome and subsequently developed a new grading scale that ranges from 0 to 5 and includes age, Hunt and Hess grade, Fisher grade, and aneurysm size. The inter-observer variability for the Ogilvy and Carter scale is very good, reflecting substantial observer agreement (kappa 0.69). However, the main limitation of this scale is that it is not generalizable to all aSAH patients as it was designed to predict surgical outcome. Most aSAH patients are now treated with endovascular coiling. Another limitation of this scale is that in some patients the location or size of the aneurysm is not known, making this scale less applicable.

The Brain Aneurysm Institute (BAI) scale [22] is another scoring system that has been developed from retrospective data and is accurate in predicting discharge outcome in aSAH patients. This score also ranges from 0 to 5 and assigns 2 points for a post-resuscitation GCS score of 8 or less, 1 point for age 70 years or older, 1 point for SAH thickness of 10 mm in any cerebral fissure or cistern, and 1 point for use of antiplatelet therapy on admission. The predictive capabilities of the BAI scale are similar to the Hunt and Hess scale. However, objectivity of the terms used in the BAI scale makes it less subjective than the Hunt and Hess scale. The area under the curve (AUC) of different aSAH prognostication scales are compared with the BAI scale in Table 4.3.

As described above, numerous grading scales have been developed in recent years; however, no single prognostic tool can predict or define all aspects of recovery and disability after aSAH. To overcome these challenges, a group of investigators interested in aSAH research collaborated to establish a large multinational network to pool individual patient data (IPD) from clinical trials and institutionally collected data sets to optimize the design and analysis of future clinical trials in aSAH. This data repository is called the Subarachnoid Hemorrhage International Trialists (SAHIT) Repository. The SAHIT score [23] was developed based on a cohort that included 10,936 patients from seven randomized controlled trials and two prospective observational hospital registries. The variables used in this model are:

- Age,
- Clinical severity on admission as measured by the WFNS scale,
- Premorbid history of hypertension,
- Volume of subarachnoid hemorrhage on computed tomography (CT) on admission (according to the Fisher grade),
- Size and location of the ruptured aneurysm, and
- Method of treatment (whether the patient had surgical clipping, endovascular coiling, or conservative treatment only).

The SAHIT score uses an online prognostic calculator algorithm that is accessible through mobile applications.

Recently, another scale has gained popularity: The Functional Recovery Expected after Subarachnoid Hemorrhage (FRESH) score [24] is the first aSAH prognostication tool to combine functional outcome with cognitive and quality of life outcomes. Witsch et al. used the Hunt and Hess and APACHE-II physiological scores on admission, age, and aneurysmal re-bleed within

Table 4.3 Comparison of different scales in prognostication of aSAH in BAI scale cohort

Scale system	Unfavorable outcome (mRS = 3–6)		Mortality (mRS = 6)	
	AUC (%)	P value	AUC (%)	P value
BAI scale	85.0	n/a	82.5	n/a
SAHIT scale	84.3	0.521	81.6	0.633
H&H scale	80.6	0.101	78.2	0.199
WFNS scale	78.5	0.001	74	0.001
Ogilvy scale	74.1	< 0.001	72.6	< 0.001

Abbreviations: aSAH: aneurysmal subarachnoid hemorrhage; AUC: area under the curve; BAI: Brain Aneurysm Institute; H&H: Hunt and Hess; mRS: modified Rankin Scale; SAHIT: aneurysmal subarachnoid hemorrhage; WFNS: World Federation of Neurosurgical Societies.

48 hours to develop the FRESH score, which showed outstanding discrimination in the derivation cohort ($n = 1,526$; AUC 90%) and moderate discrimination in the external validation cohort (with kappa 0.77).

Another major problem is the use of common outcome measures such as the modified Rankin Scale (mRS), as these scales often do not consider cognitive and behavioral/psychological consequences of aSAH. An agreed limited set of outcomes (core outcome measures) is needed to reduce selective reporting bias and allowing multiple trials to be compared or combined. To address this problem, a condition-specific aSAH Outcome Tool (SAHOT)[25] was developed in 2018 to measure changes in the patient's level of functioning. SAHOT incorporates the assessment of cognitive, emotional, and social domains that is reported by aSAH patients and their next of kin. The main advantages of this tool are its incorporation of patient-reported measures and its ability to discriminate patients with notable differences in impact of aSAH who otherwise fall within the same mRS category.

In addition to clinical and radiographic scales, it should be acknowledged that other modalities have been utilized and continue to be studied with regard to improving outcome prediction in aSAH. For example, electroencephalographic factors may prove useful in improving prognostication in this condition, and it has been shown that nonconvulsive status epilepticus in aSAH patients is associated with higher mortality.[26] In addition, a variety of findings on magnetic resonance imaging (e.g., lesions on diffusion-weighted imaging or fluid-attenuated inversion recovery lesions, measured volumes) correlate with short- and long-term outcomes [27] and additional nontraditional sequences may help with predicting outcome (e.g., arterial spin labeling [ASL], diffusion tensor imaging [DTI], blood-oxygen-level-dependent [BOLD] signal). Finally, spreading depolarizations, which are recurrent waves of neuronal and glial depolarizations, have been documented in aSAH and can worsen outcomes [28] by several putative mechanisms (e.g., enhancing metabolic demand, predisposing to epileptic discharges, activating inflammation, decreasing blood supply via vasoconstriction, disrupting the blood–brain barrier) and could thus provide a target for treatment in aSAH.

Effects of Various Treatments on the Outcome and Prognosis of aSAH

Early re-bleeding following aSAH is common, occurring at a rate up to 10% in the first 3 days with an associated worsening in prognosis. Strategies for reducing the risk of re-bleeding encompass early aneurysm repair (by way of surgical clipping or endovascular coiling) and control of extreme hypertension before securing the aneurysm.[29] Current guidelines recommend controlling blood pressure to mean systolic blood pressure (SBP) to less than 140 mmHg while awaiting definitive aneurysm treatment.[30]

Aneurysm repair should be performed early (within 72 hours based on current guidelines), since delayed treatment has been associated with a significant increase in poor outcome.[31] Overall, both surgical clipping and endovascular coiling are considered safe and are associated with low death rates. The choice between these two treatments should be based on several factors. The International Subarachnoid Aneurysm Trial (ISAT), a randomized trial comparing neurosurgical clipping with endovascular coiling, showed a benefit for endovascular treatment on the primary outcome (death or dependency at 1 year) with an absolute risk reduction of 7.4% (95% confidence interval [CI] 3.6–11.2) favoring endovascular treatment when the ruptured cerebral aneurysm was amenable to either treatment modality. However, most of the patients in ISAT had a good clinical baseline; therefore, the study is not generalizable to patients with poor-grade aSAH. Current guidelines encourage considering clipping over coiling for middle cerebral artery aneurysms. Clipping is also encouraged in patients with large (> 50 mL) intra-parenchymal hematomas, since most often these patients would require surgical removal of the hematoma as well. Other considerations based on expert opinion and observational studies recommend endovascular coiling for aneurysms of the basilar apex. Endovascular coiling may receive increased consideration in the elderly (> 70 years of age) and in those presenting with poor-grade WFNS classification (grade 4/5).[32]

It was thought that patients with Hunt and Hess grading of 5 generally had a very poor prognosis. and overall clinical practice was to offer a less aggressive treatment approach. However, in a study of aSAH patients [33] with Hunt and Hess grade 5 between 2005 and 2014, 23% (46/203) of patients had a favorable outcome (mRS score 0–2), and 67% (137/203) underwent early treatment within 72 hours. The rate of favorable outcome was similar for clipping and coil embolization (28% vs. 31%, respectively), and 49% (99/203) patients with Hunt and Hess grade 5 died before 6-month follow-up.

Hydrocephalus is another common complication of aSAH that occurs in 20–30% of patients at some time during the course of the disease. Hydrocephalus, especially when accompanied by IVH, is associated with a worse prognosis. Compared to patients without IVH, those aSAH patients with IVH have significantly higher morbidity and severe disability.[34] Current consensus among experts is that CSF diversion by way of external ventricular drain (EVD) placement or lumbar puncture is indicated in aSAH patients with a decreased level of consciousness and evidence of hydrocephalus or increased intracranial pressure. Bleeding and infection are the most common complications after EVD placement (up to 8% for each); however, if these complications are avoided, outcomes and aSAH grade can improve with EVD placement.[35]

Another complication that can have an impact on the prognosis of aSAH patients is the development of seizures and/or epilepsy. Early seizures occur in up to 18% of patients and are an independent risk factor for the development of epilepsy and poor prognosis. In a study of 872 patients from 1994 to 2000, late epilepsy occurred in 5% of aSAH patients. There was a correlation between the incidence of late epilepsy and both the presenting WFNS grade (up to 12.5% in grade 4) and the Glasgow Outcome Scale at discharge.[36] In another study,[37] development of seizures at 12 months was associated with severe disability (score ≥ 3 on the mRS and reduced quality of life on the Sickness Impact Profile).

Delayed cerebral ischemia after aSAH often leads to infarctions that are major contributors to the high case fatality and morbidity of this condition and occurs in about one-third of aSAH patients.[38] The pathogenesis of secondary ischemia has not yet been fully elucidated. Historically, vasoconstriction was thought to be the main mechanism that leads to DCI. However, cerebral infarction sometimes develops in the absence of demonstrable vasoconstriction or in a vascular territory unaffected by vasospasm. Furthermore, successful treatment of angiographic vasoconstriction does not necessarily lead to better functional outcomes.[39] Vasoconstriction was thought to be related to vasoactive agents that result in an increase of calcium in the vascular smooth-muscle cell.[40] This theory ultimately led to the development of the British Aneurysm Nimodipine Trial (BRANT).[41] The rationale was that nimodipine as a calcium channel blocker can counteract the influx of calcium in the vascular smooth-muscle cell and therefore prevent vasoconstriction. The BRANT trial showed improved outcomes in aSAH patients who were treated with nimodipine. In this trial, the nimodipine-treated patients had a decreased frequency of vasospasm, but this finding was not statistically significant. Although the exact mechanism is not known, meta-analyses of nimodipine trials show that, compared with placebo, nimodipine improves the odds of a good outcome after aSAH by 1.86 (99% CI 1.07–3.25).

Anemia is also common in aSAH patients and may be associated with poor outcome. The optimal hemoglobin goal and anemia treatment target are not well understood in aSAH. Historically, data from the randomized controlled Transfusion Requirements in Critical Care (TRICC) trial [42] showed that a restrictive transfusion threshold (< 7 g/dL) as opposed to a more liberal transfusion threshold (< 10 g/dL) is associated with decreased mortality in critically ill patients. However, patients with neurological illnesses were underrepresented in the TRICC trial, as only 4% of the cohort had a primary diagnosis of neurological abnormalities. Ayling et al. showed that, in aSAH patients, low hemoglobin (< 10 g/dL) occurring after the aneurysm-securing procedure or during the delayed cerebral ischemia (DCI) period, but not at the time of hospital admission, is associated with poor neurological outcome and death.[43] The same study also showed that patients who were transfused to keep their hemoglobin > 10 g/dL had better outcomes than those who achieved lower targets. On the other hand, data from other observational studies in the past have showed that transfusion is directly associated with adverse outcomes and higher mortality among patients with aSAH.[44,45] Due to these discrepancies, there is a need for future randomized controlled trials to address this issue; until then, an assessment of the benefits and risks of blood transfusions based on individual characteristics of each patient seems prudent.

Cognitive Impairment after aSAH

In recent years, it has become clearer that the usual outcome measures utilized in aSAH such as GCS, mRS, and National Institutes of Health Stroke Scale (NIHSS) are not adequate to predict the long-term outcome of these patients. Many patients with reasonable clinical exams or GCS scores after aSAH have cognitive deficits and poor health-related quality of life.[46] In one study,[47] the vast majority of patients (84%) had a normal NIHSS score 3 months after aSAH. However, cognitive dysfunction was much more common, with 18–42% of patients scoring in the impaired range in each of the specific neuropsychological domains that were tested. All domains of cognitive function can be affected in aSAH. However, verbal memory and motor functioning are the most prevalent domains that are impacted. Anxiety, depression, and fatigue are common in aSAH patients, with one study reporting 32% anxiety, 23% depression, and 67% fatigue in their cohort.[48] More data are needed regarding this important aspect of prognosis in aSAH patients.

Discussion

Despite the diversity of outcomes and scales, there is no definitive prognostication system in patients with aSAH. Most of the scales and grading systems that are currently being used focus on relatively short-term outcomes and are not designed to predict long-term functioning or cognitive outcomes in this population. Many also do not consider the physiological derangements that are commonly present in these patients. Older scores such as Hunt and Hess or WFNS are still the most widely used grading systems and, if consistently applied together, can reliably discriminate between favorable and unfavorable outcomes. Besides the FRESH score, few other grading systems can outperform the reliability of the Hunt and Hess or WFNS scores put together. The SAHIT scale is another good prognostication model in these patients that outperforms most of the currently existing scores. Magnetic resonance imaging, electroencephalography, and detection of spreading depolarizations could provide additional ways to assist prognostication. Cognitive impairment is a poorly studied aspect of prognosis in aSAH

patients that requires further investigations. Complications are common in the setting of aSAH, and future studies are needed to explore potential new treatments that can improve the prognosis of these patients.

As an update, new American Heart Association (AHA) and Neurocritical Care Society (NCS) aSAH guidelines were recently published. The NCS guidelines provide recommendations for measures outcomes, including the better-elucidated of antifibrinolytics prior to aneurysm treatment does not seem to affect outcome.[49] The AHA guidelines similarly discuss recommended treatments in this patient population and further recognize that patient outcomes may be affected by health inequities, such as those related to treatment access, socioeconomic status, and insurance status.[50] These guidelines also acknowledge the role that well-trained and standardized nursing can have in influencing outcomes. Further, the authors provide recommendations on predicting acute and long-term recovery; for instance, they recommend testing to screen for physical, cognitive (including presence of depression and anxiety), and quality of life deficits.[50] These screening tools can include the Glasgow Outcome Scale, the Hospital Anxiety and Depression Scale, and the EuroQol-5D, for examples.

References

1. Nieuwkamp DJ, Setz LE, Algra A, et al. Changes in case fatality of aneurysmal subarachnoid haemorrhage over time, according to age, sex, and region: a meta-analysis. *Lancet Neurol.* 2009;**8** (7):635–42.

2. Feigin VL, Rinkel GJ, Lawes CM, et al. (Risk factors for subarachnoid hemorrhage: an updated systematic review of epidemiological studies. *Stroke.* 2005;**36**(12):2773–80.

3. Etminan N, Chang, HS, Hackenberg K, et al. Worldwide incidence of aneurysmal subarachnoid hemorrhage according to region, time period, blood pressure, and smoking prevalence in the population: a systematic review and meta-analysis. *JAMA Neurol.* 2019;**76** (5):588–97.

4. Geraghty JR and Testai FD. Delayed cerebral ischemia after subarachnoid hemorrhage: beyond vasospasm and towards a multifactorial pathophysiology. *Curr Atheroscler Rep.* 2017;**19** (12):50.

5. Sabri M, Lass E, Macdonald, RL. Early brain injury: a common mechanism in subarachnoid

hemorrhage and global cerebral ischemia. *Stroke Res Treat.* 2013;**2013**:394036.

6. Suarez JI, Tarr RW, Selman WR. Aneurysmal subarachnoid hemorrhage. *N Engl J Med.* 2006;**354**(4):387–96.

7. Pickard JD, Murray GD, Illingworth R, et al. Effect of oral nimodipine on cerebral infarction and outcome after subarachnoid haemorrhage: British aneurysm nimodipine trial. *BMJ.* 1989;**298**(6674):636–42.

8. Molyneux A, Kerr R, International Subarachnoid Aneurysm Trial (ISAT) Collaborative Group. International Subarachnoid Aneurysm Trial (ISAT) of neurosurgical clipping versus endovascular coiling in 2143 patients with ruptured intracranial aneurysms: a randomized trial. *J Stroke Cerebrovasc Dis.* 2002;**11**(6):304–14.

9. Zier LS, Burack JH, Micc, G, et al. Doubt and belief in physicians' ability to prognosticate during critical illness: the perspective of surrogate decision makers. *Crit Care Med.* 2008;**36**(8):2341.

10. Frontera JA, Fernandez A, Schmidt JM, et al Defining vasospasm after subarachnoid hemorrhage: what is the most clinically relevant definition? *Stroke.* 2009;**40**(6):1963–8.

11. Wartenberg KE, Schmidt JM, Claassen, et al. Impact of medical complications on outcome after subarachnoid hemorrhage. *Crit Care Med.* 2006;**34**(3):617–23.

12. Le Roux PD, Elliott JP, Newell DW, et al. Predicting outcome in poor-grade patients with subarachnoid hemorrhage: a retrospective review of 159 aggressively managed cases. *J Neurosurg.* 1996;**85**(1):39–49.

13. Hunt WE and Hess RM. Surgical risk as related to time of intervention in the repair of intracranial aneurysms. *J Neurosurg.* 1968;**28**(1):14–20.

14. Hirai S, Ono J, Yamaura A. Clinical grading and outcome after early surgery in aneurysmal subarachnoid hemorrhage. *Neurosurgery.* 1996;**39**(3):441–6.

15. Giraldo EA, Mandrekar JN, Rubin MN, et al. Timing of clinical grade assessment and poor outcome in patients with aneurysmal subarachnoid hemorrhage. *J Neurosurg.* 2012;**117**(1):15–19.

16. Fisher CM, Kistler JP, Davis JM. Relation of cerebral vasospasm to subarachnoid hemorrhage visualized by computerized tomographic scanning. *Neurosurgery.* 1980;**6**(1):1–9.

17. Claassen J, Bernardini GL, Kreiter K, et al. Effect of cisternal and ventricular blood on risk of delayed cerebral ischemia after subarachnoid hemorrhage: the Fisher scale revisited. *Stroke.* 2001;**32**(9):2012–20.

18. Yoshimoto Y, Tanaka Y, Hoya K. Acute systemic inflammatory response syndrome in subarachnoid hemorrhage. *Stroke.* 2001;**32**(9):1989–93.

19. Claassen J, Carhuapoma JR, Kreiter K, et al. Global cerebral edema after subarachnoid hemorrhage: frequency, predictors, and impact on outcome. *Stroke.* 2002;**33**(5):1225–32.

20. Claassen J, Vu A, Kreiter KT, et al. Effect of acute physiologic derangements on outcome after subarachnoid hemorrhage. *Crit Care Med.* 2004;**32**(3):832–8.

21. Ogilvy CS and Carter BS. A proposed comprehensive grading system to predict outcome for surgical management of intracranial aneurysms. *Neurosurgery.* 1998;**42**(5):959–68.

22. Maragkos GA, Enriquez-Marulanda A. Salem MM, et al. Proposal of a grading system for predicting discharge mortality and functional outcome in patients with aneurysmal subarachnoid hemorrhage. *World Neurosurg.* 2019;**121**: e500–e510.

23. Jaja BN, Saposnik G, Lingsma HF, et al. Development and validation of outcome prediction models for aneurysmal subarachnoid haemorrhage: the SAHIT multinational cohort study. *BMJ.* 2018;**362**:k4079.

24. Witsch J, Frey HP, Patel S, et al. Prognostication of long-term outcomes after subarachnoid hemorrhage: the FRESH score. *Ann Neurol.* 2016;**80**(1):46–58.

25. Pace A, Mitchell S, Casselden E, et al. A subarachnoid haemorrhage-specific outcome tool. *Brain.* 2018;**141**(4):1111–21.

26. Kondziella D, Friberg CK, Wellwood I, et al. Continuous EEG monitoring in aneurysmal subarachnoid hemorrhage: a systematic review. *Neurocrit Care.* 2015;**22**(3):450–61.

27. Nelson SE, Sair HI, Stevens RD. Magnetic resonance imaging in aneurysmal subarachnoid hemorrhage: current evidence and future directions. *Neurocrit Care.* 2018;**29**(2):241–52.

28. Chung DY, Oka F, Ayata C. Spreading depolarizations: a therapeutic target against delayed cerebral ischemia after subarachnoid hemorrhage. *J Clin Neurophysiol.* 2016;**33**(3):196.

29. Diringer MN, Bleck TP, Hemphill JC. et al. Critical care management of patients following aneurysmal subarachnoid hemorrhage: recommendations from the Neurocritical Care Society's Multidisciplinary Consensus Conference. *Neurocrit Care.* 2011;**15**(2):211.

30. Connolly ES Jr, Rabinstein AA, Carhuapoma JR, et al. Guidelines for the management of aneurysmal subarachnoid hemorrhage: a guideline for healthcare professionals from the American Heart Association/American Stroke Association. *Stroke.* 2012;**43**(6):1711–37.

31. Dorhout Mees SM, Molyneux AJ, Kerr RS, Algra A, Rinkel GJ. Timing of aneurysm treatment after subarachnoid hemorrhage: relationship with delayed cerebral ischemia and poor outcome. *Stroke.* 2012;**43**(8):2126–9.

32. Tateshima S, Murayama Y, Gobin YP, et al. Endovascular treatment of basilar tip aneurysms using Guglielmi detachable coils: anatomic and clinical outcomes in 73 patients from a single institution. *Neurosurgery.* 2000;**47**(6):1332–42.

33. Konczalla J, Seifert V, Beck J, et al. Outcome after Hunt and Hess Grade V subarachnoid hemorrhage: a comparison of pre-coiling era (1980–1995) versus post-ISAT era (2005–2014). *J Neurosurg.* 2017;**128**(1):100–10.

34. Hayashi M, Handa Y, Kobayashi H, et al. Prognosis of intraventricular hemorrhage due to rupture of intracranial aneurysm. *Zentralbl Neurochir.* 1989;**50**(3-4):132–7.

35. Hasan D, Vermeulen M, Wijdicks EF, Hijdra A, van Gijn J. Management problems in acute hydrocephalus after subarachnoid hemorrhage. *Stroke.* 1989;**20**(6):747–53.

36. Buczacki SJ, Kirkpatrick PJ, Seeley HM, Hutchinson PJ. Late epilepsy following open surgery for aneurysmal subarachnoid haemorrhage. *J Neurol Neurosurg Psychiatry.* 2004;**75**(11):1620–2.

37. Claassen J, Peery S, Kreiter KT, et al. Predictors and clinical impact of epilepsy after subarachnoid hemorrhage. *Neurology.* 2003;**60**(2):208–14.

38. Roos YB, de Haan RJ, Beenen LFM, et al. Complications and outcome in patients with aneurysmal subarachnoid haemorrhage: a prospective hospital based cohort study in the Netherlands. *J Neurol Neurosurg Psychiatry.* 2000;**68**(3):337–41.

39. Etminan N, Vergouwen MD, Ilodigwe D, Macdonald RL. Effect of pharmaceutical treatment on vasospasm, delayed cerebral ischemia, and clinical outcome in patients with aneurysmal subarachnoid hemorrhage: a systematic review and meta-analysis. *J Cereb Blood Flow Metab.* 2011;**31**(6):1443–51.

40. Ljunggren B, Brandt L, Säveland H, et al. Outcome in 60 consecutive patients treated with early aneurysm operation and intravenous nimodipine. *J Neurosurg.* 1984;**61**(5):864–73.

41. Pickard JD, Murray GD, Illingworth R, et al. Effect of oral nimodipine on cerebral infarction and outcome after subarachnoid haemorrhage: British Aneurysm Nimodipine trial. *BMJ.* 1989;**298**(6674):636–42.

42. Hébert PC, Wells G, Blajchman MA, et al. Transfusion Requirements in Critical Care Investigators for the Canadian Critical Care Trials Group. A multicenter, randomized, controlled clinical trial of transfusion requirements in critical care. *N Eng J Med.* 1999;**340**(6):409–17.

43. Ayling OG, Ibrahim GM, Alotaibi NM, et al. Anemia after aneurysmal subarachnoid hemorrhage is associated with poor outcome and death. *Stroke.* 2018;**49**(8):1859–65.

44. Kramer AH, Gurka MJ, Nathan B, et al. Complications associated with anemia and blood transfusion in patients with aneurysmal subarachnoid hemorrhage. *Crit Care Med.* 2008;**36**(7):2070–5.

45. Kramer AH and Zygun DA. Anemia and red blood cell transfusion in neurocritical care. *Crit Care.* 2009;**13**(3):R89.

46. Hütter BO and Gilsbach JM. Which neuropsychological deficits are hidden behind a good outcome (Glasgow = I) after aneurysmal subarachnoid hemorrhage? *Neurosurgery.* 1993;**33**(6):999–1006.

47. Mayer SA, Kreiter KT, Copeland D, et al. Global and domain-specific cognitive impairment and outcome after subarachnoid hemorrhage. *Neurology.* 2002;**59**(11):1750–8.

48. Visser-Meily JA, Rhebergen ML, Rinkel GJ, van Zandvoort MJ, Post MW. Long-term health-related quality of life after aneurysmal subarachnoid hemorrhage: relationship with psychological symptoms and personality characteristics. *Stroke,* 2009;**40**(4):1526–9.

49. Treggiari MM, Rabinstein AA, Busl KM, et al. Guidelines for the neurocritical care management of subarachnoid hemorrhage. *Neurocrit Care.* 2023;**39**(1):1–28.

50. Hoh BL, Ko NU, Amin-Hanjani S, et al. 2023 Guideline for the management of patients with aneurysmal subarachnoid hemorrhage: a guideline from the American Heart Association/American Stroke Association. *Stroke.* 2023;**55**(7):e314–e370.

Chapter 5

Prognostication in Traumatic Brain Injury

Courtney Takahashi

Introduction

Traumatic brain injury (TBI) has increased in incidence and prevalence; between 2006 and 2014, the total number of emergency department visits, hospitalizations, and deaths increased by 53%.[1] More recently, hospitalizations alone have stabilized and decreased by 8%, but there is still significant disability associated with the disease.[2] Demographic data show that approximately 3 million persons in the United States (1.1% of the population) live with permanent disabilities as a result of TBI.[3] Because TBI disproportionately affects younger patients (with the potential for lost income and productivity) and males, accurate prognosis is especially crucial.[4]

Determining prognosis is difficult in every disease state, but there are special challenges to consider with TBI. Different injury patterns, such as contusions and other traumatic intra-axial hemorrhages, are all classified as TBI. Furthermore, patients may have any mix of various injuries spread among varied anatomical areas. Thus, even patients with similar diagnoses may have a wide range of clinical presentations and prognoses because of different injury patterns. The Glasgow Outcome Scale (GOS) and Extended Glasgow Outcome Scale (GOS-E) are often used to gauge patients' neurological function at the time of diagnosis, but these tools are coarse ways to judge outcome.[5] Outcomes are often dichotomized into "moderate disability or better" and "severe disability or worse."[6] Heterogeneous disease and ordinal/binary outcome scales thus make studies on prognosis challenging.

Even subspecialty experts, including neurointensivists and neurosurgeons, disagree on prognosis when presented with clinical vignettes. Both groups of physicians tend to be overly pessimistic and can overlook important information that can favorably influence the final prognosis.[7] While there are tools available to evaluate a patient's prognosis in a more objective manner, such as the International Mission for Prognosis and Analysis of Clinical Trials in TBI (IMPACT) calculator, survey results show that even populations of surgeons at Level 1 trauma centers only utilize the tool 50% of the time.[8] Hence, there is a need for more education and resources to aid with neurotrauma prognostication. This chapter is structured to examine the data currently available and to evaluate possible future ways to determine prognosis.

Admission Factors Associated with Outcomes

On admission, TBI patients can present with polytrauma (trauma involving multiple organ systems), which can make isolating the intracranial injury challenging. Despite these difficulties, some prognostic information can be gleaned from the initial neurological examination. Age is the strongest predictor of poor outcome in TBI: moving up from one age quartile to the next doubles the risk of poor outcome. Other significant factors include motor scores, particularly in patients with no movement or extensor posturing, pupillary reflex reactivity, hypoxia, and hypotension.[9–11] Admission laboratory data associated with poor outcome include higher glucose and lower hemoglobin. Head computed tomography (CT) that indicates elevated intracranial pressure and traumatic subarachnoid blood has also been associated with worse outcomes.[12,13]

Data that examine purely severe traumatic brain injury patients (Glasgow Coma Scale [GCS] score < 9) yield similar findings. Modeling from a Japanese cohort found that advanced age, absent pupillary light reflex, subarachnoid hemorrhage, elevated intracranial pressure, and midline shift were all predictors of poor prognosis.[11] Even when other injuries, such as lung and multi-injury trauma, are considered in multivariate analysis, advanced age, lower GCS, and worse injury severity scores are associated with worse functional outcomes at discharge.[14]

IMPACT and CRASH

The two largest trials of TBI patients, the International Mission on Prognosis and Analysis of Clinical Trials (IMPACT) and the Corticosteroid Randomization After Significant Head Injury (CRASH), both developed prognostic calculators to help providers determine patient outcomes.[12] The IMPACT model uses various clinical criteria at the time of admission to determine prognosis at 6 months (Table 5.1). Similarly, the CRASH model helps to predict functional outcome at 6 months and mortality risk at 14 days (Table 5.2). The IMPACT study cites up to 80% internal accuracy in predicting outcome, measured with GOS, at 6 months.[15] These calculators are the best tools available based on the large patient base in each study. [4,15,16] Large registries, using distinct prospectively collected and observational data, have externally validated the IMPACT and CRASH prediction models.[12,17] In Roozenbeek and colleagues' large external validation study, they used the IMPACT and CRASH models on data

Table 5.2 CRASH calculator characteristics

Characteristics within the first 8 hours after admission	
Country	Select country name
Age	Age in years
Glasgow Coma Score	Total score, 3–15
Pupils reactive to light	Both, one, or none
Major extracranial injury	Yes/No
On head CT: presence of petechial hemorrhages?	Yes/No
Obliteration of third ventricle or basal cisterns?	Yes/No
Subarachnoid bleeding	Yes/No
Midline shift	Yes/No
Non-evacuated hematoma	Yes/No

sets containing over 9,000 patients. Their group found that the model's highest discrimination was 0.83–0.87 (area under receiver operator curve) and worst was 0.65–0.71.[17] Other large external validation studies in countries including Spain and Singapore have also verified the applicability of the IMPACT model.[10,18] Hence, the IMPACT model performs relatively well for most TBI patients.

Surgical Decompression and Outcome

Early elevated intracranial pressures (ICP) have been associated with increased mortality and worse functional outcomes in TBI.[6,7,19] Clinicians are trained to treat elevated ICP aggressively with medical measures, serial neurological examinations, and invasive monitoring.[20] In elevated ICP cases refractory to medical management, however, surgical intervention must be considered.[21]

Surgical decompression consists of two principle steps: (1) removing part of the calvarium, and (2) opening the dura.[22] Decompression can be used to create an open area for cerebral swelling and circumvent secondary injury due to brain compression from herniation (Figure 5.1). It is most commonly considered in patients with focal traumatic lesions causing localized mass effect and in patients with diffuse injury resulting in elevated ICP.[23,24]

Table 5.1 IMPACT calculator characteristics

Admission characteristics	
Age	14–99 years
Motor score from Glasgow Coma Scale	No movement is worst, obeying is best
Pupils	Neither reactive, both reactive
Hypoxia	Present or absent
Hypotension	Present or absent
Computed tomography (CT) classification	Diffuse injury I–IV, mass lesion present or evacuated
Traumatic subarachnoid blood on CT	Present or absent
Epidural mass on CT	Present or absent
Glucose	Continuous variable
Hemoglobin	Continuous variable

85

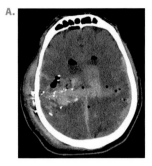

A: Gunshot wound to the head. The hyperdense areas represent blood along the bullet's trajectory in both the parenchyma and lateral ventricles.

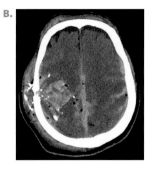

B: Bullet entry wound. Hyperdense areas depict additional intraparenchymal and subarachnoid blood.

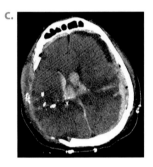

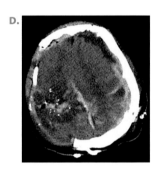

C/D: Status post right decompressive hemicraniectomy. Intraventricular blood, bullet fragments, and multiple other extra-axial hemorrhages are still present.

Figure 5.1 Surgical decompression for gunshot wound. Twenty-three-year-old male, admitted with gunshot wound to the head.

While surgical decompression may be life saving, it is unclear if it improves quality of life.[25] The Decompressive Craniectomy in Diffuse Traumatic Brain Injury (DECRA) trial was designed to determine whether early bifrontal craniectomy improved mortality and functional outcome in severe TBI patients. While early decompression did lower ICP, reduce ventilator days, and reduce hospital stay, patients ultimately suffered worse functional outcomes.[21] As a follow-up study to DECRA, the Trial of Decompressive Craniectomy for Traumatic Intracranial Hypertension (RescueICP) was designed to evaluate the role of early decompressive craniectomy in patients with ICP > 25 mmHg versus medical management. Primary outcomes were mortality and functional outcomes (measured with Extended Glasgow Outcome Scale [GOS-E]) at 6 months. Patients in the surgical arm of RescueICP had lower mortality but worsened functional outcomes, including higher rates of vegetative state and lower severe disability.[26] Table 5.3 demonstrates the stratification of outcomes in RescueICP. Both studies' results imply that while craniectomy with decompression may be life saving, it is also associated with worse long-term functional outcomes and higher rates of disability.

More specific information on prognosis after decompressive craniectomy is difficult to ascertain. While there are data to support using the CRASH and IMPACT models post-decompression, the field would still benefit from more prospective data.[27] Longer-term follow-ups in smaller cohorts indicate that patients with poor examinations prior to craniectomy tend to have poor long-term outcomes as well. Among survivors, patients in a vegetative state at discharge remained so, and most others were left with severe disabilities and inability to care for themselves.[28] Good recovery is possible,

Table 5.3 RescueICP patient outcomes at 6 months, distribution of GOS-E

GOS-E	Surgical group	Medical group
Death	26.9%	48.9%
Vegetative state	8.5%	2.1%
Lower severe disability (dependent for care)	21.9%	14.4%
Upper severe disability (independent at home)	15.4%	8.0%
Moderate disability	23.4%	19.7%
Good recovery	4.0%	6.9%

especially in younger patients; however, the means to identify these patients accurately is unclear.[29]

Markers of Futility

Fixed and Dilated Pupils: Irreversible Sign of Mortality?

Patients with GCS 3 on admission in combination with fixed and dilated pupils have traditionally been treated as "unsalvageable" because of their degree of neurological injury. Studies had reported no survivors among patients who arrived comatose with fixed and dilated pupils. [30–32] These assumptions, however, may need to be revisited. Larger multicenter studies now demonstrate mortality rates of about 48% for GCS 3 patients, implying that outcomes may be impacted by aggressive care and resuscitation.[9] More recent meta-analysis data focusing on patients who suffered from epidural and subdural hematomas have reported good outcomes in patients arriving with bilateral fixed and dilated pupils.[32,33] Particularly, rates of good outcomes are reported in 54.3% of patients suffering from epidural hematomas who receive immediate surgical evacuation. While patients with subdural hematomas experienced high mortality (66%), 6.6% of survivors reported good functional outcomes.[33] In other data that examined large trauma cohorts of severe TBI, 8/92 patients with GCS 3 and fixed and dilated pupils in the field experienced good recovery. Among the same group, 84/92 had a poor recovery. Larger

retrospective data reveal similar results; while adult mortality is high (85%), there are surviving patients. These newer data show that while fixed and dilated pupils in the comatose patient likely herald a poor prognosis, they are not the sign of universal mortality previously presumed.[34,35] Considered in total, these newer data may suggest that aggressive treatment, including surgical decompression, should be weighed as viable options even in the most severe injuries.

Persistent Vegetative State: Permanent or Recoverable?

An unfortunate but common problem after severe TBI is patients who survive in a persistent vegetative state. Persistent vegetative states (PVS) or vegetative sStates (VS) are defined by complete unawareness of self or the surrounding environment. Recently, the literature includes the term "unresponsive wakefulness syndrome" (UWS) as synonymous with vegetative state.[36] Movements are purposeless, language comprehension is absent, sleep/wake cycles may be present, and cranial nerve reflexes are variably present.[37] While the terms "vegetative state," "persistent vegetative state," and "permanent vegetative state" are occasionally used interchangeably, the traditional definitions are based on time intervals. The diagnosis of VS/UWS is based on a patient fulfilling the clinical criteria of a vegetative state (e.g., arousal but not awareness, purposeless movements) and usually implies that this condition has been present for a month or more. Persistent vegetative states are defined as clinical criteria consistent with VS/UWS on multiple serial neurological examinations for a month's duration or longer. Permanent vegetative state is considered when VS/UWS persists for more than 12 months in patients who suffered TBI and more than 3 months in patients with non-traumatic injuries.[38] These older, time-based definitions, however, are being phased out because newer data show evidence of recovery even after 1 year of VS/UWS [39]. Instead of the term "permanent vegetative state," "chronic vegetative state" is preferred, followed by the duration of the state (e.g., "chronic vegetative state for 5 months").[40]

In contrast, patients in a minimally conscious state (MCS) show some awareness of the outside world. They may be able to follow simple commands, indicate yes or no in response to a question, or show other verbal or body language clues that express true intent.[41] While this state of unawareness was previously touted as long term, patients with MCS may have better ability to recover. Studies performed in the same facility can show improved outcomes in terms of survival (67%) and recovery of consciousness (54%). These improvements likely reflect better overall hospital and rehabilitation care.[42]

Identifying signs that a patient may possibly recover from states of altered consciousness is critical for advising families and for resource allocation. While the clinical differences may seem nominal, determining whether a patient is in a persistent vegetative or minimally conscious state may be an important prognostic marker. Patients in minimally conscious states following TBI have better prognoses for emergence and recovery.[43] Hence, proper classification of altered states of consciousness may be key in gaining accurate prognostic information. While these changes are described as discrete categories, patients typically emerge slowly, progressing from MCS to post-traumatic amnesia / confusional state (PTA/CS) and finally to post-confusional / emerging independence.[44] Because the terms can be confusing, they are summarized in Figure 5.2. Intensive neurorehabilitation may help patients with prolonged states of unconsciousness to achieve better outcomes. Preliminary data in small study cohorts found that two-thirds of all patients were able to recover consciousness with intensive care. Patients may follow different recovery trajectories that include minimally conscious state, slow recovery of consciousness, and fast recovery of consciousness.[45]

Technology to Aid with Prognostication

EEG Patterns as Prognostic Markers

Long-term electroencephalogram (EEG) monitoring is common practice in traumatic brain injury patients because of blunted neurological exams and high rates of nonconvulsive seizures.[20,46] In addition to subclinical seizure detection, EEG patterns may reveal prognostic information. Patterns including alpha variability and relative fast theta power throughout EEG recordings have been associated with better outcomes.[47] Sleep architecture and patterns have also been associated with better long-term outcomes. Conversely, interictal patterns, seizures, status epilepticus, predominant delta activity, discontinuous background, and lack of sleep architecture (specifically absence of N2 transients) have been associated with lower modified Rankin Scale (mRS) scores.[48,49] EEG reactivity, particularly in comatose patients, may also be a specific marker for better outcomes.[50]

Prognostic Ability of MRI

Imaging is a key part of TBI management, especially in hospitalized patients. While magnetic resonance imaging (MRI) alone cannot determine prognosis, key features may supplement the clinician's prognostic abilities. Diffuse axonal injury (DAI) is a result of sheer force trauma and angular velocity that pathologically stretch and distort axons. Deeper structures, particularly the corpus callosum and the gray–white junction interface, are particularly susceptible to DAI.[51] Several studies have associated DAI with worse long-term outcomes. Systemic analysis has linked diffuse axonal injury, particular injury in the brainstem, to lower GOS-E scores at 6 months. [52,53] Indeed, with each increase in DAI grade, the risk of poor outcomes increases threefold.[54]

While DAI does correlate with functional outcomes, it is important to note its limitations. Other studies have not demonstrated the same robust correlation with outcomes, especially outcomes past a year.[55] Perhaps recognizing these limitations, researchers have used DAI with clinical factors to help predict long-term persistent vegetative and minimally conscious states.[56] DAI may be best used in combination with other clinical factors to build prognostic models to predict outcome.

Biomarkers in TBI

Traumatic brain injury patients suffer from both acute injuries at the time of impact and subsequent injuries from a more delayed neurodegenerative process. Axonal fiber tracts, neuronal bodies, dendrites, and oligodendrocytes are all subject to latent cellular injuries that manifest after the initial impact.[55] Because much of this injury cannot be discerned on a macroscopic level, serum markers may be a superior way to help determine a given patient's prognosis. While serum biomarkers are not consistently utilized for prognostic information outside of a research setting, many show promise in helping clinicians to predict patient outcomes (Table 5.4).

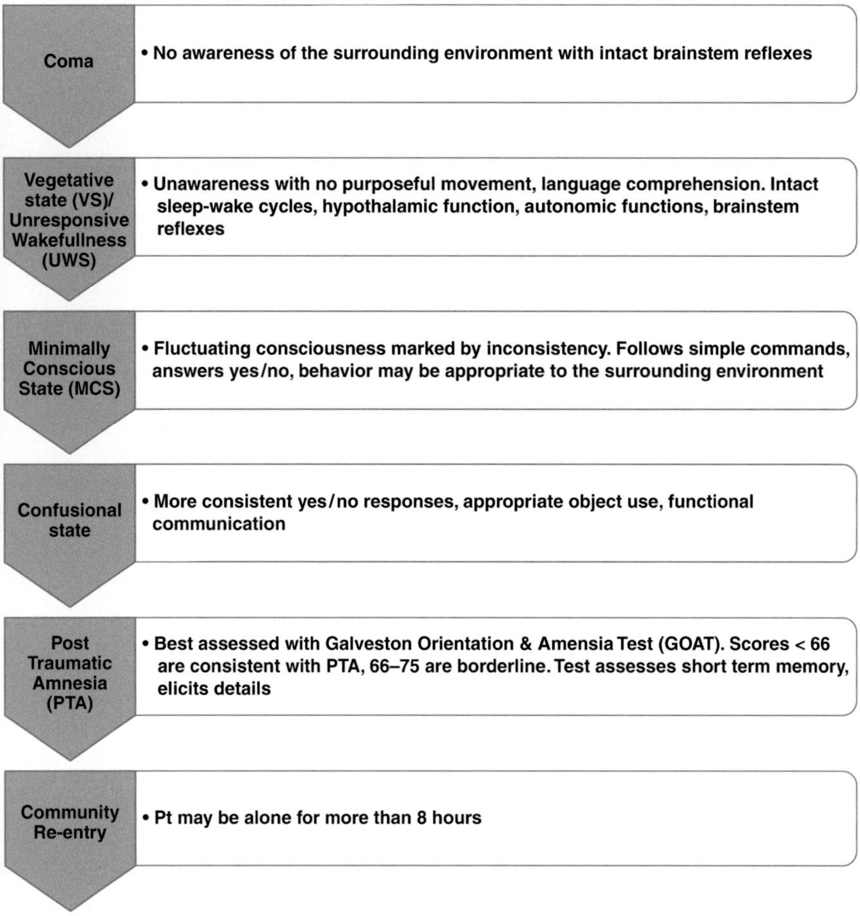

Coma	• No awareness of the surrounding environment with intact brainstem reflexes
Vegetative state (VS)/ Unresponsive Wakefullness (UWS)	• Unawareness with no purposeful movement, language comprehension. Intact sleep-wake cycles, hypothalamic function, autonomic functions, brainstem reflexes
Minimally Conscious State (MCS)	• Fluctuating consciousness marked by inconsistency. Follows simple commands, answers yes/no, behavior may be appropriate to the surrounding environment
Confusional state	• More consistent yes/no responses, appropriate object use, functional communication
Post Traumatic Amnesia (PTA)	• Best assessed with Galveston Orientation & Amensia Test (GOAT). Scores < 66 are consistent with PTA, 66–75 are borderline. Test assesses short term memory, elicits details
Community Re-entry	• Pt may be alone for more than 8 hours

Figure 5.2 Hierarchy of disorders of consciousness. Following severe traumatic brain injury, patients tend to emerge from coma slowly. Patients may arrest at any point in the recovery process.[36,44,59]

Serum biomarkers, especially in combination with clinical and imaging findings, may be key in creating better prognostic models. As yet, however, no biomarker performs reliably enough for consistent clinical use.[57,58]

Conclusion

Determining prognosis in TBI patients is still an active area of research. While some scoring systems perform reasonably well, no single algorithm is comprehensive for the care of a specific patient, and all scoring systems are impacted by the self-fulfilling prophecy of early withdrawal of life-sustaining therapies. As we are better able to define and incorporate clinical electrophysiology, neuroimaging, and biomarker information, our ability to predict functional outcomes and thus improve care will evolve as well.

Abbreviations

CRASH = Corticosteroid Randomization After Significant Head Injury

CT = computed tomography

DAI = diffuse axonal injury

DECRA = Decompressive Craniectomy in Diffuse Traumatic Brain Injury

EEG = electroencephalogram

GCS = Glasgow Coma Scale

GFAP = glial fibrillary acidic protein

GOS = Glasgow Outcome Scale

GOS-E = Extended Glasgow Outcome Scale

Table 5.4 Biomarkers with prognostic potential

Biomarker	Origin	Clinical potential	Possible pitfalls
S100B	11 kDa calcium-binding protein. Derived from astroglia [60]	Serum levels at 12–36 hours from injury may correlate with GOS at 6 months. Very high levels correlated with 100% mortality in a single study [61,62]	May be released with injury to skeletal muscle and adipose tissue, not exclusive to the brain [63]
Glial fibrillary acidic protein (GFAP)	Astroglial-associated protein [57]	Higher levels may correlate with worsened outcomes, lower levels may correlate with better outcomes on GOS-E at 6 months [64]	May need to be used in combination with other serum or biomarkers for maximum clinical utility [57]
Ubiquitin C-terminal hydrolase-L1 (UCH-L1)	Neuronal cell body cytoplasm [65]	Levels may help to distinguish mild/moderate TBI from severe, may also correlate with GOS [63]	
Neurofilament (NF) proteins	Intermediate filaments exclusive in neurons [66]	Levels may correlate with 6- and 12-month outcomes [67]	
Tau proteins	Microtubule stabilization proteins, high levels in neurons, lower levels in astrocytes and oligodendrocytes [68]	May help to predict poor outcomes in combination with GCS [69]	Limited ability to predict good outcomes [69]
Micro-RNAs	Class of non-coding RNA molecules with roles in physiological cell cycling and metabolism [70]	Elevation levels of distinct microRNA may distinguish between mild and severe TBI [65] Able to distinguish between subjects and healthy volunteers.	

ICP = intracranial pressure

IMPACT = International Mission for Prognosis and Analysis of Clinical Trials in TBI

MCS = minimally conscious state

MRI = magnetic resonance imaging

mRS = modified Rankin Scale

PVS = persistent vegetative state

RescueICP = Trial of Decompressive Craniectomy for Traumatic Intracranial Hypertension

TBI = traumatic brain injury

References

1. *Surveillance Report of Traumatic Brain Injury-Related Emergency Department Visits, Hospitalization, and Deaths – United States, 2014.* Washington, DC: US Department of Health and Human Services, Centers for Disease Control and Prevention, 2019.

2. Meschia JF, Bushnell C, Boden-Albala B, et al. Guidelines for the primary prevention of stroke: a statement for healthcare professionals from the American Heart Association/American Stroke Association. *Stroke.* 2014;**45**(12):3754–832.

3. Zaloshnja E, Miller T, Langlois JA, Selassie AW. Prevalence of long-term disability from traumatic brain injury in the civilian population of the United States, 2005. *J Head Trauma Rehabil.* 2008;**23**(6):394–400.

4. MRC CRASH Trial Collaborators. Predicting outcome after traumatic brain injury: practical prognostic models based on large cohort of international patients. *BMJ.* 2008;**336**(7641):425–9.

5. McMillan T, Wilson L, Ponsford J, et al. The Glasgow Outcome Scale – 40 years of application and refinement *Nat Rev Neurol.* 2016;**12**:477.

6. Maas AIR, Marmarou A, Murray GD, Teasdale SGM, Steyerberg EW. Prognosis and clinical trial design in traumatic brain injury: the IMPACT study. *J Neurotrauma.* 2007;**24**(2):232–8.

7. Moore NA, Brennan PM, Baillie JK. Wide variation and systematic bias in expert clinicians' perceptions of prognosis following brain injury. *Br J Neurosurg.* 2013;**27**(3):340–3.

8. Letsinger J, Rommel C, Hirschi R, Nrula R, Hawryluk GWJ. The aggressiveness of neurotrauma practitioners and the influence of the IMPACT prognostic calculator. *PLoS One*. 2017;**12**(8):e0183552.

9. Salottolo K, Carrick M, Stewart Levy A, et al. The epidemiology, prognosis, and trends of severe traumatic brain injury with presenting Glasgow Coma Scale of 3. *J Crit Care*. 2017;**38**:197–201.

10. Han JX, See AAQ, Gandhi M, King NKK. Models of mortality and morbidity in severe traumatic brain injury: an analysis of a Singapore neurotrauma database. *World Neurosurg*. 2017;**108**:885–93.e1.

11. Tasaki O, Shiozaki T, Hamasaki T, et al. Prognostic indicators and outcome prediction model for severe traumatic brain injury. *J Trauma*. 2009;**66**(2):304–8.

12. Steyerberg EW, Mushkudiani N, Perel P, et al. Predicting outcome after traumatic brain injury: development and international validation of prognostic scores based on admission characteristics. *PLoS Med*. 2008;**5**(8):e165; discussion e165.

13. Kamal VK, Agrawal D, Pandey RM. Prognostic models for prediction of outcomes after traumatic brain injury based on patients admission characteristics. *Brain Inj*. 2016;**30**(4):393–406.

14. Baum J, Entezami P, Shah K, Medhkour A. Predictors of outcomes in traumatic brain injury. *World Neurosurg*. 2016;**90**:525–9.

15. Marmarou A, IMPACT database of traumatic brain injury: design and description. *J Neurotrauma*. 2007;**24**(2):239–50.

16. Majdan M, Lingsma HF, Nieboer D., et al. Performance of IMPACT, CRASH and Nijmegen models in predicting six month outcome of patients with severe or moderate TBI: an external validation study. *Scand J Trauma Resusc Emerg Med*. 2014;**22**(1):68.

17. Roozenbeek B, Lingsman HF, Lecky FE, et al., IMPACT Study Group, CRASH Trial Collaborators, TARN. Prediction of outcome after moderate and severe traumatic brain injury: external validation of the International Mission on Prognosis and Analysis of Clinical Trials (IMPACT) and Corticoid Randomisation after Significant Head injury (CRASH) prognostic models. *Crit Care Med*. 2012;**40**(5):1609–17.

18. Egea-Guerrero JJ, Rodriguez-Rodriguez A, Gordillo-Escobar E, et al. IMPACT score for traumatic brain injury: validation of the prognostic tool in a Spanish cohort, *J Head Trauma Rehabil*. 2018;**33**(1):46–52.

19. Tucker DM, Luu PK, Pribra, H. Social and emotional self-regulation. *Ann NY Acad Sci*. 1995;**769**:213–39.

20. [No authors listed]The Brain Trauma Foundation. The American Association of Neurological Surgeons. The Joint Section on Neurotrauma and Critical Care. Glasgow coma scale score, *J. Neurotrauma*. 2000;**17**(6–7):563–71.

21. Cooper DJ, Rosenfeld JV, Murray L, et al. Decompressive craniectomy in diffuse traumatic brain injury. *N Eng J Med*. 2011;**364**(16):1493–1502.

22. Giammattei L, Messerer M, Cherian I, et al. Current perspectives in the surgical treatment of severe traumatic brain injury. *World Neurosurg*. 2018;**116**:322–8.

23. Mendelow AD, Gregson BA, Rowan EN, et al. Early Surgery versus Initial Conservative Treatment in Patients with Traumatic Intracerebral Hemorrhage (STITCHTrauma.): the first randomized trial. *J Neurotrauma*. 2015;**32**(17):1312–23.

24. Galgano M, Toshkezi G, Qiu, X, et al. Traumatic brain injury: current treatment strategies and future endeavors. *Cell Transplant*. 2017;**26**(7):1118–30.

25. Honeybul S, Gillett GR, Ho KM. Uncertainty, conflict and consent: revisiting the futility debate in neurotrauma. *Acta Neurochir (Wien)*. 2016;**158**(7):1251–7.

26. Hutchinson PJ, Kolias AG, Timofeev IS, et al. Trial of decompressive craniectomy for traumatic intracranial hypertension. *N Eng J Med*. 2016;**375**(12):1119–30.

27. Honeybul S, Ho KM. Predicting long-term neurological outcomes after severe traumatic brain injury requiring decompressive craniectomy: A comparison of the CRASH and IMPACT prognostic models. *Injury*. 2016;**47**(9):1886–92.

28. Honeybul S, Janzen C, Kruger K, Ho KM. Decompressive craniectomy for severe traumatic brain injury: is life worth living? *J Neurosurg*. 2013;**119**(6):1566–75.

29. Yatsushige H, Takasoto Y, Masoka H, et al. Prognosis for severe traumatic brain injury patients treated with bilateral decompressive craniectomy. *Acta Neurochir Suppl*. 2010;**106**:265–70.

30. Lieberman JD, Pasquale MD, Garcia R, et al. Use of admission Glasgow Coma Score, pupil size, and pupil reactivity to determine outcome for trauma patients. *J Trauma*. 2003;**55**(3):437–42; discussion 442–3.

31. Chaudhuri K, Malham GM, Rosenfeld JV. Survival of trauma patients with coma and bilateral fixed dilated pupils. *Injury*. 2009;**40**(1):28–32.

32. Tien HC, Cunha JRF, Wu SN, et al. Do trauma patients with a Glasgow Coma Scale score of 3 and bilateral fixed and dilated pupils have any chance of survival? *J Trauma*. 2006;**60**(2):274–8.

33. Scotter J, Hendrickson S, Marcus HJ, Wilson MH. Prognosis of patients with bilateral fixed dilated pupils secondary to traumatic extradural or subdural haematoma who undergo surgery: a systematic review and meta-analysis. *Emerg Med J*. 2015;**32**(8):654–9.

34. Mauritz W, Leitgeb J, Wilbacher I, et al. Outcome of brain trauma patients who have a Glasgow Coma Scale score of 3 and bilateral fixed and dilated pupils in the field. *Eur J Emerg Med*. 2009;**16**(3):153–8.

35. Emami P, Czorlich P, Fritzsche FS, et al. Impact of Glasgow Coma Scale score and pupil parameters on mortality rate and outcome in pediatric and adult severe traumatic brain injury: a retrospective, multicenter cohort study. *J Neurosurg*. 2017;**126**(3):760–7.

36. O'Donnell JC, Browne KD, Kilbaugh TJ, et al. Challenges and demand for modeling disorders of consciousness following traumatic brain injury. *Neurosci Biobehav Rev*. 2019;**98**:336–46.

37. Multi-Society Task Force on PVS. Medical aspects of the persistent vegetative state. *N Eng J Med*. 1994;**330**(21):1499–1508.

38. [No authors listed]. Practice parameters: assessment and management of patients in the persistent vegetative state (summary statement). The Quality Stardards Subcommittee of the American Academy of Neurology. *Neurology*. 1995;**45**(5):1015–18.

39. Giacino JT, Katz DK, Schiff ND, et al. Practice guideline update recommendations summary: disorders of consciousness: report of the Guideline Development, Dissemination, and Implementation Subcommittee of the American Academy of Neurology; the American Congress of Rehabilitation Medicine; and the National Institute on Disability, Independent Living, and Rehabilitation Research. *Arch Phys Med Rehabil*. 2018;**99**(9):1699–1709.

40. Giacino J. Life-sustaining treatments in vegetative state: scientific advances and ethical dilemmas. *Neurorehabilitation*. 2005;**19**(4):293–8.

41. Cranford RE. What is a minimally conscious state? *West J Med*. 2002;**176**(2):129–30.

42. Aidinoff E, Groswasser, Z, Bierman U, et al. Vegetative state outcomes improved over the last two decades. *Brain Inj*. 2018;**32**(3):297–302.

43. Noé E, Olaya J, Colomer C, et al. Current validity of diagnosis of permanent vegetative state: A longitudinal study in a sample of patients with altered states of consciousness. *Neurologia (Eng Ed)*. 2019;**34**(9):589–95.

44. Katz DI, Polyak M, Coughlan D, N ichols M, Roche A. Natural history of recovery from brain injury after prolonged disorders of consciousness: outcome of patients admitted to inpatient rehabilitation with 1–4 year follow-up. *Prog Brain Res*. 2009;**177**:73–88.

45. Eilander HJ, van Heugten CM, Wijnen VJM, et al. Course of recovery and prediction of outcome in young patients in a prolonged vegetative or minimally conscious state after severe brain injury: an exploratory study. *J Pediatr Rehabil Med*. 2013;**6**(2):73–83.

46. N. R. Temkin, S. S. Dikmen, A. J. Wilensky, et al. A randomized, double-blind study of phenytoin for the prevention of post-traumatic seizures. *N Eng J Med*. 1990;**323**(8):497–502.

47. Tolonen A, et al. Quantitative EEG parameters for prediction of outcome in severe traumatic brain injury: development study. *Clin EEG Neurosci*. 2018;**49**(4):248–57.

48. D. K. Sandsmark, M. A. Kumar, C. S. Woodward, et al. Sleep features on continuous electroencephalography predict rehabilitation outcomes after severe traumatic brain injury. *J Head Trauma Rehabil*. 2016;**31**(2):101–7.

49. Lee H, Mizrahi MA, Hartings JA, et al. Continuous electroencephalography after moderate to severe traumatic brain injury. *Crit Care Med*. 2019;**47**(4):574–82.

50. Logi F, Pasqualetti P, Tomaiuolo F. Predict recovery of consciousness in post-acute severe brain injury: the role of EEG reactivity. *Brain Inj*. 2011;**25**(10):972–9.

51. Hammoud DA and Wasserman BA. Diffuse axonal injuries: pathophysiology and imaging. *Neuroimaging Clin N Am*. 2002;**12**(2):205–16.

52. Haghbayan H, Boutin A, Laflamme M, et al. The prognostic value of MRI in moderate and severe traumatic brain injury: a systematic review and meta-analysis. *Crit Care Med*. 2017;**45**(12): e1280–e1288.

53. Woiciechowsky C and Volk HD. Increased intracranial pressure induces a rapid systemic interleukin-10 release through activation of the sympathetic nervous system. *Acta Neurochir Suppl*. 2005;**95**:373–6.

54. van Eijck MM, Schoonman GG, van der Naalt J, de Vries J, Roks G. Diffuse axonal injury after traumatic brain injury is a prognostic factor for functional outcome: a systematic review and meta-analysis. *Brain Inj*. 2018;**32**(4):395–402.

55. Humble SS, Wilson LD, Wang L, et al. Prognosis of diffuse axonal injury with traumatic brain injury. *J Trauma Acute Care Surg.* 2018;**85**(1):155–9.

56. Xu W, Kaur H, Wang X, Li H. The role of magnetic resonance imaging in the prediction of minimally conscious state after traumatic brain injury. *World Neurosurg.* 2016;94:167–73.

57. Wang KK, Yang Z, Zhu T, et al. An update on diagnostic and prognostic biomarkers for traumatic brain injury. *Expert Rev Mole Diagn.* 2018;**18**(2):165–80.

58. Di Pietro V, Ragusa M, Davies, D, et al. MicroRNAs as novel biomarkers for the diagnosis and prognosis of mild and severe traumatic brain injury. *J Neurotrauma.* 2017;**34**(11):1948–56.

59. Oberholzer M and Müri RM. Neurorehabilitation of traumatic brain injury (TBI): a clinical review. *Med Sci.* 2019;**7**(3)477.

60. Schulte S, Podlog LW, Hamson-Utley JJ, Strathmann FG, Strüder HK. A systematic review of the biomarker S100B: implications for sport-related concussion management. *J Athl Train.* 2014;**49**(6):830–50.

61. Kellermann I, Kleindienst A, Hore N, Buchfelder M, Brandner S. Early CSF and serum S100B concentrations for outcome prediction in traumatic brain injury and subarachnoid hemorrhage. *Clin Neurol Neurosurg.* 2016;**145**:79–83.

62. Thelin EP, Nelson DW, Bellander B-M. Secondary peaks of S100B in serum relate to subsequent radiological pathology in traumatic brain injury. *Neurocrit Care.* 2014;**20**(2):217–29.

63. Papa L, Silvestri S, Brophy GM, et al. GFAP outperforms S100β in detecting traumatic intracranial lesions on computed tomography in trauma patients with mild traumatic brain injury and those with extracranial lesions. *J Neurotrauma.* 2014;**31**(22):1815–22.

64. Diaz-Arrastia R, Wang KKW, Papa L, et al. Acute biomarkers of traumatic brain injury: relationship between plasma levels of ubiquitin C-terminal hydrolase-L1 and glial fibrillary acidic protein. *J. Neurotrauma.* 2014;**31**(1):19–25.

65. Liu MC, Akinyi L, Scharf D, et al. Ubiquitin C-terminal hydrolase-L1 as a biomarker for ischemic and traumatic brain injury in rats. *Eur J Neurosci.* 2010;**31**(4):722–32.

66. Posmantur R, Hayes RL, Dixon CE, Taft WC. Neurofilament 68 and neurofilament 200 protein levels decrease after traumatic brain injury. *J Neurotrauma.* 1994;**11**(5):533–45.

67. Shahim P, Gren M, Liman V, et al. Serum neurofilament light protein predicts clinical outcome in traumatic brain injury. *Sci Rep.* 2016;**6**:36791.

68. Shin RW, Iwaki T, Kitamoto T, Tateishi J. Hydrated autoclave pretreatment enhances tau immunoreactivity in formalin-fixed normal and Alzheimer's disease brain tissues. *Lab Invest.* 1991;**64**(5):693–702.

69. Liliang P-C, Liang P-C, Lu K, et al. Relationship between injury severity and serum tau protein levels in traumatic brain injured rats. *Resuscitation.* 2010;**81**(9):1205–8.

70. Li N, Long B, Han W, Yuan S, Wang K. MicroRNAs: important regulators of stem cells, *Stem Cell Res Ther.* 2017;**8**(1):110.

Prognostication in Spinal Cord Injury

Jeffrey Zimering and Konstantinos Margetis

Background, Epidemiology, and Public Health Importance

According to the National Spinal Cord Injury (SCI) Statistical Center, there are approximately 282,000 people in the United States living with SCI. The annual incidence of SCI is estimated to be 39–54 cases per million in the United States. Males account for 80% of new cases, and the average age at injury is 42 years. Motor vehicle accidents are the leading cause, followed by falls, acts of violence, and sports-related injuries. The average length of stay (LOS) in acute care hospital settings is 11 days, and the average LOS in rehabilitation centers is 35 days. Incomplete tetraplegia accounts for 45% of cases of SCI cases, followed by complete paraplegia in 20%. Less than 1% experience neurological recovery at the time of hospital discharge.[1]

Globally, the 1-year mortality rate following traumatic SCI (tSCI) remains high in developing countries, particularly in sub-Saharan Africa, where violence-related SCI rates are very high (38% of all cases). Because of missing data and incomplete reporting, it is difficult to ascertain accurate worldwide SCI incidence rates; however, the rates in Western Europe and Australia are roughly similar to those in the United States.[2]

In Iceland where all tSCI patients were treated at a single facility, the incidence of tSCI showed an increase from 2005 to 2009 due to sports-related accidents and falls in the elderly.[3] Road accidents accounted for the highest proportion of SCI (42.5%), and the 30-day mortality rate was 6.3%. Annual days of hospitalization ranged from 5.9 for AIS (American Spinal Injury Association Impairment Scale) grade A injury to 2.1 days for AIS grade D injury. The lifetime economic costs of SCI are high. In Canada, the lifetime economic burden of incomplete tetraplegia is $1.5 million, and for complete tetraplegia it is $3.0 million.[4] In a single-payer healthcare system such as the United Kingdom (UK), an estimated 1,390 new cases per year will have associated costs of roughly £1.45 billion. Seventy-one percent of the costs are directly related to healthcare, and the remainder are due to lost wages and caregiver services.[5]

The pathophysiology of acute SCI is composed of a primary mechanical injury phase involving damage to axons, blood vessels and myelin. The secondary phase is characterized by edema, inflammation, ischemia, excitotoxicity, and neuro-apoptosis. Inhibitory factors released by myelin and the post-gliotic scar interfere with axonal regeneration, contributing to the low overall complete neurological recovery rates.[6] Having validated prediction methods based on imaging, biomarkers, and neurophysiology that can accurately assess extent of axonal damage and the potential for recovery of function would be invaluable in guiding patient selection/stratification in future clinical trials of neural repair/regeneration. Due to the heterogeneity in the recovery potential of patients with the same ASIA grade of SCI, it may be important to enroll a large number of patients in randomized controlled clinical trials for potential treatments.[7] The heterogeneity in functional recovery of SCI patients may be related to genetic and environmental factors, particularly in the early post-injury phase.[7] Lack of accurate prediction of recovery is a known limitation of currently used clinical grading systems, for example, ASIA.[7] Early interventions may be beneficial, whether targeted at relieving spinal cord compression or preventing the deleterious late effects associated with the onset of the secondary injury phase.[8] Trials that evaluate the effectiveness of such interventions will need biomarkers that can predict the potential for recovery even as early as 24 hours from the SCI. In the forthcoming sections we will review the evidence of prognostication methods and models that incorporate more than one modality into the prediction of recovery following acute SCI.

Neuroprognostication in Acute Settings

Clinical Classification System

The International Standards for Neurological Classification of Spinal Cord Injury (ISNCSCI) published by the American Spinal Injury Association (ASIA) is a continually refined clinical classification system for SCI.[9] The current classification (most recent revision 2019) divides SCI into complete and incomplete injury based on whether S4–5 motor or sensory function is preserved. The injury level is next determined by motor strength in target muscles and pinprick and light touch perception at selected dermatomes. According to the classification system, an AIS (ASIA Impairment Scale) grade A injury represents complete motor and sensory injury, AIS B denotes motor complete and sensory incomplete injury, whereas AIS C and D indicate motor incomplete injuries with less than 50% versus more than 50% of key muscles maintaining antigravity strength, respectively. AIS E denotes restoration of normal neurological function.

Several studies have documented that the AIS score is a good predictor of functional outcome following SCI (Table 6.1). For AIS A injuries assessed at 72 hours post-injury, there is a low probability of neurological recovery below the level of injury. Patients who exhibit absent perianal sensation 1–2 weeks after injury are unlikely to regain a functional ambulatory status. On the other hand, most AIS D patients can expect to improve substantially, whereas recovery in AIS B and C patients is highly variable, but 60–80% can recover motor and sensory function.[10]

However, the AIS clinical scale alone has limited value in neuroprognostication. One reason is the high degree of individual variability in the capacity for meaningful recovery, which is not readily captured by assignment of an AIS grade. This shortcoming in prognosis based on clinical classification alone has spurred attempts to use other modalities in addition to the AIS grade to improve neuroprognostication.

Another limitation of the AIS grading system is that it does not incorporate early autonomic dysfunction into models that can predict the later occurrence of bowel, bladder, or other autonomically mediated functions, which are a major source of long-term complications and contribute to both morbidity and mortality. For example, cardiac autonomic dysfunction is characterized acutely by hypotension and bradyarrhythmias.[11] It can contribute to early mortality if not managed effectively. Cardiac autonomic dysfunction may preclude the use of early magnetic resonance imaging (MRI) to detect cord compression, preventing an opportunity to improve outcomes in selected patients via early surgical decompression. Late autonomic dysreflexia, which can be characterized by hypertension, is especially prevalent in patients suffering injuries about the T6 level.[11]

Table 6.1 Overview of the main SCI prognosticators

Clinical	Age, AIS, level of injury, L3 and S1 motor function and light touch sensation, hyperglycemia, infection
Imaging	BASIC score, length of injury
Biomarkers	Structural (e.g., GFAP), inflammatory, micro-RNA, proteomics
Electrophysiology	Motor evoked potentials
Effects of treatment	Timing/type of surgery, steroids (?), vasopressors/MAP goals, DVT prophylaxis, spinal cord perfusion pressure

Abbreviations: AIS = American Spinal Injury Association (ASIA) Impairment Scale; BASIC = Brain and Spinal Injury Center; GFAP = glial fibrillary acidic protein; RNA = ribonucleic acid; MAP = mean arterial pressure; DVT = deep vein thrombosis.

Therapeutic Interventions

Early therapeutic interventions can positively affect neurological outcome.[12] The most recent guidelines suggest surgery within 24 hours from injury, [13] anticoagulant thromboprophylaxis within 72 hours,[14] and specialized rehabilitation programs when patients are medically stable to improve outcomes.[15] These guidelines also suggested a 24-hour infusion of high-dose methylprednisolone initiated within 8 hours from the time of injury in adult SCI patients.[16] However, the role of steroids in SCI remains a controversial issue.[17] The principles of surgical treatment include the decompression of the neural elements and the stabilization of spine. An emerging concept in the surgical management of SCI is to perform expansile duraplasty to relieve any constricting effect that the dura might have on an edematous, injured spinal cord.[18] Maintaining the mean arterial pressure

(MAP) between 85 and 90 mmHg has been one of the treatment goals in SCI to optimize spinal cord perfusion and prevent ischemia.[19] An emerging concept is emphasizing the spinal cord perfusion pressure (SCPP) instead of MAP. The SCPP is defined as the MAP minus the cerebrospinal fluid (CSF) pressure measured via an intrathecal lumbar catheter.[20] Squair et al. [20] suggested a goal SCPP of 60–65 mmHg.

Systemic Factors

As expected, systemic comorbidities or complications can affect neurological outcomes in patients with SCI. Jaja et al. [21] showed an association of poorer neurological SCI outcomes with pneumonia, wound infection, and sepsis. When there is a need for vasopressor support, the use of dopamine is associated with a higher complication rate (e.g., atrial fibrillation, ventricular tachycardia, and troponin elevation) compared with other vasopressors.[22] Hyperglycemia at admission is also a risk factor for poor neurological outcomes.[23]

Predictive Models

Van Middendorp et al. [24] introduced an ambulation prediction rule based on parameters to predict which patients will be able to ambulate after SCI. These parameters are age (dichotomized at 65 years), the L3 and S1 motor scores and light touch sensation of dermatomes L3 and S1. A score between –10 and 40 is calculated based on these parameters, with a score of 15 being associated with an approximately 65% probability of walking independently (Table 6.2).[24] Hicks et al. [25] suggested a simplified version of van Middendorp prediction rule, which includes only three components, namely age, L3 motor score, and S1 light touch sensation. Wilson et al. [26] suggested a model to predict functional independence at one year. The model takes into account clinical factors, including the patient's age, the ASIA motor score, and the AIS grade. This model also incorporates MRI findings such as the presence of spinal cord edema or hemorrhage.[26]

Imaging

A multidisciplinary guideline committee comprising members from the AO Spine North America, AO Spine International, and the American Association and Congress of Neurological Surgeons undertook an evidence-based systematic review to determine whether the initial MRI was useful in classifying

Table 6.2 Ambulation prediction tool after traumatic SCI

	Minimum score	Maximum score
Age ≥ 65 years	−10	0
Motor score L3	0	10
Motor score S1	0	10
Light touch score L3	0	10
Light touch score S1	0	10
Total	−10	40

Source: Adapted from van Middendorp J, Hosman A, Donders A, et al. A clinical prediction rule for ambulation outcomes after traumatic spinal cord injury: a longitudinal cohort study. *Lancet.* 2011;377(9770):1004–10.

SCI severity and predicting outcome.[27] Although the quality of evidence was very low, they suggested that "MRI should be performed in adult patients with acute spinal cord injury prior to surgical intervention because it could facilitate improved clinical decision making," that is, whether the patient would benefit from early surgical decompression or not. In a prospective study by Papadopoulos et al. [28], 66/91 patients were randomized to an MRI-based imaging protocol, which resulted in emergency surgery being performed in 34 patients (54%). The MRI-protocol patients experienced significant improvement in Frankel grade compared to a control group of 25 patients who did not undergo MRI. In addition, 8 of 66 patients randomized to MRI experienced substantial improvement from a motor-complete SCI to regaining full ambulation without assistive devices, compared to no patients in the control group experiencing a similar level of improvement.

This study was cited by the guidelines committee to "suggest that MRI should be performed in adult patients in the acute period following SCI, before or after surgical intervention, to improve prediction of neurological and functional outcome."[27] The length of acute hemorrhage on MRI, the extent of cord swelling, and maximal canal compromise can help predict functional neurological recovery. With respect to implementation of the recommendations, the committee recognized cost as a barrier to widespread availability of MRI, especially in small centers and in developing countries. It was determined that potential benefit outweighed the small risks, particularly since MRI could still yield valuable prognostic information even when performed several days after acute SCI injury, which would allow time to stabilize patients with associated injuries and autonomic dysreflexia.[26]

Refinements of standard MRI techniques are an evolving area that shows promise in terms of defining microstructural characteristics that may be more predictive of functional outcomes. For example, diffusion MRI is based on water movement in axonal white matter being restricted to the direction of fibers, called anisotropy, with complete alignment of water movement having a value of 1.0 fractional anisotropy. Skinner et al. [29] reported on further refinement of diffusion-weighted imaging (DWI), called filter-probe double-diffusion encoding (FP-DDE), in predicting functional outcome compared to DWI at 48 hours post-injury in a rat model of SCI. The FP-DDE measure significantly correlated with functional outcome, and combined with functional data, for example, locomotor function, demonstrated greater prognostic value than functional data alone. The FP-DDE measure was more predictive of the number of injured axons (30 days post-injury) than DWI alone. Another advantage of FP-DDE versus DWI is the faster acquisition of data (less than 4 min) which is useful in the acute setting of SCI.[29]

In a retrospective study of 86 patients who experienced acute traumatic incomplete cervical SCI, Martinez-Perez and co-authors [30] reported that edema greater than 36 mm and facet dislocation on MRI performed 96 hours-post injury were independent predictors of poor neurological outcome regardless of the findings on initial clinical examination. In a retrospective study by Matsushita et al. of 102 patients who experienced cervical SCI, certain MRI features were found to be predictive of functional outcome.[31] When imaging was performed 2–3 days after injury, vertical diameter of T2-weighted high intensity < 45 mm was highly predictive of functional ambulation at discharge. In the group of patients who were admitted and imaged 0–1 days after injury, there was much less correlation between the vertical diameter of T2-weighted area and discharge ambulatory status.[31] Haefeli et al. [32] reported on the predictive MRI findings in 95 patients who underwent imaging within 24 hours of acute cervical SCI. They found that intrinsic measures of cord signal abnormality (obtained by axial T2 MR imaging) were the most predictive of functional outcome. Talbott et al. [33] reported on the prognostic value of the BASIC score, which grades acute cervical

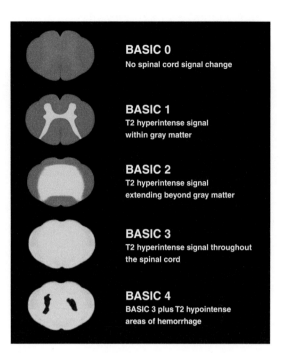

Figure 6.1 The different grades of BASIC classification.

SCI injury (based on axial T2-weighted MR patterns of intramedullary signal abnormality) into five ordinal values ranging from 0 to 4 (Figure 6.1; Table 6.3). The BASIC score highly correlated with neurological symptoms at admission and discharge, and it was able to distinguish between patients who had at least a one-grade improvement in their discharge ASIA grade compared to those patients who did not improve between admission and discharge.[33] Taken together, these data confirm the neuroprognostic importance of axial T2-weighted MRI signal abnormality in the acute phase of SCI. Magnetic resonance spectroscopy (MRS) is an emerging technique that has not yet been used in neuroprognostication following acute SCI. Like DWI, it might provide microstructural or metabolite-specific information not available through conventional MRI imaging. Finally, functional MRI (fMRI) can assess functional connectivity following SCI. In a study of patients with chronic cervical SCI, whole-brain connectivity was decreased compared to connectivity in control uninjured patients; however, sensorimotor cortex and cerebellar subnetworks showed increased connectivity in SCI patients.[34]

Biomarkers

Biomarkers in serum or CSF carry the potential of a quantitative, early indication of the extent

Table 6.3 T2-weighted MRI characteristics and cSCI severity

BASIC score	Axial T2 imaging characteristics
0	No intramedullary cord signal abnormality
1	Intramedullary T2 hyperintensity within spinal cord gray matter
2	Intramedullary T2 hyperintensity involves spinal gray and white matter, but does not involve entire transverse diameter of spinal cord
3	Intramedullary T2 hyperintensity involves entire transverse diameter of spinal cord
4	Grade 3 + discrete T2 hypointense foci = macrohemorrhage

Source: Adapted from Talbott J, Whetstone W, Reddy W, et al. The Brain and Spinal Injury Center score: a novel, simple, and reproducible method for assessing the severity of acute cervical spinal cord injury with axial T2-weighted MRI findings. *J Neurosurg Spine.* 2015;23:495–504.

of damage to neurons and glia or of the activation of the inflammatory response, and thus could potentially be valuable in neuroprognostication of functional recovery following SCI.

Yousefifard et al. [35] conducted a systematic review of evidence for the prognostic value of serum and CSF biomarkers in SCI. Sixteen human studies involving approximately 1,000 patients met the criteria for inclusion in the analysis; however, the overall quality of evidence was low. Serum levels of biomarkers that were significantly increased (within 24 hr post-injury) in non-neurologically improved versus improved SCI patients included chemokine ligand 2 (CCL-2), chemokine ligand 4 (CCL-4), tumor necrosis factor alpha (TNF-α), matrix metalloproteinase-8 (MMP-8), and the structural neurofilament protein. CSF markers of inflammatory or structural proteins that increased in the early (24 hr) interval following SCI and were increased in those patients who did not have neurological improvement included interleukin 6 (IL-6), interleukin 8 (IL-8), CCL-2, glial fibrillary acidic protein (GFAP), S100-B, and tau. Taken together, they concluded that the measurement of serum and CSF biomarkers may be useful in neuroprognostication following SCI, but more prospective longitudinal studies would be needed to improve the quality of the evidence.[35]

Neurofilaments (NF) are structural neuronal proteins that increase in serum and CSF following

SCI.[36] Hayakawa and co-authors measured phosphorylated NF-heavy chain levels in serum at both early (6 hours) and late (21 days) timepoints after SCI. They reported more than 10-fold higher levels within 24 hours of injury in ASIA A versus incomplete-injured patients. In addition, an exceptional patient who improved from ASIA A to ASIA C had an early level of pNF-H that was substantially lower than the average level in ASIA A patients.[36] More study of serum phosphorylated neurofilament heavy subunit (pNF-H) is needed to determine whether it could reliably predict a subset of ASIA A patients with a better prognosis.

Glial fibrillary acidic protein is a protein specific for glia; myelin-basic protein (MBP) and S-100b are neuronal proteins; and interleukin-8 is an inflammatory cytokine. Kwon and co-authors [37] reported that the levels of IL-8, tau, S100b, and GFAP increased in CSF between 0 and 48 hours after acute SCI and fell after 72 hours. They reported a "best-fitting" model that combined levels of S100b, GFAP, and IL-8, which had a positive predictive value of 89% in predicting acute ASIA grade A, B, or C at 24 hours post-injury. The model based on the three biomarkers also correlated with upper extremity motor recovery at 6 months following SCI.

Micro-ribonucleic acids (miRNAs) are tissue-specific regulatory factors that control RNA expression of protein translation. They are potential candidate biomarkers in human disease, although current data are largely derived from animal studies. In a rat model of SCI, more than 300 kinds of miRNA had altered expression levels, suggesting that microarray profiling of miRNA following SCI may be an important prognostic tool for future evaluation in human studies. For example, miRNA-486 and miRNA-20a are both upregulated in the acute phase (0–48 hr) following SCI and have a role in promoting neuroapoptosis. These and other miRNA might serve not only as potential biomarkers but also as novel treatment targets in SCI.[38].

In a study by Tong et al. [39] that relied on a secondary analysis of the Sygnen clinical trial of 591 patients with traumatic SCI, it was reported that higher serum albumin concentration at 1, 2, and 4 weeks was predictive of higher 52-week lower extremity motor score. One limitation of this measure is that at longer time intervals following injury the odds ratio for motor recovery progressively increases, suggesting that serum albumin is itself a marker of overall health and the occurrence of associated infections and comorbidities, which can in turn affect neurological recovery. Biomarkers predictive of meaningful recovery, which are measured at earlier times than 4 weeks post-injury, would be more useful in clinical trials involving the early application of potential neural reparative therapies.

In addition to targeted approaches to biomarker validation, a number of recent studies have undertaken an "unbiased approach" using proteomics and various types of mass spectrometry in both animal and humans. In three such studies, by Sengupta [40], Lubieniecka [41], and Moghieb [42], it was possible to correlate differential expression of certain proteins with SCI severity, complete versus incomplete-SCI patients, and alteration of expression levels in affected spinal cord segments that matched changes in human CSF. Lipidomics and metabolomics are additional strategies that could yield prognostic information. Xu et al. [43] reported that expression of polyunsaturated fatty acids containing phosphatidylcholines was a marker of microglial and astrocyte activation post-injury. Peng et al. [44] reported on a panel of metabolites that could be used to differentiate injury versus sham injury in a rat model of SCI; however, thus far the metabolomic approach has not yet been translated to human SCI.

Electrophysiology

A substantial body of literature supports the prognostic value of electrophysiological monitoring in animal models of SCI, yet there are relatively few studies in humans. Dhall et al. [45] evaluated the role of motor evoked potentials in 23 patients who suffered severe SCI (AIS A, B, or C). They reported that patients who had elicitable MEPs (during intraoperative decompression surgery performed early, that is, < 36 hours for cervical SCI) had an average improvement in AIS grade by 1.5 points compared to patients who lacked elicitable MEPs, who experienced significantly less mean improvement of 0.5 points. In addition, the absence of elicitable MEPs correlated with higher grade axial MRI findings, that is, higher BASIC score. The study was limited by its retrospective design and small sample size.[45] Spinal shock, which can occur early after cervical SCI, may have led to misclassification in a subset of patients. A practical aspect of using evoked potentials is that they are well suited for patients undergoing spinal decompression surgery, but may be difficult to perform in

an intensive care unit (ICU) setting where there is electrical interference from other devices.

Special Types of Injuries
SCIWORA

Spinal cord injury without radiological abnormality (SCIWORA) is a subset of SCI described in adults and pediatrics. Boese et al. [46] reported on 26 patients with SCIWORA who underwent MRI evaluation and were classified as either Type 1 (no detectable abnormality) or Type 2 (intraneural or extraneural abnormalities). They found that Type 1 MRI lesions were associated with significantly better functional outcome, that is, greater improvement in ASIA grade at discharge compared to patients with Type 2 MRI lesions.

Pediatric

Carroll et al. [47] reported the findings of a systematic review in 433 pediatric patients with SCIWORA. The leading cause of injury was sports related (40%), followed by falls (24%) and motor vehicle accidents (23%). An initial AIS A grade injury was associated with worse outcome compared to an adult population experiencing cervical SCIWORA. Children who presented with an initial AIS D grade injury had the highest likelihood of complete neurological recovery.

Brown–Sequard Syndrome

Brown–Sequard syndrome (BSS) is a rare form of incomplete SCI, characterized by ipsilateral weakness and loss of pain and temperature on the contralateral side below the level of injury. It is caused by hemi-cord injury with disruption of the descending lateral corticospinal tract and the ascending lateral spinothalamic tracts. Penetrating injury is a more common cause than blunt trauma; however, recovery of motor function is better compared to blunt traumatic injury. The pathophysiology of cord injury in such cases is multifactorial, including vascular insufficiency, cord compression by bone, disc or hematoma, or stretching of the cord.[48] Miranda et al. [49] reported on 10 patients with BSS following blunt trauma in order to determine whether radiological features might be predictive of motor recovery. Five of six patients with lower cervical spine fracture had a unilateral vertebral arch fracture on the same side as the hemiparesis. Seven patients had hyperintensity on T2-weighted MRI. The authors found a positive correlation between the hemi-cord edema and the initial motor deficit on admission; however, the extent of spinal cord edema did not predict neurological recovery.[49]

BSS was reported to have a more favorable prognosis for recovery than other types of incomplete SCI. Wirz et al. [50] compared the recovery potential in patients with BSS and central cord syndrome. Motor strength improved over 6 months after injury in both groups with no significant difference. Both groups experienced significant improvement in walking function, Spinal Cord Independence Measure (SCIM), a scaled score, and Somatosensory Evoked Potentials (SSEPs).

Central Cord Syndrome

Central cord syndrome (CCS) is the most common type of incomplete SCI. Trauma is the most common cause of CCS. Small lesions that affect the spinothalamic tract cause loss of pain and temperature sensation two to three segments below the level of the lesion. Large lesions can involve the anterior horn, posterior columns, corticospinal tract, and autonomic fibers in the lateral horn. Acute traumatic CCS appears as T2 hyperintensity on MRI, indicative of edema. Intramedullary hemorrhage is associated with a worse prognosis, and results in low signal intensity on gradient-echo MRI.[46] Harrop et al. [51] performed a systematic review of traumatic cervical spinal cord injury leading to CCS. CCS is clinically heterogeneous, affecting both young and older persons through fundamentally different mechanisms. In younger persons, the most common cause is traumatic injury secondary to diving accidents and motor vehicle accidents; however, in older persons a leading cause is hyperextension in a spondylotic, stenotic canal. Acute central cervical disc herniation represents a third etiological mechanism. Hyperextension leading to cervical spinal cord compression in cases of acute cervical trauma can present without any fracture on cervical spine radiographs. Early radiographic diagnosis has been shown to correlate with preservation of neurological function. Both multidetector computed tomography (CT) (to evaluate osseous structures and fracture) as well as MRI to evaluate muscle, soft tissue, and neural elements are essential for early diagnosis and prevention of neural degeneration. T2-weighted MRI can show hyperintensity as well as detect spinal cord hemorrhage, and the latter is associated with a worse prognosis. MRI is a highly sensitive method to detect spinal

instability owing to signal characteristics associated with posterior ligamentous injury.[52]

Several studies have suggested that operative decompression in CCS results in better long-term neurological recovery than medical management alone, because approximately 20–25% of the medically managed group progress to a chronic CCS syndrome due to persistent compression. Patients who presented with CCS due to acute cervical disc herniation and underwent anterior cervical decompression of the spinal cord with subsequent fusion experienced substantial improvement in neurological function, suggesting that in this particular subset of CCS early surgery is the best option.[51] On the other hand, a substantial proportion of CCS patients who do not undergo surgical decompression may also experience some spontaneous recovery of neurological function. Patient age was the main predictor of regaining functional ambulation following CCS, with older patients having a 40% chance compared to 97% of younger patients regaining the ability to ambulate with or without assistance.[53,54] Hand function is the slowest to return, and in some cases hand function may remain impaired following CCS despite the return of lower extremity and proximal upper extremity function.[55] A lack of abnormal T2-hyperintense signal in cases of traumatic cervical spine injury was predictive of full neurological recovery.[56]

Anterior Cord Syndrome

Among the incomplete cord syndromes, anterior cord syndrome has the worst prognosis.[48] These lesions do not involve the dorsal columns, allowing for intact fine touch, proprioception, and vibratory sensation. There is complete motor loss below the lesion, loss of pain and temperature, presence of orthostatic hypotension, and bowel and bladder dysfunction. The most common cause of anterior cord syndrome is anterior spinal artery (ASA) syndrome due to spinal cord ischemia or infarction. [57] Trauma is another possible cause. Children who experience cardiac malformations or trauma may be affected by anterior cord syndrome. Axial and sagittal MRI is useful in evaluating cord ischemia. T2-hyperintense signals resembling "snake eyes" is a typical finding in the anterior cord on either side of the median fissure.[48] Foo and Rossier [57] reviewed the literature on 60 cases of anterior spinal artery syndrome. They reported that about 60% of patients experienced some improvement in motor function. Prognosis was worse for arterial spinal artery thrombosis, aortic dissection, or aneurysm and angioma, and it was better in idiopathic and post-infectious cases. Partially intact pain sensation below the lesion level on initial presentation was a prognostic marker associated with better recovery of function.[57]

Posterior Cord Syndrome

Dorsal or posterior cord syndrome is caused by lesions in the posterior one-third of the spinal cord involving the dorsal columns and produces loss of vibratory, fine touch, and proprioceptive sensation. Subacute combined degeneration due to vitamin B12 deficiency and multiple sclerosis are typical causes of dorsal cord syndrome. The typical MRI T2-hyperintensity appears as an "inverted V" in dorsal cord syndrome.[48] MRI can be used to monitor response to B12 therapy in subacute combined degeneration. Posterior spinal cord ischemia is much less common than anterior spinal artery syndrome because of bilateral posterior spinal arteries and a pial vascular plexus.[48]

Conus Medullaris Syndrome

Conus medullaris syndrome (CMS) refers to injury or lesions affecting the distal (T12 through L2) portion of the spinal cord. Trauma causing cord compression is one of the possible causes, along with tumor, infection, arteriovenous shunt, and infarction. CMS typically presents with severe back pain, lower-extremity weakness, saddle anesthesia, bladder dysfunction, and impotence.[48] CT is useful in evaluating bone injury and MRI to evaluate cord and disc involvement. Early surgical intervention (based on imaging findings) has been shown to improve neurological outcome.[48]

Prognosis Based on the Anatomical Location of the Injury

Craniovertebral Dissociation

Craniocervical dislocation is associated with a high rate of mortality, severe spinal cord damage, apnea, and respiratory failure. Early recognition and prompt treatment can decrease mortality; however, discussions regarding quality of life after survival should include the potential for becoming ventilator dependent along with a lack of motor recovery. Martinez-Lage et al. [58] in their report of cases emphasized that decision making regarding surgical internal fixation needs to be individualized based in part on prognostic MRI indicators of

high cervical-level transection or whether extensive bulbo-medullary edema and hemorrhage exist.

Subaxial Cervical Spine

Cao et al. [59] reviewed the prognostic factors associated with improved neurological outcomes in 55 patients who experienced cervical SCI secondary to subaxial cervical fracture-dislocation. Thirty patients recovered spinal cord function. The patients who recovered underwent anterior cervical discectomy and fusion (ACDF) and anterior cervical corpectomy and fusion (ACCF). The surgery was performed utilizing skull traction.[59] Five patients died in the immediate postoperative period and their data were excluded from the analysis. Using multivariate regression analysis, the authors identified three factors independently predictive of worse outcomes: (1) time from injury to operation in excess of 3.8 days, (2) subaxial cervical injury classification (SLIC) score of more than 7.5, and (3) maximum spinal cord compression (MSCC) of more than 55.8%.

Thoracic and Thoracolumbar Spine

Khorasanizadeh et al. [60] performed a systematic review that showed that thoracic SCI is more likely to be associated with complete injury versus other spinal cord regions. The neurological outcomes are also worse for complete thoracic SCI compared with cervical. The potential of neurological recovery is greater for lumbar SCI, followed by cervical and thoracolumbar, while thoracic SCI has the worst potential.

Other Types of SCI Injury (Nontraumatic)
Decompression Sickness

Blatteau et al. [61] reviewed the findings in 279 cases of spinal cord decompression sickness (DCS) due to diving in a retrospective review of cases treated at hyperbaric chambers in France and Belgium. Twenty-six percent of patients had incomplete recovery after 30 days. Prognostic factors associated with worse outcome included older age at onset, greater depth of dive (> 39 m) worsening or persistence of symptoms before recompression (with hyperbaric oxygen therapy), bladder dysfunction, and higher Boussuges severity score. The Boussuges score is a weighted composite that takes into account five factors: repetitive dive, clinical course, sensory deficit, motor deficit, and bladder dysfunction (Table 6.4). Time to recompression was not

Table 6.4 Factors associated with diving-related spinal cord decompression sickness

Boussuges score	0	1	2	3	4	5	6
Clinical course before recompression							
Better		#					
Stable				#			
Worse						#	
Objective sensory deficit							
No		#					
Yes					#		
Motor impairment							
No		#					
Paresis					#		
Paraplegia							#
Hemiplegia		#		#			
Bladder dysfunction							
No		#					
Yes						#	
Repetitive dive							
No		#					
Yes			#				

Source: Adapted from Blatteau J, Gempp E, Simon O, et al. Prognostic factors of spinal cord decompression sickness in recreational diving: retrospective and multicentric analysis of 279 cases. *Neurocrit Care.* 2011;15(1):120–7.

a consistent independent predictor of recovery. Bladder dysfunction occurring early in the course of DCS was associated with a markedly increased risk of late neurological sequelae and was one of the strongest predictors of poor neurological outcome. Taken together, the Boussuges and a modified clinical severity score were useful in determining the optimal parameters of hyperbaric oxygen treatment, that is, duration and atmospheric pressure that led to improved outcomes following DCS.[61]

Aortic Surgery

Aortic aneurysm surgery can lead to nontraumatic SCI at T5–L1 levels via thoracic spinal artery occlusion. In a study of 12 patients from Japan, patients tended to be older and were more likely to have deconditioning and aspiration pneumonia and require tracheostomy support.[62] In patients undergoing thoracic abdominal aortic aneurysm surgery, prophylactic placement of a lumbar drain for cerebrospinal fluid drainage decreases intraspinal pressure and augments spinal cord perfusion, reducing the postoperative risk for spinal cord ischemic injury.[63]

Neuroprognostication over Time

Mortality

Cervical SCI is associated with increased mortality in the first 30 days after injury. Shao et al. [64] reviewed the prognostic factors associated with early mortality in 1,163 patients who experienced cervical SCI. Early mortality was observed in 9% patients. ASIA grade A injury, high cervical injury (C1–3) and no surgical intervention were independently predictive of early mortality. Early tracheostomy and better nutritional status were associated with decreased mortality. Patients with injury at or above the C3 level should undergo early tracheostomy because of the inevitable loss of diaphragmatic function resulting in respiratory failure, whereas those with C6 or lower-level injury generally do not require tracheostomy.[64]

Spinal cord injury occurring in patients with chronic kidney disease (CKD) is associated with increased early mortality. In a retrospective study by Yu et al., [65] approximately 3,300 patients with SCI and CKD were matched with 6,600 patients with SCI without CKD to determine the relative risk of early mortality. SCI with CKD had roughly twice the risk of early mortality (17%) compared to SCI without CKD. The hazard ratio of mortality was particularly high (~ 7-fold) among the SCI with CKD subgroup < 50 years old. The underlying causes of increased mortality in the SCI with CKD patients were those usually associated with increased mortality in CKD: diabetes mellitus, hypertension, coronary artery disease, and stroke. The authors concluded that patients with CKD who experience SCI will need close attention to these underlying risk factors associated with early mortality.[65]

Cervical spine fractures in the elderly are associated with increased mortality. Daneshvar et al. [66] reviewed 37 cases of cervical spine fracture resulting in SCI in patients 60 years or older. In-hospital mortality was very high, 38%. Prognostic factors associated with increased mortality were complete SCI versus incomplete SCI and injury at or above the C4 level. Age, comorbidities, and operative versus nonoperative management did not affect mortality. Respiratory failure was the leading cause of death, and complete SCI was the only predictor of no return of ambulatory function at hospital discharge.[66]

Bladder–Bowel–Sexual Function

Neurogenic bowel dysfunction (NBD) is common in SCI patients. Awad [67] reviewed the prognostic factors associated with NBD following SCI. Cervical or thoracic injuries had a higher risk of NBD compared to lumbar level of injury. Severity of injury was also predictive for NBD, as patients with ASIA A injury were at 12-fold higher risk of experiencing NBD than those with ASIA D injury. Longer duration of injury (> 10 years) and comorbid moderate-severe depression were additional predictors of NBD following SCI.

Motiei-Langroudi and Sadeghian [68] reviewed the predictors of improvement in urinary dysfunction after SCI in 103 patients who experienced SCI following traumatic vertebral fractures. About 75% of these patients were injured in a major earthquake. They found that lumbar fractures at the L 3–5 levels had the best prognosis, and thoracic fractures at the T1–10 levels had the worst prognosis.

Higher initial ASIA score was associated with better urinary and sensory outcomes. For example, approximately 86% of patients with ASIA C grade injury experienced some improvement in urinary function at follow-up, compared to only 14% of ASIA A or ASIA B patients having any improvement in long-term urinary function. Urinary function was not associated with sex, age, laminectomy, or follow-up duration or fracture level.

Infertility is common in men suffering SCI due to both erectile and ejaculatory dysfunction. Raviv and co-authors [69] reported on assistive reproductive therapy (testicular sperm aspiration), which can provide hope to men who experience infertility following SCI and substantially improve their outlook and quality of life.

Tracheostomy

The ASIA grade has been incorporated into models for predicting the need for tracheostomy in patients having C4 or higher levels of cervical cord injuries. For example, Hou et al. [70] reported that patients having ASIA grade A and any presence of respiratory complications were significantly more likely to require tracheostomy during their clinical course. The authors used the ASIA motor scoring system and determined that in patients having an admission ASIA motor score (AAMS) of 1 or complete SCI, early tracheostomy was beneficial. However, in patients with an AAMS between 2 and 22, the need for a tracheostomy was less certain and should be considered only if respiratory complications occur. For AAMS 23 and higher, they recommended "watchful waiting" to determine the possible need for tracheostomy.[70]

Pain

Chronic pain following traumatic SCI is common and difficult to manage. The International Spinal Cord Injury Pain (ISCIP) classification system is a unified classification system for pain after SCI. The main types of pain are nociceptive, neuropathic, and other types, which include pain associated with muscle spasticity. Treatment aimed at reducing spasticity may not relieve neuropathic pain. In patients with ASIA A injury, nociceptive pain response may be reduced, but nociceptive stimuli may present with increased spasticity.[71] Studies of the epidemiology of chronic pain associated with traumatic SCI indicate that prevalence is not related to gender, motor complete versus incomplete injury, or paraplegia versus tetraplegia. In addition, chronic pain is fairly stable over time, suggesting that a sudden change in pain intensity should prompt a search for additional underlying causative factors.

Gaps in Current Knowledge

An emerging concept in SCI revolves around the need to provide early treatments such as surgical decompression to aid clinical improvement and meaningful recovery of function in conjunction with the use of new assistive technologies. For example, a clinical improvement in muscle strength from 0 to 1 might not translate into a meaningful recovery. However, the development of assistive technologies such as the exoskeleton might amplify this trace movement and allow some recovery of function.[72]

A similar concept might apply to epidural electrical stimulation of the spinal cord. Three different teams recently published exciting outcomes in patients receiving this treatment.[73–75] This technique remains experimental, requires a very lengthy and intense rehabilitation process, and the stimulation parameters have not been optimized yet. However, it makes intuitive sense that it should work better in patients who have converted from complete to incomplete SCI. This is supported by one of the proposed mechanisms for such treatment, that is, reinforcement of spinal cord pathways that have survived at the level of the injury.[76]

Ongoing research on brain or peripheral stimulation alone or in combination with spinal cord stimulation [77] may lead to further study of the merit of early treatments, even if they result in trace clinical improvements. Such studies could increase our understanding of the potential of trace clinical improvements to restore function in conjunction with neuromodulation techniques.

Ongoing Research

We reviewed the main current imaging prognosticators such as morphology and extent of T2 signal abnormality in the spinal cord. Emerging imaging technologies such as higher magnetic field strengths, newer radio frequency coil designs, and suppression of the magnetic artifacts caused by spinal cord instrumentation carry promise for offering more powerful prognostication and a means for incorporating imaging biomarkers. [78] In addition, further refinement of currently existing models is anticipated. For example, the

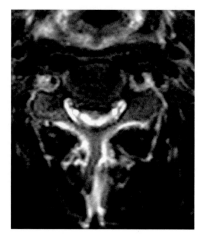

Figure 6.2 Forty-eight-year-old patient who suffered a traumatic disc herniation and rupture of the posterior tension band after a bicycle accident. Axial T2 sequence shows T2 hyperintense signal covering the majority of the spinal cord axial cross section.

BASIC Grade 2 includes cases where the spinal cord T2 hyperintense signal extends beyond the gray matter. However, in BASIC Grade 2 the T2 hyperintense signal doesn't cover the whole axial cross section of the spinal cord, which is the definition of BASIC Grade 3. There are probably subgroups within BASIC Grade 2 that carry different recovery potential. For example, Figures 6.2 and 6.3 represent an SCI case where the T2 hyperintense signal covers a significant higher proportion of the spinal cord cross section compared with the SCI case in Figures 6.4 and 6.5. Moreover, the latter case has a lower degree of T2 signal hyperintensity compared to the former case. There might be information of predictive value hidden in these differences, but the quantification of these differences would ideally require automated measurement methods.

Patient-Related Considerations

It is important to uphold shared decision making while sharing timely information about the anticipated clinical course for a patient with SCI. Often, patients with SCI can participate in decision making regarding life-sustaining procedures and rehabilitation. It is important to emphasize that recovery may take weeks to months.[79]

Conclusion

Several gaps exist in our understanding of neuroprognostication in patients with SCI. Using clinical,

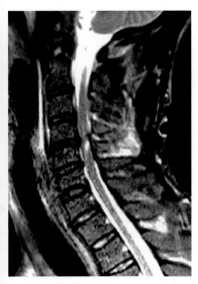

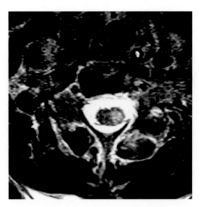

Figure 6.4 Forty-two-year-old patient who suffered C6 and C7 three-column fractures and ligamentous rupture after a fall. Axial T2 sequence showing T2 hyperintense signal extending beyond the gray matter, but limited in the left side of the spinal cord.

Figure 6.3 Same patient as in Figure 6.2. Sagittal T2 sequence shows very high intensity T2 signal at the spinal cord injury area.

References

1. [No authors listed] Spinal cord injury (SCI) 2016 facts and figures at a glance. *J Spinal Cord Med.* 2016;**39**(2):243–4.

2. Selvarajah S, Hammond ER, Haider AH, et al. The burden of acute traumatic spinal cord injury among adults in the United States: an update. *J Neurotrauma.* 2014;**31**(3):228–3.

3. Cripps RA, Lee BB, Wing P, et al. A global map for traumatic spinal cord injury epidemiology: towards a living data repository for injury prevention. *Spinal Cord.* 2011;**49**(4):493–501.

4. Knútsdóttir S, Thórisdóttir H, Sigvaldason K, et al. Epidemiology of traumatic spinal cord injuries in Iceland from 1975 to 2009. *Spinal Cord.* 2012;**50** (2):123–6.

5. McDaid D, Park AL, Gall A, Purcell M, Bacon M. Understanding and modelling the economic impact of spinal cord injuries in the United Kingdom. *Spinal Cord.* 2019;**57**(9):778–88.

6. Dukes EM, Kirshblum S, Aimetti AA, et al. Relationship of American Spinal Injury Association Impairment Scale grade to post-injury hospitalization and costs in thoracic spinal cord injury. *Neurosurgery.* 2018;**83**(3):445–51.

7. Khorasanizadeh M, Yousefifard M, Eskian M, et al. Neurological recovery following traumatic spinal cord injury: a systematic review and meta-analysis. *J Neurosurg.* 2019;**30**(5):683–99.

8. Badhiwala JH, Ahuja CS, Fehlings MG. Time is spine: a review of translational advances in spinal cord injury. *J Neurosurg Spine.* 2018;**30**(1):1–18.

9. ASIA and ISCoS International Standards Committee. The 2019 revision of the International

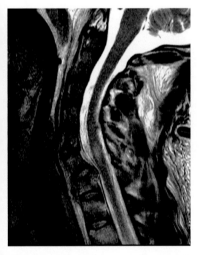

Figure 6.5 Same patient as in Figure 6.4. Sagittal T2 sequence showing T2 hyperintense signal in the spinal cord, but with lower signal intensity compared to the case in Figure 6.3.

imaging, or biomarkers alone may not help with accurate neuroprognostication in SCI. Instead, these factors may need to be combined to develop validated models for neuroprognostication. Machine learning and big data analysis could provide valuable insights into neuroprognostication in SCI. Such improvement in neuroprognostication can improve patient selection for different interventions and clinical trials.

Standards for Neurological Classification of Spinal Cord Injury (ISNCSCI) – what's new? *Spinal Cord.* 2019;57(10):815–17.

10. Krishna V, Andrews H, Varma A, et al. Spinal cord injury: how can we improve the classification and quantification of its severity and prognosis? *J Neurotrauma.* 2014;**31**(3):215–27.

11. Manogue M, Hirsh DS, Lloyd M. Cardiac electrophysiology of patients with spinal cord injury. *Heart Rhythm* 2017;**14**(6):920–7.

12. Badhiwala JH, Ahuja CS, Fehlings MG. Time is spine: a review of translational advances in spinal cord injury. *J Neurosurg Spine.* 2018;**30**:1–18.

13. Fehlings MG, Tetreault LA, Wilson JR, et al. A clinical practice guideline for the management of patients with acute spinal cord injury and central cord syndrome: recommendations on the timing (≤24 hours versus >24 hours) of decompressive surgery. *Global Spine J.* 2017;7(3_suppl):195S–202S.

14. Fehlings MG, Tetreault LA, Aarabi B, et al. A clinical practice guideline for the management of patients with acute spinal cord injury: recommendations on the type and timing of anticoagulant thromboprophylaxis. *Global Spine J.* 2017;7(3_suppl):212S–20S.

15. Fehlings MG, Tetreault LA, Aarabi B, et al. A clinical practice guideline for the management of patients with acute spinal cord injury: recommendations on the type and timing of rehabilitation. *Global Spine J.* 2017;7 (3_suppl):231S–8S.

16. Fehlings MG, Wilson JR, Tetreault LA, et al. A clinical practice guideline for the management of patients with acute spinal cord injury: recommendations on the use of methylprednisolone sodium succinate. *Global Spine J.* 2017;7(3 Suppl):203S–11S.

17. Ilyas E, Lerner DP, Ghogawala Z. Acute traumatic spinal cord injury. *Neurol Clinics.* 2021;**39**(2):471–88.

18. Zhu F, Yao S, Ren Z, et al. Early durotomy with duraplasty for severe adult spinal cord injury without radiographic abnormality: a novel concept and method of surgical decompression. *Eur Spine J.* 2019;**29**:2275.

19. Ryken TC, Hurlbert RJ, Hadley MN, et al. The acute cardiopulmonary management of patients with cervical spinal cord injuries. *Neurosurgery.* 2013;**72**:84–92.

20. Squair J, Belanger L, Tsang A, et al. Empirical targets for acute hemodynamic management of individuals with spinal cord injury. *Neurology.* 2019;**93**(12):e1205–e1211.

21. Jaja B, Jiang F, Badhiwala J, et al. Association of pneumonia, wound infection, and sepsis with clinical outcomes after acute traumatic spinal cord injury. *J Neurotrauma.* 2019;**36**(21):3044–50.

22. Inoue T, Manley G, Patel N, Whetstone W. Medical and surgical management after spinal cord injury: vasopressor usage, early surgeries, and complications. J *Neurotrauma.* 2014;**31**(3):284–91.

23. Kobayakawa K, Kumamaru H, Saiwai H, et al. Acute hyperglycemia impairs functional improvement after spinal cord injury in mice and humans. *Sci Transl Med.* 2014; **6**(256):256ra137.

24. Van Middendorp J, Hosman A, Donders A, et al. A clinical prediction rule for ambulation outcomes after traumatic spinal cord injury: a longitudinal cohort study. *Lancet.* 2011;**377**(9770):1004–10.

25. Hicks K, Zhao Y, Fallah N, et al. A simplified clinical prediction rule for prognosticating independent walking after spinal cord injury: a prospective study from a Canadian multicenter spinal cord injury registry. *Spine J.* 2017;**17** (10):1383–92.

26. Wilson J, Grossman R, Frankowski R, et al. A clinical prediction model for long-term functional outcome after traumatic spinal cord injury based on acute clinical and imaging factors. *J Neurotrauma.* 2012;**29**(13):2263–71.

27. Fehlings M, Martin A, Tetreault L, et al. Clinical practice guideline for the management of patients with acute spinal cord injury: recommendations on the role of baseline magnetic resonance imaging in clinical decision making and outcome prediction. *Global Spine J.* 2017;7(3 Suppl):221S–30S.

28. Papadopoulos S, Selden N, Quint D, et al. Immediate spinal cord decompression for cervical spinal cord injury: feasibility and outcome. *J Trauma.* 2002; **52**:323–32.

29. Skinner N, Lee S, Kurpad S, et al. Filter-probe diffusion imaging improves spinal cord injury outcome prediction. *Ann Neurol.* 2018;**84** (1):37–50.

30. Martínez-Pérez R, Cepeda S, Paredes I, Alen J, Lagares A. MRI prognostication factors in the setting of cervical spinal cord injury secondary to trauma. *World Neurosurg.* 2017;**101**:623–32.

31. Matsushita A, Maeda T, Mori E, et al. Can the acute magnetic resonance imaging features reflect neurologic prognosis in patients with cervical spinal cord injury? *Spine J.* 2017;**17**(9):1319–24.

32. Haefeli J, Mabray M, Whetstone W, et al. Multivariate analysis of MRI biomarkers for predicting neurologic impairment in cervical spinal cord injury. *Am J Neuroradiol.* 2017;**38**:648–655.

33. Talbott J, Whetstone W, Readdy W, et al. The Brain and Spinal Injury Center score: a novel, simple, and reproducible method for assessing the severity of acute cervical spinal cord injury with axial T2-weighted MRI findings. *J Neurosurg Spine.* 2015; **23**:495–504.

34. Kaushal M, Oni-Orisan A, Chen G, et al. Evaluation of whole-brain resting-state functional connectivity in spinal cord injury: a large-scale network analysis using network-based statistic. *J Neurotrauma.* 2017;**34**(6):1278–82.

35. Yousefifard M, Sarveazad A, Babahajian A, et al. Potential diagnostic and prognostic value of serum and cerebrospinal fluid biomarkers in traumatic spinal cord injury: a systematic review. *J Neurochem.* 2019;**149**(3):317–30.

36. Albayar A, Roche A, Swiatkowski P, et al. Biomarkers in spinal cord injury: prognostic insights and future potentials. *Front Neurol.* 2019;**10**:27.

37. Kwon B, Streikger F, Fallah N, et al. Cerebrospinal fluid biomarkers to stratify injury severity and predict outcome in human traumatic spinal cord injury. *J Neurotrauma.* 2017;**34**(3):567–80.

38. Rodrigues L, Moura-Neto V, E Spohr TCLS. Biomarkers in spinal cord injury: from prognosis to treatment. *Mol Neurobiol.* 2018;**55**(8):6436–48.

39. Tong B, Jutzeler C, Cragg J, et al. Serum albumin predicts long-term neurological outcomes after acute spinal cord injury. *Neurorehabil Neural Repair.* 2018;**32**(1):7–17.

40. Sengupta M, Basu M, Iswarari S, et al. CSF proteomics of secondary phase spinal cord injury in human subjects: perturbed molecular pathways post injury. *PLoS One.* 2014;**9**:e110885.

41. Lubieniecka J, Streijger F, Lee J, et al. Biomarkers for severity of spinal cord injury in the cerebrospinal fluid of rats. *PLoS One.* 2011;**6**:e19247.

42. Moghieb A, Bramlett H, Das J, et al. Differential neuroproteomic and systems biology analysis of spinal cord injury. *Mol Cell Proteomics.* 2016;**15**:2379–95.

43. Xu D, Omura T, Masaki N, et al. Increased arachidonic acid-containing phosphatidylcholine is associated with reactive microglia and astrocytes in the spinal cord after peripheral nerve injury. *Sci Rep.* 2016;**6**:26427.

44. Peng J, Zeng J, Cai B, et al. Establishment of quantitative severity evaluation model for spinal cord injury by metabolomic fingerprinting. *PLoS One.* 2014;**9**:93736.

45. Dhall S, Haefeli J, Talbott J, et al. motor evoked potentials correlate with magnetic resonance imaging and early recovery after acute spinal cord injury. *Neurosurgery.* 2018;**82**(6):870–6.

46. Boese C, Müller D, Bröer R, et al. Spinal cord injury without radiographic abnormality (SCIWORA) in adults: MRI type predicts early neurologic outcome. *Spinal Cord.* 2016;**54**(10):878–83

47. Carroll T, Smith C, Liu X, et al. Spinal cord injuries without radiologic abnormality in children: a systematic review. *Spinal Cord.* 2015;**53**(12): 842–8.

48. Kunam V, Velayudhan V, Chaudhry Z, et al. Incomplete cord syndromes: clinical and imaging review. *Radiographics.* 2018;**38**(4):1201–22.

49. Miranda P, Gomez P, Alday R, Kaen A, Ramos A. Brown-Sequard syndrome after blunt cervical spine trauma: clinical and radiological correlations. *Eur Spine J.* 2007;**16**(8):1165–70.

50. Wirz M, Zörner B, Rupp R, Dietz V. Outcome after incomplete spinal cord injury: central cord versus Brown-Sequard syndrome. *Spinal Cord.* 2010;**48** (5):407–14.

51. Harrop J, Sharan A, Ratliff J. Central cord injury: pathophysiology, management, and outcomes. *Spine J.* 2006;**6**(6 Suppl):198S–206S.

52. Song J, Mizuno J, Inoue T, Nakagawa H. Clinical evaluation of traumatic central cord syndrome: emphasis on clinical significance of prevertebral hyperintensity, cord compression, and intrame-dullary high signal intensity on magnetic resonance imaging. *Surg Neurol.* 2006;**65**(2):117–23.

53. Dai L and Jia L. Central cord injury complicating acute cervical disc herniation in trauma. *Spine.* 2000;**25**:331–6.

54. Penrod L, Hegde S, Ditunno J. Age effect on prognosis for functional recovery in acute, traumatic central cord syndrome. *Arch Phys Med Rehab.* 1990;**71**:963–8.

55. Roth E, Lawler M, Yarkony G. Traumatic central cord syndrome: clinical features and functional outcomes. *Arch Phys Med Rehab.* 1990;**71**:18–23.

56. Ishida Y and Tominaga T. Predictors of neurologic recovery in acute central cervical cord injury with only upper extremity impairment. *Spine.* 2002;**27**:1652–7.

57. Foo D and Rossier A. Anterior spinal artery syndrome and its natural history. *Paraplegia.* 1983;**21**(1):1–10.

58. Martínez-Lage J, Alarcón F, Alfaro R, et al. Severe spinal cord injury in craniocervical dislocation. Case-based update. *Childs Nerv Syst.* 2013;**29** (2):187–94.

59. Cao B, Wu Z, Liang J. Risk factors for poor prognosis of cervical spinal cord injury with subaxial cervical spine fracture-dislocation after surgical treatment: a CONSORT Study. *Med Sci Monit.* 2019;**25**:1970–5.

60. Hsieh YL, Tay J, Hsu SH, et al. Early versus late surgical decompression for traumatic spinal cord injury on neurological recovery: a systematic review and meta-analysis. *J Neurotrauma*. 2021;**38** (21):2927–36.

61. Blatteau J, Gempp E, Simon O, et al. Prognostic factors of spinal cord decompression sickness in recreational diving: retrospective and multicentric analysis of 279 cases. *Neurocrit Care*. 2011;**15** (1):120–7.

62. Ohsawa S, Tamaki M, Hirabayashi S. Medical rehabilitation of the patients with spinal cord injury caused by aortic aneurysm and its operation. Spinal Cord. 2008;**46**(2):150–3.

63. Epstein NE. Cerebrospinal fluid drains reduce risk of spinal cord injury for thoracic/ thoracoabdominal aneurysm surgery: a review. *Surg Neurol Int*. 2018;**9**:48.

64. Shao J, Zhu W, Chen X, et al. Factors associated with early mortality after cervical spinal cord injury. *J Spinal Cord Med*. 2011;**34**(6):555–62.

65. Yu S, Kuo J, Shiue Y, et al. One-year mortality of patients with chronic kidney disease after spinal cord injury: a 14-yearpopulation-based study. World Neurosurg. 2017;**105**:462–9.

66. Daneshvar P, Roffey D, Brikeet Y, Tsai E, Bailey C, Wai E. Spinal cord injuries related to cervical spine fractures in elderly patients: factors affecting mortality. *Spine J*. 2013;**13**(8):862–6.

67. Awad R. Neurogenic bowel dysfunction in patients with spinal cord injury, myelomeningocele, multiple sclerosis and Parkinson's disease. *World J Gastroenterol*. 2011;**17**(46):5035–48.

68. Motiei-Langroudi R and Sadeghian H. Traumatic spinal cord injury: long-termmotor, sensory, and urinary outcomes. *Asian Spine J*. 2017;**11** (3):412–418.

69. Raviv G, Madgar I, Elizur S, Zeilig G, Levron J. Testicular sperm retrieval and intra cytoplasmic sperm injection provide favorable outcome in spinal cord injury patients, failing conservative

70. Hou Y, Lv Y, Zhou F, et al. Development and validation of a risk prediction model for tracheostomy in acute traumatic cervical spinal cord injury patients. Eur Spine J. 2015;**24** (5):975–84.

71. Saulino M. Spinal cord injury pain. *Phys Med Rehabil Clin N Am*. 2014;**25**(2):397–410.

72. Burton A. Expecting exoskeletons for more than spinal cord injury. *Lancet Neurol*. 2018;**17** (4):302–3.

73. Angeli C, Boakye M, Morton R, et al. Recovery of over-ground walking after chronic motor complete spinal cord injury. *N Engl J Med*. 2018;**379**:1244–50.

74. Gill M, Grahn P, Calvert J, et al. Neuromodulation of lumbosacral spinal networks enables independent stepping after complete paraplegia. *Nat Med*. 2018;**24**:1677–82.

75. Wagner F, Mignardot J, Le Goff-Mignardot C, et al. Targeted neurotechnology restores walking in humans with spinal cord injury. *Nature*. 2018;**563**:65–71.

76. Angeli C, Edgerton V, Gerasimenko Y, Harkema S. Altering spinal cord excitability enables voluntary movements after chronic complete paralysis in humans. *Brain*. 2014;**137**(Pt5):1394–409.

77. James N, McMahon S, Field-Fote E, Bradbury E. Neuromodulation in the restoration of function after spinal cord injury. *Lancet Neurol*. 2018;**17** (10):905–17.

78. Freund P, Seif M, Weiskopf N, et al. MRI in traumatic spinal cord injury: from clinical assessment to neuroimaging biomarkers. *Lancet Neurol*. 2019;**18**(12):1123–35.

79. Kirshblum S, Botticello A, DeSipio G, et al. Breaking the news: a pilot study on patient perspectives of discussing prognosis after traumatic spinal cord injury. *J Spinal Cord Med*. 2016;**39**(2):155–61.

reproductive treatment. *Spinal Cord*. 2013;**51** (8):642–4.

Prognostication in Cardiac Arrest

Tobias Cronberg and Andrea O. Rossetti

Background, Epidemiology, and Public Health Importance

The global incidence of cardiac arrest (CA) outside of the hospital setting is roughly 100/100,000 person/years, but there is substantial variation between countries and continents.[1] A coronary artery occlusion is the most common cause, but CA may also be caused by a primary arrhythmia, other cardiac diseases, or be secondary to a noncardiac cause such as hypoxia or asphyxia;[2] opiate drug overdose may account for several cases, especially in the United States. Survival rates have increased during the last few decades, and approximate 10% in Europe [3] and the United States.[4] A cardiac arrest leads to an immediate interruption of perfusion of all body organs including the brain (no flow). Bystander cardiopulmonary resuscitation (CPR) will partly restore circulation (low flow), and rapid institution of bystander CPR is the most important modifiable factor for survival.[5] During the period of "no" and "low" flow until the restoration of spontaneous circulation (ROSC), the brain and all other organs are exposed to global ischemia. Depending on the time to ROSC, varying degrees of injury will develop in resuscitated patients, ranging from insignificant to severe and incompatible with survival. The brain is the organ that is most vulnerable to ischemic injury due to its high metabolic rate and very limited energy supplies. As a consequence, most patients are comatose after ROSC and in need of intensive care, including mechanical ventilation.[6] During the circulatory arrest, brain adenosine triphosphate stores are depleted, and anoxic depolarization of neuronal membranes occurs due to the cessation of energy-dependent ion pumps and loss of membrane potentials. The ensuing pathophysiological cascade is complex and involves the release of the excitatory amino acid glutamate and an increase in intracellular calcium. As oxygen is supplied during reperfusion, free radical production becomes another important mechanism.[7] Brain injury may develop rapidly if

CA (in particular the time of no flow) was long, or in a slower fashion over days and possibly even weeks. Particularly vulnerable areas are the cortical layers III, V, and VI, basal ganglia, hippocampi, and Purkinje cells of the cerebellum, while brainstem neurons are more resistant.[8] In the most severely injured patients, massive brain edema may lead to axial herniation; brain death has been reported to occur in > 10% of cardiac arrest patients [9] and is more common among patients with drug overdose.[10]

Intensive care of the post-arrest patient includes cardiac reperfusion strategies, targeted temperature management (TTM), sedation, and control of blood pressure and blood glucose levels.[11] Renal and liver function is often impaired during the first days after CA, but typically improves thereafter.

During the first 1–3 days in the intensive care unit (ICU), mortality is mainly due to multi-organ failure and cardiac causes, such as severe cardiac failure and new arrhythmias. Thereafter, most deaths occur after a decision to withdraw life-sustaining therapy (WLST) due to a presumed poor prognosis for long-term neurological recovery.[12,13] This frequent practice of WLST is probably responsible for the low rates of severe neurological disability reported in most Western countries. In settings where intensive care is continued regardless of the prognosis, severe disability is, on the other hand, very common.[14,15]

Due to the strong link between the neurological assessment of prognosis and WLST, it follows that the involved algorithms and diagnostic tools need utmost attention. Healthcare providers apparently have high expectations on the precision of the procedure, since a majority consider a $\leq 0.1\%$ false-positive rate (FPR) for WLST acceptable in this situation.[16] Premature prognostic decisions should be avoided, and a delay of at least 72 hours from CA to a conclusive discussion on prognosis is a strong recommendation in current guidelines. [11,17] Still, premature WLST for neurological reasons may be quite frequent, in particular in the United States. Propensity score matching suggests that a substantial proportion of these patients might have had a good outcome if continued care had been provided.[18,19]

Neurological prognostication after cardiac arrest has become a field of intense research over the past decade and is now integrated into international guidelines for postresuscitation care. [11,17] Repeated clinical neurological examinations of the comatose patient is the most central part of the assessment, and routine electroencephalogram (EEG) and brain computed tomography (CT) the most commonly used adjunct methods.[20] In this chapter, we will detail the currently available tools in clinical practice and discuss areas under development where clinical implementation is likely to occur within the near future. While the focus of research and guidelines has been mainly directed toward reliable identification of patients with poor prognosis, more recently, a growing interest in prognosticators of good outcome has emerged.

Neuroprognostication in Acute Settings

Clinical

Neurological examination represents an essential step for prognostication: it reflects brain function and allows integration of the results of ancillary examinations. Considering possible influence by TTM and concomitant medications, repeated assessments are recommended, especially when lingering sedation might be at play. The currently most widely used clinical scores in this context are the Glasgow Coma Scale (CGS) and the Full Outline of UnResponsiveness (FOUR).[21,22] While the former, especially the motor subscore, [23,24] is regarded as standard, it has the considerable disadvantage of routinely losing points in intubated patients, who cannot verbalize; the latter is based on eye opening, brainstem reflexes, motor reaction, and respiration. A FOUR score below 5/16 at 3–5 days seems incompatible with survival,[25] and lack of improvement within the first 3 days heralds poor prognosis with 88% specificity. [26] The Pittsburgh Cardiac Arrest Category (PCAC) is another 4-scale score, specifically designed to stratify patients early after admission using FOUR brainstem and motor subscales, and the Serial Organ Function Assessment (SOFA)

cardiovascular and respiratory subscales.[27] It has been validated and identifies most patients with poor and good outcomes;[28] there is, however, no direct comparison with the GCS or FOUR scores.

Bilateral absence of pupillary light reflexes after 72 hours represents a solid indicator of poor prognosis (FPR 0.5%, 95% confidence interval [CI]: 0–2%).[24,29–33] The lack of corneal reflexes at the same time goes in the same direction, although with lower accuracy (FPR 5%, 95% CI: 0–25%); sensitivities of these items are, however, low (globally, between 20 and 30%).[24,30,33]

Absent or extensor motor responses to stimulation at 72 hours post-arrest was an indicator of poor outcome before the TTM era;[4] nevertheless, motor reaction is clearly biased by sedatives and neuromuscular blockade and becomes less reliable in patients undergoing TTM (FPR 10–24%, 95% CI: 6–48%; sensitivity 88%).[24,30,35–37] Conversely, a localizing movement (motor score > 3) [38] is a sign indicating good prognosis (positive predictive value [PPV] 81%; 95% CI: 66–91%), and together with EEG (see below) represents one of the few available clues in this direction.[24,36]

Myoclonus was historically considered a reliable predictor of poor outcome.[34,39] However, several patients may reach a favorable prognosis despite early post-anoxic myoclonus (called "status myoclonus" if persisting more than 30 min),[40–44] a situation that may be encountered in as many as 1 in 10 patients with myoclonus.[43,45] Postanoxic myoclonus is observed in about 20% of patients; of those, 55–89% may have a concomitant epileptiform EEG;[30,43,46] in the others, it is believed that myocloni arise from subcortical structures. [47] Lacking a cortical EEG correlate is considered a poor prognostic sign. About two-thirds of patients with a post-CA epileptiform EEG (see below) exhibit myoclonic twitches. It is paramount to always consider myoclonus in a multimodal approach, integrating semiology, timing, and, most importantly, associated EEG patterns (as clinical–neurophysiological correlations are not always reliable [48,49]). Generalized myoclonic twitches lasting > 30 minutes are frequently seen together with highly malignant EEG patterns (see below) and robustly associated with poor outcome (FPR 0%, 95% CI: 0–3% [24,29,50]), especially if occurring under TTM and sedation. On the other side, brief, mostly multifocal jerks with a benign EEG background do not always herald a poor prognosis (FPR 5–11%, 95% CI: 3–26% [24,35,46,50]). This early, treatable myoclonus can represent an early form of Lance–Adams syndrome (action-induced cortical and subcortical myoclonus of various degrees in survivors of CA [47]) and should be treated with antimyoclonic compounds [50,51] (for details, see the section below on epileptiform EEG).

Electrophysiology

An electroencephalogram (EEG) is a noninvasive, widely available, real-time investigation of electrical brain activity that has been used for decades in this clinical setting;[52] importantly, EEG changes correlate with the degree of underlying neuronal injury.[53] The updated American Clinical Neurophysiology Society (ACNS) standardized guidelines for interpretation of critical care recordings,[54] whose previous version was validated in this setting,[55] allow comparisons among different environments and thus generalizability.

Hypothermia to 32–33°C, and sedative infusions of 0.1–0.2 mg/kg/hr (midazolam) or 2–3 mg/kg/hr (propofol) do not exert significant effects on EEG interpretation: prognostic accuracy seems robust [56,57] and appears even better during the first 24 hours (and during TTM) than after 2–3 days.[58–60] Of course, higher sedation may impact on EEG prognostication. EEG findings may be categorized into three main aspects.

Background activity reflects cerebral functioning: increasing brain dysfunction is paralleled by increased background slowing and decreased amplitude. Generalized suppressed (< 10 µV) background at 6–24 hours (FPR 0% [24,59, 61]), burst-suppression with synchronous epileptiform appearance at > 6 hours (FPR 0% [59, 61]), and burst-suppression with identical bursts, seen in about 10% of patients within the first 24–36 hours (FPR 0% [62, 63]), predict unfavorable outcome. "Highly malignant" patterns (suppressed or burst-suppressed EEG, with or without superimposed epileptiform discharges), display 100% specificity for poor outcome (but sensitivities as low as 5–50%) after TTM.[64] This scoring strongly correlates with other clinical, biochemical, and neurophysiological prognostic variables,[65] highlighting EEG's central role in multimodal prognostication. Conversely, a timely recovery of a continuous background as soon as 12 hours after CA (specificity 91% [61]) and normal voltage background at 24 hours (PPV 72% [59]) herald awakening. A relevant exception is "alpha-coma," characterized by an anterior, nonreactive rhythm strongly associated with poor prognosis.[66]

Epileptiform features. Sharp waves, (poly-) spikes, spikes and waves are observed in about one-third of patients in this clinical setting, [67–70] mostly as repetitive, periodic, or rhythmic patterns, and they are often labeled as status epilepticus (SE), analogous to prolonged epileptic seizures;[71] they mainly fulfill current ACNS criteria for SE.[54] While occurrence after TTM heralds a poor outcome (albeit with FPR 8% [36,60]), this trend seems more robust if repetitive epileptiform features are observed during TTM, under sedation with antiepileptic properties (FPR 2% [53,60,72]). Nevertheless, about 10% of patients with epileptiform discharges may have a chance of reaching reasonable functional outcomes, especially those with preserved brainstem reflexes, background reactivity, and somatosensory evoked potentials (SSEP).[67] In these cases, epileptiform discharges are often seen around the midline [18] and appear later (typically after TTM).[69,73] Quantitative analysis shows that patients reaching good outcomes have higher background continuity and discharge frequency, but lower discharge periodicity. [57] An EEG score has been developed and validated to identify patients with a chance of clinical improvement;[74] also, concomitant magnetic resonance imaging (MRI) findings may help clinicians in this setting.[75] The subset of patients with a potentially favorable outlook should receive anticonvulsants; we favor antimyoclonic agents, such as benzodiazepines, valproate, levetiracetam, or brivaracetam and, at times, pharmacological coma with midazolam and/or propofol; additional options include perampanel, zonisamide, or topiramate administered through the nasogastric tube. [50,51,70] The appropriate treatment duration is unknown, but it seems reasonable to limit therapy to a few (2–3) weeks. Longer durations may be indicated in selected subjects; three patients with prolonged EEG burst-suppression and epileptiform discharges, but otherwise favorable multimodal assessment, were described; they recovered several weeks after CA; all showed theta frequency of their bursts.[76]

Background reactivity is a reproducible change in frequency or amplitude after auditory, visual or noxious stimuli.[36,77] Its absence correlates with poor outcome (FPR 2%–18% [36,60,78–80]), while reactivity may indicate subsequent awakening (PPV 82%, [24,60,81,82]). An important limitation is the subjective assessment and variable inter- and intra-rater agreements. [55,83–85] A study challenged the added value of EEG reactivity to identify patients with poor prognosis, if already considering "highly malignant EEG" at 24 hours, absent brainstem reflexes, and absent cortical somatosensory responses,[85] but some methodological concerns exist.[86] In any case, a careful video-correlation and standardized stimulation protocols are recommended, as they could improve accuracy.[82,85,87] While muscle reactivity to stimuli was correlated with favorable prognosis,[88] this aspect awaits validation.

In some hospitals, continuous EEG is recorded for up to 48 hours,[58,59] but repeated standard (20 min) EEG performed within 48 hours of CA could represent an alternative for centers with limited resources, as it may offer comparable information [89] at lower costs [90] and without any measurable influence on outcome.[91] Since EEG evolves over time,[92–95] continuous or repeated assessments are strongly encouraged, particularly within the first 72 hours. Reduced montages [96,97] with even as few as two channels have been described; they are well suited for background assessment, but seem less sensitive for epileptiform transients and seizures. Also, recordings performed too early (particularly within 6 hr of CA) may overestimate the degree of brain injury; on the other hand, epileptiform features earlier than 12 hours following CA seem rare (Figure 7.1).[68]

Early latency evoked potentials result from EEG averaging of cortical responses upon repetitive electrical stimulation of the median nerve, where a negative deflection appears after about 20 ms (called N20); they are not significantly affected by the usual concomitant sedation. Bilateral N20 absence robustly correlates with unfavorable outcome (FPR 0.5%); sensitivity is, however, low (at most 49%),[23,24,30,37,79] and the positive predictive value of present N20 to predict favorable outcome is also only around 50% (95% confidence interval [CI]: 29–68%).[58,79] While a meta-analysis considering WLST triggered by SSEP results suggested that their specificity may only be 93%,[98] it seems that specificity indeed approaches 100% if technical and other issues

influencing results are eliminated.[99] At any rate, widespread SSEP availability is still suboptimal (recording tools, trained personnel), and redundancy with EEG findings, especially "benign" EEG, has been noted.[100,101] assessment of the N20 amplitude could offer additional prognostic information,[102–104] also toward good prognosis,[105] but assessment using multimodal prognostication does not seem to always confirm these findings.[106]

Imaging

Brain imaging with CT or MRI is part of the diagnostic workup for patients who remain in coma at most centers. Unfortunately, evidence supporting the use of neuroimaging for clinical decisions in these patients is still of low quality, with a high proportion of retrospective studies with high risk of selection bias.[107]

A CT scan is a rapid and readily available procedure in the emergency setting, and commonly employed on admission to rule out intracranial bleeding as a cause of the arrest in patients without an obvious cardiac etiology. Generalized edema, manifested as a reduction of gray-white matter discrimination, sulcal effacement, and reduced ventricular size, encapsulate robust signs of severe brain injury and poor prognosis (specificity 98–100%), but the sensitivity is limited to approximately 30%.[108–111]

A way to extract more information from CT is to measure the difference in attenuation between gray and white matter (GWR) in predefined regions of interest (ROI) [112,113] or in the whole brain using an automated procedure.[114] A GWR < 1.10 reliably predicts poor outcome regardless of ROI-positioning,[115] but the basal ganglia region seem superior with a pooled sensitivity of 27% and no false positives.[116] Currently, there is no consensus for the implementation of standardized GWR measurements into clinical practice.

Magnetic resonance imaging of the comatose CA patient is a lengthier procedure, necessitating compatible equipment on and around the patient, and making them less accessible in case of emergency situations during the scan. Therefore, MRI is often reserved for patients who remain comatose after sedation weaning in whom prognostication by other methods is inconclusive. Cytotoxic edema is readily detected on diffusion-weighted MRI (DWI-MRI), while vasogenic edema, which

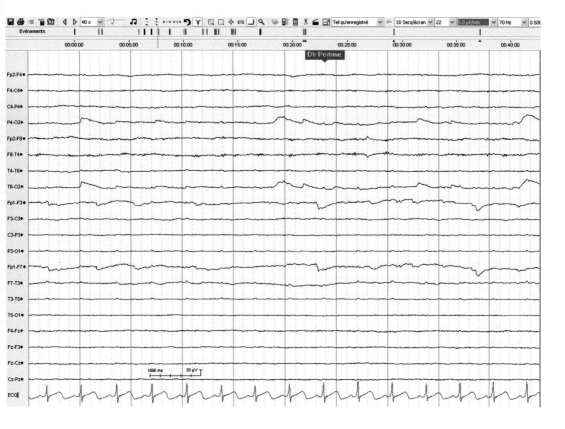

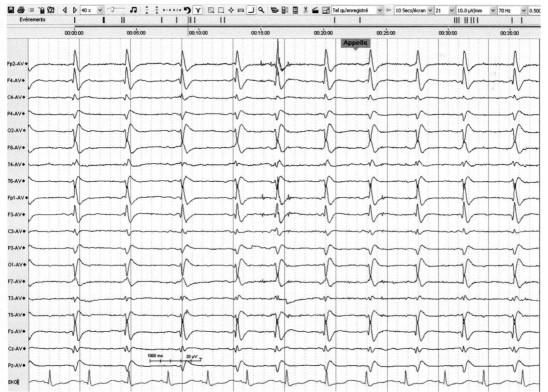

Figure 7.1 Highly malignant electroencephalogram (EEG) patterns.
(a) Suppressed EEG.
(b) Suppressed EEG with superimposed generalized periodic discharges.
(c) Burst-suppression, with superimposed generalized periodic discharges.

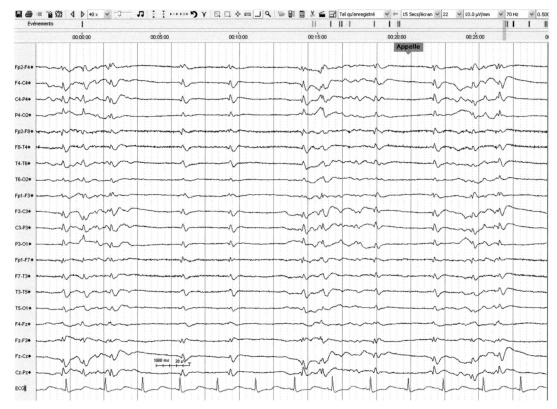

Figure 7.1 (cont.)

develops slightly later, is better visualized with T2-weighted and fluid-attenuated inversion recovery (FLAIR) sequences.[110,115] DWI changes may be detected as early as the first hours after admission, but the recommended timing is 3–5 days after arrest.[117] At this timepoint, edema is typically seen in the cortex, basal ganglia, and cerebellum, but it may later develop also in the white matter tracts.[118]

Whole-brain apparent diffusion coefficient (ADC) measurements may be a way to achieve standardization, but quantitative MRI is sensitive to imaging setup,[115] limiting comparisons between studies and clinical implementation. Another approach is the whole-brain white matter fractional anisotropy (WWM-FA), which seems superior to standard MR imaging to prognosticate patients remaining in coma 7–28 days after arrest in one large study.[119] While anoxic brain injuries on a CT or MRI are established indicators of poor prognosis and are included in current guidelines,[11,17] there are no widely adopted guidelines to classify findings from a conventional "eyeballing" assessment of the images. This may

be less problematic with CT: generalized edema on brain CT signals a very severe injury, whereas mild–moderate ischemia tends to go undetected. MRI-DWI sequences, on the other hand, are more sensitive to ischemic injury and may therefore detect more limited injuries still compatible with good outcome. Therefore, it is crucial to carefully evaluate the extent and distribution of ischemic injury and never use MRI or CT findings in isolation for decisions on level of care (Figure 7.2).

Biomarkers

Breakdown products from damaged neurons and glial cells are quantitative markers of brain injury that can be measured in the blood and cerebrospinal fluid (CSF) after CA.[120] Due to practical difficulties performing lumbar puncture in anticoagulated patients, blood borne markers are currently more in focus. Neuron-specific enolase (NSE) is the only biomarker recommended by current guidelines; [11,17] it has been used as a surrogate marker of brain injury in recent trials. NSE levels in serum correlate with EEG patterns,[53] imaging findings, (a)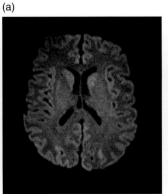

(b)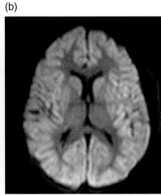

Figure 7.2 Brain MRI.

(a) Mild injury: DWI-MRI of a 45-year-old man 8 days after cardiac arrest (VF, time to ROSC 38 min) showing bilateral caudal hyperintensities. He had a good outcome with CPC 2 at 3 months.

(b) Severe injury: DWI-MRI of a 61-year-old woman 4 days after cardiac arrest (VF, time to ROSC 10–15 min) showing bilateral widespread cortical and subcortical hyperintensities. She had no cortical SSEP–N20 potentials, status epilepticus on a non-reactive EEG-background and died after withdrawal of life-sustaining therapy.

Abbreviations: CPC: cerebral performance category; DWI-MRI: diffusion-weighted magnetic resonance imaging; EEG: electroencephalogram; ROSC: restoration of spontaneous circulation; SSEP: somatosensory evoked potentials; VF: ventricular fibrillation.

[111] and the severity of histopathological injury post-mortem.[121] NSE is present in neurons, neuro-endocrine cells, erythrocytes, and platelets. Elevated levels may therefore be caused by hemolysis or neuroendocrine tumors. Hemolysis is not uncommon after CPR, and may cause elevated levels of NSE even after free hemoglobin is cleared due to its much longer half-life (≈ 24 hours); this may be particularly relevant for patients treated by extracorporeal membrane oxygenation (ECMO).[122] Levels of NSE typically increase in the first 24–48 hours after CA in patients with poor outcome: decreasing levels within this time frame should raise suspicion of hemolysis. For this reason, sampling at multiple timepoints is recommended, although a single measurement at 48 hours seems to bear similar precision on a population level. Since there is no standard for calibration, cut-off levels may vary somewhat between laboratories and analytical methods. The American Academy of Neurology (AAN) guidelines from 2006 [34] recommended a cut-off of 33 µg/L for 0% FPR, based on a single study with 231 patients.[123] The TTM-trial investigators sampled from 686 patients and found a cut-off of 48 µg/L for a 2% FPR at 48 hours.[124] A German study sampled 1,053 patients and reported a false-positive ratio of 0.5% for a cut-off of 90 µg/L (sensitivity 48%) 3 days after arrest, but using a more conservative definition of a poor outcome (cerebral performance category [CPC] 4–5) compared to other studies (CPC 3–5).[125] In the 2021 version of the European Resuscitation Council (ERC) and European Society of Intensive Care Medicine (ESICM) guidelines, a cut-off of 60 µg/L at 48 and/

or 72 hours post-arrest was introduced, since in most prior studies this would correspond to a 100% specificity.[11]

The astroglial marker S100B is used for risk stratification after head trauma. It is elevated in blood after cardiac arrest, but correlates less with long-term outcome compared to NSE.[126] Recently, more brain-specific biomarkers have been tested. Tau-protein and neurofilament light chain (NFL) are two axonal proteins that are not affected by hemolysis. Both were found superior to NSE and S100B by the TTM-investigators.[127,128] NFL appears currently the best performing biomarker and seems superior also to other diagnostic methods. However, these results need validation and standardization before clinical implementation can proceed.

Normal levels of serum biomarkers are also valuable as tools to predict a good outcome and thereby encourage prolonged care in patients who remain with indeterminate outcome after assessment according to the guideline algorithm.[11] In the TTM-trial cohort, an additional 67/190 unclassifiable patients with final good outcome were identified by normal NSE levels.[129]

Others

Currently available prognostic markers in patients after CA are not only mostly directed toward poor outcome, but also frequently challenged by subjective interpretation (e.g., clinical examination, EEG, neuroimaging) and the lack of universally accepted clear-cut threshold values (e.g., biomarkers). In this context, objective tools appear eagerly needed:

automated devices to quantify pupillary responses to light stimuli have actually been available on the market for several years. A study suggested that quantitative pupillometry correlates with neuronal injury measured by serum NSE,[130] with comparable predictive performance to EEG and SSEP, and even superior to standard clinical examination, [130–132] with a threshold of 13% (of relative pupillary response) below which poor outcome had 100% specificity. A prospective multicenter assessment confirmed these results, albeit with a different method stratifying responses into four categorical levels (defined in comparison with a database of normal subjects; a response level ≥ 3 is considered indeed a normal reaction), with level ≤ 2 being 100% specific for poor outcome.[133] The use of different pupillometry devices with different displays still precludes generalizability and routine clinical implementation; ideally, independent, prospective comparative studies using different devices should be carried out. For the time being, this quantitative approach may be used in addition to standard protocols to add valuable information in unclear situations.

Multimodal Prognostication and Suggested Algorithms

This approach is recommended in existing guidelines, but the actual meaning of the term "multimodal" may somewhat differ among them. In the much cited and discussed AAN guidelines of 2006, [34] a stepwise approach was exemplified by an algorithm in which any of a series of poor prognosis indicators suggested poor outcome with no or very low FPR. The American Heart Association (AHA) also evaluated each prognostic method separately but does not provide any algorithm. [17] The Swedish Resuscitation Council 2013 recommended a different and somewhat more complex approach, where indicators of good and poor outcome were balanced against each other. [117] In 2015, the ERC/ESICM presented an algorithm where the most robust predictors (pupillary reflexes and SSEP N20 potentials) were evaluated at 72 hours after CA, and other methods were combined after another 24 hours in the absence of sedation.[33] The ERC/ESICM 2015 algorithm was constructed to be conservative, preventing WLST in patients who may do well, and requires several criteria to be fulfilled for a statement of poor prognosis: (1) More than 72 hours should

have passed since CA; (2) Patient is unconscious with GCS Motor Response (GCS-M) score ≤ 2; (3) No serious pharmacological or metabolic confounders; (4) At least one of the most robust predictors or a combination of two of the less robust ones (≤ 96 hr) must be present. AAN, AHA, and ERC/ESICM guidelines were evaluated in a single-center context.[134] False-positive forecasts were caused by several predictors of the AHA guidelines, and the AAN algorithm had a FPR of 15% at 6 months. The ERC/ESICM algorithm led to no false-positive predictions, but had a sensitivity of only 28% to establish a "likely" poor outcome. The effect of such a cautious approach will be prolonged ICU care and further observation of patients who eventually will have a poor outcome, but will also allow time for spontaneous awakening of those destined to have a good recovery. Although late awakening exists and most late awakeners have a good outcome, the majority of patients who will awaken do so within the first few days after sedation is stopped.[135,136] A subsequent validation of the ERC 2015 algorithm in a multicenter context confirmed the high specificity (100%) but limited sensitivity (38.7%).[137] In the new guidelines on post-resuscitation care from the ERC/ESICM,[11] the prior algorithm has been updated and simplified (Figure 7.3). In the 2021 version, two indicators of a poor prognosis are mandatory, since errors are possible with all available methods. EEG-patterns have been standardized according to the ACNS terminology; suppression with or without superimposed discharges and burst-suppression are recognized as the "highly malignant patterns".

For safe and effective neuroprognostication, it is important to have a local protocol and to collect as much information as possible on all patients treated in the ICU after cardiac arrest. In addition to clinical examination, EEG, imaging (CT and/or MRI), and NSE are basic tools available at most centers. SSEP may be reserved for patients remaining in coma at 72 hours and omitted for patients with a benign EEG.

Neuroprognostication over Time

In the ICU

After sedation weaning, typically 1–2 days after the arrest, approximately half of patients will wake up within another 1–2 days and start obeying

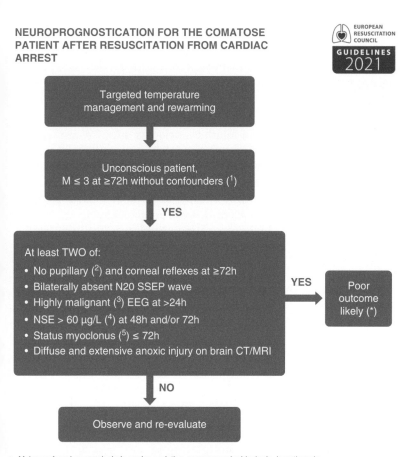

NEUROPROGNOSTICATION FOR THE COMATOSE PATIENT AFTER RESUSCITATION FROM CARDIAC ARREST

EUROPEAN RESUSCITATION COUNCIL

GUIDELINES 2021

Targeted temperature management and rewarming

Unconscious patient, M ≤ 3 at ≥72h without confounders ([1])

YES

At least TWO of:
- No pupillary ([2]) and corneal reflexes at ≥72h
- Bilaterally absent N20 SSEP wave
- Highly malignant ([3]) EEG at >24h
- NSE > 60 µg/L ([4]) at 48h and/or 72h
- Status myoclonus ([5]) ≤ 72h
- Diffuse and extensive anoxic injury on brain CT/MRI

YES → Poor outcome likely (*)

NO

Observe and re-evaluate

[1] Major confounders may include analgo-sedation, neuromuscular blockade, hypothermia, severe hypotension, hypoglycaemia, sepsis, and metabolic and respiratory derangements

[2] Use an automated pupillometer, when available, to assess pupillary light reflex

[3] Suppressed background ± periodic discharges or burst-suppression, according to American Clinical Neurophysiology Society

[4] Increasing NSE levels between 24 h–48 h or 24/48 and 72 h further support a likely poor outcome

[5] Defined as a continuous and generalised myoclonus persisting for 30 minutes or more

[*] Caution in case of discordant signs indicating a potentially good outcome (see text for details).

Figure 7.3 Algorithm for neurological prognostication recommended by the European Resuscitation Council (ERC) and the European Society for Intensive Care Medicine (ESICM) in Nolan J, et al. *Resuscitation*. 2021;161:220–69. European Resuscitation Council – www.erc.edu.

Prognostic data from multiple sources are gathered during the first days after arrest. The first assessment of prognosis occurs at ≥ 72 hours after cardiac arrest if the patient is still unconscious (Glasgow Coma Scale Motor Response (GCS-M) score [GCS-M] 1–3) and confounding factors are ruled out. At least two additional negative predictors (in addition to GCS-M 1–2) are required to conclude a likely poor neurological outcome. Many patients will need further observation without analgo-sedation and reevaluation.

commands. This group of patients rarely needs any formal prognostic assessment, since their outcome is usually good. Extubation is frequently delayed another few days due to respiratory or circulatory problems. As patients regain the capacity to communicate, they are often found to be in delirium, usually resolving within days. Cognitive problems caused by brain injury due to CA is an important risk factor for post-arrest delirium, but metabolic derangements and pharmacological side effects are modifiable

factors that always should be considered and eliminated if possible. As for all patients with delirium in the ICU, sleep and pain management are crucial. Provision of glasses and hearing aids, regular daily routines, and early mobilization are other key elements.

For patients who do not wake up after sedation weaning, a severe brain injury is the most important explanatory factor; most will ultimately have a poor outcome. Using available techniques for assessment of prognosis 72–96 hours after CA, it will be possible to conclude on the likely final outcome and make informed decisions on the level of care based on the presence of established indicators of a poor prognosis in roughly half of these patients. The rest are in need of further time for observation without the interference of analgosedation. Importantly, the usefulness of prognostic tests will decrease as time passes after the arrest: the EEG will tend to (at least partially) recover, edema to abate on imaging, and levels of blood biomarkers to decrease. Since brainstem functions usually reappear within the first days also in patients with severe brain injury, these may gradually start showing signs of "awakening" such as eye opening, yawning, and involuntary movements within the first 1–2 weeks in the context of unconscious wakefulness or vegetative state. Such signs may be difficult to interpret for relatives and clinicians. It is also important to recognize that a patient's capacity to communicate or obey commands may vary greatly during the day.

In the Long Term

The functional capacity of CA survivors is usually measured by crude outcome scales, such as the cerebral performance category, which was replaced by the modified Rankin Scale in a recent consensus document for a core outcome set after cardiac arrest (COSCA). The majority of survivors in Western countries where WLST is common practice do well in the long run, and few will need assistance in their activities of daily living (ADL). A minority nevertheless survives with severe brain injury. These patients may, for example, develop spasticity or extrapyramidal motor disturbance due to basal ganglia injury.[138] Any kind of focal neurological deficit may result from localized injury due to embolization or watershed infarctions. Although neurological function recovers most during the first 3–6 months, substantial functional improvement may still occur thereafter due to adaption.

Mild-moderate cognitive impairment occurs in approximately half of the cardiac arrest survivors. [139,140] It may be diagnosed by simple screening tests, such as the Montreal Cognitive Assessment (MoCA), or even by asking the patients how they feel.[141] Difficulties with memory, executive function, and attention/processing speed are commonly encountered. Cognitive problems limit patients' participation in societal activities

including return to work [142] and are related to anxiety and depression. It is recommended to include cognitive screening in the routine follow-up of cardiac arrest patients that is often performed within cardiological care.

Gaps in Current Knowledge

Brain injuries developing after CA are relatively homogenous, and their consequences in terms of long-term disability more predictable compared to other brain injuries. Despite this being a field of extensive research for decades, many gaps remain in our knowledge of prognostic methods. A crucial limitation of most studies is the "self-fulfilling prophecy," by which a prediction causes itself to become true. Indeed, often indicators of a poor prognosis studied were also used for decisions on WLST. Validation of prognostic tests in environments that do not perform WLST or assessments of tests not used for WSLT (ideally with masking of the treating team) are therefore of great interest. Furthermore, most data on currently recommended indicators derive from studies by experienced research centers: validation in large multicenter settings is important to test how these results translate to less experienced hands.

The multimodal approach is intuitively appealing and recommended in guidelines, but little is known about the interplay between different prognostic methods. What is the most rational sequence to perform? Which methods provide additive information, and which will only be confirmatory? Is it more cost-effective to use a stepwise approach or to perform several methods in parallel? To answer these and similar questions requires very large cohorts, preferably with all patients undergoing all tests. Since that would represent a very costly approach, "big data" analyses of overlapping results from several studies and registries is probably a more reasonable future direction.

The new and interesting methods to quantitate results of imaging and neurophysiological registrations need standardization and, similar to the new blood biomarkers, a roadmap to clinical implementation would require formal testing in large settings.

Refined knowledge of good prognosticators, reducing uncertainty for caregivers and families, is definitely needed. Finally, we still know surprisingly little about some of the most fundamental issues regarding neuroprognostication. Almost no studies focused on the lay public's expectations and opinions on prognostication and WLST after CA, or related questions regarding the correct definition of a poor outcome.

Ongoing Research

A routine blood analysis by which the amount of brain injury inflicted by an insult can be quantified is of great interest for clinicians dealing with various types of brain injury. The lack of precision and uncertainty regarding methodological standards has hampered clinical implementation so far. Recent results regarding the new, brain-specific markers NFL and tau show the potential of this approach. In the Targeted Temperature Management trial 2 (TTM2),[143] these results will be validated in a large biobank. Whether blood biomarkers can be used also to predict cognitive problems and need for rehabilitation among survivors represents a clinically relevant question. This will also be investigated in the TTM2 study, and the surviving patients will be followed for 24 months to study long-term effects of acute hypoxic-ischemic brain injury and cardio-vascular risk factors on impaired cognition, health-related quality of life, and participation in society.

Over the few last years, increasing efforts to standardize EEG interpretation have been undertaken. While the ACNS recommendations [54] offer a practical, validated approach, they do not prevent subjective assessments of some aspects, such as reactivity or "modifiers" of the principal features. Therefore, automated EEG interpretation has been pursued by several independent groups, including compressed (amplitude-integrated analysis or bispectral index) analyses. [92,94,95,144] Most results appear very promising, but the principal limitation, so far, appears to be the lack of generalizability, as each group developed its own procedure; furthermore, the possible approaches are virtually endless. It remains a hope that in the near future sustained, multicenter efforts will be made in order to improve this aspect.

References

1. Berdowski, J., R. A. Berg, J. G. Tijssen, R. W. Koster. Global incidences of out-of-hospital cardiac arrest and survival rates: systematic review of 67 prospective studies. *Resuscitation*. 2010;**81**(11):1479–87.

2. Myat, A., K. J. Song, T. Rea. Out-of-hospital cardiac arrest: current concepts. *Lancet*. 2018;**391** (10124):970–9.

3. Grasner, J. T., R. Lefering, W. Koster, et al. EuReCa ONE Collaborators. EuReCa ONE – 27 Nations, ONE Europe, ONE Registry: a prospective one month analysis of out-of-hospital cardiac arrest outcomes in 27 countries in Europe. *Resuscitation*. 2016;**105**:188–95.

4. Benjamin, E. J., M. J. Blaha, S. E. Chiuve, et al. American Heart Association Statistics and S. Stroke Statistics. Heart Disease and Stroke Statistics-2017 Update: a report from the American Heart Association. *Circulation*. 2017;**135**(10):e146–e603.

5. Sasson, C., M. A. Rogers, J. Dahl, A. L. Kellermann. Predictors of survival from out-of-hospital cardiac arrest: a systematic review and meta-analysis. *Circ Cardiovasc Qual Outcomes*. 2010;**3**(1):63–81.

6. Berg, K. M., A. V. Grossestreuer, A. Uber, P. V. Patel, M. W. Donnino. Intubation is not a marker for coma after in-hospital cardiac arrest: A retrospective study. *Resuscitation*. 2017;**119**:18–20.

7. Sanganalmath, S. K., P. Gopal, J. R. Parker, et al. Global cerebral ischemia due to circulatory arrest: insights into cellular pathophysiology and diagnostic modalities. *Mol Cell Biochem*. 2017;**426** (1–2):111–27.

8. Bjorklund, E., E. Lindberg, M. Rundgren, et al. Ischaemic brain damage after cardiac arrest and induced hypothermia – a systematic description of selective eosinophilic neuronal death. A neuropathologic study of 23 patients. *Resuscitation*. 2014;**85**(4):527–32.

9. Sandroni, C., S. D'Arrigo, C. W. Callaway, et al. The rate of brain death and organ donation in patients resuscitated from cardiac arrest: a systematic review and meta-analysis. *Intensive Care Med*. 2016;**42**(11):1661–71.

10. Ormseth, C. H., C. B. Maciel, S. E. Zhou, et al. Differential outcomes following successful resuscitation in cardiac arrest due to drug overdose. *Resuscitation*. 2019;**139**:9–16.

11. Nolan, J. P., C. Sandroni, B. W. Bottiger, et al. European Resuscitation Council and European Society of Intensive Care Medicine guidelines 2021: post-resuscitation care. *Intensive Care Med*. 2021;**47**(4):369–421.

12. Dragancea, I., M. Rundgren, E. Englund, H. Friberg, T. Cronberg. The influence of induced hypothermia and delayed prognostication on the mode of death after cardiac arrest. *Resuscitation*. 2013;**84**(3):337–342.

13. Dragancea, I., M. P. Wise, N. Al-Subaie, et al., T. T. M. t. Investigators. Protocol-driven neurological prognostication and withdrawal of life-sustaining therapy after cardiac arrest and targeted temperature management. *Resuscitation.* 2017;**117**:50–7.

14. Pachys, G., N. Kaufman, T. Bdolah-Abram, J. D. Kark. S. Einav. Predictors of long-term survival after out-of-hospital cardiac arrest: the impact of Activities of Daily Living and Cerebral Performance Category scores. *Resuscitation.* 2014;**85**(8):1052–8.

15. Kim, Y. J., S. Ahn, C. H. Sohn, et al. Long-term neurological outcomes in patients after out-of-hospital cardiac arrest. *Resuscitation.* 2016;**101**:1–5.

16. Steinberg, A., C. W. Callaway, R. M. Arnold, et al. Prognostication after cardiac arrest: Results of an international, multi-professional survey. *Resuscitation.* 2019;**138**:190–7.

17. Callaway, C. W., M. W. Donnino, E. L. Fink, et al. Part 8: Post-Cardiac Arrest Care: 2015 American Heart Association Guidelines Update for Cardiopulmonary Resuscitation and Emergency Cardiovascular Care. *Circulation.* 2015;**132**(18 Suppl 2):S465–82.

18. Elmer, J., C. Torres, T. P. Aufderheide, et al., C. Resuscitation Outcomes Consortium. Association of early withdrawal of life-sustaining therapy for perceived neurological prognosis with mortality after cardiac arrest. *Resuscitation.* 2016;**102**:127–35.

19. May, T. L., R. Ruthazer, R. R. Riker, et al. Early withdrawal of life support after resuscitation from cardiac arrest is common and may result in additional deaths. *Resuscitation.* 2019;**139**:308–13.

20. Friberg, H., T. Cronberg, M. W. Dunser, et al. Survey on current practices for neurological prognostication after cardiac arrest. *Resuscitation.* 2015;**90**:158–62.

21. Wijdicks, E. F., W. R. Bamlet, B. V. Maramattom, E. M. Manno, R. L. McClelland. Validation of a new coma scale: the FOUR score. *Ann Neurol.* 2005;**58**(4):585–93.

22. Wijdicks, E. F. Clinical scales for comatose patients: the Glasgow Coma Scale in historical context and the new FOUR Score. *Rev Neurol Dis.* 2006;**3**(3):109–17.

23. Sandroni, C., A. Cariou, F. Cavallaro, et al. Prognostication in comatose survivors of cardiac arrest: an advisory statement from the European Resuscitation Council and the European Society of Intensive Care Medicine. *Intensive Care Med.* 2014;**40**(12):1816–31.

24. Rossetti, A. O., A. A. Rabinstein, M. Oddo. Neurological prognostication of outcome in patients in coma after cardiac arrest. *Lancet Neurol.* 2016;**15**:597–609.

25. Fugate, J. E., A. A. Rabinstein, D. O. Claassen, R. D. White, E. F. Wijdicks. The FOUR score predicts outcome in patients after cardiac arrest. *Neurocrit Care.* 2010;**13**(2):205–10.

26. Weiss, N., M. Venot, F. Verdonk, et al. Daily FOUR score assessment provides accurate prognosis of long-term outcome in out-of-hospital cardiac arrest. *Rev Neurol (Paris).* 2015;**171**(5):437–44.

27. Rittenberger, J. C., S. A. Tisherman, M. B. Holm, F. X. Guyette, C. W. Callaway. An early, novel illness severity score to predict outcome after cardiac arrest. *Resuscitation.* 2011;**82**(11):1399–1404.

28. Coppler, P. J., J. Elmer, L. Calderon, et al. Post Cardiac Arrest Service. Validation of the Pittsburgh Cardiac Arrest Category illness severity score. *Resuscitation.* 2015;**89**:86–92.

29. Fugate, J. E., E. F. Wijdicks, J. Mandrekar, et al. Predictors of neurologic outcome in hypothermia after cardiac arrest. *Ann Neurol.* 2010;**68**(6):907–14.

30. Bouwes, A., J. M. Binnekade, M. A. Kuiper, et al. Prognosis of coma after therapeutic hypothermia: a prospective cohort study. *Ann Neurol.* 2012;**71**(2):206–12.

31. Greer, D. M., J. Yang, P. D. Scripko, et al. Clinical examination for prognostication in comatose cardiac arrest patients. *Resuscitation.* 2013;**84**(11):1546–51.

32. Golan, E., K. Barrett, A. S. Alali, et al. Predicting neurologic outcome after targeted temperature management for cardiac arrest: systematic review and meta-analysis. *Crit Care Med.* 2014;**42**(8):1919–30.

33. Sandroni, C., A. Cariou, F. Cavallaro, et al. Prognostication in comatose survivors of cardiac arrest: an advisory statement from the European Resuscitation Council and the European Society of Intensive Care Medicine. *Resuscitation.* 2014;**85**(12):1779–89.

34. Wijdicks, E. F., A. Hijdra, G. B. Young, C. L. Bassetti, S. Wiebe. Practice parameter: prediction of outcome in comatose survivors after cardiopulmonary resuscitation (an evidence-based review):report of the Quality Standards Subcommittee of the American Academy of Neurology. *Neurology.* 2006;**67**(2):203–10.

35. Al Thenayan, E., M. Savard, M. Sharpe, L. Norton, B. Young. Predictors of poor neurologic outcome

after induced mild hypothermia following cardiac arrest. *Neurology*. 2008;**71**(19):1535–7.

36. Rossetti, A. O., M. Oddo, G. Logroscino, P. W. Kaplan. Prognostication after cardiac arrest and hypothermia: a prospective study. *Ann Neurol*. 2010;**67**(3):301–7.

37. Samaniego, E. A., M. Mlynash, A. F. Caulfield, I. Eyngorn, C. A. Wijman. Sedation confounds outcome prediction in cardiac arrest survivors treated with hypothermia. *Neurocrit Care*. 2011;**15**(1):113–19.

38. Schefold, J. C., C. Storm, A. Kruger, C. J. Ploner, D. Hasper. The Glasgow Coma Score is a predictor of good outcome in cardiac arrest patients treated with therapeutic hypothermia. *Resuscitation*. 2009;**80**(6):658–61.

39. Wijdicks, E. F., J. E. Parisi, F. W. Sharbrough. Prognostic value of myoclonus status in comatose survivors of cardiac arrest. *Ann Neurol*. 1994;**35** (2):239–43.

40. Bisschops, L. L., N. van Alfen, S. Bons, J. G. van der Hoeven, C. W. Hoedemaekers. Predictors of poor neurologic outcome in patients after cardiac arrest treated with hypothermia: a retrospective study. *Resuscitation*. 2011;**82**(6):696–701.

41. Bouwes, A., D. van Poppelen, J. H. Koelman, et al. Acute posthypoxic myoclonus after cardiopulmonary resuscitation. *BMC Neurol*. 2012;**12**:63.

42. Lucas, J. M., M. N. Cocchi, J. Salciccioli, et al. Neurologic recovery after therapeutic hypothermia in patients with post-cardiac arrest myoclonus. *Resuscitation*. 2012;**83**(2):265–9.

43. Seder, D. B., K. Sunde, S. Rubertsson, et al. Neurologic outcomes and postresuscitation care of patients with myoclonus following cardiac arrest. *Crit Care Med*. 2015;**43**(5):965–72.

44. Lybeck, A., H. Friberg, A. Aneman, et al., T. T.-t. Investigators. Prognostic significance of clinical seizures after cardiac arrest and target temperature management. *Resuscitation*. 2017;**114**:146–51.

45. Sandroni, C., F. Cavallaro, C. W. Callaway, et al. Predictors of poor neurological outcome in adult comatose survivors of cardiac arrest: a systematic review and meta-analysis. Part 2: patients treated with therapeutic hypothermia. *Resuscitation*. 2013;**84**(10):1324–38.

46. Dhakar, M. B., A. Sivaraju, C. B. Maciel, et al. Electro-clinical characteristics and prognostic significance of post anoxic myoclonus. *Resuscitation*. 2018;**131**:114–20.

47. Hallett, M. Physiology of human posthypoxic myoclonus. *Mov Disord*. 2000;**15**(Suppl 1):8–13.

48. van Zijl, J. C., M. Beudel, J. J. Elting, et al. The inter-rater variability of clinical assessment in post-anoxic myoclonus. *Tremor Other Hyperkinet Mov (N Y)*. 2017;**7**:470.

49. van Zijl, J. C., M. Beudel, B. M. de Jong, et al. The interrelation between clinical presentation and neurophysiology of posthypoxic myoclonus. *Ann Clin Transl Neurol*. 2018;**5**(4):386–96.

50. Elmer, J., J. C. Rittenberger, J. Faro, et al. S. Pittsburgh Post-Cardiac Arrest. Clinically distinct electroencephalographic phenotypes of early myoclonus after cardiac arrest. *Ann Neurol*. 2016;**80**(2):175–84.

51. Aicua Rapun, I., J. Novy, D. Solari, M. Oddo, A. O. Rossetti. Early Lance-Adams syndrome after cardiac arrest: prevalence, time to return to awareness, and outcome in a large cohort. *Resuscitation*. 2017;**115**:169–72.

52. Synek, V. M. Value of a revised EEG coma scale for prognosis after cerebral anoxia and diffuse head injury. *Clin Electroencephalogr*. 1990;**21** (1):25–30.

53. Rossetti, A. O., E. Carrera, M. Oddo. Early EEG correlates of neuronal injury after brain anoxia. *Neurology*. 2012;**78**(11):796–802.

54. Hirsch, L. J., M. W. K. Fong, M. Leitinger, et al. American Clinical Neurophysiology Society's Standardized Critical Care EEG Terminology: 2021 version. *J Clin Neurophysiol*. 2021;**38** (1):1–29.

55. Westhall, E., I. Rosen, A. O. Rossetti, et al. Interrater variability of EEG interpretation in comatose cardiac arrest patients. *Clin Neurophysiol*. 2015;**126**(12):2397–404.

56. Stecker, M. M., A. T. Cheung, A. Pochettino, et al. Deep hypothermic circulatory arrest: I. effects of cooling on electroencephalogram and evoked potentials. *Ann Thorac Surg*. 2001;**71**(1):14–21

57. Ruijter, B. J., M. van Putten, W. M. van den Bergh, S. C. Tromp, J. Hofmeijer. Propofol does not affect the reliability of early EEG for outcome prediction of comatose patients after cardiac arrest. *Clin Neurophysiol*. 2019;**130**(8):1263–70.

58. Hofmeijer, J., T. M. Beernink, F. H. Bosch, et al. Early EEG contributes to multimodal outcome prediction of postanoxic coma. *Neurology*. 2015;**85**(2):137–43.

59. Sivaraju, A., E. J. Gilmore, C. R. Wira, et al. Prognostication of post-cardiac arrest coma: early clinical and electroencephalographic predictors of outcome. *Intensive Care Med*. 2015;**41**(7): 1264–72.

60. Rossetti, A. O., D. F. Tovar Quiroga, E. Juan, et al. Electroencephalography predicts poor and good

outcomes after cardiac arrest: a two-center study. *Crit Care Med.* 2017;**45**(7):e674–e682.

61. Ruijter, B. J., M. C. Tjepkema-Cloostermans, S. C. Tromp, et al. Early EEG for outcome prediction of postanoxic coma: a prospective cohort study. *Ann Neurol.* 2019;**86**(2):203–14.

62. Hofmeijer, J., M. C. Tjepkema-Cloostermans, M. J. van Putten. Burst-suppression with identical bursts: a distinct EEG pattern with poor outcome in postanoxic coma. *Clin Neurophysiol.* 2014;**125**(5):947–54.

63. Barbella, G., J. Novy, P. Marques-Vidal, M. Oddo, A. O. Rossetti. Prognostic role of EEG identical bursts in patients after cardiac arrest: multimodal correlation. *Resuscitation.* 2020;**148** 140–4.

64. Westhall, E., A. O. Rossetti, A. F. van Rootselaar, et al., T. T.-t. investigators. Standardized EEG interpretation accurately predicts prognosis after cardiac arrest. *Neurology.* 2016;**86**(16):1482–90.

65. Beuchat, I., D. Solari, J. Novy, M. Oddo, A. O. Rossetti. Standardized EEG interpretation in patients after cardiac arrest: correlation with other prognostic predictors. *Resuscitation.* 2018;**126**:143–6.

66. Berkhoff, M., F. Donati, C. Bassetti. Postanoxic alpha (theta) coma: a reappraisal of its prognostic significance. *Clin Neurophysiol.* 2000;**111**(2):297–304.

67. Rossetti, A. O., M. Oddo, L. Liaudet, P. W. Kaplan. Predictors of awakening from postanoxic status epilepticus after therapeutic hypothermia. *Neurology.* 2009;**72**(8):744–9.

68. Legriel, S., J. Hilly-Ginoux, M. Resche-Rigon, et al. Prognostic value of electrographic postanoxic status epilepticus in comatose cardiac-arrest survivors in the therapeutic hypothermia era. *Resuscitation.* 2013;**84**(3):343–50.

69. Backman, S., E. Westhall, I. Dragancea, et al. Electroencephalographic characteristics of status epilepticus after cardiac arrest. *Clin Neurophysiol.* 2017;**128**(4):681–8.

70. Beretta, S., A. Coppo, E. Bianchi, et al. Neurologic outcome of postanoxic refractory status epilepticus after aggressive treatment. *Neurology.* 2018;**91**(23):e2153–e2162.

71. Trinka, E., H. Cock, D. Hesdorffer, et al. A definition and classification of status epilepticus – report of the ILAE Task Force on Classification of Status Epilepticus. *Epilepsia.* 2015;**56**(10):1515–23.

72. Sadaka, F., D. Doerr, J. Hindia, K. P. Lee, W. Logan. Continuous electroencephalogram in comatose postcardiac arrest syndrome patients treated with therapeutic hypothermia: outcome prediction study. *J Intensive Care Med.* 2015;**30**(5):292–6.

73. Westhall, E., I. Rosen, M. Rundgren, et al. Time to epileptiform activity and EEG background recovery are independent predictors after cardiac arrest. *Clin Neurophysiol.* 2018;**129**(8):1660–8.

74. Barbella, G., J. W. Lee, V. Alvarez, et al. Prediction of regaining consciousness despite an early epileptiform EEG after cardiac arrest. *Neurology.* 2020;**94**(16):e1675–e1683.

75. Beuchat, I., A. Sivaraju, E. Amorim, et al. MRI-EEG correlation for outcome prediction in postanoxic myoclonus: a multicenter study. *Neurology.* 2020;**95**(4):e335–e341.

76. Forgacs, P. B., O. Devinsky, N. D. Schiff. Independent functional outcomes after prolonged coma following cardiac arrest: a mechanistic hypothesis. *Ann Neurol.* 2020;**87**(4):618–32.

77. Admiraal, M. M., A. F. van Rootselaar, J. Horn. International consensus on EEG reactivity testing after cardiac arrest: towards standardization. *Resuscitation.* 2018;**131**:36–41.

78. Al Thenayan, E., M. Savard, M. D. Sharpe, L. Norton, B. Young. Electroencephalogram for prognosis after cardiac arrest. *J Crit Care.* 2010;**25**(2):300–4.

79. Oddo, M. and A. O. Rossetti. Early multimodal outcome prediction after cardiac arrest in patients treated with hypothermia. *Crit Care Med.* 2014;**42**(6):1340–7.

80. Juan, E., J. Novy, T. Suys, M. Oddo, A. O. Rossetti. clinical evolution after a non-reactive hypothermic EEG following cardiac arrest. *Neurocrit Care.* 2015;**22**:403–8.

81. Rossetti, A. O., L. A. Urbano, F. Delodder, P. W. Kaplan, M. Oddo. Prognostic value of continuous EEG monitoring during therapeutic hypothermia after cardiac arrest. *Crit Care.* 2010;**14**(5):R173.

82. Tsetsou, S., M. Oddo, A. O. Rossetti. Clinical outcome after a reactive hypothermic EEG following cardiac arrest. *Neurocrit Care.* 2013;**19**(3):283–6.

83. Noirhomme, Q., R. Lehembre, R. Lugo Zdel, et al. Automated analysis of background EEG and reactivity during therapeutic hypothermia in comatose patients after cardiac arrest. *Clin EEG Neurosci.* 2014;**45**(1):6–13.

84. Duez, C. H. V., M. Q. Ebbesen, K. Benedek, et al. Large inter-rater variability on EEG-reactivity is improved by a novel quantitative method. *Clin Neurophysiol.* 2018;**129**(4):724–30.

85. Admiraal, M. M., A. F. van Rootselaar, J. Hofmeijer, et al. Electroencephalographic

reactivity as predictor of neurological outcome in postanoxic coma: a multicenter prospective cohort study. *Ann Neurol.* 2019;**86**(1):17–27.

86. Lee, J. W. EEG reactivity in coma after cardiac arrest: is it enough to wake up the dead? *Epilepsy Curr.* 2019;**19**(6):369–71.

87. Fantaneanu, T. A., B. Tolchin, V. Alvarez, et al. Effect of stimulus type and temperature on EEG reactivity in cardiac arrest. *Clin Neurophysiol.* 2016;**127**(11):3412–17.

88. Caporro, M., A. O. Rossetti, A. Seiler, et al. Electromyographic reactivity measured with scalp-EEG contributes to prognostication after cardiac arrest. *Resuscitation.* 2019;**138**:146–52.

89. Alvarez, V., A. Sierra-Marcos, M. Oddo. A. O. Rossetti. Yield of intermittent versus continuous EEG in comatose survivors of cardiac arrest treated with hypothermia. *Crit Care.* 2013;**17**(5):R190.

90. Crepeau, A. Z., J. E. Fugate, J. Mandrekar, et al. Value analysis of continuous EEG in patients during therapeutic hypothermia after cardiac arrest. *Resuscitation.* 2014;**85**(6):785–79.

91. Rossetti, A. O., K. Schindler, R. Sutter, et al. Continuous vs routine electroencephalogram in critically ill adults with altered consciousness and no recent seizure: a multicenter randomized clinical trial. *JAMA Neurol.* 2020;**77**(10):1225–32.

92. Rundgren, M., E. Westhall, T. Cronberg, I. Rosen, H. Friberg. Continuous amplitude-integrated electroencephalogram predicts outcome in hypothermia-treated cardiac arrest patients. *Crit Care Med.* 2010;**38**(9):1838–44.

93. Cloostermans, M. C., F. B. van Meulen, C. J. Eertman, H. W. Hom, M. J. van Putten. Continuous electroencephalography monitoring for early prediction of neurological outcome in postanoxic patients after cardiac arrest: a prospective cohort study. *Crit Care Med.* 2012;**40**(10):2867–75.

94. Oh, S. H., K. N. Park, Y. M. Kim, er al. The prognostic value of continuous amplitude-integrated electroencephalogram applied immediately after return of spontaneous circulation in therapeutic hypothermia-treated cardiac arrest patients. *Resuscitation.* 2013;**84** (2):200–5.

95. Oh, S. H., K. N. Park, Y. M. Shon, et al. Continuous amplitude-integrated electroencephalographic monitoring is a useful prognostic tool for hypothermia-treated cardiac arrest patients. *Circulation.* 2015;**132** (12):1094–1103.

96. Tjepkema-Cloostermans, M. C., J. Hofmeijer, H. W. Hom, F. H. Bosch, M. van Putten.

Predicting outcome in postanoxic coma: are ten EEG electrodes enough? *J Clin Neurophysiol.* 2017;**34**(3):207–12.

97. Backman, S., T. Cronberg, I. Rosen, E. Westhall. Reduced EEG montage has a high accuracy in the post cardiac arrest setting. *Clin Neurophysiol.* 2020;**131**(9):2216–23.

98. Amorim, E., M. M. Ghassemi, J. W. Lee, et al. Estimating the false positive rate of absent somatosensory evoked potentials in cardiac arrest prognostication. *Crit Care Med.* 2018;**46**(12): e1213–e1221.

99. Rothstein, T. L. SSEP retains its value as predictor of poor outcome following cardiac arrest in the era of therapeutic hypothermia. *Crit Care.* 2019;**23**(1):327.

100. Fredland, A., S. Backman, E. Westhall. Stratifying comatose postanoxic patients for somatosensory evoked potentials using routine EEG. *Resuscitation.* 2019;**143**:17–21.

101. Beuchat, I., J. Novy, G. Barbella, M. Oddo, A. O. Rossetti. EEG patterns associated with present cortical SSEP after cardiac arrest. *Acta Neurol Scand.* 2020;**142**(2):181–6.

102. Endisch, C., C. Storm, C. J. Ploner, C. Leithner. Amplitudes of SSEP and outcome in cardiac arrest survivors: a prospective cohort study. *Neurology.* 2015;**85**(20):1752–60.

103. Carrai, R., M. Scarpino, F. Lolli, et al. Early-SEPs' amplitude reduction is reliable for poor-outcome prediction after cardiac arrest? *Acta Neurol Scand.* 2019;**139**(2):158–65.

104. Oh, S. H., K. N. Park, S. P. Choi, et al. Beyond dichotomy: patterns and amplitudes of SSEPs and neurological outcomes after cardiac arrest. *Crit Care.* 2019;**23**(1):224.

105. Scarpino, M., F. Lolli, G. Lanzo, et al. SSEP amplitude accurately predicts both good and poor neurological outcome early after cardiac arrest; a post-hoc analysis of the ProNeCA multicentre study. *Resuscitation.* 2021;**163**:162–71.

106. Barbella, G., J. Novy, P. Marques-Vidal, M. Oddo, A. O. Rossetti. Added value of somato-sensory evoked potentials amplitude for prognostication after cardiac arrest. *Resuscitation.* 2020;**149**:17–23.

107. Hahn, D. K., R. G. Geocadin, D. M. Greer. Quality of evidence in studies evaluating neuroimaging for neurologic prognostication in adult patients resuscitated from cardiac arrest. *Resuscitation.* 2014;**85**(2):165–72.

108. Inamasu, J., S. Miyatake, M. Suzuki, et al. Early CT signs in out-of-hospital cardiac arrest survivors: temporal profile and prognostic significance. *Resuscitation.* 2010;**81**(5):534–8.

109. Wu, O., L. M. Batista, F. O. Lima, et al. Predicting clinical outcome in comatose cardiac arrest patients using early noncontrast computed tomography. *Stroke.* 2011;**42**(4):985–992.

110. Greer, D. M., O. Wu. Neuroimaging in cardiac arrest prognostication. *Semin Neurol.* 2017;**37** (1):66–74.

111. Moseby-Knappe, M., T. Pellis, I. Dragancea, et al., T. T.-t. Investigators. Head computed tomography for prognostication of poor outcome in comatose patients after cardiac arrest and targeted temperature management. *Resuscitation.* 2017;**119**:89–94.

112. Metter, R. B., J. C. Rittenberger, F. X. Guyette, C. W. Callaway. Association between a quantitative CT scan measure of brain edema and outcome after cardiac arrest. *Resuscitation.* 2011;**82**(9):1180–5.

113. Gentsch, A., C. Storm, C. Leithner, et al. Outcome prediction in patients after cardiac arrest: a simplified method for determination of gray-white matter ratio in cranial computed tomography. *Clin Neuroradiol.* 2015;**25**(1):49–54.

114. Hanning, U., P. B. Sporns, P. Lebiedz, et al. Automated assessment of early hypoxic brain edema in non-enhanced CT predicts outcome in patients after cardiac arrest. *Resuscitation.* 2016;**104**:91–4.

115. Keijzer, H. M., C. W. E. Hoedemaekers, F. J. A. Meijer, et al. Brain imaging in comatose survivors of cardiac arrest: pathophysiological correlates and prognostic properties. *Resuscitation.* 2018;**133**:124–36.

116. Na, M. K., W. Kim, T. H. Lim, et al. Gray matter to white matter ratio for predicting neurological outcomes in patients treated with target temperature management after cardiac arrest: a systematic review and meta-analysis. *Resuscitation.* 2018;**132**:21–8

117. Cronberg, T., M. Brizzi, L. J. Liedholm, et al. Neurological prognostication after cardiac arrest-Recommendations from the Swedish Resuscitation Council. *Resuscitation.* 2013;**84** (7):867–72.

118. Greer, D., P. Scripko, J. Bartscher, et al. Serial MRI changes in comatose cardiac arrest patients. *Neurocrit Care.* 2011;**14**(1):61–7.

119. Velly, L., V. Perlbarg, T. Boulier, et al. Use of brain diffusion tensor imaging for the prediction of long-term neurological outcomes in patients after cardiac arrest: a multicentre, international, prospective, observational, cohort study. *Lancet Neurol.* 2018;**17**(4):317–26.

120. Stammet, P. blood biomarkers of hypoxic-ischemic brain injury after cardiac arrest. *Semin Neurol.* 2017;**37**(1):75–80.

121. Cronberg, T., M. Rundgren, E. Westhall, et al. Neuron-specific enolase correlates with other prognostic markers after cardiac arrest. *Neurology.* 2011;**77**(7):623–30.

122. Sahai, S. K., T. Majic, J. Patel, et al. Neurological prognostication of cardiac arrest in an era of extracorporeal membrane oxygenation. *Neurohospitalist.* 2017;**7**(1):35–8.

123. Zandbergen, E. G., A. Hijdra, J. H. Koelman, et al. Prediction of poor outcome within the first 3 days of postanoxic coma. *Neurology.* 2006;**66**(1):62–8.

124. Stammet, P., O. Collignon, C. Hassager, et al.; T. T.-T. Investigators. Neuron-specific enolase as a predictor of death or poor neurological outcome after out-of-hospital cardiac arrest and targeted temperature management at 33 degrees C and 36 degrees C. *J Am Coll Cardiol.* 2015;**65**(19): 2104–14.

125. Streitberger, K. J., C. Leithner, M. Wattenberg, et al. Neuron-specific enolase predicts poor outcome after cardiac arrest and targeted temperature management: a multicenter study on 1,053 patients. *Crit Care Med.* 2017;**45**(7):1145–51.

126. Stammet, P., J. Dankiewicz, N. Nielsen, et al. Target Temperature Management after Out-of-Hospital Cardiac Arrest Trial. Protein S100 as outcome predictor after out-of-hospital cardiac arrest and targeted temperature management at 33 degrees C and 36 degrees C. *Crit Care.* 2017;**21** (1):153.

127. Mattsson, N., H. Zetterberg, N. Nielsen, et al. Serum tau and neurological outcome in cardiac arrest. *Ann Neurol.* 2017;**82**(5):665–75.

128. Moseby-Knappe, M., N. Mattsson, N. Nielsen, et al. Serum neurofilament light chain for prognosis of outcome after cardiac arrest. *JAMA Neurol.* 2019;**76**(1):64–71.

129. Moseby-Knappe, M., N. Mattsson-Carlgren, P. Stammet, et al. Serum markers of brain injury can predict good neurological outcome after out-of-hospital cardiac arrest. *Intensive Care Med.* 2021;**47** (9):984–94.

130. Solari, D., A. O. Rossetti, L. Carteron, et al. Early prediction of coma recovery after cardiac arrest with blinded pupillometry. *Ann Neurol.* 2017;**81** (6):804–10.

131. Suys, T., P. Bouzat, P. Marques-Vidal, et al. Automated quantitative pupillometry for the prognostication of coma after cardiac arrest. *Neurocrit Care.* 2014;**21**(2):300–8.

132. Heimburger, D., M. Durand, L. Gaide-Chevronnay, et al. Quantitative pupillometry and transcranial Doppler measurements in patients treated with hypothermia after cardiac arrest. *Resuscitation.* 2016;**103**:88–93.

133. Oddo, M., C. Sandroni, G. Citerio, et al. Quantitative versus standard pupillary light reflex for early prognostication in comatose cardiac arrest patients: an international prospective multicenter double-blinded study. *Intensive Care Med.* 2018;**44**(12):2102–11.

134. Zhou, S. E., C. B. Maciel, C. H. Ormseth, et al. Distinct predictive values of current neuroprognostic guidelines in post-cardiac arrest patients. *Resuscitation.* 2019;**139**: 343–50.

135. Gold, B., L. Puertas, S. P. Davis, et al. Awakening after cardiac arrest and post resuscitation hypothermia: are we pulling the plug too early? *Resuscitation.* 2014;**85**(2):211–14.

136. Lybeck, A., T. Cronberg, A. Aneman, et al. Time to awakening after cardiac arrest and the association with target temperature management. *Resuscitation.* 2018;**126**:166–71.

137. Moseby-Knappe, M., E. Westhall, S. Backman, et al. Performance of a guideline-recommended algorithm for prognostication of poor neurological outcome after cardiac arrest. *Intensive Care Med.* 2020;**46**(10):1852–62.

138. Peskine, A., C. Picq, P. Pradat-Diehl. Cerebral anoxia and disability. *Brain Inj.* 2004;**18** (12):1243–54.

139. Moulaert, V. R., J. A. Verbunt, C. M. van Heugten, D. T. Wade. Cognitive impairments in survivors of out-of-hospital cardiac arrest: a systematic review. *Resuscitation.* 2009;**80**(3):297–305.

140. Lilja, G., N. Nielsen, H. Friberg, et al. Cognitive function in survivors of out-of-hospital cardiac arrest after target temperature management at 33 degrees C versus 36 degrees C. *Circulation.* 2015;**131**(15):1340–9.

141. Juan, E., M. De Lucia, V. Beaud, et al. How do you feel? Subjective perception of recovery as a reliable surrogate of cognitive and functional outcome in cardiac arrest survivors. *Crit Care Med.* 2018;**46**(4):e286–e293.

142. Lilja, G., N. Nielsen, J. Bro-Jeppesen, et al. Return to work and participation in society after out-of-hospital cardiac arrest. *Circ Cardiovasc Qual Outcomes.* 2018;**11**(1):e003566.

143. Dankiewicz, J., T. Cronberg, G. Lilja, et al., T. T. M. T. Investigators. Hypothermia versus normothermia after out-of-hospital cardiac arrest. *N Engl J Med.* 2021;**384**(24):2283–94.

144. Riker, R. R., P. C. Stone Jr, T. May, et al. Initial bispectral index may identify patients who will awaken during therapeutic hypothermia after cardiac arrest: a retrospective pilot study. *Resuscitation.* 2013;**84**(6):794–7.

Prognostication in Neuroinfectious Disease

Anna M. Cervantes-Arslanian and Pria Anand

Introduction

Patients with neurological infections are often critically ill, requiring cardiopulmonary support and prolonged admission to the Neurointensive Care Unit (Neuro-ICU). In recent years, the pathogens and manifestations of neurological infections have expanded in the setting of both immunosuppressive medications and globalization. Despite advances in antimicrobial therapy, however, the morbidity and mortality of these infections remains high. Outcomes following neurological infections are variable, determined by host factors, pathogen factors, and the specific syndrome. In this chapter, we will review outcomes following neurological infections of the central nervous system (CNS) in critically ill patients, focusing on the most commonly encountered diagnoses, including meningitis, abscess, and encephalitis.

Bacterial Infections of the CNS

Acute Bacterial Meningitis

Acute bacterial meningitis (ABM) is a life-threatening emergency characterized by a purulent infection of the subarachnoid space and often accompanied by inflammation of meninges, brain parenchyma, and cerebrovasculature.[1] Adoption and widespread use of conjugate vaccinations (specifically *Haemophilus influenzae*) have shifted the burden of illness in acute bacterial meningitis from children to adults. Despite shifts in epidemiology, meningitis remains an important public health challenge. The World Health Organization (WHO) convened a panel in March 2019 to create a global strategy to "defeat meningitis by 2030."[2] The incidence of ABM is not uniform; countries within the "meningitis belt" in the Sahel region of Africa are disproportionately affected, with 1,000 per 100,000 people in the region affected per year, compared to 1–2 per 100,000 in the United Kingdom, Western Europe, and the United States.[3]

In high-income countries, mortality has dropped from 25% [4] to 5.5–17%.[5–7] In low- and middle-income countries (LMIC), mortality from ABM remains extremely high, with a case fatality rate of 22% in Ethiopia [8] and 54% in Malawi.[9] The number of deaths globally is estimated to be 380,000 per year.[10] For those who survive hospitalization with ABM, 20% develop long-term disabling sequelae, with hearing loss being the most common. Motor deficits, seizures, visual deficits, and cognitive impairment are also commonly noted. The risk of disability following ABM is three times greater in LMIC than high-income countries.[11]

Several factors have been identified as key determinants of prognosis in ABM, including pathogen and host factors, stage of infection at presentation, neurological examination at presentation, and the development of neurological sequelae during infection.

Pathogens

Historically, meningitis was most often a childhood disease, with *Haemophilus influenzae* the most common pathogen.[12] In large part due to a successful vaccination strategy for *H. influenzae*, today most cases of ABM are caused by *Streptococcus pneumoniae* and *Neisseria meningitis*. Studies have consistently shown a higher mortality with pneumococcal meningitis than with meningococcal meningitis, and neurological complications are also more common in survivors of pneumococcal meningitis.[12–14] (See Case Study 8.1 and Case Study 8.2.)

Host Factors

Several Host Factors influence prognosis in ABM. In children, infants have a higher mortality than older children.[12] In adults, elderly patients (> 65 years of age) have worse outcomes than younger patients, even when controlling for comorbidities.[15,16] Comorbidities leading to immunocompromise increase the likelihood of poor outcome – in particular diabetes mellitus, alcoholism, and infection with human immunodeficiency virus (HIV).[17,18]

Case Study 8.1 A 52-year-old gentleman presented with fevers, seizure, and altered mental status requiring intubation. MRI revealed (A) a left-sided subdural fluid collection with restricted diffusion suggestive of a subdural empyema and (B) pachymeningeal thickening and enhancement suggestive of meningitis. Cerebrospinal fluid (CSF) analysis revealed a neutrophilic pleocytosis with a positive *Streptococcus pneumoniae* polymerase chain reaction (PCR). He was treated with broad-spectrum antibiotics and steroids before narrowing to ceftriaxone for a 6-week course. At follow-up 1 month after the conclusion of antibiotics, he remained in a skilled nursing facility. He was able to walk independently, with resolution of his seizures and improvement in his mental status to baseline.

(A)　　　　　　　　　(B)

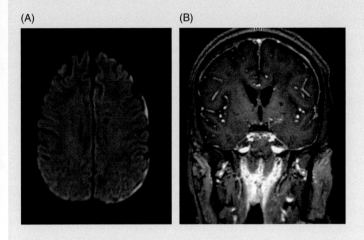

Case Study 8.2 A 39-year-old gentleman presented with fever and headache, with rapidly worsening mental status following presentation requiring intubation. A head CT showed A) and B) diffuse cerebral edema and complete effacement of the cerebral sulci. He was started on broad-spectrum antibiotics, steroids, and hyper-osmolar therapy. CSF was obtained following placement of an external ventricular drain (EVD), with a positive PCR for *Neisseria meningitis*. After 3 days of antibiotic therapy, his mental status had improved, and he was able to be successfully extubated. After 4 days of antibiotic therapy, his EVD was clamped and removed. He completed 2 weeks of antibiotics, and at follow-up 2 months later was living independently and reported complete recovery to his previous baseline, with no deficits noted on neurological examination.

(A)　　　　　　　　　(B)

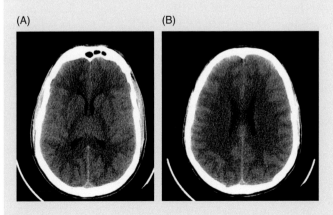

Systemic Factors

Studies have shown that delayed initiation of antibiotics at the time of presentation with ABM is strongly associated with poor outcome (neurological deficit at hospital discharge) and death.[19,20] Thus, guidelines recommend starting antibiotics as soon as possible when ABM is suspected (no later than 1 hour after arrival to the hospital) without waiting for testing such as head computed tomography (CT) or lumbar puncture. Delayed CSF sterilization after 24 hours of antibiotics is also associated with development of neurological complications and worse outcomes (defined as a neurological complications at discharge or Glasgow Outcome Scale [GOS] of 1–4).[8,21,22] Variability in CSF clearance is likely due to differences in the initial CSF infectious burden, levels of antigen present prior to initiation of treatment,[23] and host inflammatory response.

Signs of systemic illness at admission are also associated with worse outcomes. One multi-center retrospective study of 269 patients with ABM in Connecticut hospitals between 1970 and 1995 found that hypotension at admission (systolic blood pressure [SBP] ≤ 90 mmHg) was a key factor in predicting poor outcomes (neurological deficit at discharge or death).[20] Similarly, an analysis of patients with Glasgow Coma Scale (GCS) score of 3 (30 of the 1,083) in the MeninGene prospective observational study in the Netherlands showed the outcome was uniformly fatal if signs of septic shock (SBP < 90 mmHg, diastolic blood pressure [DBP] < 60 mmHg, or heart rate [HR] > 120 bpm) were present on arrival.[24] Persistent fever (lasting greater than 2 days after admission) was associated with unfavorable outcomes (GOS 1–4) in a prospective study of 90 patients in Ethiopia from 2013 to 2015.[8] Paradoxically, a low CSF white blood cell (WBC) count (< 1,000 cells/mm^3) has also been associated with worsened prognosis.[25]

Neurological Exam at Presentation

The neurological exam at the time of presentation with ABM plays an important role in determining prognosis. The presence of focal neurological deficits at admission portends a worse prognosis.[26] The strongest predictor of outcomes in ABM is the patient's level of consciousness at admission, with lower levels of consciousness at arrival increasing the risk of death.[27] In a single-center retrospective study of 493 episodes of ABM in 445 adults over a 27-year period (1962–1988) in Massachusetts, 49%

of patients who presented obtunded (unresponsive or responsive only to pain) died compared to 16% of those who were alert or lethargic.[4] Level of arousal is most commonly described using the Glasgow Coma Scale (Table 8.1). In a prospective study of 100 patients, those presenting with a GCS score ≤ 8 had significantly higher mortality than those presenting with a GCS ≥12 (62.5% vs. 9.3%).[28] Recent data suggest that the Full Outline of Unresponsiveness (FOUR) score (Table 8.1) is comparable to the historically widely used GCS score with regard to the ability to predict unfavorable outcomes, including death, in ABM. In addition, the FOUR score allowed for better distinction amongst patients with lower scores on the GCS, as the FOUR score provides greater neurological detail than GCS and is useful in intubated patients whose verbal scores on the GCS are unreliable.[29,30]

In the MeninGene Study, the majority of patients arriving with minimal GCS were found to have poor outcomes (77% with severe disability and 60% with death). All patients with GCS 3 and bilateral absence of pupillary light (8 of 25) or corneal (7 of 9) responses died. Despite the preponderance of poor outcomes, 12 of 30 (40%) survived, and 7 patients (23%) made a full recovery.[24]

Treatment of ABM before it progresses to moderate or severe impairment of consciousness is important. In one study, early administration of antibiotics only showed a benefit in outcomes when administered before the GCS deteriorated to 10.[31]

Neurological Sequelae

Seizures

Many studies have found that seizures in community-acquired ABM are associated with increased risk of in-hospital mortality or neurological deficits at discharge.[4,16,20] Roughly 17% of patients with community-acquired ABM develop seizures.[32] Infection with S. pneumoniae, comorbid alcohol abuse or diabetes, and abnormal imaging demonstrating infarction all increased the risk for seizures. [33]

Stroke

Stroke is a common complication of ABM. The highest risk of ischemic stroke occurs with S. pneumonia, where roughly a third of patients are affected, compared to 15–25% with other bacteria.[34–36] Stroke may occur at any time during the course of infection, and often occurs

Table 8.1 Glasgow Coma Scale (GCS) and Full Outline of Unresponsiveness (FOUR) scoring

	FOUR score	GCS score
Eye response	4 – Eyelids open or opened, tracking, or blinking to command 3 - Eyelids open but not tracking 2 - Eyelids closed but open to loud voice 1 - Eyelids closed but open to pain 0 - Eyelids remain closed with pain	4 - Opens eyes spontaneously 3 - Opens eyes in response to voice 2 - Opens eyes in response to pain 1 - Does not open eyes
Motor response	4 - Thumbs-up, fist, or peace sign 3 - Localizing to pain 2 - Flexion response to pain 1 - Extension response to pain 0 - No response to pain or generalized myoclonus status	6 - Obeys commands 5 - Localizes to painful stimuli 4 - Withdrawal to painful stimuli 3 - Flexion to painful stimuli 2 - Extension to painful stimuli 1 - Makes no movements
Brainstem reflexes	4 - Pupil and corneal reflexes present 3 - One pupil wide and fixed 2 - Pupil or corneal reflexes absent 1 - Pupil and corneal reflexes absent 0 - Absent pupil, corneal, and cough reflex	
Respiration	4 - Not intubated, regular breathing pattern 3 - Not intubated, Cheyne–Stokes breathing pattern 2 - Not intubated, irregular breathing 1 - Breathes above ventilator rate 0 - Breathes at ventilator rate or apnea	
Verbal response		5 - Oriented, converses normally 4 - Confused, disoriented 3 - Words 2 - Makes sounds 1 - Makes no sounds

despite initiation of appropriate antibiotic therapy. Increased age at presentation, reduced level of consciousness on admission, and low CSF WBC count have all been associated with increased risk of stroke.[37] In the Dutch Meningitis Cohort Study of 696 episodes of ABM, 174 were complicated by ischemic stroke. Unfavorable neurological outcomes (GOS 1–4) were seen in 108 of 174 (62%) of patients with ABM and stroke. Mortality was also increased in this cohort (55 of 174 patients (32%), compared with 88 of 522 (17%) without stroke). Death was more likely to be attributable to a neurological cause in patients with stroke. Stroke also increased the risk for cardiorespiratory failure.[35]

Sparse literature exists to guide prevention and therapy of stroke. A small retrospective study identified 22 children from the Canadian Pediatric Ischemic Stroke Registry with ABM and ischemic stroke over a 15-year period. In this group, 8 patients received either aspirin or heparin, and no cases were complicated by intracranial bleeding. Eight of the 22 children had recurrent strokes, 4 of whom had been treated with aspirin.[38] One study from India randomized 118 patients with tuberculous meningitis (TBM) to aspirin 150 mg or placebo to look at primary prevention of stroke. Thirty-three percent of patients developed stroke, but aspirin did not significantly decrease the risk. In this group, aspirin did significantly improve 3-month mortality, and no patients developed adverse bleeding effects.[39]

Acute vasculitis may develop in the setting of ABM, leading to stroke as well as delayed post-infectious vasculopathy. Case reports cite benefits of steroids, but the role for treatment with steroids or other immunomodulatory

129

therapies is unclear.[40,41] Some centers advocate monitoring ABM patients with transcranial Doppler routinely to assess for increased cerebral blood flow velocities, indicative of vessel narrowing.[42]

Hydrocephalus

In ABM, CSF protein increases as a result of breakdown of the blood–brain barrier. This can lead to increased CSF viscosity and decreased absorption of CSF through the arachnoid villi, resulting in communicating hydrocephalus. Increased CSF protein is a risk factor for developing hydrocephalus and an independent risk factor for mortality.[43] Studies have shown increasing mortality in ABM, with increases in the ventricle-to-brain ratio on imaging independent of the clinical diagnosis of hydrocephalus.[43]

Clinically observed hydrocephalus is a potentially devastating complication of ABM. There is wide variation in estimates of the incidence of hydrocephalus, ranging from 3 to 21% of patients. [44–46] In the Netherlands Reference Laboratory for Bacterial Meningitis (NRLBM), a prospective nationwide cohort study that captures 90% of ABM patients' CSF samples nationwide, hydrocephalus was diagnosed in 26 of 577 episodes (4.5%). The majority of these patients (69%) were diagnosed at admission. Clinical characteristics (age, presence of headache, meningismus, GCS, and causative bacteria) were similar between patients with and without hydrocephalus, but the outcomes greatly varied. Unfavorable outcomes (GOS 1–4) were seen in 18 of the 26 patients with hydrocephalus (69%), compared to 179 of the 547 patients (33%) without hydrocephalus. Mortality was similarly increased, with a rate of 46% in those with hydrocephalus and 17% of those without. The majority of cases (95%) of hydrocephalus were classified as communicating hydrocephalus, with one case classified as obstructive secondary to an intracerebral hemorrhage. It should be noted that only 6 of the 26 patients with hydrocephalus in this study underwent surgical treatment with external ventricular drainage (EVD).[44] In a Taiwanese retrospective study, 136 patients were identified with ABM over a 16-year period. Twenty-eight of these patients (21%) were found to have hydrocephalus. In their study, increased age and decreased level of consciousness on presentation were risk factors for the development of hydrocephalus. Mortality was 50%. *Klebsiella pneumoniae* was the most

commonly isolated organism from this cohort, but did not appear to increase the risk of developing hydrocephalus, and more likely reflects the higher incidence in Taiwan. Of the seven patients with EVD placement, four went on to survive with normal neurological outcomes.[46]

Therapeutic Considerations
Steroids

Animal studies have shown that outcomes in bacterial meningitis are related to the severity of inflammation in the subarachnoid space.[47] Attempts to attenuate the host inflammatory response via treatment with steroids have been evaluated in multiple trials. A Cochrane meta-analysis in 2015 found that overall, corticosteroids (most commonly dexamethasone 10 mg every 6 hours for 4 days) reduced hearing loss and neurological sequelae, but did not affect mortality in all-comers. In subanalyses, mortality was specifically reduced in pneumococcal meningitis. It appears that the beneficial effects of steroids are seen in high-income countries only.[48]

Intracranial Hypertension

The pathophysiology of elevated intracranial pressure (ICP) in ABM is complex and multifactorial. Pathogen-specific toxins and the host inflammatory response can lead to disruption of the blood–brain barrier, cerebral edema, CSF outflow obstruction (and resultant hydrocephalus), loss of cerebral autoregulation, and vasculitis leading to subsequent thrombosis, infarction, hemorrhage, or venous congestion.[49] Elevated ICP is associated with increased risk of neurological disability and death, regardless of cause. Despite early recognition of symptoms and appropriate antimicrobial therapy, some ABM patients still worsen neurologically. Substantial morbidity and mortality in ABM may be due to undertreatment of intracranial hypertension. Empiric treatment for intracranial hypertension has been attempted in several studies. The majority of these studies have looked at the use of glycerol as a routine adjunct therapy in ABM, with no clear benefit.[50]

Elevated ICP is more prevalent among patients who present with lower GCS scores and is associated with higher mortality. Targeted therapy of elevated ICP in ABM has been shown to improve outcomes. [51] Yet, the use of ICP monitors in ABM has been quite limited and is not part of any existing guidelines. This may be due to the fact that the majority of

ABM patients are not admitted to a Neuro-ICU, and medical intensive care units may focus more on systemic resuscitation than on cerebral-specific resuscitation and care. The routine use of ICP monitors has been protocoled in some institutions, and regular use in selected populations has been associated with improved outcomes. Specifically, several studies showed that the implementation of an ICP-targeted treatment protocol in a Neuro-ICU was associated with a reduction in mortality and unfavorable outcomes including hearing loss and neurological impairment leading to disability.[7,49,52] Another study found that cerebral perfusion pressure-targeted therapy was superior to an ICP-alone strategy in decreasing 90-day mortality among ABM patients.[53] The use of an EVD gives the additional benefit of allowing CSF drainage, which may also be used for ICP reduction and has specifically been shown to improve overall outcomes in many patients with ABM. The use of ICP monitors has demonstrated that significant intracranial hypertension may accompany ABM, and that with treatment, good outcomes still may be obtained: in one study, 28 patients out of 52 made a full recovery despite ICPs up to 40 mmHg.[54]

Other Adjunctive Therapies

The routine use of prophylactic AEDs, acetaminophen, and intravenous immunoglobulins (IVIg) have been shown not to be of benefit in ABM.[19] Additionally, although the presence of fever worsens the neurological prognosis in multiple conditions, including stroke and traumatic brain injury, this is less clear in ABM. An open-label, multicenter, randomized trial of moderate hypothermia (32–34°C for 48 hr) in comatose patients with ABM (77% pneumococcus) in France was stopped early due to excess mortality in the treatment group (25 of 49, 51%) compared with control group (15 of 49, 31%). It remains unknown whether target temperature management/normothermia confers any benefit.

Risk Scoring Systems

Many risk scoring systems have been published, but unfortunately none has performed well enough to use for individual patient management.[27] For research purposes, the Weisfelt score has been identified as the best instrument for scientific research on risk stratification in community-acquired ABM in high-income countries, but is not reliable in LMIC.[55] The Weisfelt score uses age, tachycardia (> 120 bpm), GCS, cranial nerve palsy, low CSF

leukocyte count (< 1,000 cells/mm^3), and positive CSF Gram stain (Table 8.2).

Bacterial Meningitis in Neurosurgical Patients

One to 7% of neurosurgical procedures are complicated by infection, though some procedures, such as placement of an EVD, are associated with higher rates of infection (2–22%) than other procedures, such as craniotomy (5–8%) and spinal surgery (6%).[56] The most frequent pathogens implicated in EVD-related meningitis are different than in community-acquired meningitis. Most commonly, skin flora such as *Staphylococcus* species (*S. aureus, S. epidermidis*) or *Propionibacterium acnes* are the causative agents, with some contribution of gram-negative pathogens. CSF leaks in post-operative and trauma, patients as well as prolonged duration of EVD catheter placement, are strong risk factors for development of meningitis. The symptoms of bacterial meningitis may be hard to distinguish from the underlying neurological/neurosurgical pathology. The course of meningitis may also be more indolent. As much as 50% of this population of patients with EVD-associated infections may experience subsequent neurological complications.[57] The use of prophylactic antibiotics is controversial. On one hand, studies have shown decreased infection when used around the time of placement.[58] On the other, ongoing antibiotic therapy for the duration of EVD catheter placement may not necessarily decrease rates of meningo-ventriculitis, and may allow for selection of more virulent gram-negative organisms.[59]

Brain Abscess and Empyema

Bacterial pathogens may also lead to a focal collection of pus within the brain parenchyma (abscess) or between the arachnoid and dura mater (subdural empyema). Classically, patients present with headache, fever, and focal neurological deficits. Intracranial suppurative infections may be due to contiguous infection from otitis/mastoiditis (33%), sinusitis (10%), meningitis (6%), or odontogenic sources (5%); hematogenous spread from a distant source (33%); head trauma (13%); or prior neurosurgical procedures (9%).[60] These infections are quite rare, estimated at 0.3 to 1.3 per 100,000 people per year, but can be considerably higher in certain risk groups, including patients with HIV/AIDS,[61] in whom outcomes are often worse.

Table 8.2 Weisfelt score for risk stratification in community-acquired acute bacterial meningitis

Age (years)	Points
20	0
30	2
40	4
50	6
60	8
70	10
80	12

Tachycardia (heart rate greater than 120 beats/minute)	Points
No	0
Yes	10

Cranial nerve palsy	Points
No	0
Yes	9

Cerebrospinal fluid (CSF) leukocyte count	Points
High	0
Low (<1,000 cells/mm^3)	13

CSF Gram stain	Points
Gram-negative cocci	0
No bacteria	1
Other bacterial species	2
Gram-positive cocci	12

Total points (sum of all point values from above variables)	Estimated probability of an unfavorable outcome
0	3.2
5	5.1
10	8.2
15	13
20	20
25	29
30	40
35	52
40	64
45	75
50	83
55	89
60	93
65	96

Overall, outcomes with brain abscess are variable. Similar to ABM, impaired consciousness, seizures, and focal neurological deficits at presentation are associated with unfavorable outcomes (death or long-term disability).[62] A high number of survivors develop epilepsy. When abscess is complicated by rupture into the ventricular system with resultant ventriculitis and hydrocephalus, the mortality greatly increases from 27% to 85%.[60] Yet, overall mortality has greatly improved, from 40% in the 1950s to 5–10% in 2014, and a large number of survivors make a full recovery (33% in the 1950s vs. 64–70% in 2014).[62,63]

Viral Infections of the CNS

Encephalitis

Encephalitis describes direct inflammation of the brain parenchyma and can occur with or without concomitant meningitis. Although encephalitis can result from a primary inflammatory process, worldwide, infection is the most common cause of acute encephalitis.[64–66] Infectious encephalitides may be either primary, characterized by viral invasion of the central nervous system, or post-infectious, with inflammation occurring after resolution of the infection. In the acute setting, patients with infectious encephalitis often require prolonged intensive care. Encephalitis may be complicated by seizures, including refractory status epilepticus, as well as cerebral edema, and in the post-acute setting, survivors of infectious encephalitis may suffer from neurocognitive sequelae or epilepsy.[67–69]

The modern study of epidemic encephalitis began with descriptions of encephalitis lethargica by Constantin von Economo in 1917, following his examination of several patients at the University of Vienna who had presented with marked lethargy, ocular dysmotility, psychiatric symptoms, fever, and movement disorders.[70] The epidemic persisted into the 1930s, and the prognosis was grim: one in three patients died during the acute phase of the illness, and half of survivors were left with permanent neurological deficits, including parkinsonism and akinetic mutism.

A century later, descriptions of infectious encephalitis related to a diverse range of etiologies have grown exponentially, with more than 100 infectious species identified as causative agents of encephalitis, with variable rates of survival and long-term morbidity (Table 8.3). In contemporary clinical practice, both emerging infections, such as Zika virus, and reemerging infections, such as measles virus, are of particular clinical relevance.

Challenges and Limitations

Prognostication following encephalitis is challenging, limited by the diverse range of etiologies and by the frequency of cryptogenic encephalitis, seen in up to half of cases.[64,71] Directed therapy is often delayed because of diagnostic uncertainty, and historical studies often fail to distinguish between infectious and autoimmune etiologies of encephalitis.

In the acute critical care setting, few studies have examined survivorship at the population level with a focus on infectious encephalitis. A retrospective study of 103 patients hospitalized with acute encephalitis in a US tertiary care center (37% with confirmed infectious etiologies) found a mortality rate of 19%.[67] Mortality was significantly associated with the presence of cerebral edema, status epilepticus, and thrombocytopenia. Among survivors, 36% had mild disability at last follow-up, with a favorable outcome associated with infectious rather than autoimmune encephalitis, and poor outcome associated with a need for ventilator support.

Studies of long-term outcomes following infectious encephalitis are similarly limited. A 3-year prospective study in France examined 176 surviving patients with a history of infectious encephalitis who survived their hospitalization, and found that 5% died of delayed complications related to their encephalitis.[69] Sixty-one percent survived without sequelae, 18% were mildly impaired, 14% were

Table 8.3 Pathogens that cause encephalitis

Sporadic pathogens	
Herpesviruses	Herpes simplex virus type 1 and 2, varicella zoster, Epstein–Barr, and cytomegalovirus viruses and human herpes viruses type 6 and 7
Enteroviruses	Coxsackie, echo, enterovirus 70 and 71, parechovirus, and polio viruses
Paramyxovirus	Measles and mumps viruses
Others	Influenza, adenovirus, parvovirus, lymphocytic choriomeningitis, and rubella viruses
Geographically restricted pathogens	
Americas	West Nile, La Crosse, St. Louis, Rocio, Powassan encephalitis, Venezuelan encephalitis, eastern and western equine encephalitis, Colorado tick fever, dengue, and rabies viruses
Europe/Middle East	West Nile, Toscana, rabies, and dengue viruses
Africa	West Nile, rabies, Rift Valley fever, dengue, and Chikungunya viruses
Asia	Japanese encephalitis, West Nile, Murray Valley encephalitis, dengue, Nipah, Chikungunya, and rabies viruses
Australia	Murray Valley encephalitis, Japanese encephalitis, dengue, and Kunjin viruses

severely impaired, and 1% remained in a vegetative state. Neurocognitive deficits at follow-up included difficulties in concentration, behavioral and speech disorders, and memory loss. One-quarter of those who were previously employed had not returned to work.

A Swedish study of 71 children who were hospitalized with acute encephalitis, half with a confirmed infectious etiology, found that 60% of children ages 5 and over, and 45% of children under age 5, at the time of encephalitis had persistent symptoms, including personality changes, poor memory, noise sensitivity, and poor concentration.[68] Among those reporting complete recovery, the majority recovered within 6 months of hospitalization. Risk factors for persisting symptoms included admission to an ICU during the acute phase of illness, abnormal electroencephalogram (EEG) findings, and the presence of fever. Ten percent of the children developed epilepsy after recovery from their acute encephalitis.

Studies describing mortality and outcomes following all-cause encephalitis are useful in counseling and prognostication given the frequency of cryptogenic encephalitis. However, mortality rates and recovery following acute infectious encephalitis vary based on the infectious pathogen and promptness of initiation of directed therapy. For instance, established rabies encephalitis is overwhelmingly fatal, while other forms of viral encephalitis carry a more favorable prognosis.[72]

Herpesviruses

Herpes Simplex Virus

Despite widely available antiviral therapy, herpes simplex virus (HSV) is the most common cause of fatal encephalitis worldwide. The mortality rate in untreated HSV encephalitis is 70%, and fewer than 3% of untreated patients return to full independence. [73,74] In the 1980s, two trials demonstrated reduced mortality in patients treated with acyclovir, with 80% survival; however, half of survivors suffered from permanent neurological disability, typically cognitive and other memory impairments.[75,76] Factors contributing to the likelihood of a full functional recovery included younger age and higher GCS in the acute setting. However, the literature has suffered from a relative paucity of studies on outcomes following HSV encephalitis in the post-acyclovir era (see Case Study 8.3).

A 2002 retrospective multicenter study of 93 adults with HSV encephalitis treated with acyclovir found that at 6 months, 15% had died and 20% had severe disability. Factors associated with poor prognosis included a delay of acyclovir initiation of 2 or more days.[77] A larger 2007 Swedish study of 236 patients with a laboratory-confirmed diagnosis of HSV-1 encephalitis followed patients for a median of 4.3 years per patient.[78] One-year mortality was 14%, with an overall mortality rate of 25%. Of the survivors, 87% were readmitted to the hospital, most often for epilepsy, with a 60- to 90-fold increase in epilepsy risk compared with that of the general population. Neuropsychiatric sequelae were evident in 22% of survivors, and the incidence of venous thromboembolism, including pulmonary embolism, was 5–14 times higher than that of the general population.

As a result of the particular predilection of HSV for the temporal lobe and limbic structures, specific neuropsychiatric deficits seen in survivors of HSV encephalitis include anterograde amnesia and Klüver–Bucy syndrome, characterized by diminished ability to visually recognize objects, loss of normal anger and fear responses, and inappropriate sexual behaviors.[79–81] Electroencephalography has been found to aid in prognostication following acute HSV encephalitis in the intensive care unit. In a study of 76 hospitalized patients who underwent EEG monitoring during acute encephalitis, having a normal EEG was an independent predictor of survival adjusting for confounders such as coma, cerebral edema, and mechanical ventilation.[82]

Several recent studies have suggested that in some patients, sequelae and recurrence of HSV encephalitis despite treatment may be related to post-viral autoimmune encephalitis. A 2017 prospective study of 51 patients with HSV encephalitis found that 27% developed autoimmune encephalitis with positive neuronal antibodies (64% with anti-N-methyl-D-aspartate receptor antibodies).[83] Of the patients who did not develop recurrent encephalitis, 30% still developed antibodies. Autoimmune encephalitis most often presented within 2 months after treatment, and symptoms were age-dependent, with a worse outcome in young children. Patients who develop autoimmune encephalitis are likely to have recurrent epilepsy or neuropsychiatric symptoms that may be mitigated by immunotherapy.

Case Study 8.3 A 76-year-old gentleman presented with seizure activity and respiratory failure requiring intubation. Initial MRI showed (A) T2-FLAIR hyperintensities of the bilateral temporal lobes. Lumbar puncture revealed a lymphocytic pleocytosis and positive herpes simplex virus (HSV) 1 PCR. He was started on acyclovir. Repeat MRI 3 days into admission revealed worsening, extensive confluent T2/FLAIR signal hyperintensities involving (B) the bilateral mesial temporal lobes and (C) extending throughout the bilateral cerebral hemispheres, with multiple areas of diffusion restriction involving D) the gyri and E) right more than left temporal lobes. At the conclusion of a 21-day course of acyclovir, he continued to demonstrate ongoing status epilepticus and autonomic lability.

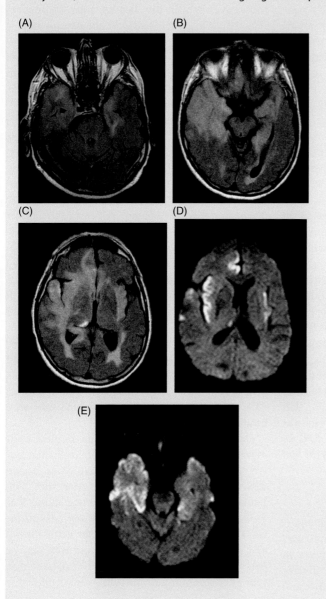

(A)　(B)　(C)　(D)　(E)

Varicella Zoster Virus

Varicella zoster virus (VZV) has been described in association with two distinct forms of encephalitis: acute cerebellar ataxia in children younger than 15 and diffuse encephalitis seen in both adults and young children. Although cerebellar ataxia is typically self-limited and followed by complete recovery, diffuse encephalitis can manifest with a range of clinical features and carries a particularly poor prognosis in older and immunocompromised patients. Mortality rates approach 10% in patients with diffuse VZV encephalitis, with long-term neurological sequelae reported in 15%.[84–86] Patients with VZV encephalitis may also have a concomitant VZV vasculitis involving the intra- and extracranial vessels, characterized by vessel wall damage and transmural granulomatous inflammation. Approximately 1 in 15,000 cases of primary VZV infection are associated with subsequent stroke; the risk of stroke is highest in those with ophthalmic-distribution VZV, particularly within the first 3 months after infection and up to 1 year.[87–89]

Although CSF VZV PCR is incompletely sensitive for diagnosis, studies suggest that quantitative PCR may correlate with the severity and duration of encephalitis.[90] In addition to sequelae of stroke, survivors of VZV encephalitis may continue to suffer from neuropsychiatric symptoms, cranial neuropathy, and epilepsy.[91] One case series of 20 patients with VZV encephalopathy without vasculopathy found that 15% died during the acute phase of infection, and 45% were discharged with deficits that included cognitive impairment and sensorimotor deficits.[92] At follow-up 3 years later, 13% of the initial survivors were deceased, and 41% had moderate to severe sequelae.

Arboviruses

In recent years, the emergence and re-emergence of a number of arthropod-borne viruses (arboviruses) have brought these infections to public attention. Arboviruses are a diverse group of viruses transmitted by mosquito and tick vectors. Neurotropic arboviruses can cause severe encephalitis and other diseases of the central nervous system. Although outcomes vary by virus, across arbovirus encephalitides, roughly half of survivors suffer permanent neurological damage.[93]

West Nile Virus

In 1999, West Nile virus (WNV), a little-known flavivirus, caused a cluster of 62 cases of meningoencephalitis and acute flaccid paralysis in New York City.[94] In the United States, WNV remains the most common neurotropic arbovirus, although less than 1% of infected patients develop neurological disease. Among patients with neuroinvasive WNV, the fatality rate approaches 10%, while in patients with WNV encephalitis, it is 20%.[95] Risk factors for developing neuroinvasive disease include immunodeficiency, extremes of age, and underlying diabetes mellitus. Death in the acute setting is most often a result of respiratory failure or cardiac complications.

Studies of functional outcomes among survivors of symptomatic WNV are limited by small sample sizes, and often focus on deficits resulting from acute flaccid paralysis rather than encephalitis. One study of 49 patients with WNV-associated fever, meningitis, or encephalitis, followed up 13 months after diagnosis, found ongoing self-reported deficits related to fatigue, memory, weakness, and word-finding disability, with an overall sense of poor physical health.[96] Neuropsychological testing showed abnormalities of motor skills, attention, and executive functions. A later study of 116 patients both with and without neuroinvasive disease, followed up 18 months after initial presentation, found that concentration difficulties and confusion were more common among patients with neuroinvasive disease than those with isolated WNV fever.[97] Among patients hospitalized with WNV encephalitis in Colorado, 75% required some amount of assisted care after hospitalization for acute illness.[98]

Movement disorders and extrapyramidal findings are common following WNV encephalitis, but are transient in many patients. However, a case series of 16 patients observed after the 2002 Louisiana epidemic of WNV infection found that 38% continued to display tremors and parkinsonism 8 months after resolution of the acute illness, and a study in North Dakota found that new or persistent tremor was reported in 20% of patients 1 year after resolution of the initial illness.[96,99]

Zika Virus

In 2014, following several large outbreaks of Zika viral infection with accompanying neurological symptoms, the World Health Organization declared the disease a global crisis. Like WNV, Zika virus is a flavivirus, closely related to dengue virus. As has WNV, Zika virus has been described as a human pathogen for decades, but has only manifested with outbreaks in recent years. Given the rarity of encephalitis and the relatively recent awareness of neurological Zika infection, studies regarding long-term outcomes are relatively lacking. Guillain–Barré syndrome (GBS) is the most commonly described neurological manifestation, but in a study of Zika viral infection during the French West Indies 2016 outbreak, 21% of patients were found to have encephalitis or encephalomyelitis.[100] Among all infected patients, 37% required ICU care and 24% required mechanical ventilation, more often in patients with GBS. At 14 months, three patients were deceased, one with encephalitis. Twenty-five percent of survivors had residual disability, more severe in patients with positive Zika virus PCR in urine, plasma, or CSF.

Powassan Virus

Powassan virus is a rare tick-borne flavivirus in North America, though it is being seen with increasing incidence. Encephalitis is present in the majority of neuroinvasive cases. Approximately 10–15% of neuroinvasive cases are fatal, and half of the nonfatal cases develop severe neurological sequelae, including memory loss and weakness.[101,102] A series of eight cases of Powassan virus encephalitis in New England included two patients who died during their acute illness, with findings of brain herniation. Of the survivors, two had severe residual deficits, with one patient who had purposeful movement only in the left upper extremity and could only intermittently follow simple, one-step commands, and one patient with persistent headaches, cerebellar dysarthria, delayed motor function, and incoordination 18 months after acute presentation. Four patients were described as having a favorable recovery, including two who returned to work and had normal neuroimaging and examinations at follow-up.[101] Large-scale studies are needed to better characterize long-term outcomes following Powassan virus encephalitis.

Japanese Encephalitis Virus

Japanese encephalitis virus is the most common cause of arboviral epidemic encephalitis worldwide, with 70,000 cases and 15,000 deaths reported annually.[103] In patients with neurological disease, symptoms include decreased mental status and sometimes coma. Up to 85% of patients will develop seizures during their illness, and worse outcomes, defined as either death or inability to independently perform activities of daily living at follow-up, are associated with multiple seizures, prolonged seizures, or status epilepticus.[104] Prominent extrapyramidal signs, including masked facies, tremor, hypertonia, choreoathetosis, and dystonia, are also common. [105–107] The case fatality rate of Japanese encephalitis is 30%, with an additional 50% of patients experiencing long-term neurological and functional sequelae.[108,109]

Paramyxoviruses

Measles Virus

Measles is a highly contagious viral infection. Although routine vaccination of children in the United States has largely eliminated endemic infection, measles remains an important cause of morbidity and mortality in children worldwide, and outbreaks still occur in the United States among unvaccinated individuals. In the setting of international travel and variable rates of vaccination, 704 cases of measles were reported to the Centers for Disease Control and Prevention (CDC) between January 1, 2019, and April 26, 2019, the highest rate in a single year since 1994 and since measles was declared eliminated within the country in 2000.[110]

Acute encephalitis is a rare complication of measles infection, occurring in 0.1% of cases.[111] The mortality rate of acute measles encephalitis is 10–15%, with 25% of survivors sustaining permanent neurological sequelae. Measles inclusion body encephalitis (MIBE) can also develop in the subacute setting, seen within the first year of infection. MIBE is characteristically seen in immunocompromised patients, and has been described in patients with malignancies, HIV infection, kidney transplantation, stem cell transplantation, and autoimmune illnesses. The mortality of this syndrome approaches 100%.[112,113] Subacute sclerosing panencephalitis (SSPE), most often seen in children, occurs years after initial infection and is progressive and overwhelmingly fatal. Measles infection at an early age is a risk factor for the development of SSPE. Symptoms typically progress through stages that include insidious neurological symptoms followed by myoclonus, autonomic dysfunction, and ultimately brain death.[114]

Acute disseminated encephalomyelitis (ADEM) may occur as a post-infectious, autoimmune

137

response to the measles virus in 0.1% of patients, presenting during the recovery phase.[115] ADEM following measles infection is associated with 10–20% mortality, compared with 7% in patients with ADEM due to other causes. Survivors often suffer from residual neurological deficits, including epilepsy and neuropsychiatric disorders.[116]

Mumps Virus

Mumps was formerly a leading cause of encephalitis, though routine vaccination has rendered mumps encephalitis virtually eradicated. In addition to diffuse encephalitis, patients may present with cerebellitis or cerebellar ataxia.[117] Mumps encephalitis carries a mortality rate of less than 5%, and the majority of patients recover completely.[118]

Coronavirus Disease 2019

Neurological manifestations of severe acute respiratory syndrome coronavirus 2 (SARS-CoV-2) infection are common regardless of the severity of illness. Among hospitalized patients, encephalopathy occurs frequently, in up to 55% of those who are critically ill, [119] while other serious complications such as stroke or seizure occur in less than 5%. For patients with COVID-19 infection, serious neurological manifestations, including encephalopathy, are associated with higher rates of ICU admission, increased disability, and higher mortality. Acute encephalitis due to SARS-CoV-2 is rare, reported in less than 0.5% of hospitalized patients.[120] Neither neuropathology nor CSF studies suggest widespread neuroinvasion, suggesting the majority of cases of encephalitis are para-infectious or immune mediated encephalitis. The mortality for SARS-CoV-2 associated encephalitis is 15%.[121]

Conclusion

Neurological infections, including meningitis, abscess, and encephalitis, are commonly encountered in the Neuro-ICU as well as other intensive care units. Tremendous advances have been made in treatment, but the prognosis for many of these infections remains highly variable. More research is needed to better understand prevention and optimal therapy of both the primary infection and secondary neurological complications in order to improve survival and functional outcomes

References

1. LaPenna PA, Roos KL. Bacterial infections of the central nervous system. *Sem Neurol.* 2019;**39** (03):334–42.

2. World Health Organization. Defeating meningitis by 2030: developing a global roadmap. 2019.

3. Thigpen MC, Whitney SG, Messonnier NE, et al. Bacterial meningitis in the United States, 1998–2007. *N Engl J Med.* 2011;**364**(21):2016–25.

4. Durand M, Calderwood S, Weber D, et al. Acute bacterial meningitis in adults: a review of 493 episodes. *N Engl J Med.* 1993;**328**:21–8.

5. Buchholz G, Koedel U, Pfister H-W, Kastenbauer S, Klein M. Dramatic reduction of mortality in pneumococcal meningitis. *Crit Care.* 2016;**20** (1):312.

6. Bijlsma MW, Brouwer MC, Kasanmoentalib ES, et al. Community-acquired bacterial meningitis in adults in the Netherlands, 2006–14: a prospective cohort study. *Lancet Infect Dis.* 2016;**16**(3): 339–47.

7. Glimåker M, Brink M, Naucler P, Sjölin J. Betamethasone and dexamethasone in adult community-acquired bacterial meningitis: a quality registry study from 1995 to 2014. *Clin Microbiol Infect.* 2016;**22**(9):814.e1–814.e7.

8. Gudina EK, Tesfaye M, Wieser A, Pfister H-W, Klein M. Outcome of patients with acute bacterial meningitis in a teaching hospital in Ethiopia: a prospective study. *PLoS One.* 2018;**13**(7): e0200067.

9. Wall EC, Mukaka M, Scarborough M, et al. Prediction of outcome from adult bacterial meningitis in a high-hiv-seroprevalence, resource-poor setting using the Malawi Adult Meningitis Score (MAMS). *Clin Infect Dis.* 2017;**64**(4):413–19.

10. Zunt JR, Kassebaum NJ, Blake N, et al. Global, regional, and national burden of meningitis, 1990–2016: a systematic analysis for the Global Burden of Disease Study 2016. *Lancet Neurol.* 2018;**17**(12):1061–82.

11. Edmond K, Clark A, Korczak VS, et al. Global and regional risk of disabling sequelae from bacterial meningitis: a systematic review and meta-analysis. *Lancet Infect Dis.* 2010;**10**(5):317–28.

12. Wiebe R, Crast FW, Hall R, Bass J. Clinical factors relating to prognosis of bacterial meningitis. *South Med J.* 1972;**65**(3):257–64.

13. Bohr V, Hansen B, Jessen O, et al. Eight hundred and seventy-five cases of bacterial meningitis. Part I of a three-part series: clinical data, prognosis, and the role of specialised hospital departments. *J Infect.* 1983;7(1):21–30.

14. Pfister H-W. Spectrum of complications during bacterial meningitis in adults: results of a prospective clinical study. *Arch Neurol*. 1993;**50**(6):575.

15. Cabellos C, Verdaguer R, Olmo M, et al. Community-acquired bacterial meningitis in elderly patients: experience over 30 years. *Medicine*. 2009;**88**(2):115–19.

16. Lai W-A, Chen S-F, Tsai N-W, et al. Clinical characteristics and prognosis of acute bacterial meningitis in elderly patients over 65: a hospital-based study. *BMC Geriatr*. 2011;**11**(1):91.

17. Weisfelt M, de Gans J, van der Ende A, van de Beek D. Community-acquired bacterial meningitis in alcoholic patients. *PLoS One*. 2010;**5**(2):e9102.

18. van Veen KEB, Brouwer MC, van der Ende A, van de Beek D. Bacterial meningitis in diabetes patients: a population-based prospective study. Sci Rep. 2016;**6**(1):36996.

19. van de Beek D, Cabellos C, Dzupova O, et al. ESCMID guideline: diagnosis and treatment of acute bacterial meningitis. *Clin Microbiol Infect*. 2016;**22**:S37–62.

20. Aronin SI. Community-acquired bacterial meningitis: risk stratification for adverse clinical outcome and effect of antibiotic timing. *Ann Intern Med*. 1998;**129**(11):862.

21. Lebel MH, McCracken GH Jr. Delayed cerebrospinal fluid sterilization and adverse outcome of bacterial meningitis in infants and children. *Infect Dis Newsletter*. 1990;**9**(1):7–8.

22. Schaad U, Suter S, Gianella-Borradori A, et al. A comparison of ceftriaxone and cefuroxime for the treatment of bacterial meningitis in children. *N Engl J Med*. 1990;**322**(3):141–7.

23. Tunkel AR, Hartman BJ, Kaplan SL, et al. Practice guidelines for the management of bacterial meningitis. *Clin Infect Dis*. 2004;**39**(9):1267–84.

24. Lucas MJ, Brouwer MC, van der Ende A, van de Beek D. Outcome in patients with bacterial meningitis presenting with a minimal Glasgow Coma Scale score. *Neurol Neuroimmunol Neuroinflamm*. 2014;**1**(1):e9.

25. van de Beek D, de Gans J, Spanjaard L, et al. Clinical features and prognostic factors in adults with bacterial meningitis. *N Engl J Med*. 2004;**351**(18):1849–59.

26. Flores-Cordero JM, Amaya-Villar R, Rincón-Ferrari MD, et al. Acute community-acquired bacterial meningitis in adults admitted to the intensive care unit: clinical manifestations, management and prognostic factors. *Inten Care Med*. 2003;**29**(11):1967–73.

27. Bijlsma MW, Brouwer MC, Bossuyt PM, et al. Risk scores for outcome in bacterial meningitis: Systematic review and external validation study. *J Infect*. 2016;**73**(5):393–401.

28. Schutte C-M, van der Meyden CH. A prospective study of Glasgow Coma Scale (GCS), age, CSF-neutrophil count, and CSF-protein and glucose levels as prognostic indicators in 100 adult patients with meningitis. *J Infect*. 1998;**37**(2):112–15.

29. van Ettekoven CN, Brouwer MC, Bijlsma MW, Wijdicks EFM, van de Beek D. The FOUR score as predictor of outcome in adults with bacterial meningitis. *Neurology*. 2019;**92**(22):e2522–6.

30. Wijdicks EFM, Bamlet WR, Maramattom BV, Manno EM, McClelland RL. Validation of a new coma scale: the FOUR score. *Ann Neurol*. 2005;**58**(4):585–93.

31. Lu C-H, Huang C-R, Chang W-N, et al. Community-acquired bacterial meningitis in adults: the epidemiology, timing of appropriate antimicrobial therapy, and prognostic factors. Clin Neurol Neurosurg. 2002;**104**(4):352–8.

32. Zoons E, Weisfelt M, de Gans J, Spanjaard L. Seizures in adults with bacterial meningitis. *Neurology*. 2008;**70**(22):2109–15.

33. Larsen FTBD, Brandt CT, larsen L, et al. Risk factors and prognosis of seizures in adults with community-acquired bacterial meningitis in Denmark: observational cohort studies. *BMJ Open*. 2019;**9**(7):e030263.

34. Kastenbauer S, Pfister H-W. Pneumococcal meningitis in adults: spectrum of complications and prognostic factors in a series of 87 cases. *Brain*. 2003;**126**(5):1015–25.

35. Schut ES, Lucas MJ, Brouwer MC, et al. Cerebral infarction in adults with bacterial meningitis. *Neurocrit Care*. 2012;**16**(3):421–7.

36. Pfister H-W, Borasio GD, Dirnagl U, Bauer M, Einhaupl KM. Cerebrovascular complications of bacterial meningitis in adults. *Neurology*. 1992;**42**(8):1497.

37. Shulman JG, Cervantes-Arslanian AM. Infectious etiologies of stroke. *Semin Neurol*. 2019;**39**(4):482–94.

38. Boelman C, Shroff M, Yau I, et al. Antithrombotic therapy for secondary stroke prevention in bacterial meningitis in children. *J Pediatr*. 2014;**165**(4):799–806.

39. Misra UK, Kalita J, Nair PP. Role of aspirin in tuberculous meningitis: a randomized open label placebo controlled trial. *J Neurol Sci*. 2010;**293**(1–2):12–17.

40. Pugin D, Copin J-C, Goodyear M-C, Landis T, Gasche Y. Persisting vasculitis after pneumococcal meningitis. *Neurocrit Care*. 2006;**4**(3):237–40.

41. Czartoski T. Postinfectious vasculopathy with evolution to moyamoya syndrome. *J NeurolNeurosurgPsychiatry*. 2005;**76**(2):256–9.

42. Ries S, Schminke U, Fassbender K, et al. Cerebrovascular involvement in the acute phase of bacterial meningitis. *J Neurol*. 1996;**244**(1):51–5.

43. Sporrborn JL, Knudsen GB, Sølling M, et al. Brain ventricular dimensions and relationship to outcome in adult patients with bacterial meningitis. *BMC Infect Dis*. 2015;**15**(1):367.

44. Soemirien Kasanmoentalib E, Brouwer MC, van der Ende A, van de Beek D. Hydrocephalus in adults with community-acquired bacterial meningitis. *Neurology*. 2010;**75**(10):918–23.

45. Bodilsen J, Schønheyder HC, Nielsen H. Hydrocephalus is a rare outcome in community-acquired bacterial meningitis in adults: a retrospective analysis. *BMC Infect Dis*. 2013;**13**(1):321.

46. Wang K-W, Chang W-N, Chang H-W, Wang H-C, Lu C-H. Clinical relevance of hydrocephalus in bacterial meningitis in adults. *Surg Neurol*. 2005;**64**(1):61–5.

47. Mook-Kanamori BB, Geldhoff M, van der Poll T, van de Beek D. Pathogenesis and pathophysiology of pneumococcal meningitis. *Clin Microbiol Rev*. 2011;**24**(3):557–91.

48. Brouwer MC, McIntyre P, Prasad K, van de Beek D. Corticosteroids for acute bacterial meningitis. *Cochrane Database Syst Rev*. 2015;**2015**(9): CD004405

49. Tariq A, Aguilar-Salinas P, Hanel RA, Naval N, Chmayssani M. The role of ICP monitoring in meningitis. *Neurosurg Focus*. 2017;**43**(5):E7.

50. Wall EC, Ajdukiewicz KM, Bergman H, Heyderman RS, Garner P. Osmotic therapies added to antibiotics for acute bacterial meningitis. *Cochrane Database Syst Rev*. 2018;**2**(2): CD008806.

51. Lindvall P, Ahlm C, Ericsson M, et al. Reducing intracranial pressure may increase survival among patients with bacterial meningitis. *Clin Infect Dis*. 2004;**38**:384–90.

52. Grande P-O, Myhre EB, Nordstrom C-H, Schliamser S. Treatment of intracranial hypertension and aspects on lumbar dural puncture in severe bacterial meningitis. *Acta Anaesthesiol Scand*. 2002;**46**(3):264–70.

53. Kumar R, Singhi S, Singhi P, et al. Randomized controlled trial comparing cerebral perfusion pressure–targeted therapy versus intracranial pressure–targeted therapy for raised intracranial pressure due to acute cns infections in children. *Crit Care Med*. 2014;**42**(8):1775–87.

54. Glimåker M, Johansson B, Halldorsdottir H, et al. Neuro-intensive treatment targeting intracranial hypertension improves outcome in severe bacterial meningitis: an intervention-control study. *PLoS One*. 2014;**9**(3):e91976.

55. Weisfelt M, van de Beek D, Spanjaard L, Reitsma JB, de Gans J. A risk score for unfavorable outcome in adults with bacterial meningitis. *Ann Neurol*. 2008;**63**(1):90–7.

56. Sader E, Moore J, Cervantes-Arslanian AM. Neurosurgical Infections. *Semin Neurol*. 2019;**39**:1–8.

57. Weisfelt M, van de Beek D, Spanjaard L, de Gans J. Nosocomial bacterial meningitis in adults: a prospective series of 50 cases. *J Hosp Infect*. 2007;**66**(1):71–8.

58. Sonabend AM, Korenfeld Y, Crisman C, et al. Prevention of ventriculostomy-related infections with prophylactic antibiotics and antibiotic-coated external ventricular drains: a systematic review. *Neurosurgery*. 2011;**68**(4):996–1005.

59. Lyke KE, Obasanjo OO, Williams MA, et al. Ventriculitis Complicating Use of Intraventricular Catheters in Adult Neurosurgical Patients. *Clin Infect Dis*. 2001;**33**(12):2028–33.

60. Brouwer MC, Tunkel AR, McKhann GM, van de Beek D. Brain abscess. *N Eng J Med*. 2014;**371**(5):447–56.

61. Kastenbauer S, Pfister H-W, Wispelwey B, Scheld WM. Brain abscess. In *Infections of the Central Nervous System*. 3rd ed. Philadelphia: Lippincott Williams & Wilkins; 2004:479–507.

62. Widdrington JD, Bond H, Schwab U, et al. Pyogenic brain abscess and subdural empyema: presentation, management, and factors predicting outcome. *Infection*. 2018;**46**(6):785–92.

63. Brouwer MC, Coutinho JM, van de Beek D. Clinical characteristics and outcome of brain abscess: systematic review and meta-analysis. *Neurology*. 2014;**82**(9):806–13.

64. Glaser CA, Gilliam S, Schnurr D, et al. In search of encephalitis etiologies: diagnostic challenges in the California Encephalitis Project, 1998–2000. *Clin Infect Dis*. 2003;**36**(6):731–42.

65. Tunkel AR, Glaser CA, Bloch KC, et al. The management of encephalitis: clinical practice guidelines by the Infectious Diseases Society

of America. *Clin Infect Dis*. 2008;**47** (3):303–27.

66. Chaudhuri A, Kennedy PGE. Diagnosis and treatment of viral encephalitis. *Postgrad Med J*. 2002;**78**(924):575–83.

67. Thakur KT, Motta M, Asemota AO, et al. Predictors of outcome in acute encephalitis. *Neurology*. 2013;**81**(9):793–800.

68. Fowler A, Stodberg T, Eriksson M, Wickstrom R. Long-term outcomes of acute encephalitis in childhood. *Pediatrics*. 2010;**126**(4):e828–35.

69. Mailles A, Stahl J. Infectious encephalitis in France in 2007: a national prospective study. *Clin Infect Dis*. 2009;**49**(12):1838–47.

70. Lutters B, Foley P, Koehler PJ. The centennial lesson of encephalitis lethargica. *Neurology*. 2018;**90**(12):563–7.

71. Granerod J, Tam CC, Crowcroft NS, et al. Challenge of the unknown: a systematic review of acute encephalitis in non-outbreak situations. *Neurology*. 2010;**75**(10):924–32.

72. World Health Organization. WHO Expert Consultation on Rabies: WHO TRS No. 982. Second report. World Health Organization technical report series. 2013.

73. Whitley RJ. Herpes simplex virus infections of the central nervous system: encephalitis and neonatal herpes. *Drugs*. 1991;**42**(3):406–27.

74. Whitley RJ. Herpes simplex encephalitis: adolescents and adults. *Antiviral Res*. 2006;**71**(2–3):141–8.

75. Whitley RJ, Alford CA, Hirsch MS, et al. Vidarabine versus acyclovir therapy in herpes simplex encephalitis. *N Engl J Med*. 1986;**314** (3):144–9.

76. Sköldenberg B, Alestig K, Burman L, et al. Acyclovir versus vidarabine in herpes simplex encephalitis. Randomised multicentre study in consecutive Swedish patients. *Lancet*. 1984;**2** (8405):707–11.

77. Raschilas F, Wolff M, Delatour F, et al. Outcome of and prognostic factors for herpes simplex encephalitis in adult patients: results of a multicenter study. *Clin Infect Dis*. 2002;**35** (3):254–60.

78. Hjalmarsson A, Blomqvist P, Skoldenberg B. Herpes simplex encephalitis in Sweden, 1990–2001: incidence, morbidity, and mortality. *Clin Infect Dis*. 2007;**445**(7):875–80.

79. Grydeland H, Walhovd KB, Westlye LT, et al. Amnesia following herpes simplex encephalitis: diffusion-tensor imaging uncovers reduced integrity of normal-appearing white matter. *Radiology*. 2010;**257**(3):74–81.

80. Gordon B, Selnes OA, Hart J, Hanley DF, Whitley RJ. Long-term cognitive sequelae of acyclovir-treated herpes simplex encephalitis. *Arch Neurol*. 1990;**47**(6):646–7.

81. Hart RP, Kwentus JA, Frazier RB, Hormel TL. Natural history of Klüver-Bucy syndrome after treated herpes encephalitis. *South Med J*. 1986;**79** (11):1376–8.

82. Sutter R, Kaplan PW, Cervenka MC, et al. Electroencephalography for diagnosis and prognosis of acute encephalitis. *Clin Neurophysiol*. 2015;**126**(8):1524–31.

83. Armangue T, Spatola M, Vlagea A, et al. Frequency, symptoms, risk factors, and outcomes of autoimmune encephalitis after herpes simplex encephalitis: a prospective observational study and retrospective analysis. *Lancet Neurol*. 2018;**17** (9):760–72.

84. Kleinschmidt-Demasters BK, Amlie-Lefond C, Gilden DH. The patterns of varicella zoster virus encephalitis. *Hum Pathol*. 1996;**27** (9):927–38.

85. Fleisher G, Henry W, Mcsorley M, Arbeter A, Plotkin S. Life-threatening complications of varicella. *Am J Dis Child*. 1981;**135**(10):896–9.

86. Preblud SR. Age-specific risks of varicella complications. *Pediatrics*. 1981;**68**(1):14–17.

87. Lin HC, Chien CW, Ho J Der. Herpes zoster ophthalmicus and the risk of stroke: a population-based follow-up study. *Neurology*. 2010;**74** (10):792–7.

88. Sreenivasan N, Basit S, Wohlfahrt J, et al. The short- and long-term risk of stroke after herpes zoster – a nationwide population-based cohort study. *PLoS One*. 2013;**8**(7):e69156.

89. Langan SM, Minassian C, Smeeth L, Thomas SL. Risk of stroke following herpes zoster: A self-controlled case-series study. *Clin Infect Dis*. 2014;**58**(11):1497–503.

90. Rottenstreich A, Oz ZK, Oren I. Association between viral load of varicella zoster virus in cerebrospinal fluid and the clinical course of central nervous system infection. *Diagn Microbiol Infect Dis*. 2014;**79**(2):174–7.

91. Becerra JCL, Sieber R, Martinetti G, et al. Infection of the central nervous system caused by varicella zoster virus reactivation: a retrospective case series study. *Int J Infect Dis*. 2013;**17**(7):e529–34.

92. De Broucker T, Mailles A, Chabrier S, et al. Acute varicella zoster encephalitis without evidence of primary vasculopathy in a case-series of 20 patients. *Clin Microbiol Infect*. 2012;**18**(8):808–19.

93. Lyons JL. Viral meningitis and encephalitis. *Continuum (Minneap Minn)*. 2018;**24** (5):1284–97.

94. Nash D, Mostashari F, Fine A, et al. The outbreak of West Nile virus infection in the New York City area in 1999. *N Engl J Med*. 2001;**344**(24):1807–14.

95. Sejvar JJ, Haddad MB, Tierney BC, et al. Neurologic manifestations and outcome of West Nile virus infection. *JAMA*. 2003;**290**(4):511–15.

96. Carson PJ, Konewko P, Wold KS, et al. Long-term clinical and neuropsychological outcomes of West Nile virus infection. *Clin Infect Dis*. 2006;**43**(6):723–30.

97. Haaland KY, Sadek J, Pergam S, et al. Mental status after West Nile virus infection. *Emerg Infects Dis*. 2006;**12**(8):1620–2.

98. Bode A V., Sejvar JJ, Pape WJ, Campbell GL, Marfin AA. West Nile virus disease: a descriptive study of 228 patients hospitalized in a 4-county region of Colorado in 2003. *Clin Infect Dis*. 2006;**42**(9):1234–40.

99. Sejvar JJ, Haddad MB, Tierney BC, et al. Neurologic manifestations and outcome of West Nile virus infection. *JAMA*. 2003;**290** (4):511–15.

100. Lannuzel A, Fergé J-L, Lobjois Q, et al. Long-term outcome in neuroZika: when biological diagnosis matters. *Neurology*. 2019;**92**(21): e2406–e2420.

101. Piantadosi A, Rubin DB, McQuillen DP, et al. Emerging cases of Powassan virus Encephalitis in New England: clinical presentation, imaging, and review of the literature. *Clin Infect Dis*. 2015;**62**(6):707–13.

102. Ebel GD. Update on Powassan virus: emergence of a North American tick-borne flavivirus. *Annu Rev Entomol*. 2010;**55**:95–110.

103. Sejvar JJ. Zika virus and other emerging arboviral central nervous system infections. *Continuum (Minneap Minn)*. 2018;**24**(5):1512–34.

104. Kalita J, Misra UK. EEG in Japanese encephalitis: a clinico-radiological correlation. *Electroencephalogr Clin Neurophysiol*. 1998;**105** (3):238–43.

105. Kalita J, Misra UK. Markedly severe dystonia in Japanese encephalitis. *Mov Disord*. 2000;**15** (6):1168–72.

106. Misra UK, Kalita J. Spectrum of movement disorders in encephalitis. *J Neurol*. 2010;**257** (12):2052–8.

107. Jang H, Boltz DA, Webster RG, Smeyne RJ. Viral parkinsonism. *Biochim Biophy Acta*. 2009;**1792** (7):714–21.

108. Murgod UA, Muthane UB, Ravi V, Radhesh S, Desai A. Persistent movement disorders following Japanese encephalitis. *Neurology*. 2001;**57** (12):2313–15.

109. Misra UK, Kalita J. Prognosis of Japanese encephalitis patients with dystonia compared to those with parkinsonian features only. *Postgrad Med J*. 2002;**78**(918):238–41.

110. Patel M, Lee AD, Redd SB, et al. Increase in measles cases – United States, January 1–April 26, 2019. *MMWR Morb Mortal Wkly Rep*. 2019;**68** (17):402–4.

111. Fisher DL, Defres S, Solomon T. Measles-induced encephalitis. *QJM*. 2015;**108**(3):177–82.

112. Baldolli A, Dargère S, Cardineau E, et al. Measles inclusion-body encephalitis (MIBE) in a immunocompromised patient. *J Clin Virol*. 2016;**81**:43–6.

113. Freeman AF. A new complication of stem cell transplantation: measles inclusion body encephalitis. *Pediatrics*. 2004;**114**(5):e657–60.

114. Anlar B. Subacute sclerosing panencephalitis and chronic viral encephalitis. *Handb Clin Neurol*. 2013;**112**:1183–9.

115. Johnson RT. Measles encephalomyelitis clinical and immunologic studies. *Pediatr Infect Dis J*. 1984;**310**(3):137–41.

116. Tenembaum S, Chamoles N, Fejerman N. Acute disseminated encephalomyelitis: a long-term follow-up study of 84 pediatric patients. *Neurology*. 2002;**59**(8):1224–31.

117. Cohen HA, Ashkenazi A, Nussinovitch M, et al. Mumps-associated acute cerebellar ataxia. *Am J Dis Child*. 1992;**146**(8):930–1.

118. Koskiniemi M, Donner M, Pettay O. Clinical appearance and outcome in mumps encephalitis in children. *Acta Pædiatr Scand*. 1983;**72**(4):603–9.

119. Pun BT, Badenes R, Heras LA, et al. Prevalence and risk factors for delirium in critically ill patients with COVID-19 (COVID-D): a multicentre cohort study. *Lancet Respir Med*. 2021;**9**:239–50.

120. Cervantes-Arslanian AM, Venkata C, Anand P, et al. Neurologic manifestations of severe acute respiratory syndrome coronavirus 2 infection in hospitalized patients during the first year of the COVID-19 pandemic. *Crit Care Explor*. 2022;**4** (4):e0686.

121. Pilotto A, Masciocchi S, Volonghi I, et al. Clinical presentation and outcomes of severe acute respiratory syndrome coronavirus 2-related encephalitis: the ENCOVID multicenter study. *J Infect Dis*. 2021;**223**:28–37.

Prognostication in Neuromuscular Disease

Christopher L. Kramer and Alejandro A. Rabinstein

Introduction

Prognostication in patients with acute neuromuscular disorders presenting to the intensive care unit (ICU) can be challenging, even for experienced providers. The various neuromuscular conditions that result in severe limb and respiratory weakness are heterogeneous with regard to their pathophysiology, natural history, and response to therapy. Furthermore, many patients with respiratory weakness require ventilatory support and can have relatively protracted ICU and hospital stays where systemic complications, such as delirium, hospital-acquired infections (particularly in immunosuppressed patients), deep venous thromboses and thromboembolism, sedation requirements, pre-existing diagnoses, affective disorders, and immobilization may all confound the ability to predict long-term recovery. Yet, outcome data on some of the most common etiologies of neuromuscular weakness in the ICU, including myasthenia gravis (MG), Guillain–Barré syndrome (GBS), ICU-acquired weakness (ICUAW), and amyotrophic lateral sclerosis (ALS) is available and can aid tremendously in guiding prognostication when taken in the context of the individual patient's unique clinical condition. Accurate assessment of prognosis is particularly important for patients with neuromuscular weakness, as many of these conditions can improve substantially with treatment and time – in appropriate cases, severely affected patients and their families often require support and encouragement during the acute phase of the illness when weakness is at its nadir, communicating with the patient is difficult, uncertainty is high, and hope may be low. Conversely, prognostication in patients with neuromuscular weakness due to a degenerative condition, such as ALS, may be instrumental in determining goals of care that may result in palliation and limitation of invasive therapies. Accordingly, in this chapter, we will examine the factors that contribute to prognosis in the aforementioned conditions that may result in neuromuscular respiratory failure.

Prognostication in Myasthenia Gravis

Myasthenia gravis is a disorder of the neuromuscular junction characterized by fatigable weakness due to autoantibody binding against the post-synaptic acetylcholine receptor (AChR) or one of the proteins responsible for docking of the AChR to the cell membrane.[1,2] This weakness most commonly occurs in the facial and bulbar muscles as well as the limb muscles, where the weakness is typically most pronounced proximally.[3–5] The respiratory muscles are commonly involved, particularly in more severe cases – the term "myasthenic crisis" has been coined to characterize patients with an acute exacerbation of MG who require ventilatory assistance.[6] To classify and communicate disease severity, the Myasthenia Gravis Foundation of America (MGFA) has developed a I–V grading scale depicting the spectrum of weakness; note that patients requiring mechanical ventilation are considered grade V (Table 9.1). Women in early adulthood and older men are more commonly afflicted with MG, and the disorder typically follows a relapsing–remitting course, where symptoms can often be well controlled between exacerbations.[1] Exacerbations are most commonly triggered by infections, though virtually any trigger of inflammation and many medications are also implicated.[7]

Aggressive immunotherapy has the potential to improve exacerbation or crisis symptoms relatively rapidly as, unlike many other acute neuromuscular

Table 9.1 Myasthenia Gravis Foundation of America Clinical Grading Scale

Class I	Any ocular muscle weakness; may have weakness of eye closure. All other muscle strength is normal
Class II	Mild weakness affecting muscles other than ocular muscles; may also have ocular muscle weakness of any severity Sub-class IIa: Predominantly affecting limb, axial muscles, or both. May also have lesser involvement of oropharyngeal muscles Sub-class IIb: Predominantly affecting oropharyngeal, respiratory muscles, or both. May also have lesser or equal involvement of limb, axial muscles, or both
Class III	Moderate weakness affecting muscles other than ocular muscles; may also have ocular muscle weakness of any severity Sub-class IIIa: Predominantly affecting limb, axial muscles, or both. May also have lesser involvement of oropharyngeal muscles Sub-class IIIb: Predominantly affecting oropharyngeal, respiratory muscles, or both. May also have lesser or equal involvement of limb, axial muscles, or both
Class IV	Severe weakness affecting muscles other than ocular muscles; may also have ocular muscle weakness of any severity Sub-class IVa: Predominantly affecting limb, axial muscles, or both. May also have lesser involvement of oropharyngeal muscles Sub-class IVb: Predominantly affecting oropharyngeal, respiratory muscles, or both. May also have lesser or equal involvement of limb, axial muscles, or both. The use of a feeding tube without intubation places the patient in class IVb
Class V	Defined as intubation, with or without mechanical ventilation, except when employed during routine postoperative management

Obtained with permission from Howard J. *Myasthenia Gravis: A Manual for the Health Care Provider.* Myasthenia Gravis Foundation of America, 2009: 24. Online at: www.myasthenia.org/LinkClick.aspx?fileticket=JsLyvMFcDh8%3d&tabid=125.

disorders, minimal neuronal or muscle loss occurs during disease exacerbations (though simplification of the post-synaptic membrane can occur with chronic disease) and progressive removal of the offending antibody allows the function of the neuromuscular junction to return in parallel.[2,6,8] Accordingly, the overall prognosis of acute neuromuscular weakness secondary to MG is relatively good. In fact, the in-hospital mortality associated with MG has declined substantially over the past several decades, likely due to advances in immunotherapy and intensive and neurointensive care, and is generally estimated at 5–12%, though some higher and lower figures have been reported.[4,9–15] As MG is a rare condition overall and patients presenting in crisis represent but a fraction of all MG patients, most studies describing prognosis related to MG exacerbation/crisis are either small, single-center studies or large registries, both of which present limitations on the data they provide.[9] The most commonly reported factors associated with poor prognosis in patients presenting with an acute exacerbation of MG are, as alluded to above, respiratory failure and age. Interestingly, neither the presence of a thymoma nor the type of antibody appears to affect prognosis.

Respiratory Failure

Approximately 15–20% of patients with MG will experience myasthenic crisis, commonly within the first 2 years of diagnosis.[7] For some, crises may be recurrent events, and 20% of patients may present in crisis as their first disease manifestation.[7,9] Crisis has also been reported to be more common in older and male patients.[9,10] One study demonstrated the disparity in outcome between patients hospitalized for myasthenia exacerbation and found the mortality of patients in crisis was over four times greater than noncrisis patients.[10] The type of ventilation used (invasive vs. noninvasive) does not have a significant impact on outcome or mortality, but has been associated with reduced duration of ventilation and ICU and hospital length of stay as well as pulmonary complications.[9,16,17] Noninvasive ventilation (NIV) is more likely to fail in patients with MGFA class III–IV symptoms prior to crisis, as well as in patients with infection (primarily pneumonia).[9] Interestingly, one study for patients in crisis is typically 1–2 weeks; mechanical ventilation is considered prolonged when > 15 days. [9,13,18] Older patients, those with late-onset MG, higher pre-hospital MGFA class, those with three or more chronic comorbidities (especially cardiac disease and diabetes), and patients with pneumonia or who require cardiopulmonary resuscitation during admission are at a higher risk for prolonged ventilation.[9,18] Reintubation is also associated with prolonged duration of mechanical ventilation and ICU stay, occurring in as many as 25% of patients requiring invasive ventilation for myasthenic crisis. [18,19] Conversely, patients with early onset MG, thymus hyperplasia, and a successful trial of non-invasive ventilation are at lower risk of prolonged intubation.[9] Additionally, patients with prolonged ventilation were observed to be more likely to receive combination immunotherapy with both IVIG and PLEX.[9] Up to 20% of patients require mechanical ventilation at discharge, and these patients tend to be older, have higher MGFA scores prior to presentation, and have multiple medical comorbidities (especially cardiac disease and diabetes).[9,14]

Age

Age has also been consistently associated in studies with poor outcome in patients hospitalized for myasthenia exacerbation/crisis. One recent study reported no deaths in patients admitted under 40 years of age. However, mortality rates increased by each decade thereafter.[10]

Complications, Comorbidities, and Outcome

While only multiple medical comorbidities and severe systemic complications such as the need for cardiopulmonary resuscitation, sepsis, and acute respiratory distress syndrome (ARDS) have independently been shown to be associated with mortality, nearly all systemic complications including pneumonia, atelectasis, delirium, and urinary tract infections have been associated with length of ventilation and hospital and ICU stay.[9] With the notable exception of patients with an incomplete disease response to immunotherapy, if severe systemic complications can be avoided, the functional outcome even for crisis patients can be quite good.[10,12] In one study, 78% of patients presenting in crisis were discharged home.[10] Another study's results were not as optimistic,

with approximately 50% of crisis patients being discharged to a rehabilitation facility; however, 50% of patients at a median follow-up of 10 weeks were at home living independently or with mild assistance.[9]

Prognosis of Guillain–Barré Syndrome

Guillain–Barré syndrome (GBS) has a monophasic course and uniformly improves over time after reaching a nadir or variable severity and then a plateau of variable duration. It can be acutely fatal due to respiratory failure, dysautonomia, or secondary systemic complications, but mortality has decreased considerably over recent decades thanks primarily to better critical care.[20] Recovery from severe cases is often slow and sometimes incomplete.[20,21] Prognostic studies on GBS have focused on two main endpoints: need for mechanical ventilation and functional outcome, often defined as recovery of independent ambulation at 6 months.

Respiratory Failure

The rapidity of progression of the weakness, the presence of weakness in facial and bulbar muscles and the severity of appendicular weakness are prognostic indicators of respiratory failure. The Erasmus GBS Respiratory Insufficiency Score (EGRIS) incorporates these factors into a simple tool that predicts the need for mechanical ventilation within the first week of hospitalization with very good accuracy (area under the curve [AUC] 0.84 on the derivation cohort of 397 patients and AUC 0.82 on a separate validation cohort of 191 patients) (Table 9.2).[22]

Bedside pulmonary function tests can also assist in identifying patients at high risk of respiratory failure that will require ventilatory assistance. Vital capacity < 20 mL/kg, maximal inspiratory worse than –30 cmH$_2$O, maximal inspiratory pressure < 40 cmH$_2$O, or decrease of any of these parameters by more than 30% have been shown to predict the need for mechanical ventilation.[23] Demyelinating features and a proximal/distal compound muscular amplitude potential ratio of the common peroneal nerve below 55% on electrophysiological studies have also been reported to be more common in patients with GBS who eventually need

Table 9.2 The Erasmus Guillain–Barré Syndrome Respiratory Insufficiency Score (EGRIS)

Factor	Categories	Score
Days between onset of weakness and hospital admission	> 7 days	0
	4–7 days	1
	≤ 3 days	2
Facial or bulbar weakness at hospital admission	Absent	0
	Present	1
Medical Research Counsel sum score at hospital admission	60–51	0
	50–41	1
	40–31	2
	30–21	3
	≤ 20	4
EGRIS		0–7

Table 9.3 Erasmus Guillain–Barré Syndrome Outcome Score (EGOS)

Factor	Categories	Score
Age at onset (years)	≤ 40	0
	41–60	0.5
	> 60	1
Diarrhea (within previous 4 weeks)	Absent	0
	Present	1
GBS disability score* (at 2 weeks)	0–1	1
	2	2
	3	3
	4	4
	5	5
EGOS		1–7

*GBS disability score: 0 = healthy; 1 = minor symptoms and capable of running; 2 = able to walk ≥ 10 meters without assistance but unable to run; 3 = able to walk 10 meters across an open space with help; 4 = bedridden or chair-bound; 5 = requiring assisted ventilation for at least part of the day.

mechanical ventilation, but these associations are not fully validated.[24]

Functional Outcome

Multiple factors have been reported to influence prognosis in patients with GBS. These include older age; shorter interval between symptom onset and admission; greater degree of weakness (i.e., lower Medical Research Council [MRC] muscle strength grading scale sum score) at day 7; preceding diarrhea (typically associated with the axonal form of GBS); nerve inexcitability, severe conduction block, or very reduced amplitude of distal compound muscle action potentials on electrophysiological studies; and some chemical biomarkers (such as various serum interleukins and IgG1 subclass of anti-GM1 antibodies).[21,25] The chances of independent ambulation at 6 months can be estimated using the Erasmus GBS Outcome Score (EGOS) at 2 weeks (Table 9.3).[26] A modified version of EGOS (mEGOS) can be applied upon hospital admission or at 7 days (Table 9.4).[27] While axonal GBS is typically considered to be associated with worse prognosis, some patients with findings of acute axonal disease may experience a rapid recovery, likely from restoration of transient conduction block in the absence of axonal degeneration.[28] Prolonged mechanical ventilation is associated with worse prognosis, but meaningful functional recovery is possible even among patients who remain ventilator-dependent for months; in such cases, recovery may continue for years.[29]

There is scant information on the main determinants of quality of life, long-term disability (beyond independent ambulation) and reinsertion into the workplace among GBS patients. Fatigue, persistent weakness, and pain are common complaints even long after the acute course of the disease. GBS recurrence is distinctly uncommon, and its presumed occurrence should prompt considering the diagnosis of chronic inflammatory polyradiculoneuropathy.

Table 9.4 Modified Erasmus Guillain–Barré Syndrome Outcome Score (mEGOS)

Factor	Categories	Score
Age at onset (years)	≤ 40	0
	41–60	0.5
	> 60	1
Diarrhea (within previous 4 weeks)	Absent	0
	Present	1
Medical Research Counsel sum score	51–60	0
	41–50	3
	31–40	6
	0–30	9
EGOS		1–12

Prognostication in ICU-Acquired Weakness

The diagnosis of ICU-acquired weakness (ICUAW) is a clinical one, made when a critically ill patient develops a summative score of < 48 on the MRC muscle strength grading scale.[30] However, the pathophysiology underlying the clinical syndrome is much more complex and is thought to arise from a combination of muscle atrophy and critical illness polyneuropathy (CIP), critical illness myopathy (CIM), or a proportionate mix of CIP and CIM, termed critical illness neuromyopathy (CINM).[31] Patients typically develop limb weakness (which is distal initially in CIP and proximal in CIM), facial weakness, and/or respiratory weakness (which, interestingly, may not be proportional to the degree of appendicular weakness).[32–34] Additionally, a stocking/glove sensory neuropathy and reduced or absent reflexes may occur, characteristically with CIP. The illness is extremely common and is estimated to occur in 40–70% of critically ill patients, particularly those with risk factors.[35] The most prominent of these risk factors associated with ICUAW are also associated with the presence and severity of systematic inflammation (e.g., sepsis, Acute Physiology And Chronic Health Evaluation (APACHE) score, multi-organ failure), and it is speculated that the axonal polyneuropathy in CIP and the muscle inexcitibility from the sodium channelopathy and myosin degradation in CIP are secondary to the deleterious downstream effects of inflammation.[36] No disease-modifying treatment is available, though early mobilization has been associated with a reduction in the emergence of ICUAW, as well as mortality, in critically ill patients.[37–39] Patients with ICUAW have been found to have longer ICU and hospital stays, spend more days on mechanical ventilation, and have a reduced quality of life and higher ICU, hospital, and 1-year mortality.[30,31,35,36] However, the precise causal relationship between ICUAW and death has been debated in the literature and speculation exists as to whether the higher mortality observed in patients with ICUAW is merely an epiphenomenon of the underlying disease severity. A recent propensity matched cohort refutes this notion, though, observing 13% mortality (30% in patients with ICUAW and 17% without) one year after discharge in patients with ICUAW, while the ICU and hospital mortality between the matched cohorts did not differ.[40] The cause of death in these patients with chronic weakness related to ICUAW is speculated to be secondary to residual dysphagia, difficulty clearing secretions, respiratory weakness, and other medical issues associated with immobility, including venous thromboembolism and skin ulcers. However, the debate continues – while a recent study supported the observation that ICUAW is independently associated with higher mortality in a comparative cohort of patients in

the post-ICU setting (28% vs. 11%), most deaths occurred on admission or during the remainder of the hospital course and no difference in post-hospital mortality was apparent in patients with ICUAW relative to controls (in-hospital mortality 22% in the ICUAW group vs. 5% in the control group [p = 0.01], but post-hospital discharge mortality was 9% and 6% [p = 0.71], respectively).[41] Patients with poorer outcomes tend to be older, have a higher portion of CIP, and have more severe weakness. Survivors, however, typically enjoy some degree of clinical recovery, and it may take up to 1 or 2 years before a plateau in clinical improvement occurs.[42]

Age

One study analyzed the impact of ICUAW on patients 65 years and older and found that the mortality rate post-ICU discharge is over twice the value typically reported in trials incorporating adults of all ages at 51%.[43] Clinical reserve may be limited in the elderly due to age-related accumulation of medical comorbidities and polypharmacy, which may make them more vulnerable to complications prior to hospital discharge. Additionally, the threshold to transition the goals of care to comfort measures may be lower in older patients. However, it remains unsettled as to whether age, and the associated concept of frailty, predisposes an individual to ICUAW and to what degree its development influences mortality.[35] Clinical frailty is categorized by the degree of attributable disability, includes sarcopenia, and afflicted individuals have higher mortality rates independently.[44] The presence and degree of preexisting frailty and its effect on ICUAW are inadequately studied and should be a focus of future research in ICUAW.

Presence of Critical Illness Polyneuropathy

As the weakness in critical illness polyneuropathy (CIP) is due to axonal degeneration while muscle inexcitability due to dysfunction of muscle membrane sodium channels underlies at least part of the mechanism responsible for weakness in CIM, speculation existed as to whether the motor deficits seen in CIP were associated with a poorer prognosis given the longer time required for axonal regeneration (as opposed to myocyte regeneration).[31] Additionally, while pathological changes that

147

disrupt the cellular architecture (such as muscle fiber and preferential myosin degeneration) do occur in CIM, the sodium channelopathy and decreased muscle excitability, which also occur in the disease and can substantially contribute to weakness, are thought to be reversible.[45,46] A number of small studies have shown a correlation between the presence of CIP and long-term functional outcome, with patients afflicted with CIP or CINM having more prolonged or incomplete recoveries.[47–50]

Severity of Weakness

The persistence of limb weakness upon ICU discharge is associated with 1-year mortality.[40] In particular, some studies have correlated lower MRC scores on ICU discharge with the risk of death.[41] Furthermore, a couple of recent studies have investigated the effect diaphragm weakness has on outcome, as ICUAW may manifest both with and without substantial involvement of the respiratory muscles.[34,51] Similarly, critically ill patients can develop diaphragmatic weakness, termed ICU-acquired diaphragm dysfunction (ICUDD), both with and without appendicular weakness. Interestingly, one study found that ICUAW, but not ICUDD, was associated with ICU mortality. However, ICU mortality increased substantially in patients with both ICUAW and ICUDD (39%) relative to patients with ICUAW alone (13%).[34] Another study found similar mortality rates for patients with ICUAW with and without diaphragm dysfunction (36% and 21%) and found a prevalence of 63% of patients in their cohort with evidence of diaphragm dysfunction.[51]

Functional Status

Significantly longer than controls, the median duration of ICU and hospital stay for patients with ICUAW is approximately 2 and 3 weeks, respectively. [34,40,51] Furthermore, patients with ICUAW are more likely to be discharged to a long-term care facility or rehabilitation unit and less likely to be discharged home.[40,41] Similar to mortality, patients with lower MRC scores carry a higher burden of disability.[41] However, recovery of strength does occur with time – a prospective study showed a decline in the presence of weakness in their cohort from 36% at hospital discharge to 22% at 3 months, to 4–14% at 1 year, and 9% at 2 years.[42] Yet, the

quality of life of patients with ICUAW can suffer due to persistent generalized weakness, fatigue, and pain, the latter of which may be related to involvement of the small nerve fibers.[30,41] ICUAW remains a cornerstone of post-ICU syndrome, which encompasses all the residual disability survivors of critical illness face, along with long-term cognitive impairment and affective disorders.[53]

Prognostication in Amyotrophic Lateral Sclerosis

Amyotrophic lateral sclerosis (ALS) is a degenerative disorder affecting approximately 1 in 400 people that causes limb and respiratory weakness with the characteristic combination of upper and lower motor neuron findings due to involvement of the motor cortex, brainstem, and anterior horn cells. [54] Variation exists among several subtypes that are stratified according to the area of the body that is initially affected and whether upper motor neuron or lower motor neuron symptoms predominate. ALS is a uniformly fatal disease, with the cause of death commonly related to respiratory complications, thromboembolism, or failure to thrive, which usually occur approximately 3–5 years after the initial diagnosis.[55] Older patients, those with familial disease inheritance, and those with early bulbar and/or respiratory involvement typically have shorter survival times.[56] Currently, the only treatment options for the disease are riluzole and edaravone, though these only confer a survival benefit of several months.[57]

Most patients with ALS often have an established diagnosis and are admitted to the ICU in the setting of a respiratory infection, aspiration event, or other systemic complication, or to monitor respiratory status after an elective procedure. In this setting, supportive care is often administered commensurate with the reason for admission, and goals of care are addressed given the relentlessly progressive nature of the condition. A recent observational study of 90 patients with ALS admitted to an ICU with a mean interval from diagnosis of 26.5 months found a median ICU stay of 4 days and a median hospital stay of 10 days. Mortality was 20% in the ICU and 33% overall in the hospital. At the 3 months and 1 year follow-up, the mortality of the cohort was 46% and 71%, respectively. Additionally, the study found that patients with more severe respiratory acidosis and higher simplified acute physiology scores on

Table 9.5 Summary of prognostic characteristics of conditions commonly causing acute neuromuscular respiratory failure

Illness	Hospital mortality	Length of stay	Functional outcome	Factors associated with poor outcome
Myasthenia gravis	5–14%	– If required, typically spend 1–2 weeks on mechanical ventilation – All systemic complications, reintubation, and higher pre-hospital MGFA class can prolong LOS – The use of NIV in selected patients can reduce ICU LOS	– Prognosis is generally good – 50% may require rehabilitation, but often return to baseline	– Respiratory failure – Older age – Severe systemic complications – Multiple medical comorbidities
Guillain–Barré syndrome	1–18%	– If required, typically spend weeks to months on mechanical ventilation	– Calculating mEGOS at 7 days or EGOS at 14 days can predict functional outcome	– Respiratory failure – Older age – Severe systemic complications – Multiple medical comorbidities
ICU-acquired weakness	22%	– ICU LOS typically 2 weeks – Hospital LOS typically 3 weeks	– Most patients improve, though up to 9% may remain weak at 2 years – Contributes to post-ICU syndrome	– Older age – CIP – Severity of weakness – Respiratory failure
Amyotrophic lateral sclerosis	– 20% in ICU – 33% during hospital stay overall	– Median ICU stay of 4 days and a median hospital stay of 10 days	– Relentlessly progressive course, though NIV, tracheostomy, and PEG tube insertion may prolong survival	– More severe respiratory acidosis – Higher admission simplified acute physiology scores – Older age – Early bulbar/respiratory involvement – Familial inheritance

Abbreviations: CIP: critical illness polyneuropathy; ICU: intensive care unit; LOS: length of stay; MGFA: Myasthenia Gravis Foundation of America; mEGOS: Modified Erasmus Guillain–Barré Syndrome Outcome Score; EGOS: Erasmus Guillain–Barré Syndrome Outcome Score; NIV: noninvasive ventilation; PEG: percutaneous endoscopic gastrostomy.

admission, in particular, had higher mortality rates.[58]

Not uncommonly, a discussion may be required with ALS patients who present to ICU that were not previously on noninvasive ventilation (NIV) or who did not have a tracheostomy or percutaneous endoscopic gastrostomy (PEG) feeding tube placed prior to admission regarding the need to place one. While the American Academy of Neurology has guidelines regarding when to consider placing such devices using respiratory parameters such as peak cough expiratory flow, sniff nasal pressure, abnormal nocturnal oximetry, forced vital capacity, minimal inspiratory pressure as well as clinical factors, the decision to institute NIV long term or place a tracheostomy or PEG tube may be challenging in the acute setting in the ICU, as some of the tests to measure respiratory function may not be available in the inpatient setting and because the values obtained from the tests may be falsely low, especially in the setting of acute pulmonary pathology.[57] Discussion with the patient's primary outpatient neurologist or pulmonologist to better assess the trajectory of the patient's disease prior to admission may offer additional perspectives, which may be helpful in the decision process, if one is required. NIV has been proven to prolong survival by months to over a year in patients with ALS, particularly in those with bulbar disease, and may also improve quality of life.[59–61] Tracheostomy placement can prolong survival up to several years and PEG placement has also been associated in several trials with prolonged survival.[57,62,63] However, prior to performing procedures, particularly tracheostomy and PEG, it is imperative to have a discussion with the patient and family to ensure that prolonged survival, at times at the expense of quality of life, is in line with the patient's wishes.

Conclusion

While the conditions that commonly precipitate acute neuromuscular respiratory failure vary substantially, all share some similar characteristics with regard to prognostication. Older age, weakness severity, respiratory failure, systemic complications, and medical comorbidities are shared to some degree among all patients presenting to the ICU with acute weakness secondary to MG, GBS, ICUAW, or ALS as being associated with a poorer prognosis (see Table 9.5). Nonetheless, with the exception of ALS, all patients have the potential for substantial improvement in their functional status with time and rehabilitation. Even with ALS, treatment options exist to prolong survival if consistent with the patient's wishes. Therefore, while patients presenting with acute neuromuscular weakness may have a protracted hospital course or appear quite ill on initial presentation, the majority of patients will improve with current therapies over time. In patients with a potentially favorable outcome, giving hope and encouragement to patients and families is warranted and sometimes necessary to instill in them a drive to survive and participate in therapy.

References

1. Gilhus NE. Myasthenia gravis. *N Engl J Med.* 2016;**375**(26):2570–81.

2. Hocker S. Primary acute neuromuscular respiratory failure. *Neurol Clin.* 2017;**35**(4):707–21.

3. Greene-Chandos D, Torbey M. Critical care of neuromuscular disorders. *Continuum (Minneap Minn).* 2018;**24**(6):1753–75.

4. Drachman DB. Myasthenia gravis. *Semin Neurol.* 2016;**36**:419–24.

5. Nicolle MW. Myasthenia gravis and Lambert–Eaton myasthenic syndrome. *Continuum (Minneap Minn).* 2016;**22**:1978–2005.

6. Wijdicks EFM. Management of acute neuromuscular disorders. *Handb Clin Neurol.* 2017;**140**(3):229–37

7. Kalita J, Kohat AK, Misra UK. Predictors of outcome of myasthenic crisis. *Neurol Sci.* 2014;**35**(7):1109–14.

8. Barth D, Nabavi Nouri M, Ng E, Nwe P, Bril V. Comparison of IVIg and PLEX in patients with myasthenia gravis. *Neurology.* 2011;**76**:2017–23

9. Neumann B, Angstwurm K, Mergenthaler P, Kohler S. Myasthenic crisis demanding mechanical ventilation: a multicenter analysis of 250 cases. *Neurology.* 2020;**94**(3):e299–e313.

10. Alshekhlee A, Miles JD, Katirji B, Preston DC, Kaminski HJ. Incidence and mortality rates of myasthenia gravis and myasthenic crisis in US hospitals. *Neurology.* 2009;**72**:1548–54.

11. Thomas CE, Mayer SA, Swarup R, et al. Myasthenic crisis: clinical features, mortality, complications, and risk factors for prolonged intubation. *Neurology.* 1997;**48**:1253–60.

12. Spillane J, Hirsch NP, Kullmann DM, Taylor C, Howard RS. Myasthenia gravis: treatment of acute

severe exacerbations in the intensive care unit results in a favourable long-term prognosis. *Eur J Neurol.* 2014;**21**:171–3.

13. Ramos-Fransi A, Rojas-Garc´ıa R, Segovia S, et al. Myasthenia gravis: descriptive analysis of life-threatening events in a recent nationwide registry. *Eur J Neurol.* 2015;**22**:1056–61.

14. O'Riordan JI, Miller DH, Mottershead JP, Hirsch NP, Howard RS. The management and outcome of patients with myasthenia gravis treated acutely in a neurological intensive care unit. *Eur J Neurol.* 1998;**5**:137–42.

15. Damian MS, Ben-Shlomo Y, Howard R, et al. The effect of secular trends and specialist neurocritical care on mortality for patients with intracerebral haemorrhage, myasthenia gravis and Guillain-Barre syndrome admitted to critical care: an analysis of the Intensive Care National Audit & Research. *Intens Care Med.* 2013;**39**:1405–12.

16. Wu JY, Kuo PH, Fan PC, et al. The role of non - invasive ventilation and factors predicting extubation outcome in myasthenic crisis. *Neurocrit Care.* 2009;**10**(1):35–42.

17. Seneviratne J, Mandrekar J, Wijdicks EF, Rabinstein AA. Noninvasive ventilation in myasthenic crisis. *Arch Neurol.* 2008;**65**:54–8.

18. Liu Z, Yao S, Zhou Q, et al. Predictors of extubation outcomes following myasthenic crisis. *J Int Med Res.* 2016;**44**(6):1524–1533.

19. Rabinstein AA, Mueller-Kronast N. Risk of extubation failure in patients with myasthenic crisis. *Neurocrit Care.* 2005;**3**:213–5.

20. Van den Berg B, Bunschote C, van Doorn PA, Jacobs BC. Mortality in Guillain-Barre syndrome. *Neurology.* 2013;**80**(18):1650–4.

21. Rajabally YA and Uncini A. Outcome and its predictors in Guillain-Barre syndrome. *J Neurol Neurosurg Psychiatry.* 2012;**83**(7):711–18.

22. Walgaard C, Lingsma HF, Ruts L, et al. Prediction of respiratory insufficiency in Guillain-Barre syndrome. *Ann Neurol.* 2010;**67**(6):781–7.

23. Lawn ND, Fletcher DD, Henderson RD, Wolter TD, Wijdicks EF. Anticipating mechanical ventilation in Guillain-Barre syndrome. *Arch Neurol.* 2001;**58**(6):893–8.

24. Durand M-C., Porcher R, Orlikowski D, et al. Clinical and electrophysiological predictors of respiratory failure in Guillain-Barré syndrome: a prospective study. *Lancet Neurol.* 2006;**5**(12):1021–18.

25. Verma R. Chaudhari TS, Raut TP, Garg RK. Clinico-electrophysiological profile and predictors of functional outcome in Guillain-Barre syndrome (GBS). *J Neurol Sci.* 2013;**335**(1–2):105–11.

26. Van Koningsveld R, Steyerberg EW, Hughes RAC, et al. A clinical prognostic scoring system for Guillain-Barré syndrome. *Lancet Neurol.* 2007;**6**(7):589–94.

27. Walgaard C, Lingsma HF, Ruts L, et al. Early recognition of poor prognosis in Guillain-Barre syndrome. *Neurology.* 2011;**76**(11):968–75.

28. Kuwabara S, Mori M, Ogawara K, Hattori T, Yuki N. Indicators of rapid clinical recovery in Guillain-Barré syndrome. *J Neurol Neurosurg Psychiatry.* 2001;**70**(4):560–2.

29. van den Berg B, Storm EF, Garssen MJP, et al. Clinical outcome of Guillain-Barré syndrome after prolonged mechanical ventilation. *J Neurol Neurosurg Psychiatry.* 2018;**89**(9):949–54.

30. Hermans G, Van den Berghe G. Clinical review: intensive care unit acquired weakness. *Crit Care.* 2015;**19**:274.

31. Kramer CL. ICU-acquired weakness. *Neurol Clin.* 2017;**35**(4):723–36.

32. Batt J, dos Santos CC, Cameron JI, Herridge MS. Intensive care unit-acquired weakness: clinical phenotypes and molecular mechanisms. *Am J Respir Crit Care Med.* 2013;**187**:238–46.

33. Jung B, Moury PH, Mahul M, et al. Diaphragmatic dysfunction in patients with ICU-acquired weakness and its impact on extubation failure. *Intensive Care Med.* 2016;**42**:853–61.

34. Saccheri C, Morawiec E, Delemazure J, et al. ICU-acquired weakness, diaphragm dysfunction and long-term outcomes of critically ill patients. *Ann Intensive Care.* 2020;**10**(1):1.

35. Jolley SE, Bunnell AE, Hough CL. ICU-acquired weakness. *Chest* 2016;**150**:1129–40.

36. Kress JP, Hall JB. ICU-acquired weakness and recovery from critical illness. *N Engl J Med.* 2014;**370**:1626–35.

37. Hermans G, De Jonghe B, Bruyninckx F, Van den Berghe G. Interventions for preventing critical illness polyneuropathy and critical illness myopathy. *Cochrane Database Syst Rev.* 2014:**2014**(1):CD006832.

38. Kayambu G, Boots R, Paratz J. Physical therapy for the critically ill in the ICU: a systematic review and meta-analysis. *Crit Care Med.* 2013;**41**:1543–54.

39. Burtin C, Clerckx B, Robbeets C, et al. Early exercise in critically ill patients enhances short-term functional recovery. *Crit Care Med.* 2009;**37**:2499–505.

40. Hermans G, Van Mechelen H, Clerckx B, et al. Acute outcomes and 1-year mortality of intensive care unit-acquired weakness. A cohort study and propensity-matched analysis. *Am J Respir Crit Care Med.* 2014;**190**:410–20.

41. Wieske L, Dettling-Ihnenfeldt DS, Verhamme C, et al. Impact of ICU-acquired weakness on post-ICU physical functioning: a follow-up study. *Crit Care.* 2015;**19**:196.

42. Fan E, Dowdy DW, Colantuoni E, et al. Physical complications in acute lung injury survivors: a two-year longitudinal prospective study. *Crit Care Med.* 2014;**42**(4):849–59.

43. Sacanella E, Perez-Castejon JM, Nicolas JM, et al. Functional status and quality of life 12 months after discharge from a medical ICU in healthy elderly patients: a prospective observational study. *Crit Care.* 2011;**15**:R105.

44. Montgomery CL, Rolfson DB, Bagshaw SM. Frailty and the association between long-term recovery after intensive care unit admission. *Crit Care Clin.* 2018;**34**(4):527–47.

45. Allen DC, Arunachalam R, Mills KR. Critical illness myopathy: further evidence from muscle-fiber excitability studies of an acquired channelopathy. *Muscle Nerve.* 2008;**37**(1):14–22.

46. Kramer CL, Boon AJ, Harper CM, Goodman BP. Compound muscle action potential duration in critical illness neuromyopathy. *Muscle Nerve.* 2018;**57**(3):395–400.

47. Guarneri B, Bertolini G, Latronico N. Long-term outcome in patients with critical illness myopathy or neuropathy: the Italian multicentre CRIMYNE study. *J Neurol Neurosurg Psychiatry.* 2008;**79**:838–41.

48. Intiso D, Amoruso L, Zarrelli M, et al. Long-term functional outcome and health status of patients with critical illness polyneuromyopathy. *Acta Neurol Scand.* 2011;**123**:211–19.

49. Koch S, Wollersheim T, Bierbrauer J, et al. Long-term recovery in critical illness myopathy is complete, contrary to polyneuropathy. *Muscle Nerve.* 2014;**50**:431–6.

50. Koch S, Spuler S, Deja M, et al. Critical illness myopathy is frequent: accompanying neuropathy protracts ICU discharge. *J Neurol Neurosurg Psychiatry.* 2011;**82**(3):287–93.

51. Dres M, Jung B, Molinari N, et al. Respective contribution of intensive care unit-acquired limb muscle and severe diaphragm weakness on weaning outcome and mortality: a post hoc analysis of two cohorts. *Crit Care.* 2019;**23**(1):370.

52. Needham DM, Dinglas VD, Morris PE, et al. Physical and cognitive performance of patients with acute lung injury 1 year after initial trophic versus full enteral feeding. EDEN trial follow-up. *Am J Respir Crit Care Med.* 2013;**188**:567–76.

53. Harvey MA, Davidson JE. Postintensive care syndrome: right care, right now . . . and later. *Crit Care Med.* 2016;**44**:381–5.

54. Chiò A, Logroscino G, Traynor BJ, et al. Global epidemiology of amyotrophic lateral sclerosis: a systematic review of the published literature. *Neuroepidemiology.* 2013;**41**(2):118–30.

55. Forsgren L, Almay BG, Holmgren G, Wall S. Epidemiology of motor neuron disease in northern Sweden. *Acta Neurol Scand.* 1983;**68**(1):20–9.

56. Kiernan MC, Vucic S, Cheah BC, et al. Amyotrophic lateral sclerosis. *Lancet.* 2011;**377** (9769):942–55.

57. Miller RG, Jackson CE, Kasarskis EJ, et al. Practice parameter update: the care of the patient with amyotrophic lateral sclerosis: drug, nutritional, and respiratory therapies (an evidence-based review): report of the Quality Standards Subcommittee of the American Academy of Neurology. *Neurology.* 2009;**73**(15):1218–26.

58. Mayaux J, Lambert J, Morélot-Panzini C, et al. Survival of amyotrophic lateral sclerosis patients after admission to the intensive care unit for acute respiratory failure: an observational cohort study. *J Crit Care.* 2019;**50**:54–8.

59. Berlowitz DJ, Howard ME, Fiore JF Jr, et al. Identifying who will benefit from non-invasive ventilation in amyotrophic lateral sclerosis/motor neurone disease in a clinical cohort. *J Neurol Neurosurg Psychiatry.* 2016;**87**(3):280–6.

60. Radunovic A, Annane D, Rafiq MK, Brassington R, Mustfa N. Mechanical ventilation for amyotrophic lateral sclerosis/motor neuron disease. *Cochrane Database Syst Rev.* 2017;**2017**(10):CD004427.

61. Bourke SC, Tomlinson M, Williams TL, et al. Effects of non-invasive ventilation on survival and quality of life in patients with amyotrophic lateral sclerosis: a randomised controlled trial. *Lancet Neurol.* 2006;**5**(2):140–7.

62. Sancho J, Servera E, Díaz JL, et al. Home tracheotomy mechanical ventilation in patients with amyotrophic lateral sclerosis: causes, complications and 1-year survival. *Thorax.* 2011;**66** (11):948–52.

63. Hayashi N, Atsuta N, Yokoi D, et al. Prognosis of amyotrophic lateral sclerosis patients undergoing tracheostomy invasive ventilation therapy in Japan. *J Neurol Neurosurg Psychiatry.* 2020;**91** (3):285–90.

Chapter 10

Prognostication in Status Epilepticus

Katlyn Nemani and Ariane Lewis

Background, Epidemiology, and Public Health Importance

Status epilepticus (SE) is a neurological emergency with a mortality rate of 20–30%.[1] SE can have long-term consequences such as neuronal death, neuronal injury, and alteration of neuronal networks.[2] Severe neurological or cognitive sequelae have been reported in 11–16% of survivors.[3] The annual direct inpatient cost of SE is estimated to be over $4 billion in the United States.[4]

There is an estimated global incidence of 12.6 episodes of SE per 100,000 person-years.[5] However, it is worth noting that the definition of the clinical and electrographic findings consistent with SE have changed over time and can vary depending on which definition is being used. Additionally, there are multiple different semiologies of SE. The most commonly accepted definition for convulsive SE is either 5 minutes or more of continuous seizure activity or two or more discrete seizures between which there is incomplete recovery of consciousness.[6] Definitions of nonconvulsive SE are more controversial, with one common definition being "a range of conditions in which greater than 30 minutes of seizure activity results in nonconvulsive clinical symptoms,"[7] and another specifying "when electrographic seizure activity persists for greater than 30 minutes in the absence of visible convulsions."[8] A unified definition proposed by the Neurocritical Care Society defines SE as 5 minutes or longer of continuous and/or electrographic seizure activity, or recurrent seizure activity without recovery between seizures.[3]

The Commission of Classification and Terminology of the International League Against Epilepsy (ILAE) and the Commission on Epidemiology revised their definition of SE in 2015 to specify both when treatment should be started and when long-term consequences develop based on seizure type.[2] For generalized convulsive SE, they note that treatment should be initiated after 5 minutes, and long-term damage begins after 30 minutes. Contrastingly, for focal SE with impaired awareness, they specify that treatment should begin after 10 minutes and long-term damage begins after 60 minutes. The timepoints proposed were based on limited data and are "general approximations meant for operational purposes only," and the disclaimer was provided that "the timing and onset of cerebral damage will vary considerably in different circumstances."[2] The timepoints for other forms of SE were not defined due to a lack of data.

Defining the timepoint after which SE leads to neuronal damage is important when considering prognostication after SE. However, the likelihood of poor outcome is dependent on a number of factors in addition to seizure duration. In this chapter, we review the evidence to help guide neuroprognostication after SE in the acute setting based on clinical, imaging, biomarker, and electrophysiological data and functional, cognitive, and behavioral outcomes over time.

Neuroprognostication in Acute Settings

Clinical

Etiology

The prognosis of SE is largely dependent on its underlying cause. Under the most recent ILAE classification system, causes are classified as known (i.e., symptomatic) or unknown (i.e., cryptogenic).[2] Known causes are subdivided based on temporal relationship to SE and can be acute (e.g., stroke, intoxication, encephalitis), remote (e.g., post-traumatic, post-encephalitic, post-stroke), or progressive (e.g., brain tumor, Lafora disease, dementias). However, while defined electroclinical syndromes (e.g., myoclonic status in Dravet syndrome) are acknowledged to be known causes of SE by the ILAE, the ILAE classification system does not include a relapsing-remitting temporal category. The terms "idiopathic" or "genetic" do not explain the underlying etiology of SE in this classification system, as patients with a genetic epilepsy syndrome (e.g., juvenile myoclonic epilepsy) can be symptomatic due to a variety of causes (e.g., inappropriate antiepileptic drug treatment or drug intoxication). The terms "unknown" or "cryptogenic" SE strictly indicate unknown cause. The mortality rate of SE of cryptogenic etiology is estimated to be 5–20%, whereas the mortality rate of SE of a known cause is 0–100%, depending on etiology of SE.[9]

Most cases of SE are attributed to an acute symptomatic etiology, and the outcome of this type of SE is reported to be worse than the outcome of SE due to other etiologies.[10] Contrastingly, SE due to remote symptomatic etiology has been associated with lower mortality.[11]

However, there is a lot of heterogeneity within groups based on specific disease processes. When comparing all patients with SE due to acute symptomatic etiology, those with SE in the setting of acute hypoxia have the worst prognosis. This is particularly evident if the SE is myoclonic.[9] In these cases, mortality is on the order of 60–100%, and survivors are left with severe neurological morbidity.[12–15] Because of this, patients with SE who have anoxic injuries are often excluded from analyses and clinical scoring systems. On the other hand, SE due to subtherapeutic antiepileptic drug levels or alcohol abuse has a relatively good prognosis, with mortality rates less than 10%.[9]

Age

The outcome of SE varies with age. Elderly patients (defined as older than 60 or 65 years in most studies) have the worst outcomes, with mortality rates up to 50%,[16–20] while children have the best outcomes, with mortality rates between 3–5%.[21] However, many studies do not control for seizure duration or etiology when comparing age groups.[17,20,22] A retrospective study of 197 adults comparing younger patients (< 65 years) to older patients found that differences in mortality rates were not statistically significant and that functional outcomes did not significantly differ in cases with acute symptomatic etiology (52.7% vs. 45.7%), but were worse in elderly patients with remote symptomatic and cryptogenic etiologies (33.3% vs. 12%).[23] However, this study excluded

post-hypoxic SE, which may have lowered the mortality rate of the elderly group. Another retrospective study of 420 patients that included post-hypoxic SE found that age > 65 was the strongest independent predictor of mortality (odds ratio [OR] = 2.55) and a strong negative predictor for return to independence.[16]

Semiology

The backbone of the clinical classification of SE based on two main criteria: the presence or absence of prominent motor symptoms (e.g., convulsive vs. nonconvulsive) and the degree of impaired consciousness.[2] Subtypes within both categories include generalized and focal seizures.

Presence or absence of motor features (convulsive SE vs nonconvulsive SE): While convulsive status epilepticus (CSE) is easily identified clinically, there is no single clinical sign or symptom that has been shown to be specific for a diagnosis of nonconvulsive status epilepticus (NCSE). The inability to distinguish NCSE from other causes of confusion can lead to delays in diagnosis and treatment. In a large randomized trial comparing treatment regimens for SE, 30-day mortality was significantly higher for patients with NCSE (65%) compared to patients with convulsive SE (27%).[24] However, this study was conducted prior to the introduction of the new ILAE terminology and included patients with NCSE with coma (previously referred to as "subtle status"). This group has consistently poor outcomes across studies, which may be related to the underlying etiology. A more recent retrospective study found a case fatality rate of 27.6% in patients with NCSE without coma compared to a 3.5% fatality rate in patients with motor symptoms.[20] However, the study did not control for duration or etiology of SE, and these may have been the main contributors to outcome. Several other studies have shown similar outcomes between patients with NCSE and patients with SE with motor features when controlling for duration of seizures and etiology.[19,25,26]

Degree of consciousness impairment: There is conflicting data regarding the role of level of consciousness in predicting outcome after SE. Consciousness was established as an independent predictor of mortality in a retrospective analysis of 96 patients with SE,[11] but a prospective study of 154 patients by the same group did not find a significant relationship between consciousness impairment and outcome.[27] An interaction between consciousness and seizure type was proposed as a possible explanation. Another retrospective study did not find a relationship between level of consciousness and mortality within different semiological groups (generalized convulsive SE, focal motor SE, NCSE).[28] Contrastingly, a large prospective trial of 298 patients found a Glasgow Coma Scale score ≤ 8 to be a strong predictor of disability and mortality after SE, regardless of semiology and etiology.[19] The difference in findings across the two latter studies may be attributed to the exclusion of post-anoxic patients in the retrospective trial, as other trials have demonstrated that there is no relationship between comatose NCSE and outcome in this patient population.[29]

It is important to note that the new ILAE SE classification does not include a modifier for consciousness impairment under "focal motor seizures," which were previously subdivided into "simple partial seizures" and "complex partial seizures." Because impairment of consciousness can only be studied in patients with focal motor SE (as all patients with generalized SE have impaired consciousness), the new classification system will restrict further investigation into the prognostic value of level of consciousness to patients with NCSE in studies that adhere to the ILAE classification system alone. Some have argued that a modifier indicating impairment of consciousness should be added to the new classification system, citing evidence that focal motor SE with impaired consciousness shows a higher mortality rate than focal motor SE without impaired consciousness. [30] However, the study referenced did not control for etiology and duration of seizures.

Generalized versus focal: When comparing patients with clinically generalized versus focal SE, the comparison must be restricted to patients with motor symptoms, as this distinction is rarely clinically evident in patients with NCSE. Outcomes for generalized convulsive SE vary considerably between studies (mortality rates of 7–26%) depending on characteristics of the population studied.[30] Patients with focal motor SE are heterogeneous, and prognosis in this population is largely dependent on the underlying lesion. One recent study comparing patients with focal and generalized SE reported mortality rates (after

a mean follow-up time of 8 months) of 59.7% in patients with focal motor SE, compared to 31.1% in patients with generalized convulsive SE.[31] Focal seizures in this study were mostly secondary to focal lesions, including stroke and tumors.

Duration

The duration of SE is associated with outcome. Refractory SE is commonly defined as SE refractory to treatment with first-line benzodiazepines and a second-line antiepileptic drug (phenytoin, valproic acid, levetiracetam, and phenobarbital). [32] Refractory SE is associated with increased mortality,[33] increased hospital length of stay, and functional disability.[33,34]

Clinical Scoring Systems

Three prognostic scores to predict mortality due to SE before hospital discharge have been proposed to date: the Status Epilepticus Severity Score (STESS), the Epidemiology-based Mortality score in Status Epilepticus (EMSE), and the modified STESS (mSTESS). All three scoring systems exclude patients with SE from cerebral anoxia due to perceived invariably poor prognosis. A brief description of each scoring system is provided below. See Table 10.1 for details regarding score calculation and a comparison of the positive and negative predictive value for death for each score.

STESS: This was the first prognostic score designed to estimate in-hospital mortality after SE. Because the etiology of SE is often unknown at the time of presentation, the STESS optimizes clinical utility by substituting seizure history as a surrogate for seizure etiology. The STESS is determined based on four variables that are evaluated upon admission: (1) level of consciousness, (2) worst seizure type, (3) age, and (4) history of seizures. While the STESS reliably identifies SE patients who will survive, it has a low positive predictive value for death and cannot be used to justify withdrawal of life-sustaining therapies.[27]

EMSE: Unlike the STESS, the EMSE assigns scores based on previously published epidemiological data within the source population. It can be adapted in different regions of the world to prognosticate outcome based on the etiology and comorbidity pattern of SE, such as malaria or neurocysticercosis. Four factors are taken into account: etiology, age, comorbidity, and electroencephalography (EEG) pattern.

155

Table 10.1 Clinical scoring systems for neuroprognostication after status epilepticus

Score	Calculation	Excluded variable	Negative predictive value	Positive predictive value
STESS	1. **Level of consciousness** (awake/somnolent 0 pt; stuporous/comatose 1 pt) 2. **Worst seizure type** (focal nonconvulsive seizures without coma 0 pt; convulsive seizures 1 pt; nonconvulsive seizures with coma 2 pt) 3. **Age** (age ≥ 65 2 pt) 4. **History of seizures** (no history of seizure 1 pt)	Etiology of SE (seizure history used as a surrogate)	STESS ≥ 3: 88% [35]	STESS ≥ 3: 32% [35]
EMSE	1. **Etiology** (CNS-anomalies 2 pt; drug reduction/withdrawal, poor compliance 2 pt; multiple sclerosis 5 pt; remote cerebrovascular disease/brain injury 7 pt; hydrocephalus 8 pt; alcohol abuse 10 pt; drug overdose 11 pt; head trauma 12 pt; cryptogenic 12 pt; brain tumor 16 pt; sodium imbalance 17 pt; metabolic disorders 22 pt; acute cerebrovascular disease 26 pt; acute CNS infection 33 pt; anoxia 65 pt) 2. **Age** (21–30 yrs 1 pt; 31–40 yrs 2 pt; 41–50 yrs 3 pt; 51–60 yrs 5 pt; 61–70 yrs 7 pt; 71–80 yrs 8 pt; > 80 yrs 10 pt) 3. **Comorbidity** (myocardial infarction, CHF, peripheral vascular disease, cerebrovascular disease, dementia, chronic pulmonary disease, connective tissue disease, ulcer disease, diabetes 10 pt; hemiplegia, moderate or severe renal disease, diabetes with end organ damage, any tumor 20 pt; moderate or severe liver disease 30 pt; metastatic solid tumor or AIDS 60 pt) 4. **EEG pattern** (spontaneous burst suppression 60 pt; ASIDs 40 pt; LPDs 40 pt; GPDs 40pt; no LPDs, GPDs, or ASIDs 0 pt)	Seizure semiology	EMSE ≥ 64: 100% [28]	EMSE ≥ 64: 69% [28]
mSTESS	1. **Level of consciousness** (awake/somnolent 0 pt; stuporous/comatose 1 pt) 2. **Worst seizure type** (focal nonconvulsive seizures without coma 0 pt; convulsive seizures 1 pt; nonconvulsive seizures with coma 2 pt) 3. **Age** (age ≥ 70 2 pt) 4. **History of seizures** (no history of seizure 1 pt) 5. **Modified Rankin Scale** (0, 0 pt; 1–3, 1 pt; ≥ 4, 2 pt)	Etiology of SE	mSTESS > 4: 87% [35]	mSTESS > 4: 58% [35]

Abbreviations: ASID: after status ictal discharges; CHF: congestive heart failure; CNS: central nervous system; EEG: electroencephalography; GPD: generalized periodic discharges; LPD: lateralized epileptiform discharges.

[28] The EMSE does not use seizure semiology to prognosticate. This might represent an advantage given changing seizure classifications, but excluding this may make this score less valuable given that aspects of seizure semiology that could have prognostic value are not considered. Another potential disadvantage of the EMSE is that it may be difficult to obtain quickly given the need to review the EEG pattern.

mSTESS: The mSTESS added the modified Rankin Scale (mRS) to the STESS and raised the cutoff age from 65 to 70 years.[35] The purpose of adding the mRS was to incorporate an easy and fast tool that would serve as a proxy for different comorbidities leading to a more accurate prediction of mortality. The increased cut-off for age decreased the ceiling effect of patients older than age 65 without a history of epilepsy. However, neither the STESS nor the mSTESS take the etiology of SE into account, and this can have a major impact on outcome.[9]

Imaging

During seizures, there is an increase in metabolic demand (with increased glucose utilization and oxygen extraction) which is coupled with an increase in cerebral blood flow to maintain cellular energy status. Perfusion magnetic resonance imaging (MRI) and magnetic resonance angiography can show evidence of seizure-related blood flow changes, including increased prominence of blood vessels and ictal hyperperfusion in the region of epileptic discharges.[36] In SE, despite increased blood flow, the persistently high demand for glucose and oxygen cannot be met, so tissue hypoxia and neuronal injury develops.

The most commonly encountered MRI alterations in SE are restricted diffusion and hyperintensities on T2-weighted and fluid-attenuated inversion recovery (FLAIR) sequences, representing a continuum of cytotoxic edema (corresponding to restricted diffusion) and vasogenic edema (increased diffusion-weighted imaging [DWI] and increased T2 without decreased apparent diffusion coefficient [ADC] signal).[37] Animal studies of induced seizures suggest that these MRI findings are the result, not the cause, of seizures.[38] Nonetheless, it is often challenging to determine whether MRI changes are the cause or consequence of SE, because (1) prospective human studies are lacking, in part due to the variability in occurrence of these findings and the range of forms of SE; and (2) it is rare to have pre-ictal baseline imaging.[39] Acute/subacute MRI changes are frequently transitory in nature.[40] However, some patients with SE have irreversible changes such as cortical laminar necrosis, mesial temporal sclerosis, and focal brain atrophy, which are associated with chronic epilepsy.[41,42]

Because it is difficult to distinguish cause and effect in acute MRI changes in patients with SE, neuroimaging has little utility in routine prognostic evaluation. However, MRI does provide an opportunity to assess the underlying etiology of new onset SE (e.g., tumor, stroke, autoimmune/inflammatory conditions) – which, as previously noted, impacts outcome.

Biomarkers

As discussed above, there are a variety of prognostic indicators for patients with SE, but, as of yet, there are neither molecular biomarkers that are generalizable across all patients with SE nor biomarkers that are specific to SE. Nonetheless, some studies have looked at biomarkers after SE (see Table 10.2). Neuron-specific enolase (NSE) has been shown to

Table 10.2 Molecular biomarkers that may be useful for neuroprognostication after status epilepticus

Biomarker	Source	Evidence
Albumin	Serum	Lower levels independently associated with refractory SE and death in a prospective trial of 135 patients [84]
High-mobility group box protein 1 (HMGB1)	Plasma	Predicts development of epilepsy in rats with electrically induced SE; no human trials [47]
Neuron-specific enolase (NSE)	Serum and cerebral spinal fluid (CSF)	Higher levels correlate with longer seizure duration and worse outcome, but studies are limited and sample sizes are small [43,49]
Procalcitonin	Serum	Increase associated with high mortality and low Glasgow Outcome Scale in an observational cohort study of 91 patients [50]
T-tau protein	CSF	Increase associated with higher risk of developmental disability and chronic epilepsy in a small retrospective study [46]

be elevated after SE.[43] Although NSE has value in predicting neurological outcome after traumatic brain injury[44] and hypoxic–ischemic injury,[45] there is insufficient evidence supporting its use as an independent predictor following SE. A small retrospective study found that SE patients with a higher t-tau protein level in their cerebrospinal fluid had a higher risk of developing disability and chronic epilepsy compared to patients with lower t-tau levels,[46] but this finding has not yet been replicated or studied prospectively. High-mobility group box protein 1 (HMGB1) has been shown to predict epilepsy development after SE in animal models, but its utility as a biomarker of epileptogenesis in humans has yet to be determined.[47]

Systemic inflammation can influence epileptic activity and the course of SE.[48] Epileptic activity during SE can cause systemic inflammatory reactions that are reflected in changes in cytokine levels (IL-1β, IL-2, IL-6, and tumor necrosis factor), increased numbers of circulating immune cells, and disruption of the blood–brain barrier.[49] Procalcitonin, an acute phase protein, was associated with unfavorable outcome in SE in one study; notably, it was not related to infection.[50] Another study found an association between low serum albumin, a negative acute-phase protein that is decreased in inflammatory states, at the onset of SE to be associated with refractory SE and death regardless of seizure severity.[51]

These studies show promise with regard to prediction of outcome in SE, but biomarkers are not ready for prime-time prognostication.

Electrophysiology

In 2012, the American Clinical Neurophysiology Society introduced Standardized Critical Care EEG Terminology that clearly defines rhythmic and periodic patterns (RPPs) and EEG background features. [52] Most data on the association between EEG patterns and clinical outcome were published before the introduction of this terminology. Data derived from studies using the old terminology are included in the sections below, but the EEG patterns are classified based on the current terminology.

Electrographic Seizure Characteristics

With the creation of the new terminology, the definition of unequivocal electrographic seizures (generalized spike-wave discharges at 3/s or faster or clearly evolving discharges of any type that

reach a frequency of > 4/s, whether focal or generalized) did not change.[52]

A number of electrographic seizure characteristics including ictal location,[53,54] number of seizures per hour,[54,55] and ictal continuity[53] have been found to have no relationship to outcome in patients with SE. Seizure duration, however, is associated with higher morbidity and mortality,[56–58] worse functional outcome,[59] and increased risk of subsequent epilepsy.[60]

Rhythmic and Periodic Patterns ("Interictal EEG" according to Old Terminology)

The American Clinical Neurophysiology Society's 2012 EEG terminology uses two terms to classify interictal discharges: the first corresponds to localization of the waveform pattern (generalized, lateralized, bilateral independent, or multifocal) and the second denotes the type of waveform and interval between discharges (periodic discharges, rhythmic delta activity, and spike and wave/sharp and wave). Periodic is defined as "repetition of a waveform with relatively uniform morphology and duration with a quantifiable inter-discharge interval between consecutive waveforms and recurrence of the waveform at nearly regular intervals."[52]

Periodic discharges across all distributions (generalized, lateralized, bilateral, and multifocal) have been associated with an increased risk of refractory SE which, as discussed above, is associated with increased mortality, increased hospital length-of-stay, and functional disability.[22,33,34,61] One study found increased morbidity and mortality associated with periodic lateralized epileptiform discharges (now referred to as LPDs) in SE when controlling for etiology. [62] However, other studies have not found periodic discharges to be a risk factor for mortality when controlling for the etiology of SE.[22,55] Periodic discharges (as opposed to rhythmic patterns) are more often associated with structural lesions – the most common being cerebrovascular disease, followed by tumors and infections [16] – which may contribute to their association with refractory SE and poor outcome in some studies.

Background EEG

The American Clinical Neurophysiology Society's 2012 EEG terminology classifies the background

EEG pattern according to nine components: symmetry, posterior dominant "alpha" rhythm, predominant background EEG frequency, anterior–posterior gradient, variability, reactivity, voltage, stage II sleep transients, and continuity.[52]

A prospective study of continuous EEG after SE that included a comprehensive review of seizures, rhythmic/periodic patterns, and background activity found that the only EEG features that were significantly associated with outcome were (1) the absence of a posterior-dominant rhythm (PDR), which had a significant relationship to mortality, and (2) changes in stage II sleep pattern, which had a significant relationship with complete recovery.[55] An absent PDR increased the likelihood of mortality with an odds ratio of 9.8. The description of stage II sleep (categorized as absent, present and abnormal, or present and normal) predicted the likelihood of complete recovery, with an increased odds ratio of 2.59 for each step up in these categories. The presence of a PDR and sleep spindles may be electrographic markers of an intact thalamocortical system, which is likely to play an important role in recovery.[63]

Neuroprognostication over Time

Long-term outcome after SE encompasses multiple domains, including functional and cognitive deficits, quality of life, and development of subsequent epilepsy. As with prognostication in the acute setting, etiology of SE is the main determinant of long-term outcome. However, additional factors including demographics, neuroimaging and EEG characteristics, and treatment interventions correlate with outcome (see Table 10.3).

Functional

Most studies of adults with SE focus on functional, rather than cognitive, outcomes using standardized scales like the modified Rankin Scale (mRS) and the Glasgow Outcome Scale (GOS). The mRS is a 6-point disability scale (0 = no residual symptoms, 1 = no significant disability, 2 = slight disability, 3 = moderate disability [requiring some external help], 4 = moderately severe disability [unable to walk or function without assistance], 5 = severe disability [bedridden, requires continuous care], 6 = dead).[64] The GOS is a global scale for functional outcome that ranks patients on a 5-point scale: dead, persistent vegetative state, severe disability, moderate disability, or good

Table 10.3 Factors associated with poor long-term outcome after status epilepticus

Predictors of poor long-term outcome
Focal neurological signs [64]
Longer SE duration [10,59,64]
Intubation [71]
Nonconvulsive SE [31]
Older age [17,64]
Refractory SE [17,64]
Sepsis [59]

recovery.[65] Patients with post-anoxic brain injury are typically excluded from studies assessing functional outcome due to poor prognosis.

Demographic and Clinical Variables

A prospective trial of 248 patients with convulsive SE identified 5 factors independently associated with a poor 90-day functional outcome (defined as GOS score 5): longer seizure duration, progression to refractory status epilepticus, presence of a cerebral insult, older age, and focal neurological signs at time of presentation.[64] A retrospective trial of patients with refractory SE found that shorter SE duration (with duration of 10 days as a significant cut-off point) was associated with better long-term outcome (mRS 0–2), while STESS score ≥ 3 and sepsis were associated with poor outcome.[59]

Electrophysiological and Imaging Characteristics

A multicenter retrospective study of patients with prolonged refractory status epilepticus (PRSE, defined as SE that persisted despite at least 1 week of induced coma) found that reactivity on initial EEG and normal neuroimaging (CT or MR) were associated with improved clinical outcome (mRS 0–3) at 6 months post-PRSE.[66] Notably, patients with abnormal imaging may have had underlying pathology that predated PRSE, as there was insufficient data to determine whether the findings were representative of injury acquired due to SE.

Treatment Interventions

A multicenter retrospective study of patients with PRSE found that poor outcome after 1 year (defined as mRS 4–6) was associated with the use of vasopressors to treat hypotension due to

159

medications used to treat SE, sepsis, or other causes.[67] It could not be determined whether poor outcome was related to a deleterious effect of vasopressors or the underlying disease process that precipitated hypotension, but the latter was felt to be more likely.

Other studies have demonstrated an association between poor long-term outcomes and the use of intravenous anesthetic drugs, particularly pentobarbital [68,69] and thiopental,[69] though, again, the indication for these medications is a confounding factor.

A multicenter randomized controlled trial evaluating the effect of hypothermia for neuroprotection in patients with convulsive SE found that hypothermia added to standard care was not associated with significantly better 90-day functional outcomes.[70]

END-IT score

While the STESS, mSTESS, and EMSE are used to predict mortality before hospital discharge, they do not predict functional outcome after discharge. A new prognostic tool was designed to predict functional outcome for patients with convulsive SE 3 months after discharge. Consistent with other scoring systems for patients with SE, patients with cerebral anoxia were excluded due to the high mortality rate.

This 6-point clinical score is named END-IT, an acronym of five independent predictors of poor functional outcome defined as mRS of 3–6 (Encephalitis, NCSE [determined based on continuous video-EEG monitoring following convulsive SE], Diazepam resistance, Image abnormalities, and Tracheal intubation).[71] Four points are determined based on the presence or absence of encephalitis, NCSE, diazepam resistance, and intubation. The final two points are determined based on neuroimaging findings; unilateral lesions are given one point and bilateral lesions are given two points. The cut-off point of 3/6 produced the optimal sensitivity and specificity for the prediction of an unfavorable outcome. Of note, the median age of the sample group was 25.5 years, compared to a median age over 60 in the cohorts used to validate the STESS, EMSE, and mSTESS.

It is interesting to note the history behind the selection of the etiological, SE severity, and comorbidity data included in END-IT. Encephalitis was the only etiological factor incorporated into the score because it was the most frequent cause of acute symptomatic SE in the study population. Four variables related to refractoriness of SE were analyzed (resistance to diazepam, SE duration, drug-induced coma, and the use of three or more types of antiepileptic medications), but only diazepam resistance was identified as an independent risk factor for unfavorable outcome. To determine the relationship between comorbidity and outcome, a comparison of outcome and both Charlson's Comorbidity Index and intubation was performed, but only intubation was independently related to unfavorable outcome.

Cognitive

There is very little research assessing cognitive sequelae after SE in adults. In one study of only 15 patients, there was no cognitive decline (measured by IQ and Weschler Adult Intelligence Scale) seen after 3 years in patients with SE of various durations and etiologies.[72] In children, the underlying etiology for SE is the main factor associated with long-term cognitive outcome.[73] Age < 1 year at the time of SE has also been associated with worse cognitive sequelae.[74]

Behavioral

There is a lack of research on long-term psychiatric or behavioral sequelae of status epilepticus in adults. In children, both SE and less prolonged seizures (lasting greater than 10 seconds but less than 30 minutes) are associated with worse adaptive behavior and worse behavioral-emotional problems, but a difference in behavioral outcomes between patients with SE and less prolonged seizures has not been found.[75] While it seems plausible that SE may produce secondary brain injury that affects neurobehavioral outcomes, this conclusion cannot be verified, as there is insufficient data from prospective trials comparing behavioral measures before and after SE that control for the underlying etiology and allow for the identification of prognostic risk factors.

Subsequent Epilepsy

A study that included both adults and children with SE found a rate of new symptomatic epilepsy in 87.5% of patients with refractory SE, compared to 22% in patients without.[76] Refractory SE was likely a proxy for the underlying cause of SE, given that, as with all other long-term outcome measures after SE, the main predictor of subsequent epilepsy is the underlying SE etiology.[73] This is often a confounder when assessing the predictive value of age, seizure type, and drug response. Notably, rates of subsequent epilepsy in patients who survive an episode of cerebral anoxia with associated SE are particularly high.[77]

Gaps in Current Knowledge

There are a number of limitations to assessing prognostic factors in patients with SE. One reason it is challenging to compare outcome data across the existing literature is the fact that the electroclinical definitions and classifications of SE have evolved with time. Additionally, study populations and designs are heterogeneous. Because etiology of SE has been identified as the most important prognostic indicator across studies, research comparing patients with the same underlying etiology is needed to quantify the independent contribution of other risk factors in predicting prognosis.

There is a lack of prospective trials comparing imaging, electrographic characteristics, biomarkers, and cognitive assessments at pre-ictal baseline and serially over time. It would be ideal to collect pre-ictal baseline imaging to differentiate lesions that are the consequence of SE from those that cause it. The same holds true for determining the direct impact of SE on cognition, behavior, and functional status. Defining the causal relationship between SE and these outcomes is necessary before SE-specific variables with prognostic significance can be identified.

Ongoing Research

In order to improve clinical care and outcomes for patients with SE, more research is needed to identify modifiable risk factors and treatment interventions. Class I evidence supports using a benzodiazepine as the first-line agent in SE, but there is weaker evidence guiding the choice of second-line agents and third-line therapies (anesthetic medication).[78] The comparable effectiveness of these medications at controlling SE and their impact on secondary outcomes is not yet clear. The Established Status Epilepticus Treatment Trial (ESETT) is currently under way to compare the effectiveness of three second-line therapies (fosphenytoin, valproic acid, and levetiracetam), including secondary outcome measures and mortality rates. The results of

this study may help inform the selection of a second-line treatment to optimize outcomes.[79]

In animal models, prognostic biomarkers that can predict the development of epilepsy after induced SE have been identified. These include serum markers (increased HMGB1),[80] MRI abnormalities (reduced T2 relaxation in the amygdala and thalamus),[81] and behavioral phenotypes (slow rate of learning and accelerated forgetting).[82] These preclinical studies are being translated into human trials focusing on one epilepsy etiology at a time.[83]

Hopefully, with the passage of time, additional research will allow us to (1) optimize our interventions to improve SE outcomes, and (2) provide families with better neuroprognostication after SE in both the acute and long-term settings.

References

1. Prasad M, Krishnan PR, Sequeira R, Al-Roomi K. Anticonvulsant therapy for status epilepticus. *Cochrane Database Syst Rev.* 2014;**2014**(9): CD003723.

2. Trinka E, Cock H, Hesdorffer D, et al. A definition and classification of status epilepticus – report of the ILAE Task Force on Classification of Status Epilepticus. *Epilepsia.* 2015;**56**:1515–23.

3. Brophy GM, Bell R, Claassen J, et al. Guidelines for the evaluation and management of status epilepticus. *Neurocrit Care.* 2012;**17**:3–23.

4. Betjemann J, Betjemann JP, Lowenstein DH. Status epilepticus in adults. *Lancet Neurol.* 2015;**14**:615–39.

5. Lv R-J, Wang Q, Cui T, Zhu F, Shao X-Q. Status epilepticus-related etiology, incidence and mortality: a meta-analysis. *Epilepsy Res.* 2017.;**136**:12–17.

6. Vanhaerents S, Gerard EE. Epilepsy emergencies: status epilepticus, acute repetitive seizures, and autoimmune encephalitis. *Continuum (Minneap Minn).* 2019;**25**:454–76.

7. Walker M, Cross H, Smith S, et al. Nonconvulsive status epilepticus: Epilepsy Research Foundation workshop reports. *Epileptic Disord.* 2005;**7**:253–96.

8. Husain AM. Treatment of Recurrent Electrographic Nonconvulsive Seizures (TRENdS) Study. *Epilepsia.* 2013;**54**:84–88.

9. Neligan A. Frequency and prognosis of convulsive status epilepticus of different causes. *Arch Neurol.* 2010;**67**:931–40.

161

10. Logroscino G, Hesdorffer DC, Cascino GD, et al. Long-term mortality after a first episode of status epilepticus. *Neurology.* 2002;**58**:537–41.

11. Rossetti AO, Hurwitz S, Logroscino G, Bromfield EB. Prognosis of status epilepticus: role of aetiology, age, and consciousness impairment at presentation. *J Neurol Neurosurg Psychiatry.* 2006;**77**:611–15.

12. Dragancea I, Backman S, Westhall E, et al. Outcome following postanoxic status epilepticus in patients with targeted temperature management after cardiac arrest. *Epilepsy Behav.* 2015;**49**:173–7.

13. Vignatelli L, Tonon C, D'Alessandro R, Bologna Group for the Study of Status Epilepticus. Incidence and short-term prognosis of status epilepticus in adults in Bologna, Italy. *Epilepsia.* 2003;**44**:964–8.

14. Youn CS, Callaway CW, Rittenberger JC, Post Cardiac Arrest Service. Combination of initial neurologic examination and continuous EEG to predict survival after cardiac arrest. *Resuscitation.* 2015;**94**:73–9.

15. Koubeissi M, Alshekhlee A. In-hospital mortality of generalized convulsive status epilepticus: a large US sample. *Neurology.* 2007;**69**:886–93.

16. Li H-T, Wu T, Lin W-R, et al. Clinical correlation and prognostic implication of periodic EEG patterns: a cohort study-NC-ND license. *Epilepsy Res.* 2017;**131**:44–50.

17. Kantanen A-M, Reinikainen M, Parviainen I, Kälviäinen R. Long-term outcome of refractory status epilepticus in adults: a retrospective population-based study. *Epilepsy Res.* 2017;**133**:13–21.

18. Mert Atmaca M, Bebek N, Baykan B, Gökyiğit A, Gürses C. Predictors of outcomes and refractoriness in status epilepticus: a prospective study. *Epilepsy Behav.* 2017;**75**:158–64.

19. Baysal-Kirac L, Feddersen B, Einhellig M, Rémi J, Noachtar S. Does semiology of status epilepticus have an impact on treatment response and outcome? *Epilepsy Behav.* 2018;**83**:81-6.

20. Leitinger M, Trinka E, Giovannini G, et al. Epidemiology of status epilepticus in adults: a population-based study on incidence, causes, and outcomes. *Epilepsia.* 2019;**60**:53–62.

21. Raspall-Chaure M, Chin RFM, Neville BG, Scott RC. Outcome of paediatric convulsive status epilepticus: a systematic review. *Lancet Neurol.* 2006;**5**:769–79.

22. Atmaca MM, Bebek N, Baykan B, Gökyiğit A, Gürses C. Predictors of outcomes and refractoriness in status epilepticus: a prospective study. *Epilepsy Behav.* 2017;**75**:158–64.

23. Yoshimura H, Matsumoto R, Ueda H, et al. Status epilepticus in the elderly: comparison with younger adults in a comprehensive community hospital. *Seizure.* 2018;**61**:23–9.

24. Treiman DM, Meyers PD, Walton NY, et al. A comparison of four treatments for generalized convulsive status epilepticus. *N Engl J Med.* 1998;**339**:792–8.

25. Towne AR, Pellock JM, Ko D, DeLorenzo RJ. Determinants of mortality in status epilepticus. *Epilepsia.* 1994;**35**:27–34.

26. Pollak L, Gandelman-Marton R, Margolin N, Boxer M, Blatt I. Clinical and electroencephalographic findings in acutely ill adults with non-convulsive vs convulsive status epilepticus. *Acta Neurol Scand.* 2014;**129**:405–11.

27. Rossetti AO, Logroscino G, Milligan TA, et al. Status Epilepticus Severity Score (STESS): a tool to orient early treatment strategy. *J Neurol.* 2008;**255**:1561–6.

28. Leitinger M, Höller Y, Kalss G, et al. Epidemiology-based mortality score in status epilepticus (EMSE). *Neurocrit Care.* 2015;**22**:273–82.

29. Sutter R, Marsch S, Fuhr P, Rüegg S. Mortality and recovery from refractory status epilepticus in the intensive care unit: a 7-year observational study. *Epilepsia.* 2013;**54**:502–11.

30. Rossetti AO, Trinka E, Stähli C, Novy J. New ILAE versus previous clinical status epilepticus semiologic classification: analysis of a hospital-based cohort. *Epilepsia.* 2016;**57**:1036–41.

31. Horváth L, Fekete I, Molnár M, et al. The outcome of status epilepticus and long-term follow-up. *Front Neurol.* 2019;**10**:427.

32. Hocker S, Tatum WO, LaRoche S, Freeman WD. Refractory and super-refractory status epilepticus – an update. *Curr Neurol Neurosci Rep.* 2014;**14**:452.

33. Novy J, Logroscino G, Rossetti AO. Refractory status epilepticus: a prospective observational study. *Epilepsia.* 2010;**51**:251–6.

34. Mayer SA, Claassen J, Lokin J, et al. Refractory status epilepticus: frequency, risk factors, and impact on outcome. *Arch Neurol.* 2002;**59**:205–10.

35. González-Cuevas M, Santamarina E, Toledo M, et al. A new clinical score for the prognosis of status epilepticus in adults. *Eur J Neurol.* 2016;**23**:1534–40.

36. Leonhardt G, de Greiff A, Weber J, et al. Brain perfusion following single seizures. *Epilepsia.* 2005;**46**:1943–9.

37. Yu J-T, Tan L. Diffusion-weighted magnetic resonance imaging demonstrates parenchymal pathophysiological changes in epilepsy. *Brain Res Rev.* 2008;**59**:34–41.

38. Prichard JW, Neil JJ. Diffusion-weighted MRI: periictal studies. *Adv Neurol.* 2000;**83**:279–84.

39. Grillo E. Postictal MRI abnormalities and seizure-induced brain injury: notions to be challenged. *Epilepsy Behav.* 2015;**44**:195–9.

40. Cianfoni A, Caulo M, Cerase A, et al. Seizure-induced brain lesions: a wide spectrum of variably reversible MRI abnormalities. *Eur J Radiol.* 2013;**82**:1964–72.

41. Pohlmann-Eden B, Gass A, Peters CNA, et al. Evolution of MRI changes and development of bilateral hippocampal sclerosis during long lasting generalised status epilepticus. *J Neurol Neurosurg Psychiatry.* 2004;**75**:898–900.

42. Huang Y-C, Weng H-H, Tsai Y, et al. Periictal magnetic resonance imaging in status epilepticus. *Epilepsy Res.* 2009;**86**:72–81.

43. DeGiorgio CM, Correale JD, Gott PS, et al. Serum neuron-specific enolase in human status epilepticus. *Neurology.* 1995;**45**:1134–7.

44. Thelin EP, Jeppsson E, Frostell A, et al. Utility of neuron-specific enolase in traumatic brain injury; relations to S100B levels, outcome, and extracranial injury severity. *Crit Care.* 2016;**20**:285.

45. Vondrakova D, Kruger A, Janotka M, et al. Association of neuron-specific enolase values with outcomes in cardiac arrest survivors is dependent on the time of sample collection. *Crit Care.* 2017;**21**:172.

46. Monti G, Tondelli M, Giovannini G, et al. Cerebrospinal fluid tau proteins in status epilepticus. *Epilepsy Behav.* 2015;**49**:150–4.

47. Nath YN, Shaikh MF, Chakraborti A, et al. HMGB1: a common biomarker and potential target for TBI, neuroinflammation, epilepsy, and cognitive dysfunction. *Front Neurosci.* 2018;**12**:628.

48. Ethemoglu O, Ay H, Koyuncu I, Gönel A. Comparison of cytokines and prooxidants/ antioxidants markers among adults with refractory versus well-controlled epilepsy: a cross-sectional study. *Seizure.* 2018;**60**:105–9.

49. Sutter R, Kaplan PW, Rüegg S. Outcome predictors for status epilepticus – what really counts. *Nat Rev Neurol.* 2013;**9**:525–34.

50. Sutter R, Valença M, Tschudin-Sutter S, Rüegg S, Marsch S. Procalcitonin and mortality in status epilepticus: an observational cohort study. *Crit Care.* 2015;**19**:361.

51. Sutter R, Grize L, Fuhr P, Rüegg S, Marsch S. Acute-phase proteins and mortality in status epilepticus. *Crit Care Med.* 2013;**41**:1526–33.

52. Hirsch LJ, LaRoche SM, Gaspard N, et al. American Clinical Neurophysiology Society's Standardized Critical Care EEG Terminology. *J Clin Neurophysiol.* 2013;**30**:1–27.

53. Nei M, Lee J-M, Shanker VL, Sperling MR. The EEG and prognosis in status epilepticus. *Epilepsia.* 1999;**40**:157–163.

54. Shneker BF, Fountain NB. Assessment of acute morbidity and mortality in nonconvulsive status epilepticus. *Neurology.* 2003;**61**:1066–73.

55. Alvarez V, Drislane FW, Brandon Westover M, Dworetzky BA, Lee JW. Characteristics and role in outcome prediction of continuous EEG after status epilepticus: a prospective observational cohort HHS Public Access. *Epilepsia.* 2015;**56**:933–41.

56. Phabphal K, Limapichat K, Sathirapanya P, Setthawatcharawanich S, Geater A. Clinical characteristics, etiology and long-term outcome of epilepsia partialis continua in adult patients in Thailand. *Epilepsy Res.* 2012;**100**:179–87.

57. Power KN, Gramstad A, Gilhus NE, Engelsen BA. Prognostic factors of status epilepticus in adults. *Epileptic Disord.* 2016;**18**:297–304.

58. Vilella L, González Cuevas M, Quintana Luque M, et al. Prognosis of status epilepticus in elderly patients. *Acta Neurol Scand.* 2018;**137**:321–8.

59. Madžar D, Geyer A, Knappe RU, et al. Association of seizure duration and outcome in refractory status epilepticus. *J Neurol.* 2016;**263**:485–91.

60. Santamarina E, Gonzalez M, Toledo M, et al. Prognosis of status epilepticus (SE): relationship between SE duration and subsequent development of epilepsy. *Epilepsy Behav.* 2015;**49**:138–40.

61. Tian F, Su Y, Chen W, et al. RSE prediction by EEG patterns in adult GCSE patients. *Epilepsy Res.* 2013;**105**:174–82.

62. Jaitly R, Sgro JA, Towne AR, Ko D, DeLorenzo RJ. Prognostic value of EEG monitoring after status epilepticus: a prospective adult study. *J Clin Neurophysiol.* 1997;**14**:326–34.

63. Tennant KA, Taylor SL, White ER, Brown CE. Optogenetic rewiring of thalamocortical circuits to restore function in the stroke injured brain. *Nat Commun.* 2017;**8**:15879.

64. Legriel S, Azoulay E, Resche-Rigon M, et al. Functional outcome after convulsive status epilepticus. *Crit Care Med.* 2010;**38**:2295–303.

65. Jennett B, Bond M. Assessment of outcome after severe brain damage: a practical scale. *Lancet.* 1975;**305**:480–4.

66. Kilbride RD, Reynolds AS, Szaflarski JP, Hirsch LJ. Clinical outcomes following prolonged refractory status epilepticus (PRSE). *Neurocrit Care.* 2013;**18**:374–85.

67. Lai A, Outin HD, Jabot J, et al. Functional outcome of prolonged refractory status epilepticus. *Crit Care*. 2015;**19**:199.

68. Ferlisi M, Shorvon S. The outcome of therapies in refractory and super-refractory convulsive status epilepticus and recommendations for therapy. *Brain*. 2012;**135**:2314–28.

69. Bellante F, Legros B, Depondt C, et al. Midazolam and thiopental for the treatment of refractory status epilepticus: a retrospective comparison of efficacy and safety. *J Neurol*. 2016;**263**:799–806.

70. Legriel S, Lemiale V, Schenck M, et al. Hypothermia for neuroprotection in convulsive status epilepticus. *N Engl J Med*. 2016;**375**:2457–67.

71. Gao Q, Ou-Yang T, Sun X, et al. Prediction of functional outcome in patients with convulsive status epilepticus: the END-IT score. *Crit Care*. 2016;**20**:46.

72. Adachi N, Kanemoto K, Muramatsu R, et al. intellectual prognosis of status epilepticus in adult epilepsy patients: analysis with Wechsler Adult Intelligence Scale-Revised. *Epilepsia*. 2005;**46**:1502–9.

73. Sculier C, Gaínza-Lein M, Sánchez Fernández I, Loddenkemper T. Long-term outcomes of status epilepticus: a critical assessment. *Epilepsia*. 2018;**59**:155–69.

74. Tabarki B, Yacoub M, Selmi H, et al. Infantile status epilepticus in Tunisia. Clinical, etiological and prognostic aspects. *Seizure*. 2001;**10**:365–9.

75. Abend NS, Wagenman KL, Blake TP, et al. Electrographic status epilepticus and neurobehavioral outcomes in critically ill children. *Epilepsy Behav*. 2015;**49**:238.

76. Holtkamp M, Othman J, Buchheim K, Meierkord H. Predictors and prognosis of refractory status epilepticus treated in a neurological intensive care unit. *J Neurol Neurosurg Psychiatry*. 2005;**76**:534–9.

77. Hesdorffer DC, Logroscino G, Cascino G, Annegers JF, Hauser WA. Risk of unprovoked seizure after acute symptomatic seizure: effect of status epilepticus. *Ann Neurol*. 1998;**44**:908–12.

78. Hill CE, Parikh AO, Ellis C, Myers JS, Litt B. Timing is everything: where status epilepticus treatment fails. *Ann Neurol*. 2017;**82**:155–65.

79. Falco-Walter JJ, Bleck T. Treatment of established status epilepticus. *J Clin Med*. 2016;**5**:49.

80. Fu L, Liu K, Wake H, et al. Therapeutic effects of anti-HMGB1 monoclonal antibody on pilocarpine-induced status epilepticus in mice. *Sci Rep*. 2017;**7**:1179.

81. Choy M, Dube CM, Patterson K, et al. A novel, noninvasive, predictive epilepsy biomarker with clinical potential. J Neurosci. 2014;**34**:8672–84.

82. Pascente R, Frigerio F, Rizzi M, et al. Cognitive deficits and brain myo-Inositol are early biomarkers of epileptogenesis in a rat model of epilepsy. *Neurobiol Dis*. 2016;**93**:146–55.

83. Pitkänen A, Ekolle Ndode-Ekane X, Lapinlampi N, Puhakka N, Virtanen AI. Epilepsy biomarkers – toward etiology and pathology specificity. *Neurobiol Dis*. 2019;**123**:42–58.

84. Sutter R, Grize L, Fuhr P, Rüegg S, Marsch S. Acute-phase proteins and mortality in status epilepticus: a 5-year observational cohort study. *Crit Care Med*. 2013;**41**:1526–33.

Prognostication in Fulminant Hepatic Failure

Alexandra S. Reynolds and Thomas D. Schiano

Background and Epidemiology

Acute liver failure (ALF), a liver injury developing over 26 weeks or less with evidence of coagulopathy and encephalopathy, disproportionately affects young, healthy adults with high resultant mortality.[1] ALF results in cerebral dysfunction, which can range from minor encephalopathy to coma, and is associated with high neurological morbidity due to higher grade hepatic encephalopathy (HE), cerebral edema, and elevated intracranial pressure (ICP),[2,3] although other complications including seizures may contribute.[4]

While ALF is considered a rare syndrome, with an estimated annual incidence of 1–5 cases per million people yearly,[5] there appears to be a trend toward increasing numbers of hospitalizations for ALF, including up to a 30% increase in the United States over a 4-year period.[6] Etiologies of ALF vary geographically; in developed countries, the majority of cases are caused by toxic ingestions, autoimmune hepatitis, or hepatitis B, while cases in developing countries most commonly are caused by hepatitis A, B, or E.[7] ALF etiologies appear in Table 11.1. The etiology of the ALF can influence both treatment options and prognosis.

Patients with ALF often present with evidence of acute kidney injury, hemodynamic instability, vasodilatory shock, and infection. Overall mortality has improved from > 80% to approximately 33% in the United States over the past quarter century, but the most common cause of death remains multi-organ failure.[8]

The neurological presentation of ALF begins with mild encephalopathy and frontal dysfunction, which can include apathy, attentional deficits, and impaired judgment.[9] The concept of minimal encephalopathy, which may not be evident unless diligently screened for with more complex testing, has evolved to represent a Grade 0 encephalopathy.[10] As encephalopathy progresses, personality changes increase and

Table 11.1 Etiologies of acute liver failure

Category	Main etiologies
Viruses	Hepatitis A (HAV) Hepatitis B (HBV) Hepatitis E (HEV) Herpes simplex (HSV) Varicella zoster (VZV) Cytomegalovirus (CMV) Epstein–Barr (EBV) Dengue
Drugs and toxins	Acetaminophen Isoniazid Ecstasy Iron supplementation Herbal medications Wild mushrooms Weight loss drugs
Vascular	Budd–Chiari Hypoxemia
Pregnancy	Hemolysis, elevated liver enzymes, and low platelets (HELLP) Acute fatty liver of pregnancy
Hematological/ oncological	Lymphoma Malignancy Hemophagocytic lymphohistiocytosis (HLH)
Other	Wilson disease Autoimmune hepatitis

level of consciousness decreases. In addition to encephalopathy, patients may exhibit seizures, asterixis, clonus, hypertonia, multifocal myoclonus, and an exaggerated startle response.[4,11] As patients develop worsening encephalopathy, their risk of cerebral edema increases as well. Cerebral edema can be mild, but it may cause intracranial hypertension, which accounts for up to 25% of all deaths from ALF.[12]

Importantly, it is thought that HE itself is reversible with liver transplantation or spontaneous improvement in liver function. A great deal of research has centered on the development of prognostic scores that can predict the need for

Table 11.2 West Haven Criteria for Hepatic Encephalopathy

Grade 1	Minimal lack of awareness, anxiety or euphoria, shortened attention span, impairment of calculations
Grade 2	Disorientation for time or place, lethargy or apathy, subtle personality changes, inappropriate behavior
Grade 3	Somnolence to stupor but responsiveness to stimuli, gross disorientation, confusion
Grade 4	Coma

liver transplantation or death, but there are little data on neurological prognosis once ALF has resolved.

Neuroprognostication in the Acute Setting

Clinical Scoring Systems

Hepatic encephalopathy is graded using the West Haven criteria (Table 11.2).[13] More recently, work using the Psychometric Hepatic Encephalopathy Score has revealed minimal, or Grade 0, encephalopathy, which can be detected with more complex bedside testing.[10] The presence of worsening degrees of HE is associated with worse outcomes,[14] which may persist even after liver transplantation.[3]

The presence of cerebral edema has also been linked to worse post-transplant neurological outcomes.[15] Elevated intracranial pressure (ICP) occurs in up to 75–90% of patients with grade 3 or 4 HE,[16,17] and most neurological morbidity and mortality is due to elevated ICP. Rigorous monitoring for signs of elevated ICP is warranted in this patient population, although there are no clear guidelines on how to do this, and there are significant variabilities in transplant center protocols.[18]

Several scoring systems have been developed to predict mortality or need for liver transplantation in the ALF population (Table 11.3), but only two include stage of HE. The King's College Criteria is used to predict need for liver transplantation in ALF, and notably uses the presence of high grade HE in its prediction scale for ALF resulting from acetaminophen toxicity, and the timing to development of HE in its non-acetaminophen-induced toxicity prediction model.[19] More recently there has been interest in incorporating the dynamics of the neurological exam and lab values into the development of a more accurate score.[14,20]

Imaging

Computed tomography (CT) of the head can be a helpful tool in the critically ill ALF patient. While CT has poor sensitivity in the detection of cerebral edema and can lag behind clinical changes consistent with elevated ICP,[21] the presence of sulcal effacement, blurring of the gray–white junction, or narrowing of the ventricles or cisterns may suggest cerebral edema. Because many patients with ALF are young, they may already have full brains, which may result in suboptimal assessment of subtle edema, or overestimation of edema when it does not exist; in these cases, obtaining a baseline CT head prior to decompensation can be helpful (Figure 11.1A). CT can also be helpful in detecting multicompartmental hemorrhage (Figure 11.1B, C) or large ischemic stroke, both of which may occur in ALF.

Because cerebral edema is primarily cytotoxic in ALF,[22] MRI changes can be seen on diffusion-weighted imaging (DWI) with concurrent decreases in the apparent diffusion coefficient (ADC) maps.[23] These changes can appear quite similar to the changes of acute hyperammonemia,[24] even in the absence of very high serum ammonia levels (Figure 11.2).[25] More complex MR spectroscopy (MRS) imaging can distinguish ALF from acute-on-chronic and chronic liver failure,[26] but the clinical utility of these scans is limited.

In the unstable ALF patient, insonation of the optic nerve sheath with ultrasound for measurement of the optic nerve sheath diameter (ONSD) can be helpful in estimating whether there is elevated ICP (Figure 11.3). The optic nerve is surrounded by a space contiguous with the intracranial subarachnoid space, and the optic nerve sheath is an extension of the intracranial dura. When elevated ICP is transmitted forward, the optic nerve sheath distends, with a maximal distension 3 mm behind the globe.[27] The diameter of the optic nerve sheath 3 mm posterior to the globe has been shown to correlate with invasively measured ICP in a variety of disease processes, with a cut-off of anywhere from 5 to 6 mm corresponding to an elevated ICP.[28] Further, the ONSD dynamically and rapidly responds to changes in ICP,[29,30] making it a useful real-time bedside tool. A recent study in adult ALF patients showed

Table 11.3 Prognostic scoring systems

King's College Criteria		Modified King's College criteria	Model for End-stage Liver Disease (MELD)	MELD – Na
Acetaminophen toxicity	**Non-acetaminophen toxicity**			
pH < 7.3 OR INR > 6.5, serum creatinine > 3.4 mg/dL, and grade 3–4 HE	INR > 6.5 OR 3 of these 5: 1. Age < 10 or > 40 years 2. Cause is nonA, nonB hepatitis or idiosyncratic drug reaction 3. Duration of jaundice before HE > 7 days 4. INR > 3.5 5. Serum bilirubin > 17.5 mg/dL	Arterial lactate > 3.5 mmol/L after early (4 h) resuscitation pH < 7.3 OR Lactate > 3.0 mmol/L after 12 h fluid resuscitation	Serum creatinine (mg/dL)* Bilirubin (mg/dL) INR	Serum creatinine (mg/dL)* Bilirubin (mg/dL) INR Sodium (mEq/L)

* Patients who have been dialyzed twice in the past 7 days are automatically set to Cr 4 mg/dL.

Abbreviations: INR: international normalized ratio; HE: hepatic encephalopathy.

that the median highest ONSD did not reliably detect concurrent ICP elevation measured with invasive ICP monitors,[31] but given that the baseline ONSD can vary between patients,[27] it is possible that a trend of values is more reliable than an absolute value. Case series have described using the ONSD in monitoring for the development of cerebral edema during liver transplant surgery for ALF, [32,33] which guided modification of the patient's positioning and administration of hyperosmolar therapies intraoperatively.

Biomarkers

The most utilized scoring system using serum biomarkers to predict need for transplant and mortality is the Model for End-stage Liver Disease (MELD) score (Table 11.3), which originally was used to predict mortality of cirrhotics. Subsequently, it has been validated in ALF as well,[34] and has been modified to incorporate the serum sodium concentration as the MELD-Na score.[35] The serum laboratory markers that it incorporates are liver-specific values (total bilirubin and the International Normalized Ratio [INR]), as well as renal function (creatinine) and sodium. These scores have not only been validated in the severity of liver dysfunction, but have also been shown to determine the reversibility of HE and brain dysfunction, even after liver transplantation.[3]

Hyperammonemia is a known complication of ALF, and in some animal models is thought to be directly responsible for astrocyte swelling and the activation of proinflammatory cascades. [22] Other data suggest that while ammonia itself may not directly cause cytotoxic edema, it may result in downstream effects that trigger changes in cerebral blood flow or either direct or indirect cellular toxicity.[36] Persistently elevated arterial ammonia levels have been associated with greater rates of complications and higher mortality,[37] although it is unclear if this is a causal relationship or whether ammonia in this setting is a marker of the degree of hepatic injury. While hyperammonemia alone does not appear to directly lead to HE or the development of cerebral edema,[38] elevated ICP has been shown to be more likely present in patients with very elevated arterial ammonia,[39,40] and a reduction of serum ammonia using renal replacement therapy has been shown to both decrease serum ammonia and result in better outcomes among patients with high grade HE.[41] One study identified that 60% of patients with an admission arterial ammonia > 200 μmol/L developed elevated ICP within 10 days of admission, compared with 30% of those with an ammonia of 100–200 μmol/L and 20% with an ammonia < 100 μmol/L.[40] Thus, an arterial ammonia may help stratify those

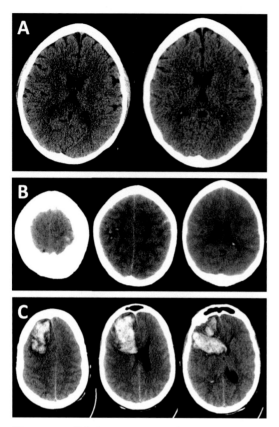

Figure 11.1 CT findings in acute liver failure.
(A) Subtle cerebral edema (right) with decreased gray–white differentiation and sulcal effacement, particularly posteriorly. This is more obvious in comparison to a baseline head CT (left) obtained 3 days earlier. (B) Moderate to severe cerebral edema with diffuse sulcal effacement and blurring of the gray–white junction, along with petechial intracerebral hemorrhages and high cortical subarachnoid hemorrhage. (C) Large right frontal intraparenchymal hemorrhage with resultant right-to-left midline shift, trapping of the left lateral horn, and cerebral edema.

patients at risk for developing significant cerebral edema with resultant elevated ICP.

There may be potentiation of the neurotoxic effect of ammonia by the presence of systemic infection or inflammation. Some studies have found worsening HE with greater degree of systemic inflammatory response syndrome [42,43] or with development of a confirmed infection.[43] Other studies have found a correlation between inflammatory cytokines and elevated ICP,[44] potentially via effects on cerebral blood flow.[45]

Elevated pre-transplant serum lactate has been shown to be associated with need for transplant and mortality.[20,46–48] While work on animal models has suggested that exposure of the brain

to high levels of lactate may induce cell injury and cerebral edema,[49] there does not yet seem to be evidence to support this in the published literature. Studies have found increased concentrations of brain lactate in the absence of cerebral edema in patients with ALF, and it is not yet clear if this is due to elevated serum lactate crossing the blood–brain barrier or a change in brain metabolism.[50]

Higher serum phosphorus levels have also been shown to be predictive of both need for liver transplant and mortality,[51,52] but there are no data suggesting prognostic benefit for neurological-specific outcome.

Electrophysiology

Continuous EEG (cEEG) monitoring can be helpful in managing ALF by recognizing seizures, evaluating HE, and monitoring for elevated ICP.[53] Seizures, either focal or generalized, may occur at any point throughout the course of ALF, and can be provoked by the hypothetical epileptogenesis of acute hyperammonemia and resultant glutamine toxicity,[36] or from the many metabolic issues that occur in ALF including hyponatremia and hypoglycemia. The true incidence of seizures is difficult to assess due to confounding from other common movement disorders that may occur (such as asterixis, myoclonus, and clonus) as well as the potential for solely electrographic seizures. Two studies found a rate of electrographic seizures as high as 25%,[54,55] but true rates may differ depending on the criteria for obtaining EEG and the duration of EEG monitoring.

Continuous EEG has been shown to be able to prompt treatment of elevated ICP in ALF patients more quickly than relying on the clinical exam alone.[56,57] Changes in EEG patterns have been shown to correlate with HE grade,[58,59] and potentially with overall outcome.[59] There seems to be good evidence to suggest that standardized measures from cEEG may be useful in predicting an ALF patient's clinical course, but which specific electrographic parameters to use is still debated.

Others

Intraparenchymal ICP Monitoring

Invasive ICP monitors are the gold standard for accurate ICP measurement in neurological disease processes, but their use is highly controversial in the ALF population.[60] ALF results in coagulopathy, the degree of which may not be accurately

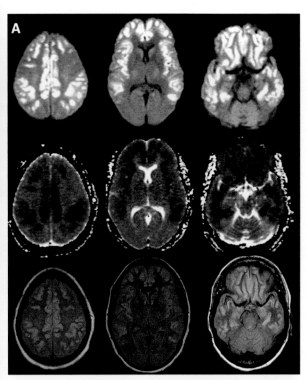

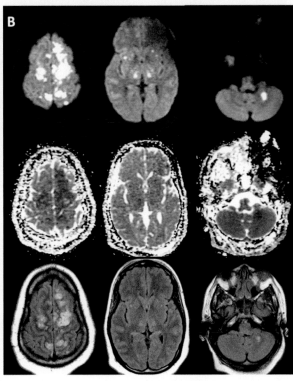

Figure 11.2 MRI findings in acute liver failure. (A) Diffusion-weighted imaging (DWI) (top row), apparent diffusion coefficient (ADC) (middle row), and fluid-attenuated inversion recovery (FLAIR) (bottom row) images in a patient with acute hyperammonemia. (B) DWI (top row), ADC (middle row), and FLAIR (bottom row) images in an ALF patient with ischemic strokes.

measured by conventional laboratory tests.[61] There is a 5–15% risk of fatal hemorrhage after ICP monitor placement,[61–63] and another 4–15% risk of non-fatal hemorrhage.[61,64,65] True rates are difficult to establish given varying strategies for reversal of coagulopathy, varying

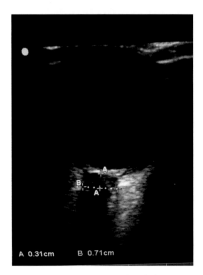

Figure 11.3 Optic nerve sheath diameter.
Ultrasound of the eye with measurement of elevated optic nerve sheath diameter of 7.1 mm (B) at 3 mm behind the globe (A).

compartments of ICP monitor placement, and lack of consistency in performing post-placement imaging to diagnose intraparenchymal hemorrhage. Many centers will reverse coagulopathy at the time of placement and removal, but it is unclear whether coagulopathy needs to be aggressively managed for the duration of the time the monitor remains in place. Further, given dynamic fibrinolysis that occurs intraoperatively during liver transplantation,[66] it is unclear whether the risks of maintaining an ICP monitor intraoperatively outweigh the benefits.

While patients with invasive ICP monitors have higher rates of treatment for elevated ICP,[67] there has been a lack of strong evidence showing any association with improved survival.[63,64] Multimodal monitoring via the same burr-hole in the form of brain tissue oxygenation and cerebral blood flow monitoring may help in determining appropriate systemic blood pressure goals,[68] but there is some evidence of regional differences in cerebral blood flow in ALF,[69,70] which may make interpretation of data from a small region of the brain more difficult.

Transcranial Doppler

Transcranial Doppler (TCD) uses ultrasound to measure flow velocities through major intracranial vessels (Figure 11.4). As elevations in ICP result in increased extramural pressure, flow velocities increase, waveform morphology changes, and the pulsatility index (PI), a ratio of the difference between the peak systolic and end diastolic velocities to the mean flow velocity, also increases.[71] The cerebral perfusion pressure, and thus the ICP, can be calculated based on increase of flow velocities and the arterial blood pressure, although several different calculations have been used with varying accuracy.[72–74] In one study of 16 patients with ALF and epidural ICP monitors, various aspects of the TCD including velocity, waveform analysis and PI were evaluated as a means of dividing patients into subsets of ICP ranges (< 20, 20–30, > 30 mmHg).[75] TCD values could be used to correctly classify which group the patient belonged to only 53–67% of the time. Another study in ALF patients exploring the relationship between the PI and invasively measured ICP did not show a reliable correlation, but demonstrated that a calculated ICP using an estimated cerebral perfusion pressure from TCD flow velocities indeed correlated with measured ICP. [31] Two small case series of ALF patients have shown that patients with higher PIs were more likely to deteriorate neurologically or die while awaiting spontaneous improvement in their liver function or transplantation than those patients having normal PI.[76,77]

Jugular Bulb Oximetry

By retrograde catheterization of the internal jugular vein into the intracerebral jugular bulb, real time jugular venous oximetry (JvO_2) allows for estimation of the average oxygen consumption of the brain by calculating the arteriovenous oxygen difference. This difference can in turn help assess CBF and the cerebral metabolic state.[78] Jugular bulb oximetry has been described in monitoring patients with various other types of brain injury.[79] To date, studies evaluating jugular bulb oximetry in fulminant liver failure have shown the possible utility of this technique to monitor cerebral blood flow in patients at baseline and during hyperventilation [80] and hypothermia.[81] Additionally, one group reported the utility of monitoring JvO_2 while treating a patient with ALF and neurological decompensation.[82] Overall, there is some evidence to suggest the usefulness of the jugular bulb oximeter as a component of a multimodal monitoring platform, but there is not yet sufficient evidence to reliably correlate its measurements with ICP.

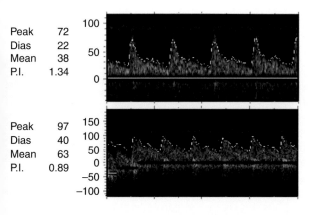

Peak	72
Dias	22
Mean	38
P.I.	1.34

Peak	97
Dias	40
Mean	63
P.I.	0.89

Figure 11.4 Transcranial Dopplers. Transcranial Dopplers insonating the right middle cerebral artery of a patient with global cerebral edema before (top) and after (bottom) treatment with hypertonic saline. Clinically the patient's pupils became reactive after treatment. Note the change in the waveform morphology as well as the pulsatility index (PI) after treatment.

Neuroprognostication over Time

Until recently, outcomes after ALF were measured primarily as survival to hospital discharge, and little research has gone into longer term outcomes. In particular, it is unclear whether the changes seen with HE are completely reversible with spontaneous improvement in liver function or with transplantation, or whether more permanent deficits remain.[83]

Further, secondary neurological injury can occur after liver transplantation and can either worsen prognosis or impair rehabilitation from the primary injury.[84] Complications such as seizures and posterior reversible encephalopathy syndrome (PRES) can arise as a result of using calcineurin inhibitors post-transplant. Intraoperatively and immediately postoperatively, changes in blood pressure and coagulation factors can result in ischemic and hemorrhagic strokes, and fluid and osmotic shifts can result in osmotic demyelination syndrome. Additionally, chronic immunosuppression can predispose patients to central nervous system infections, and prolonged intensive care unit stays can result in critical illness myoneuropathy.

Functional Outcomes

A recent study has looked at self-reported functional outcomes in long-term adult survivors of ALF by questionnaires at 1–2 years post-hospitalization.[85] This study found that, compared to controls from the U.S. general population, ALF survivors reported lower quality-of-life scores due to impaired physical health and activity limitations, both after liver transplant and after spontaneous recovery. A single-center retrospective study found that patients with pre-transplant moderate to severe cerebral edema were more likely to die within the first year or to have permanent gait and speech deficits requiring assisted living.[86]

Cognitive Outcomes

There are limited data on the persistence of cognitive deficits long term, and the existing studies primarily focus on post-transplant patients, in whom immunosuppressive medications may represent a confounding factor. A small study of seven ALF patients who required transplantation were compared to age-matched chronic liver disease patients who also required transplantation.[87] Both groups complained of memory difficulties after transplantation, but ALF patients specifically complained of more concentration difficulties, which were confirmed on limited neuropsychiatric testing. Another study of 12 patients who were 10 years out from liver transplantation for a variety of indications (including chronic liver failure) found global cognitive impairment in all patients in the absence of affective disorders.[88]

Behavioral Outcomes

While little about behavioral outcomes has been studied, there is some preliminary work on psychosocial factors that affect adherence, and therefore long-term viability of transplanted organs.[89] Work on all ALF patients suggest that patients with spontaneous recovery after acetaminophen overdose have the worst self-reported quality-of-life scores and worse self-reported mental health scores, which may be attributable to a higher rate of premorbid substance use disorders or psychiatric disease.[90] It is unknown whether these psychosocial factors are due to preexisting behaviors or are

171

a result of more permanent behavioral changes that occur due to longer-lasting brain injury as a result of elevated ICP and HE.

Gaps in Current Knowledge

The neurological monitoring and prognostication of patients with ALF remains a field with many unanswered questions and the pressing need for answers. It is still difficult to predict who will develop cerebral edema and elevated ICP, and even among transplantation centers there is no consistent monitoring paradigm or trigger for transfer to a higher level of care.[18] Furthermore, once the neurological exam becomes more limited with higher-grade HE, and with confounding metabolic issues like renal failure, sepsis, and hypoglycemia, identification of elevated ICP can be difficult. Cerebral edema is known to occur in patients with acute-on-chronic [91] and chronic liver failure.[92] but risk factors in those disease processes are also unknown.

The optimal neurological monitoring scheme of ALF patients is still unknown. Invasive ICP monitoring is still considered the gold standard, but given the potential of intracranial hemorrhage there has been a strong interest recently in protocolizing the noninvasive monitoring of patients to detect cerebral edema and elevated ICP.[93] However, given the lack of high-quality data, further multicenter trials are necessary in order to evaluate what combination of noninvasive monitors is most accurate and what the optimal frequency and duration of monitoring is. Choosing which patients may benefit from invasive monitoring is still most frequently a multidisciplinary discussion on a case-by-case basis.

In addition, there is no evidence-based guidance for intraoperative neuromonitoring for liver transplant patients. Significant fluid shifts can occur intraoperatively, which may precipitate elevations in ICP.[17,65] In fact, in one study of 22 patients with ALF who had ICP monitor placement, 82 episodes of elevated ICP occurred in 21 patients, with 5% occurring during the operative course and 20% occurring post-transplant.[17] Few studies have investigated the role of noninvasive monitoring intraoperatively, but given the physiological changes that occur in the anhepatic phase intraoperatively and then with engraftment, it appears wise to continue monitoring of patients through the intraoperative and postoperative period until the neurological exam improves.

Treatment of elevated ICP in ALF largely is extrapolated from the literature on primary brain injury. There are some very limited data on ALF-specific data on the use of indomethacin to lower ICP,[94] though this has not been confirmed in a large cohort of patients. Further, given known differences in autoregulation in ALF patients, spontaneous hyperventilation to a goal CO_2 of as low as 25–30 is felt to be acceptable in this patient population.[68–70,81] Further elucidating mechanisms of cerebral edema in the ALF patient may lead to the development of disease-specific therapies to prevent or treat cerebral edema and elevated ICP.

Optimal timing of initiation of renal replacement therapy has also been an interesting topic of debate. There are some preliminary data that continuous veno-venous hemofiltration is associated with ammonia clearance [95] and may be associated with a reduced risk of cerebral edema.[41] Certainly, initiation of a standard hemodialysis session should be avoided in cases of ALF given the risk of rapid osmotic shifts resulting in rapid development of cerebral edema, but perhaps early initiation of renal replacement therapy can prevent or mitigate the effects of cerebral edema.

The long-term outcomes of ALF survivors, either via spontaneous improvement in liver function or with transplantation, remain unknown. There are some small studies suggesting impairment in functional, cognitive, and behavioral/psychiatric realms, but the true incidence and degree of impairment need to be characterized further. One difficulty is the rapid onset of HE in ALF, precluding standardized testing prior to neurological decompensation. However, given the relatively young and healthy population that suffers from ALF, any long-term deficits could likely be attributed to their illness. Further characterizing the burden of these impairments may also help with more targeted rehabilitation therapies for this patient population.

Ongoing Research

The U.S. Acute Liver Failure Study Group (ALFSG) is a multicenter consortium that has been prospectively enrolling patients since 1998, and importantly has been collecting serum samples. Several biomarker studies are ongoing internationally, but there are no ongoing trials registered with ClinicalTrials.gov focusing on neurological issues in ALF.

In summary, there are little data to guide prognostication of patients in ALF. The ideal monitoring protocol is not agreed upon and there are inconsistent criteria used to determine candidacy for transplantation. There remains a lot of work to be done to optimally treat this small but very sick group of patients. Targeted ICP therapies may help reduce mortality from neurological causes, while an accurate assessment of long-term deficits may help to reduce morbidity in those who have spontaneous recovery of liver function or are able to receive a transplant.

References

1. European Association for the Study of the Liver. EASL Clinical Practical Guidelines on the management of acute (fulminant) liver failure. *J Hepatol.* 2017;**66**(5):1047–81.

2. Bernal W, Wendon J. Acute liver failure. *N Engl J Med.* 2013;**369**(26):2525–34.

3. Sarici KB, Karakas S, Otan E, et al. Can patients who develop cerebral death in fulminant liver failure despite liver transplantation be previously forseen? *Transplant Proc.* 2017;**49**(3):571–4.

4. Datar S, Wijdicks EF. Neurologic manifestations of acute liver failure. *Handb Clin Neurol.* 2014;**120**:645–59.

5. Bower WA, Johns M, Margolis HS, Williams IT, Bell BP. Population-based surveillance for acute liver failure. *Am J Gastroenterol.* 2007;**102**:2459–63.

6. Hirode G, Vittinghoff E, Wong RJ. Increasing burden of hepatic encephalopathy among hospitalized adults: an analysis of the 2010–2014 national inpatient sample. *Dig Dis Sci.* 2019;**64**(6):1448–57.

7. Stravitz RT, Lee WM. Acute liver failure. *Lancet.* 2019;**394**:869–81.

8. Riordan SM & Williams R. Perspectives on liver failure: past and future. *Semin Liver Dis.* 2008;**28** (2):137–41.

9. Ferenci P, Lockwood A, Mullen K, et al. Hepatic encephalopathy – definition, nomenclature, diagnosis, and quantification: final report of the working party at the 11th World Congresses of Gastroenterology, Vienna, 1998. *Hepatology.* 2002;**35** (3):716–21.

10. Weissenborn K, Ennen JC, Schomerus H, Ruckert N, Hecker H. Neuropsychological characterization of hepatic encephalopathy. *J Hepatol.* 2001;**34**(5):768–73.

11. Shawcross DL, Wendon JA. The neurological manifestations of acute liver failure. *Neurochem Int.* 2012;**60**(7):662–71.

12. Stravitz RT, Kramer DJ. Management of acute liver failure. *Nat Rev Gastroenterol Hepatol.* 2009;**6** (9):542–53.

13. Atterbury CE, Maddrey WC, Conn HO. Neomycin-sorbitol and lactulose in the treatment of acute portal-systemic encephalopathy: a controlled, double-blind clinical trial. *Am J Dig Dis.* 1978;**23**(5):398–406.

14. Kumar R, Shalimar HS, Sharma H, et al. Prospective derivation and validation of early dynamic model for predicting outcome in patients with acute liver failure. *Gut.* 2012;**61**(7):1068–75.

15. Tan WF, Steadman RH, Farmer DG, et al. Pretransplant neurological presentation and severe posttransplant brain injury in patients with acute liver failure. *Transplantation.* 2012;**94**(7):768–74.

16. Munoz SJ, Mortiz MJ, Bell R, et al. Factors associated with severe intracranial hypertension in candidates for emergency liver transplantation. *Transplantation.* 1993;**55**:1071–4.

17. Raschke RA, Curry SC, Rempe S, et al. Results of a protocol for the management of patients with fulminant liver failure. *Crit Care Med.* 2008;**36**;2244–8.

18. Rabinowich L, Wendon J, Bernal W, Shibolet O. Clinical management of acute liver failure: results of an international multi-center survey. *World J Gastroenterol.* 2016;**22**(33):7595–603.

19. O'Grady JG, Alexander GJ, Hayllar KM, Williams R. Early indicators of prognosis in fulminant hepatic failure. *Gastroenterology.* 1989;**97**(2):439–45.

20. Bernal W, Wang Y, Maggs J, et al. Development and validation of a dynamic outcome prediction model for paracetamol-induced acute liver failure: a cohort study. *Lancet Gastroenterol Hepatol.* 2016;**1**(3):217–25.

21. Munoz SJ, Robinson M, Northrup B, et al. Elevated intracranial pressure and computed tomography of the brain in fulminant hepatocellular failure. *Hepatology.* 1991;**13**(2):209–12.

22. Rama Rao KV, Jayakumar AR, Norenberg MD. Brain edema in acute liver failure: mechanisms and concepts. *Metab Brain Dis.* 2014;**29**(4):927–36.

23. Ranjan P, Mishra AM, Kale R, Saraswat VA, Gupta RK. Cytotoxic edema is responsible for raised intracranial pressure in fulminant hepatic failure: in vivo demonstration using diffusion-weighted MRI in human subjects. *Metab Brain Dis.* 2005;**20**(3):181–92.

24. Pulivarthi S, Gurram MK. Magnetic resonance imaging of brain findings in hyperammonemic encephalopathy. *J Neurosci Rural Pract.* 2016;**7** (3):469–71.

25. Fridman V, Galetta SL, Pruitt AA, Levine JM. MRI findings associated with acute liver failure. *Neurology*. 2009;**72**(24):2130–1.

26. Chavarria L, Cordoba J. Magnetic resonance imaging and spectroscopy in hepatic encephalopathy. *J Clin Exp Hepatol*. 2015;**5**(Suppl 1):S69–74.

27. Hansen HC, Helmke K. The subarachnoid space surrounding the optic nerves. An ultrasound study of the optic nerve sheath. *Surg Radiol Anat*. 1996;**18**(4):323–8.

28. Dubourg J, Javouhey E, Geeraerts T, Messerer M, Kassai B. Ultrasonography of optic nerve sheath diameter for detection of raised intracranial pressure: a systematic review and meta-analysis. *Intensive Care Med*. 2011;**37**(7):1059–68.

29. Hansen HC, Helmke K. Validation of the optic nerve sheath response to changing cerebrospinal fluid pressure: ultrasound findings during intrathecal infusion tests. *J Neurosurg*. 1997;**87**(1):34–40.

30. Launey Y, Nesseler N, Le Maquet P, Malledant Y, Sequin P. Effect of osmotherapy on optic nerve sheath diameter in patients with increased intracranial pressure. *J Neurotrauma*. 2014;**31**(10):984–8.

31. Rajajee V, Williamson CA, Fontana RJ, Courey AJ, Patil PG. Noninvasive intracranial pressure assessment in acute liver failure. *Neurocrit Care*. 2018;**29**(2):280–90.

32. Kim YK, Seo H, Yu J, Hwang GS. Noninvasive estimation of raised intracranial pressure using ocular ultrasonography in liver transplant recipients with acute liver failure – a report of two cases. *Korean J Anesthesiol*. 2013;**64**(5):451–5.

33. Krishnamoorthy V, Beckmann K, Mueller M, Sharma D, Vavilala MS. Perioperative estimation of the intracranial pressure using the optic nerve sheath diameter during liver transplantation. *Liver Transpl*. 2013;**19**(3):246–9.

34. Zaman MB, Hoti E, Qasim A, et al. MELD score as a prognostic model for listing acute liver failure patients for liver transplantation. *Transplant Proc*. 2006;**38**(7):2097–8.

35. Kim WR, Biggins SW, Kremers WK, et al. Hyponatremia and mortality among patients on the liver-transplant waiting list. *N Engl J Med*. 2008;**359**(10):1018–26.

36. Butterworth RF. Pathophysiology of brain dysfunction in hyperammonemic syndromes: the many faces of glutamine. *Mol Genet Metab*. 2014;**113**(1–2):113–17.

37. Kumar R, Shalimar, Sharma H, et al. Persistent hyperammonemia is associated with complications and poor outcomes in patients with acute liver failure. *Clin Gastroenterol Hepatol*. 2012;**10**(8):925–31.

38. Bemeur C, Cudalbu C, Dam G, et al. Brain edema: a valid endpoint for measuring hepatic encephalopathy? *Metab Brain Dis*. 2016;**31**(6):1249–58.

39. Clemmesen JO, Larsen FS, Kondrup J, Hansen BA, Ott P. Cerebral herniation in patients with acute liver failure is correlated with arterial ammonia concentration. *Hepatology*. 1999;**29**(3):648–53.

40. Bernal W, Hall C, Karvellas CJ, et al. Arterial ammonia and clinical risk factors for encephalopathy and intracranial hypertension in acute liver failure. *Hepatology*. 2007;**46**(6):1844–52.

41. Cardoso FS, Gottfried M, Tujios S, Olson JC, Karvellas CJ, US Acute Liver Failure Study Group. Continuous renal replacement therapy is associated with reduced serum ammonia levels and mortality in acute liver failure. *Hepatology*. 2018;**67**(2):711–20.

42. Rolando N, Wade J, Davalos M, et al. The systemic inflammatory response syndrome in acute liver failure. *Hepatology*. 2000;**32**(4 Pt 1):734–9.

43. Vaquero J, Polson J, Chung C, et al. Infection and the progression of hepatic encephalopathy in acute liver failure. *Gastroenterology*. 2003;**125**(3):755–64.

44. Wright G, Shawcross D, Olde Damink SW, Jalan R. Brain cytokine flux in acute liver failure and its relationship with intracranial hypertension. *Metab Brain Dis*. 2007;**22**(3–4):375–88.

45. Jalan R, Olde Damink SW, Hayes PC, Deutz NE, Lee A. Pathogenesis of intracranial hypertension in acute liver failure: inflammation, ammonia and cerebral blood flow. *J Hepatol*. 2004;**41**(4):613–60.

46. Bernal W, Donaldson N, Wyncoll D, Wendon J. Blood lactate as an early predictor of outcome in paracetamol-induced acute liver failure: a cohort study. *Lancet*. 2002;**359**(9306):558–63.

47. Bernal W. Lactate is important in determining prognosis in acute liver failure. *J Hepatol*. 2010;**53**(1):209–210.

48. Michard B, Artzner T, Lebas B, et al. Liver transplantation in critically ill patients: Preoperative predictive factors of post-transplant mortality to avoid futility. *Clin Transplant*. 2017;**31**(12):e13115.

49. Ott P, Vilstrup H. Cerebral effects of ammonia in liver disease: current hypotheses. *Metab Brain Dis*. 2014;**29**(4):901–11.

50. Rose CF. Increase brain lactate in hepatic encephalopathy: cause or consequence? *Neurochem Int*. 2010;**57**(4):389–94.

51. Baquerizo A, Anselmo D, Shackleton C, et al. Phosphorus as an early predictive factor in patients with acute liver failure. *Transplantation.* 2003;**75**(12):2007–14.

52. Chung HS, Lee YJ, Jo YS. Proposal for a new predictive model of short-term mortality after living donor liver transplantation due to acute liver failure. *Ann Transplant.* 2017;**22**:101–7.

53. Guerit JM, Amantini A, Fischer C, et al. Neurophysiological investigations of hepatic encephalopathy: ISHEN practice guidelines. *Liver Int.* 2009;**29**(6):789–96.

54. Ellis AJ, Wendon JA, Williams R. Subclinical seizure activity and prophylactic phenytoin infusion in acute liver failure: a controlled clinical trial. *Hepatology.* 2000;**32**(3):536–41.

55. Bhatia V, Batra Y, Acharya SK. Prophylactic phenytoin does not improve cerebral edema or survival in acute liver failure – a controlled clinical trial. *J Hepatol.* 2004;**41**(1):89–96.

56. Trewby PN, Casemore C, Williams R. Continuous bipolar recording of the EEG in patients with fulminant hepatic failure. *Electroencephalogr Clin Neurophysiol.* 1978;**45**(1):107–10.

57. Davenport A, Bramley PN. 1993. Cerebral function analyzing monitor and visual evoked potentials as a noninvasive method of detecting cerebral dysfunction in patients with acute hepatic and renal failure treated with intermittent machine hemofiltration. *Renal Fail.* 1993;**15**(4):515–22.

58. Van der Rijt C, Schalm SW. Quantitative EEG analysis and survival in liver disease. *Electroencephalogr Clin Neurophysiol.* 1985;**61**(6):502–4.

59. Stewart J, Sarkela M, Koivusalo AM, et al. Frontal electroencephalogram variables are associated with the outcome and stage of hepatic encephalopathy in acute liver failure. *Liver Transpl.* 2014;**20**(10):1256–65.

60. Fortea JI, Banares R, Vaquero J. Intracranial pressure in acute liver failure: to bolt or not to bolt – that is the question. *Crit Care Med.* 2014;**42**(5):1304–5.

61. Maloney PR, Mallory GW, Atkinson JL, Wijdicks EF, Rabinstein AA, Van Gompel JJ. Intracranial pressure monitoring in acute liver failure: institutional case series. *Neurocrit Care.* 2016;**25**(1):86–93.

62. Blei AT, Olafsson S, Webster S, Levy R. Complications of intracranial pressure monitoring in fulminant hepatic failure. *Lancet.* 1993;**341**(8838):157–8.

63. Karvellas CJ, Fix OK, Battenhouse H, et al. Outcomes and complications of intracranial pressure monitoring in acute liver failure: a retrospective cohort study. *Crit Care Med.* 2014;**42**(5):1157–67.

64. Vaquero J, Fontana RJ, Larson AM, et al. 2005. Complications and use of intracranial pressure monitoring in patients with acute liver failure and severe encephalopathy. *Liver Transpl.* 2005;**11**(12):1581–9.

65. Rajajee V, Fontana RJ, Courey AJ, Patil PG. Protocol based invasive intracranial pressure monitoring in acute liver failure: feasibility, safety and impact on management. *Crit Care.* 2017;**21**(1):178.

66. Kang YG, Martin DJ, Marquez J, et al. Intraoperative changes in blood coagulation and thrombelastographic monitoring in liver transplantation. *Anesth Analg.* 1985;**64**(9):888–96.

67. Kamat P, Kunde S, Vos M, et al. Invasive intracranial pressure monitoring is a useful adjunct in the management of severe hepatic encephalopathy associated with pediatric acute liver failure. *Pediatr Crit Care Med.* 2012;**13**(1):e33–38.

68. Larsen FS, Ejlersen E, Hansen BA, et al. Functional loss of cerebral blood flow autoregulation in patients with fulminant hepatic failure. *J Hepatol.* 1995;**23**(2):212–17.

69. Strauss GI, Hogh P, Moller K, Regional cerebral blood flow during mechanical hyperventilation in patients with fulminant hepatic failure. *Hepatology.* 1999;**30**(6):1368–73.

70. Larsen FS, Strauss G, Moller K, Hansen BA. Regional cerebral blood flow autoregulation in patients with fulminant hepatic failure. *Liver Transpl.* 2000;**6**(6):795–800.

71. Werner C, Kochs E, Rau M, Schulte Esch J. Transcranial Doppler sonography as a supplement in the detection of cerebral circulatory arrest. *J Neurosurg Anesthesiol.* 1990;**2**(3):159–65.

72. Aaslid R, Lundar T, Lindegaard KF, Nornes H. Estimation of cerebral perfusion pressure from arterial blood pressure and transcranial Doppler recordings. In Miller JD, Teasdale GM, Rowan JO, editors. *Intracranial Pressure VI.* Berlin: Springer, 1986; 226–9.

73. Chan KH, Miller JD, Dearden NM, Andrews PJ, Midgley S. The effect of changes in cerebral perfusion pressure upon middle cerebral artery blood flow velocity and jugular bulb venous oxygen saturation after severe brain injury. *J Neurosurg.* 1992;**77**(1):55–61.

74. Edouard AR, Vanhille E, Le-Moigno S, Benhamou D, Mazoit JX. Non-invasive assessment of cerebral perfusion pressure in brain injured patients with moderate intracranial hypertension. *Br J Anaesth.* 2005;**94**(2):216–21.

75. Aggarwal S, Brooks DM, Kang Y, Linden PK, Patzer JF. Noninvasive monitoring of cerebral perfusion pressure in patients with acute liver failure using transcranial Doppler ultrasonography. *Liver Transpl.* 2008;14(7):1048–57.

76. Kawakami M, Koda M, Murawaki Y. Cerebral pulsatility index by transcranial Doppler sonography predicts the prognosis of patients with fulminant hepatic failure. *Clin Imaging.* 2010;34(5):327–31.

77. Abdo A, Perez-Bernal J, Hinojosa R, et al. Cerebral hemodynamics patterns by transcranial Doppler in patients with acute liver failure. *Transplant Proc.* 2015;47(9):2647–9.

78. Paschoal FM Jr, Nogueira RC, Ronconi Kde A, et al. Multimodal brain monitoring in fulminant hepatic failure. *World J Hepatol.* 2016;8(22):915–23.

79. Steiner LA, Andrews PJ. Monitoring the injured brain: ICP and CBF. *Br J Anaesth.* 2006;97(1):26–38.

80. Strauss GI, Møller K, Holm S, et al. Transcranial doppler sonography and internal jugular bulb saturation during hyperventilation in patients with fulminant hepatic failure. *Liver Transpl.* 2001;7(4):352–8.

81. Jalan R, Olde Damink SW, Deutz NE, Hayes PC, Lee A. Restoration of cerebral blood flow autoregulation and reactivity to carbon dioxide in acute liver failure by moderate hypothermia. *Hepatology.* 2001;34(1):50–4.

82. Kim Y, Kim CK, Jung S, Ko SB. Brain oxygen monitoring via jugular venous oxygen saturation in a patient with fulminant hepatic failure. *Korean J Crit Care Med.* 2016;31:251–5.

83. Moore KA. Liver transplantation: what do we really know about the long-term impact? *Liver Transpl.* 2003;9(11):1149–51.

84. Weiss N, Thabut D. Neurological complications occurring after liver transplantation: role of risk factors, hepatic encephalopathy, and acute (on chronic) brain injury. *Liver Transpl.* 2019;25(3):469–87.

85. Rangnekar AS, Ellerbe C, Durkalski V, et al. Quality of life is significantly impaired in long-term survivors of acute liver failure and particularly in acetaminophen-overdose patients. *Liver Transpl.* 2013;19(9):991–1000.

86. Chan G, Taqi A, Marotta P, et al. Long-term outcomes of emergency liver transplantation for acute liver failure. *Liver Transpl.* 2009;15(12):1696–1702.

87. Jackson EW, Zacks S, Zinn S, et al. Delayed neuropsychologic dysfunction after liver transplantation for acute liver failure: a matched, case–controlled study. *Liver Transpl.* 2002;8(10):932–6.

88. Lewis MB, Howdle PD. Cognitive dysfunction and health-related quality of life in long-term liver transplant survivors. *Liver Transpl.* 2003;9(11):1145–8.

89. Alsina A, Alsina A, Athienitis A, et al. Is fulminant hepatic failure the nemesis for liver transplant centers? A two decade psychosocial and long-term outcome study. *Am Surg.* 2018;84(7):1197–1203.

90. Rangnekar AS, Ellerbe C, Durkalski V, et al. Quality of life is significantly impaired in long-term survivors of acute liver failure and particularly in acetaminophen-overdose patients. *Liver Transpl.* 2013;19(9):991–1000.

91. Wright G, Sharifi Y, Jover-Cobos M, Jalan R. The brain in acute on chronic liver failure. *Metab Brain Dis.* 2014;29(4):965–73.

92. Cudalbu C, Taylor-Robinson SD. Brain edema in chronic hepatic encephalopathy. *J Clin Exp Hepatol.* 2019;9(3):362–82.

93. Reynolds AS, Brush B, Schiano TD, Reilly KJ, Dangayach NS. Neurological monitoring in acute liver failure. *Hepatology.* 2019;70(5):1830–5.

94. Tofteng F, Larsen FS. The effect of indomethacin on intracranial pressure, cerebral perfusion and extracellular lactate and glutamate concentrations in patients with fulminant hepatic failure. *J Cereb Blood Flow Metab.* 2004;24(7):798–804.

95. Slack AJ, Auzinger G, Willars C, et al. Ammonia clearance with haemofiltration in adults with liver disease. *Liver Int.* 2014;34(1):42–8.

Chapter 12

Prognostication in Post-Intensive Care Syndrome

Natalie Kreitzer, Neha S. Dangayach, and Brandon Foreman

Introduction

The first intensive care units (ICUs) were established in the 1950s in the wake of a pandemic in order to rescue patients with respiratory failure from certain death, launching an entirely new field referred to today as critical care medicine.[1] The mortality associated with critical illness has improved substantially over the decades,[2,3] and long-term patient- and family-centered outcomes have emerged as important new targets for intervention. The *post-intensive care syndrome* (PICS) was defined in 2012 [2] as a constellation of cognitive, mental health, or physical impairments that occur after treatment in the ICU and persist well beyond discharge (Figure 12.1). A key feature of PICS is that these symptoms lead to a quality of life that is worse than expected based on the patient's initial acute illness.[2,4] PICS may be overlooked during or shortly after hospital discharge, when success means simply surviving a critical illness, but these symptoms may result in substantial long-term disability months or even years later in one-half or more patients with critical illness.[5] More recently, PICS-Family (PICS-F) has been defined as the acute and chronic psychological effects of critical illness on the *families* of patients, and may impact as many as 30% of patients' family members.[6] An understanding of the risks for PICS, and its domain-specific impact particularly in patients with acute brain injuries, is the subject of this chapter.

Symptoms of PICS after Intensive Care

Mental Health Impairments

Mental health impairment that may develop after recovery from intensive care includes new and persistent anxiety, depression, sleep impairment, or post-traumatic stress disorder (PTSD). Those at highest risk include patients of younger age,[7–9] female gender,[10–12] and those with prior psychiatric history with a relative risk (RR) of developing mental health impairment of 3.9 (95% confidence interval [CI]: 1.5–6.5).[13] Specific risk factors for post-intensive care depression include, hypoglycemia,[13] sepsis,[10] acute respiratory distress syndrome (ARDS),[14,15] sedation,[8,13,16,17] delirium,[7] restraints, and agitation.[16,18] At 12 months, the prevalence of depression in ICU survivors without preexisting depression is 30%, and even higher in those with preexisting depression.[19] Similarly, a diagnosis of anxiety disorder has been reported in 16–62% of ICU survivors. No differences in the prevalence of anxiety have been shown among survivors from different types of ICUs,[20] however. PTSD, defined as a response to a life-altering or life-threatening event that persists for more than 4 weeks and includes avoidance of trauma triggers, physiological hyperarousal, re-experiencing and negative thoughts about the experience,[21] occurs in 25–44% of ICU survivors according to a meta-analysis of 36 different studies. One in five patients were found to have PTSD even a year after their illness.[22]

The diagnosis of impairments in mental health tends to rely on patient-reported instruments based on formal diagnostic criteria as outlined by the DSM 5.[23] Screening tools used for depression and anxiety include the Patient Health Questionnaire-9, Hospital Acquired Anxiety Depression Scale (HADS), and Beck's Depression Inventory. PTSD can be screened using the PTSD Checklist (PCL-5) or the Impact of Events Scale-Revised (IES-R). The HADS and IES-R tools specifically have been endorsed as core outcome measurements in survivors of ARDS based on a Delphi consensus process.[24]

The proportion of patients with mental health impairment after neurocritical illness is high and mirrors the general critical care population. After

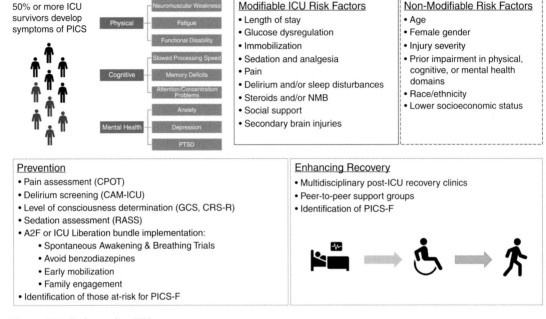

50% or more ICU survivors develop symptoms of PICS

Physical
- Neuromuscular Weakness
- Fatigue
- Functional Disability

Cognitive
- Slowed Processing Speed
- Memory Deficits
- Attention/Concentration Problems

Mental Health
- Anxiety
- Depression
- PTSD

Modifiable ICU Risk Factors
- Length of stay
- Glucose dysregulation
- Immobilization
- Sedation and analgesia
- Pain
- Delirium and/or sleep disturbances
- Steroids and/or NMB
- Social support
- Secondary brain injuries

Non-Modifiable Risk Factors
- Age
- Female gender
- Injury severity
- Prior impairment in physical, cognitive, or mental health domains
- Race/ethnicity
- Lower socioeconomic status

Prevention
- Pain assessment (CPOT)
- Delirium screening (CAM-ICU)
- Level of consciousness determination (GCS, CRS-R)
- Sedation assessment (RASS)
- A2F or ICU Liberation bundle implementation:
  - Spontaneous Awakening & Breathing Trials
  - Avoid benzodiazepines
  - Early mobilization
  - Family engagement
- Identification of those at-risk for PICS-F

Enhancing Recovery
- Multidisciplinary post-ICU recovery clinics
- Peer-to-peer support groups
- Identification of PICS-F

Figure 12.1 Understanding PICS.
A2 F = ABCDEF Bundle; CAM-ICU = Confusion Assessment Method – ICU; CPOT = critical care pain observation tool; CRS-R = Coma Recovery Score-Revised; ICU = intensive care unit; GCS = Glasgow Coma Scale; NMB = neuromuscular blockade; PICS = post-intensive care syndrome; PICS-F = post-intensive care unit family; RASS = Richard Agitation and Sedation Score.

ICH, depression occurs in about 20%,[25,26] and in a systematic review of patients with subarachnoid hemorrhage, a weighted proportion of 28.1% of patients exhibited depression even several years following injury.[27] In some cases, risks for impairments in mental health may be even higher than in the general critical care population. For instance, patients who experience traumatic brain injury (TBI) have a higher prevalence of mental health impairments *prior* to injury. In a meta-analysis, the pooled prevalence of pre-TBI depression and anxiety were 13% and 19%, respectively; yet, after injury, the prevalence of depression and anxiety increased to 43% and 36%, respectively, over the years following injury.[28]

Post-traumatic stress disorder is increasingly recognized after sudden brain injuries. Across the spectrum of TBI, PTSD occurs in an estimated 15.6% of patients according to one meta-analysis. In this study, there were no differences in the rates of PTSD among those with mild vs moderate to severe TBI, and the pooled prevalence of PTSD after TBI was *twice* that of control patients or those with non-brain trauma.[29] After mild TBI, those with less education, certain race/ethnicity

groups, prior psychiatric history, and injury from assault have higher rates of PTSD. Risk factors for PTSD after moderate to severe TBI have been less well studied, although a seemingly shorter degree of post-traumatic amnesia or memory of the event are related to the development of PTSD,[28] which could result in less PTSD for those requiring critical care with more severe injuries. After ischemic stroke, 23% of patients have PTSD within the year.[30] Similarly, about one-quarter of patients with SAH have PTSD,[31] which persists even 3 years following the injury [32] and impacts quality of life.[33] Rates of PTSD may be lower after ICH, in which a 6.5% incidence has been reported.[34]

The most studied mental health impairment after brain injury is often considered a separate entity: post-stroke depression (PSD). PSD has an estimated prevalence of 33% across the stroke population, including ischemic and hemorrhage stroke. PSD has been associated with higher mortality, worse disability, and more increased cognitive impairment.[35] While the putative mechanisms behind PSD are thought to involve the vascular injury itself, its risk factors – which include female gender, older age, prior personal or family history of mental health impairment, and severity of stroke [36] – overlap substantially between this condition and other PICS-related impairments, highlighting difficulties in disentangling brain injury from the impact of critical care itself.

Larger or multiple strokes predict PSD, but no differences in the proportion of patients with PSD have been shown based on the type or location of stroke, although underlying volume of white matter disease may enhance the risk. [35] Lack of post-stroke social support may play an important role in the development of depression as well. However, factors related to intensive care that may impact the development of mental health impairment after neurological injury have been understudied.

Cognitive Impairments

The impact of critical illness on cognition has come into focus in the last 20 years,[37] and it has become clear that cognitive impairment after intensive care occurs independent of age and disease process. In a nested case–control cohort from the Mayo Clinic, nearly 2.5% of patients admitted to the ICU developed new and persistent cognitive dysfunction, which was associated with "brain failure," a term that encompasses delirium as well as disorders of consciousness (e.g., coma) independent of a diagnosis of sepsis.[38] A recent Delphi consensus statement endorsed assessment of cognitive function as a core domain associated with PICS.[39]

Cognitive impairment encompasses multiple domains: executive functioning, memory, attention, language processing, and visuospatial abilities. The majority of the existing literature has leveraged multiple assessments to gauge cognition from objective tests to patient-reported batteries, and the Mini-Mental Status Exam and the Trail Making Test were the most commonly used.[37] Tests that assess global cognition include the multidimensional Repeatable Battery for the Assessment of Neuropsychological Status (RBANS) [40] and the Patient-Reported Outcomes Measurement Information System (PROMIS) cognitive function batteries, which are subjectively reported. Most recently, recommendations from the general critical care community recommend a revision of the Montreal Cognitive Assessment (MoCA) without visual tasks (MoCA-BLIND) for objectively assessing cognitive function after respiratory failure.[24]

The neurologically critically ill experience a high prevalence of cognitive dysfunction. In a feasibility study of follow-up after neurocritical care, only 223/496 (45.0%) survivors contacted were able to participate in cognitive testing, of whom 20% had scores consistent with cognitive impairment.[41] After acute ischemic stroke, between 35 and 90% experience cognitive dysfunction 3 months after injury, depending on the assessment used.[42] After hemorrhagic stroke, 37% experienced a decline in their Mini-Mental Status scores over several years following their injury.[43] After subarachnoid hemorrhage (SAH), more than one-third (36%) had global cognitive scores based on the Telephone Interview for Cognitive Skills (modified) that were ≥ 2 standard deviations below normal at 3 months after injury. [44] These cognitive deficits may remain for years. [45] TBI in particular impacts cognition, with up to 60% reporting cognitive dysfunction even 3–5 years after injury.[46]

In survivors of both general and neurological critical illness, secondary brain injuries may play a role in the development of cognitive dysfunction. Delirium is clearly implicated in patients with respiratory failure and shock, and similarly, patients with ICH who experience delirium experience significantly lower patient-reported applied executive functioning, independent of their initial National Institutes of Health Stroke Scale [47] at 28 days following injury. Seizures occur frequently in the neurocritically ill, and in a study of patients with SAH, seizure burden (the duration of seizure activity) was independently associated with decreases in cognition at 3 months.[48] Similar associations between cognitive impairment and seizures or ictal–interictal patterns have been described after moderate to severe TBI.[49] In some cases, this may be confounded by findings that phenytoin and levetiracetam, used to prevent seizures, may impact cognitive outcome after hemorrhagic stroke.[50,51] The impact of other secondary brain injury patterns that may affect both the general critical care population and the neurocritically ill is less clear, although early evidence suggests there may be an association between autoregulatory dysfunction and delirium,[52] for instance.

Importantly, cognitive ability after neurocritical illness may be impacted not only by the critical illness but also by the underlying neurological injury itself. After SAH, predictive models of functional outcome and cognitive function contain similar underlying clinical variables, suggesting shared impact.[53] In survivors of TBI, the Extended Glasgow Outcome Scale (GOS-E), a widely used functional outcome scale, modestly corresponds to both cognitive and emotional health.[54] Importantly, not all patients who experience critical illness are able to complete cognitive assessments, leading to a selection bias favoring those with milder injuries, excluding those who die or who have injuries to regions of the brain that do not affect language or other sensory functions necessary to participate in testing. With mortality rates between 25 and 40%,[41] studies of patients with neurocritical illness face significant statistical limitations when considering functional outcome alone,[55] no less so than when comparing outcomes with more challenging assessments such as cognition.

Physical Impairments

Physical impairments after critical illness are composed of activity limitations that occur in ICU survivors who did not have neuromuscular disability prior to their hospitalization. Much of the work done to characterize the physical impairments associated with PICS is from ARDS survivors. Weakness secondary to critical illness and reduced respiratory function are commonly reported after critical illness, with ICU-acquired weakness (ICUAW) present in approximately 40% of critically ill adult patients.[56] Most commonly, this is a result of critical illness myopathy, followed by critical illness neuromyopathy, and then critical illness polyneuropathy.[57] Patients with these physical impairments have increased morbidity and mortality both in-hospital and at 1 year when compared to those who do not experience critical care-associated physical impairments.[58]

Risk factors for the development of ICUAW include female gender, sepsis or systemic inflammatory response syndrome (SIRS), a high catabolic state, multiorgan failure, a long period of mechanical ventilation, increased immobility, hyperglycemia, glucocorticoids, and use of neuromuscular blocking agents.[59] The most severe form of ICUAW, quadriparesis, is also an independent risk factor for prolonged ventilator weaning, which compounds both weakness and the development of other risk factors for PICS such as delirium.[60] The muscle impairments

associated with ICUAW may partially resolve several weeks after critical illness; however, motor function may continue to be impaired for several months or years.[61]

The measurement of physical impairment is complex and may involve pulmonary function testing or electrophysiological assessments,[37] some of which require specialists to perform and interpret. Simpler tests, such as hand grip strength, have been closely associated with decreased respiratory strength and reduced exercise capacity, both common after critical illness, even up to 12 months following admission.[62,63] The 6-minute walk test is endorsed as a quantitative measure of physical functioning based on recommendations, but no consensus-based test has been identified.[24] Less direct assessments involve questions related to activities of daily living (ADL) or restrictions in activity, and include commonly used scales such as the GOS-E, the modified Rankin Scale (mRS), the Barthel Index, or the Functional Independence Measure (FIM), among many others.[37] Using these methods, around one-third of ICU survivors require assistance in at least one ADL, such as bathing, dressing, toileting, transferring, or feeding 3 months after critical illness.[64]

Physical impairment after neurocritical care is common in part due to the primary brain injury. After stroke, the severity of the stroke-related symptoms correlates with quality of life, [53,65,66] as does functional disability after TBI, [67] and studies have shown that functional outcome scales such as the mRS tend to correlate predominantly with mobility.[68] A challenge in defining physical impairment related to PICS in the neurocritical care population is understanding which impairments might be attributable to intensive care vs the structural brain injury. Future studies to better understand measures that may prevent additional physical impairments in neurocritical care survivors are needed.

Factors during Intensive Care Related to the Development of PICS

Delirium

Delirium is a clinical diagnosis defined by *the Diagnostic and Statistical Manual of Mental Disorders* (DSM-5) [69] and characterized by the following: (1) a disturbance in attention and awareness, (2) over a short period of time, acutely changing from baseline and fluctuating in severity, (3) with an additional cognitive disturbance. These disturbances cannot be explained by preexisting neurocognitive disorders (e.g., dementia), and by definition patients with disorders of consciousness such as coma cannot be considered delirious. Delirium encompasses several phenotypes, including patients with agitation and those with decreased motor movements despite characteristic alterations in attention and awareness. Hypoactive delirium may be more difficult to recognize compared to agitated delirium.[70]

Delirium is remarkably common in the ICU setting. In a meta-analysis including 4,550 ICU patients, the overall pooled prevalence of delirium was 31%.[71] In a systematic review of 7 studies encompassing nearly 1,200 patients with neurocritical illness, the median prevalence of delirium was between 11 and 37%.[72] In a pooled analysis of the Modifying the Incidence of Delirium (MIND-ICU) and Bringing to light the Risk factors And Incidence of Neuropsychological dysfunction (BRAIN-ICU) studies, the following etiologies of delirium were described: hypoxic, sedative-associated, metabolic, septic, and unclassified.[73] A single delirium phenotype was present in only 1,355 (32%) of 4,187 participant-delirium days, whereas two or more phenotypes were present during 2,832 (68%) delirium days.

The underlying pathophysiology of delirium is not clear, although emerging evidence suggests that impaired connectivity within functional brain networks may play a role.[74] In a normal state of health, several networks, including the default mode network and task positive networks, serve as the basis of focused awareness. Electrophysiological studies have shown that in patients with sepsis who experience delirium, background slowing of the scalp electroencephalogram (EEG) was increased.[75] Similar to patients undergoing anesthesia,[76] a case–control study of patients with delirium found decreased network integration suggested by increased connectivity within the theta band and abnormal alpha band connectivity on scalp EEG.[77]

In a review of 68 studies, clinical risk factors for delirium included several factors that modify baseline brain network connectivity: age, underlying medical comorbidities (e.g., the American Society of Anesthesiologists Physical Status Classification), and preexisting dementia. Risk factors that subsequently impact brain connectivity include emergency surgery or trauma, admission injury severity (i.e., the Acute Physiology And Chronic Health Evaluation [APACHE] score), prior coma, use of benzodiazepines, and transfusion of blood products.[78] In a meta-analysis of 22 trials of nonpharmacological interventions for preventing delirium,[79] multicomponent approaches with attention to nutrition and hydration, oxygenation, medication review, assessment of mood, and bowel and bladder care were found to reduce the incidence of delirium.

The assessment of delirium is aided by several bedside scales, including the Confusion Assessment Method for the ICU (CAM-ICU) [80] and the Intensive Care Delirium Screening Checklist (ICDSC).[81] Direct comparison of these two in the medical intensive care population has suggested that the CAM-ICU has superior summary receiver operating characteristics compared with the ICDSC (0.97 vs. 0.89, respectively). The CAM-ICU also demonstrated better sensitivity to detect hypoactive delirium (57% vs. 32% for the ICDSC).[82] In neurocritically ill patients, assessments may be confounded by changes in level of arousal or focal deficits, such as aphasia, and severely limit the sensitivity of both formal and bedside testing. In a study of patients with intracerebral hemorrhage undergoing comprehensive assessment of delirium, core features of delirium such as inattention and disorientation were often unable to be assessed without a nonverbal method of screening. In this setting, the ICDSC outperformed the CAM-ICU with a sensitivity of 77% and specificity of 97% (compared to 68% and 88%, respectively).[83] Bedside methods that may infer the presence of delirium outside of these formal evaluations include asking a patient to state the months of year backwards, which yields an 83% sensitivity and 91% specificity for delirium; however, many patients cannot perform this cognitively challenging task, and others have chosen simpler tasks such as counting backwards from 20 to 1 within 30 seconds, which is easy to quantify and follow day to day.[84]

The recognition of delirium is increasingly important as a marker of vulnerability and in addition to being a risk for developing PICS, delirium has been associated with important short-term outcomes such as ventilator time, ICU stay, cost, and mortality.[85] Merely the act of assessing for delirium may reduce in-hospital mortality.[86] The BRAIN-ICU study included 821 patients with respiratory failure or shock, of whom the majority experienced delirium. Nearly one-third of these patients experienced persistent cognitive impairment similar to that experienced by patients with moderate traumatic brain injury.[40] A follow-up study of these same patients found that one-third developed at least mild depressive symptoms 1 year following their illness, primarily related to somatic symptoms rather than cognitive-affective symptoms. Controlling for age, educational level, baseline comorbidities, injury severity, and sedation, the duration of delirium was independently associated with depression (point estimate [PE] 2.31, 95% CI: 1.25 to 4.27) and the mental component of quality of life based on the Short Form-36 (PE –5.79, 95% CI: –10.26 to –1.31).[87] In the neurocritical care population, delirium similarly impacts ICU length of stay, hospital length of stay, functional independence, and cognition,[72] and likely plays a role in the development of PICS symptoms after recovery from critical illness. Despite challenges in applying diagnostic tools to the neurocritical care population, one study reported the incidence of delirium after stroke to be as high as 10–48%.[88]

Agitation and the Use of Sedation

Sedation is commonly used in the ICU as a method of addressing anxiety and discomfort in the setting of mechanical ventilation. The nonspecific symptoms of being physically or mentally uncomfortable may manifest as restlessness or agitation, which results in attempts to remove care-related equipment and even frank combativeness irrespective of a patient's premorbid cognitive abilities. Motor agitation can be described using several scales, including the Riker Sedation-Agitation Scale (SAS), which ranges from 1 to 7,[89] and the Richmond Agitation-Sedation Scale (RASS), which ranges from +4 to –5.[90] SAS and RASS have also been correlated with delirium measurements, suggesting at link between the two.[91] Both delirium and the depth, type and duration of sedation are important modifiable risk factors for PICS.

While the definition of "light" sedation is not uniform, a meta-analysis performed as part of the Society of Critical Care Medicine's Clinical Practice Guidelines for the Prevention and Management of Pain, Agitation/Sedation, Delirium, Immobility, and Sleep Disruption in Adult Patients in the ICU (PADIS) guidelines found low-quality evidence that targeting a RASS –2 to +1 was associated with a shorter time to extubation and reduced the rates of tracheostomy, but this did not alter the incidence of delirium, depression, or PTSD.[78] Rather than depth of sedation, the *agent* used for sedation may play a larger role: benzodiazepines have been clearly linked with delirium and cognitive dysfunction.[40] Compared with benzodiazepines, the use of dexmedetomidine for sedation reduced the odds for delirium (relative risk 0.71, 95% CI: 0.61–0.83) [92] in one study, although pooled analyses have not confirmed this effect.[78] The Maximizing the Efficacy of Sedation and Reducing Neurological Dysfunction and Mortality in Septic Patients with Acute Respiratory Failure (MENDS) 2 study found no difference in outcomes among mechanically ventilated sepsis patients receiving light sedation using dexmedetomidine versus propofol.[93] Further, in the Sedation Practice in Intensive Care Evaluation (SPICE) III study, patients receiving dexmedetomidine as the sole sedative agent had more hypotension and bradycardia compared to patients receiving propofol or midazolam sedation as part of standard care.[94] In patients with acute brain injuries, less is known about the effects of different sedative agents on delirium and the development of PICS.

Pain

Critically ill patients experience moderate to severe pain at rest and even during standard ICU procedures like turning in bed, suctioning as well as during invasive procedures such as arterial line placement or removal of chest tubes.[95,96] There are several consequences of untreated pain in the ICU, such as psychological distress, delirium, and prolonged hospitalization.[78] In a cohort study of 5,176 medical ICU patients, higher intensities of self-reported pain were associated with younger age, female gender, history of prior surgery, higher number of comorbidities, and history of anxiety and depression.[97] In patients undergoing cardiac surgery, patients with a history of preexisting depression or anxiety were more likely to report higher intensities of pain.[98] In an international study, a history of prior opioid use was a further risk factor for procedural pain.[96]

The assessment of pain can be challenging in critically ill patients, particularly in patients who cannot verbalize their pain or follow commands.

For those who *are* able to verbalize pain, several validated scales have been studied, such as the Visual Analog Scale, the Numerical Rating Scale (NRS), or the Wong-Baker FACES scale. In the ICU setting, NRS may have better sensitivity and specificity compared to the Visual Analog Scale.[99] For patients who are not able to speak, the critical care pain observation tool (CPOT) [100,101] and the behavioral rating scale (BRS) have been validated [102,103] in populations experience brain injuries or neurosurgery. In addition, several studies have been conducted to understand the utility of physiological variables such as heart rate or blood pressure but found that these variables could not be used reliably as surrogate markers of pain or pain intensity.[104–107] The Neurocritical Care Society has endorsed the PADIS guidelines,[78] which recommend frequent assessment of pain in the ICU using a validated scale; however, no studies have assessed the validity of a unified scale across the neurocritical care population.

Immobility

ICU-acquired weakness develops in 25–50% of critical care survivors[108] and negatively impacts long-term survival and quality of life.[58,109,110] Critical illness leads to a catabolic state that predisposes to muscle breakdown and weakness. Deconditioning and critical illness myopathy, neuropathy, and polymyoneuropathy contribute to ICUAW in critical care survivors. One of the most important risk factors for ICUAW is bedrest.[109,111] Early mobilization has been shown to improve outcomes after critical illness.[78] Early mobilization can be challenging in critically ill patients due to hemodynamic instability, mechanical ventilation, other devices for mechanical circulatory or oxygenation support such as extracorporeal membrane oxygenation (ECMO), intra-aortic balloon pumps, ventricular assist devices, and continuous renal replacement therapy. Further, PICS risk factors such as delirium, sedation, and agitation all impact a patient's ability to participate in early mobilization,[112] potentially worsening the development of PICS symptoms.

Despite these challenges, several studies have described multidisciplinary protocols for ambulation and provided guidance to maintain safety while ambulating critically ill patients.[113] The role of early mobilization in neurocritical care has not been well studied, and randomized controlled trials (RCTs) are lacking. While potential benefits have been identified in retrospective cohort studies, some evidence suggests that inpatients with ischemic stroke could develop worse outcomes with very early, aggressive mobilization provided within the first 24 hours after injury.[114]

Sleep

High-quality sleep plays a critical role in consolidating memories, regulating the immune system, and coordinating neuroendocrine functions.[115] Effective sleep consists of four divided stages based on EEG findings: stage N1 and N2 are classified as light sleep, while stage N3 and rapid eye movement sleep (REM) are classified as deep sleep.[116] Abnormalities in sleep, by contrast, are thought to increase the risk of a broad range of adverse health effects, including cardiovascular disease, depression, cognitive impairment, seizures, and even overall mortality.[117] Critical care is highly disruptive of sleep for numerous reasons and can serve as a precursor for the development of PICS. The 2018 PADIS guidelines acknowledged this by adding sleep as an integral component of their clinical practice guidelines.

Sleep derangements are common during critical illness. During intensive care, the amount of total sleep time is not necessarily decreased, but the amount of time in light sleep is increased and the amount of time in deep sleep is decreased.[118] Furthermore, sleep in the ICU is fragmented compared to the normal circadian sleep rhythm due to noise, painful stimulation or procedures, psychological factors, ventilator or respiratory factors, medications, restricted movement and inability to get comfortable in the hospital bed, and frequent examinations.[78] Mechanical ventilation is a leading risk factor for sleep fragmentation in critically ill patients because of associated pressure support, ventilator asynchrony, or ventilator alarms.[119] Daytime sleep may be increased due to bedrest or sedation, and nighttime sleep is often reduced due to alarms or nursing duties.[120] Additionally, unusual, atypical, or dissociated sleep, defined as a lack of cyclic organization and the absence of K complexes and sleep spindles in stage N2 of sleep is reported in patients who receive sedation.[118]

Yet, sleep has an impact on the development of delirium and therefore outcome. Delirium is the most notable proximal related effect of poor sleep in the ICU, although a causal link between lack of sleep and delirium has not been established. Higher rates of daytime sleeping and lower amounts of REM sleep have been associated with higher rates of delirium,[121] but delirium itself leads to inability to accurately assess sleep quality. Subjective sleep quality measures, used in many studies of sleep in the ICU, are likely unreliable. [78] In contrast, better sleep quality has been associated with lower rates of delirium in the ICU. [122] Based on these links, several studies have sought to find solutions to improve sleep quality in the ICU,[123–125] but evidence is still lacking to guide best practices.

Potential interventions to improve sleep include using assist control ventilation rather than synchronized intermittent mandatory ventilation at night or pressure support modes, but this is only a conditional recommendation with low quality of evidence per the PADIS guidelines.[78] Noninvasive, low-cost interventions such as noise and light reduction or earplugs may improve sleep quality in the ICU,[126, 127] although they have only been evaluated in small RCTs. Dexmedetomidine may improve sleep architecture and sleep efficiency, as demonstrated in a small RCT.[128, 129] In a large double-blind randomized controlled trial of elderly patients undergoing cardiac surgery, those who received dexmedetomidine had lower levels of pain and improved sleep, but no difference in rates of delirium.[130] Multicomponent protocols that include combinations of noise and light reduction, ear plugs, music, pharmacological agents, or minimization of overnight interruptions have been studied; however, these studies are at high risk of bias, but given their low risk, are conditionally recommended with very low quality of evidence by the Society of Critical Care Medicine.[78]

Neurological injury requiring critical care likely compounds the problems associated with poor sleep quality, so patients in the neurointensive care unit may be particularly at risk of deleterious effects of poor sleep. In a study comparing critically ill patients with and without neurological injury, those with a neurological injury had worse circadian rhythm disturbances compared to those without.[131] In a study using polysomnography to test the effect of noninvasive eye masks and melatonin in the neurointensive care unit, nearly two-thirds exhibited sleep that was unscorable using standard criteria.[132] Another study including patients with moderate to severe TBI monitored with actigraphy acutely after injury found that derangement of consolidated night rest and day activity was associated with worse severity of injury, longer ICU stay, and worse disability after injury. Faster improvement in normal rest-activity cycles predicted recovery, highlighting the role of brain injuries in sleep cycle disturbances.[133] In addition, the use of hourly neurochecks is a specific intervention used in the neurointensive care unit to identify acute neurological deteriorations. Retrospective studies have suggested that beyond the first 24–48 hours, the frequency of neurochecks may be implicated in sleep disturbance, delirium, or even outcome and perhaps should be decreased.[134]

Family and Caregiver PICS (PICS-F)

Family members of critically ill patients are at high risk of developing PICS-F, which is defined as the acute and chronic psychological effects of having a loved one in the ICU. Family members are faced with a multitude of challenges due to critical illness, including difficulty with food, housing, or basic medical care for themselves. Many caregivers are forced to move homes, delay education, or even file for bankruptcy after a family member's critical illness.[135] The stressors associated with a family member's ICU admission can acutely lead to a cluster of adverse psychological outcomes such as depression, anxiety, and post-traumatic stress disorder, or complicated grief; however, the symptoms of PICS-F can persist for more than 4 years. [6] Although intensivists are not responsible directly for the health of family members, improving quality of care of families of patients in the ICU may improve the outcomes of their patients as these psychological repercussions may decrease a family member's ability to fully provide caregiving functions after hospitalization.[6]

Not surprisingly, family members of patients who die in the ICU are at the highest risk of psychological stress. Indeed, 20–51% of family members of patients who die in the ICU meet criteria for at least one psychiatric illness,[136] and the prevalence of major depressive disorder in family members between 3 and 12 months is 27%.[137] Psychiatric illness is most common in bereaving family members when the patient is a spouse, if the family member is experiencing additional stressors after their loss, more acute illness (defined as the patient having been ill less than 5 years prior to death), and importantly, for families who felt the patient's physician was not comforting.[137,138] In one study of bereaved family members of patients who died in the ICU, those who perceived that the physician was *not* comforting had a higher risk of psychiatric illness compared to those who felt the physician was comforting.[137]

For families of ICU survivors, critical illness does not end at discharge from the ICU. After hospitalization, family members are tasked with informal caregiving jobs. Not surprisingly, informal caregiving is often associated with decreased physical and emotional health when the patient does not recover fully.[139–141] Although there is disagreement on the term "caregiver burden" within the caregiver research community and how this term should be utilized, informal caregivers are frequently involved in tasks related to multiple aspects of the survivor's care.[142] Chronically critically ill patients who are younger and whose relatives are younger have a lower health-related quality of life.[138,143] Younger patients and their partners likely have more emotional interdependence to one another, and therefore may be at risk to develop the symptoms of PICS-F as they are commonly challenged by occupational disability, financial burdens, and caring for minor children. This is in contrast with older dyads who are less likely to have as many adverse effects from a family member with critical illness. [144,145]

There are several nonmodifiable risk factors for the development of PICS-F that may be recognized early during ICU admission, including female gender, younger age, family members of a younger patient, families with lower educational levels, spouses of patients, patients with more comorbidities, or an unmarried parent of a critically ill child. [6] Screening for caregivers at high risk of PICS-F during the ICU admission may reduce poor outcomes in caregivers of critical illness survivors. [146] Further, nurses or social workers can provide consistent support to families and reduce conflict between families and medical personnel, and may improve family satisfaction.[147] These measurements have the potential to be integrated into the rounding and discharge processes of ICU patients.

Inclusion of families in decision-making processes and care of the patient may positively affect the long-term outcomes of family members.[6] In a qualitative study examining the effects of family members in the ICU, their presence was considered emotionally protective to patients undergoing prolonged mechanical ventilation, provided the patient reported a good relationship with the family member prior to his or her critical illness. The ability of family members to provide reassurance to loved ones is another reason to support families of critically ill patients.[148,149] However, further study is needed in those with neurocritical illness, given the high likelihood of cognitive dysfunction or challenges associated with patients who experience disorders of consciousness.

The health and wellness outcomes of both the patient and caregiver influence one another, and the best approaches to risk mitigation may involve the patient/caregiver dyad as an interdependent unit.[150] Psychological diseases such as PTSD and health-related quality of life may be diminished for both the patient *and* caregiver.[139] Specialized therapy known as "dyadic coping" may be utilized after critical illness, representing a new direction to improve relationship quality after critical illness, [144] and interventions developed on the basis of qualitative feedback from dyads and nurses to improve interpersonal communication and boost resiliency such as "Recovering Together"[151] are promising. The concept of PICS-F should be recognized as part of the care that ICU survivors receive within multidisciplinary post-ICU follow-up clinics. Alternatively, family physicians of informal caregivers of former ICU patients should be aware of PICS-F symptoms and screen family caregivers for anxiety, depression, and poor health-related quality of life.[152]

Summary and Recommendations

ICU survivorship is fraught with challenges for providers, patients, and families. Lengthy rehabilitation, the risks of medical complications such as recurrent infections, pressure ulcers, chronic respiratory failure, venous thromboembolic events, and re-admission to acute care impact both the general critical care population and particularly those with neurocritical illness. While PICS and PICS-F have been increasingly well-characterized in those surviving ARDS or sepsis, knowledge about this disorder among neurocritical care survivors is limited. Several risk factors have been identified that may increase the likelihood of long-term mental health, cognitive, or physical impairment: younger age, preexisting cognitive or psychiatric impairments, higher severity of underlying illness, longer length of ICU stay or duration of mechanical ventilation, sedation, immobilization, hyperglycemia, and delirium have been associated with the development of PICS in the general critical care population. However, PICS in patients with neurocritical care has not been defined, and additional risk factors, such as the location of structural injury or the duration of disorders of consciousness, may play a pivotal role in the development of these symptoms and ultimately impact quality of life. A recent review [153] and executive summary [154] have highlighted the need to study PICS and PICS-F in the neurocritical care population.

In the absence of studies dedicated to those with neurocritical illness, it may be reasonable to extrapolate key practices from the existing PICS literature. First, the ICU Liberation Bundle (or ABCDEF bundle, which includes spontaneous awakening trials, spontaneous breathing trials, choice of analgesia, screening and preventing delirium, early mobilization) should be implemented across the population.[155] Second, patients at risk for PICS or PICS-F should be identified, and both patients and their loved ones should receive education about these unintended consequences of critical care, allowing for preparation of survivors for the new state of "normal." Finally, multidisciplinary clinic models for critical care recovery clinics or post-ICU clinics form an important component to recognition and management of PICS and PICS-F. A recent meta-analysis showed that post-ICU recovery clinics can help reduce PTSD and depression among ICU survivors.[156] Peer-to-peer support programs should be encouraged, as these can similarly reduce PTSD and depression among ICU survivors.[157] The Society of Critical Care Medicine's THRIVE collaborative (www.sccm.org/MyICUCare/THRIVE) and more recently, the Critical and Acute Illness Recovery Organization (CAIRO) (https://sites.google.com/umich.edu/cairo/home) provide opportunities for collaboration and application of lessons learned about PICS from the general critical care literature to survivors of neurocritical care. Future studies focused on the needs of those with neurocritical illness are needed so that effective, targeted strategies can be developed to prevent and treat PICS and PICS-F in these patients.

References

1. Vincent JL. Critical care – where have we been and where are we going? *Crit Care*. 2013;**17**(Suppl 1):S2.

2. Needham DM, Davidson J, Cohen H, et al. Improving long-term outcomes after discharge from intensive care unit: report from a stakeholders' conference. *Crit Care Med*. 2012;**40**(2):502–9.

3. Needham DM, Kamdar BB, Stevenson JE. Rehabilitation of mind and body after intensive care unit discharge: a step closer to recovery. *Crit Care Med*. 2012;**40**(4):1340–1.

4. Davidson J, Hopkins RO, Louis D, Iwashyna TJ. Post-intensive Care Syndrome: Society of Critical Care Medicine; 2013. Available from: www.sccm.org/MyICUCare/THRIVE/Post-intensive-Care-Syndrome.

5. Marra A, Pandharipande PP, Girard TD, et al. Co-occurrence of post-intensive care syndrome problems among 406 survivors of critical Illness. *Crit Care Med*. 2018;**46**(9):1393–401.

6. Davidson JE, Jones C, Bienvenu OJ. Family response to critical illness: postintensive care syndrome-family. *Crit Care Med*. 2012;**40**(2):618–24.

7. Davydow DS, Gifford JM, Desai SV, Needham DM, Bienvenu OJ. Posttraumatic stress disorder in general intensive care unit survivors: a systematic review. *Gen Hosp Psychiatry*. 2008;**30**(5):421–34.

8. Girard TD, Shintani AK, Jackson JC, et al. Risk factors for post-traumatic stress disorder symptoms following critical illness requiring mechanical ventilation: a prospective cohort study. *Crit Care*. 2007;**11**(1):R28.

9. Cuthbertson BH, Hull A, Strachan M, Scott J. Post-traumatic stress disorder after critical illness requiring general intensive care. *Intensive Care Med*. 2004;**30**(3):450–5.

10. Davydow DS, Hough CL, Langa KM, Iwashyna TJ. Depressive symptoms in spouses of older patients with severe sepsis. *Crit Care Med*. 2012;**40**(8):2335–41.

11. Chung CR, Yoo HJ, Park J, Ryu S. Cognitive impairment and psychological distress at discharge from intensive care unit. *Psychiatry Investig*. 2017;**14**(3):376–9.

12. Hopkins RO, Weaver LK, Collingridge D, et al. Two-year cognitive, emotional, and quality-of-life

outcomes in acute respiratory distress syndrome. *Am J Respir Crit Care Med.* 2005;**171**(4):340–7.

13. Dowdy DW, Dinglas V, Mendez-Tellez PA, et al. Intensive care unit hypoglycemia predicts depression during early recovery from acute lung injury. *Crit Care Med.* 2008;**36**(10):2726–33.

14. Mikkelsen ME, Christie JD, Lanken PN, et al. The adult respiratory distress syndrome cognitive outcomes study: long-term neuropsychological function in survivors of acute lung injury. *Am J Respir Crit Care Med.* 2012;**185**(12):1307–15.

15. Hopkins RO, Key CW, Suchyta MR, Weaver LK, Orme JF Jr. Risk factors for depression and anxiety in survivors of acute respiratory distress syndrome. *Gen Hosp Psychiatry.* 2010;**32**(2): 147–55.

16. Jones C, Backman C, Capuzzo M, et al. Precipitants of post-traumatic stress disorder following intensive care: a hypothesis generating study of diversity in care. *Intensive Care Med.* 2007;**33**(6):978–85.

17. Jones C, Griffiths RD, Humphris G, Skirrow PM. Memory, delusions, and the development of acute posttraumatic stress disorder-related symptoms after intensive care. *Crit Care Med.* 2001;**29** (3):573–80.

18. Samuelson KA, Lundberg D, Fridlund B. Stressful memories and psychological distress in adult mechanically ventilated intensive care patients – a 2-month follow-up study. *Acta Anaesthesiol Scand.* 2007;**51**(6):671–8.

19. Adhikari NKJ, Tansey CM, McAndrews MP, et al. Self-reported depressive symptoms and memory complaints in survivors five years after ARDS. *Chest.* 2011;**140**(6):1484–93.

20. Myhren H, Ekeberg O, Toien K, Karlsson S, Stokland O. Posttraumatic stress, anxiety and depression symptoms in patients during the first year post intensive care unit discharge. *Crit Care.* 2010;**14**(1):R14.

21. Yehuda R. Post-traumatic stress disorder. *N Engl J Med.* 2002;**346**(2):108–14.

22. Parker AM, Sricharoenchai T, Raparla S, et al. Posttraumatic stress disorder in critical illness survivors: a metaanalysis. *Crit Care Med.* 2015;**4b3**(5):1121–9.

23. Choi KW, Shaffer KM, Zale EL, et al. Early risk and resiliency factors predict chronic posttraumatic stress disorder in caregivers of patients admitted to a neuroscience ICU. *Crit Care Med.* 2018;**46**(5):713–9.

24. Needham DM, Sepulveda KA, Dinglas VD, et al. Core outcome measures for clinical research in acute respiratory failure survivors. An

International Modified Delphi Consensus Study. *Am J Respir Crit Care Med.* 2017;**196**(9):1122–30.

25. Christensen MC, Mayer SA, Ferran JM, Kissela B. Depressed mood after intracerebral hemorrhage: the FAST trial. *Cerebrovasc Dis.* 2009;**27**(4): 353–60.

26. Francis BA, Beaumont J, Maas MB, et al. Depressive symptom prevalence after intracerebral hemorrhage: a multi-center study. *J Patient Rep Outcomes.* 2018;**2**(1):55.

27. Tang WK, Wang L, Kwok Chu Wong G, et al. Depression after subarachnoid hemorrhage: a systematic review. *J Stroke.* 2020;**22**(1):11–28.

28. Scholten AC, Haagsma JA, Cnossen MC, et al. Prevalence of and risk factors for anxiety and depressive disorders after traumatic brain injury: a systematic review. *J Neurotrauma.* 2016;**33** (22):1969–94.

29. Van Praag DLG, Cnossen MC, Polinder S, Wilson L, Maas AIR. Post-traumatic stress disorder after civilian traumatic brain injury: a systematic review and meta-analysis of prevalence rates. *J Neurotrauma.* 2019;**36** (23):3220–32.

30. Edmondson D, Richardson S, Fausett JK, et al. Prevalence of PTSD in survivors of stroke and transient ischemic attack: a meta-analytic review. *PLoS One.* 2013;**8**(6):e66435.

31. Hutter BO, Kreitschmann-Andermahr I. Subarachnoid hemorrhage as a psychological trauma. *J Neurosurg.* 2014;**120**(4):923–30.

32. Visser-Meily JM, Rinkel GJ, Vergouwen MD, et al. Post-traumatic stress disorder in patients 3 years after aneurysmal subarachnoid haemorrhage. *Cerebrovasc Dis.* 2013;**36**(2): 126–30.

33. Noble AJ, Baisch S, Schenk T, et al. Posttraumatic stress disorder explains reduced quality of life in subarachnoid hemorrhage patients in both the short and long term. *Neurosurgery.* 2008;**63** (6):1095–105.

34. Garton A, Gupta VP, Pucci JU, Couch CK, Connolly ES, Jr. Incidence and predictors of post-traumatic stress symptoms in a cohort of patients with intracerebral hemorrhage. *Clin Neurol Neurosurg.* 2020;**190**:105657.

35. Medeiros GC, Roy D, Kontos N, Beach SR. Post-stroke depression: A 2020 updated review. *Gen Hosp Psychiatry.* 2020;**66**:70–80.

36. Shi Y, Yang D, Zeng Y, Wu W. Risk factors for post-stroke depression: a meta-analysis. *Front Aging Neurosci.* 2017;**9**:218.

37. Turnbull AE, Rabiee A, Davis WE, et al. Outcome measurement in ICU survivorship research from

1970 to 2013: a scoping review of 425 publications. *Crit Care Med.* 2016;**44**(7):1267–77.

38. Sakusic A, O'Horo JC, Dziadzko M, et al. Potentially modifiable risk factors for long-term cognitive impairment after critical illness: a systematic review. *Mayo Clin Proc.* 2018;**93** (1):68–82.

39. Turnbull AE, Sepulveda KA, Dinglas VD, et al. core domains for clinical research in acute respiratory failure survivors: an international Modified Delphi Consensus Study. *Crit Care Med.* 2017;**45**(6):1001–10.

40. Pandharipande PP, Girard TD, Ely EW. Long-term cognitive impairment after critical illness. *N Engl J Med.* 2014;**370**(2):185–6.

41. Schlichter E, Lopez O, Scott R, et al. Feasibility of nurse-led multidimensional outcome assessments in the neuroscience intensive care unit. *Crit Care Nurse.* 2020;**40**(3):e1–e8.

42. Gottesman RF, Hillis AE. Predictors and assessment of cognitive dysfunction resulting from ischaemic stroke. *Lancet Neurol.* 2010;**9** (9):895–905.

43. Benedictus MR, Hochart A, Rossi C, et al. Prognostic factors for cognitive decline after intracerebral hemorrhage. *Stroke.* 2015;**46** (10):2773–8.

44. Mayer SA, Kreiter KT, Copeland D, et al. Global and domain-specific cognitive impairment and outcome after subarachnoid hemorrhage. *Neurology.* 2002;**59**(11):1750–8.

45. Al-Khindi T, Macdonald RL, Schweizer TA. Cognitive and functional outcome after aneurysmal subarachnoid hemorrhage. *Stroke.* 2010;**41**(8):e519–36.

46. Dikmen SS, Machamer JE, Powell JM, Temkin NR. Outcome 3 to 5 years after moderate to severe traumatic brain injury. *Arch Phys Med Rehabil.* 2003;**84**(10):1449–57.

47. Naidech AM, Beaumont JL, Rosenberg NF, et al. Intracerebral hemorrhage and delirium symptoms. Length of stay, function, and quality of life in a 114-patient cohort. *Am J Respir Crit Care Med.* 2013;**188**(11):1331–7.

48. De Marchis GM, Pugin D, Meyers E, et al. Seizure burden in subarachnoid hemorrhage associated with functional and cognitive outcome. *Neurology.* 2016;**86**(3):253–60.

49. Foreman B, Lee H, Mizrahi MA, et al. Seizures and cognitive outcome after traumatic brain injury: a post hoc analysis. *Neurocrit Care.* 2022;**36**(1):130–8.

50. Naidech AM, Kreiter KT, Janjua N, et al. Phenytoin exposure is associated with functional and cognitive disability after subarachnoid hemorrhage. *Stroke.* 2005;**36**(3):583–7.

51. Naidech AM, Beaumont J, Muldoon K, et al. Prophylactic seizure medication and health-related quality of life after intracerebral hemorrhage. *Crit Care Med.* 2018;**46**(9):1480–5.

52. Chan B, Butler E, Frost SA, Chuan A, Aneman A. Cerebrovascular autoregulation monitoring and patient-centred outcomes after cardiac surgery: a systematic review. *Acta Anaesthesiol Scand.* 2018;**62**(5):588–99.

53. Witsch J, Frey HP, Patel S, et al. Prognostication of long-term outcomes after subarachnoid hemorrhage: the FRESH score. *Ann Neurol.* 2016;**80**(1):46–58.

54. Nelson LD, Ranson J, Ferguson AR, et al. Validating multidimensional outcome assessment using the TBI common data elements: an analysis of the TRACK-TBI pilot sample. *J Neurotrauma.* 2017;**34**(22):3158–72.

55. Colantuoni E, Scharfstein DO, Wang C, et al. Statistical methods to compare functional outcomes in randomized controlled trials with high mortality. *BMJ.* 2018;**360**:j5748.

56. Appleton RT, Kinsella J, Quasim T. The incidence of intensive care unit-acquired weakness syndromes: a systematic review. *J Intensive Care Soc.* 2015;**16**(2):126–36.

57. Inoue S, Hatakeyama J, Kondo Y, et al. Post-intensive care syndrome: its pathophysiology, prevention, and future directions. *Acute Med Surg.* 2019;**6**(3):233–46.

58. Hermans G, Van Mechelen H, Clerckx B, et al. Acute outcomes and 1-year mortality of intensive care unit-acquired weakness. A cohort study and propensity-matched analysis. *Am J Respir Crit Care Med.* 2014;**190**(4):410–20.

59. Kress JP, Hall JB. ICU-acquired weakness and recovery from critical illness. N Engl J Med. 2014;**370**(17):1626–35.

60. De Jonghe B, Bastuji-Garin S, Durand M-C, et al. Respiratory weakness is associated with limb weakness and delayed weaning in critical illness. *Crit Care Med.* 2007;**35**(9):2007–15.

61. Guarneri B, Bertolini G, Latronico N. Long-term outcome in patients with critical illness myopathy or neuropathy: the Italian multicentre CRIMYNE study. *J Neurol Neurosurg Psychiatry.* 2008;**79** (7):838–41.

62. Fan E, Cheek F, Chlan L, et al. An official American Thoracic Society Clinical Practice guideline: the diagnosis of intensive care unit-acquired weakness in adults. *Am J Respir Crit Care Med.* 2014;**190**(12):1437–46.

63. Solverson KJ, Grant C, Doig CJ. Assessment and predictors of physical functioning post-hospital discharge in survivors of critical illness. *Ann Inten Care.* 2016;6(1):1–8.

64. Brummel NE, Jackson JC, Pandharipande PP, et al. Delirium in the intensive care unit and subsequent long-term disability among survivors of mechanical ventilation. *Crit Care Med.* 2014;42 (2):369.

65. Christensen MC, Mayer S, Ferran JM. Quality of life after intracerebral hemorrhage: results of the Factor Seven for Acute Hemorrhagic Stroke (FAST) trial. *Stroke.* 2009;40(5):1677–82.

66. Dhamoon MS, Moon YP, Paik MC, et al. Quality of life declines after first ischemic stroke. The Northern Manhattan Study. *Neurology.* 2010;75 (4):328–34.

67. Kosty J, Macyszyn L, Lai K, et al. Relating quality of life to Glasgow outcome scale health states. *J Neurotrauma.* 2012;29(7):1322–7.

68. Naidech AM, Beaumont JL, Berman M, et al. Dichotomous "good outcome" indicates mobility more than cognitive or social quality of life. *Crit Care Med.* 2015;43(8):1654–9.

69. American Psychiatric Association. *Diagnostic and Statistical Manual of Mental Disorders: DSM-5.* 5th ed. Arlington, VA: APA, 2013.

70. Hayhurst CJ, Marra A, Han JH, et al. Association of hypoactive and hyperactive delirium with cognitive function after critical illness. *Crit Care Med.* 2020;48(6):e480–e8.

71. Krewulak KD, Stelfox HT, Leigh JP, Ely EW, Fiest KM. Incidence and prevalence of delirium subtypes in an adult ICU: a systematic review and meta-analysis. *Crit Care Med.* 2018;46(12):2029–35.

72. Patel MB, Bednarik J, Lee P, et al. Delirium monitoring in neurocritically ill patients: a systematic review. *Crit Care Med.* 2018;46 (11):1832–41.

73. Girard TD, Thompson JL, Pandharipande PP, et al. Clinical phenotypes of delirium during critical illness and severity of subsequent long-term cognitive impairment: a prospective cohort study. *Lancet Respir Med.* 2018;6 (3):213–22.

74. Maldonado JR. Delirium pathophysiology: an updated hypothesis of the etiology of acute brain failure. *Int J Geriatr Psychiatry.* 2018;33 (11):1428–57.

75. Nielsen RM, Urdanibia-Centelles O, Vedel-Larsen E, et al. Continuous EEG monitoring in a consecutive patient cohort with sepsis and delirium. *Neurocrit Care.* 2020;32(1):121–30.

76. Numan T, Slooter AJC, van der Kooi AW, et al. Functional connectivity and network analysis during hypoactive delirium and recovery from anesthesia. *Clin Neurophysiol.* 2017;128(6):914–24.

77. Fleischmann R, Traenkner S, Kraft A, et a. Delirium is associated with frequency band specific dysconnectivity in intrinsic connectivity networks: preliminary evidence from a large retrospective pilot case–control study. *Pilot Feasibility Stud.* 2019;5:2.

78. Devlin JW, Skrobik Y, Gelinas C, et al. Clinical practice guidelines for the prevention and management of pain, agitation/sedation, delirium, immobility, and sleep disruption in adult patients in the ICU. *Crit Care Med.* 2018;46 (9):e825–e73.

79. Burton JK, Craig LE, Yong SQ, et al. Non-pharmacological interventions for preventing delirium in hospitalised non-ICU patients. *Cochrane Database Syst Rev.* 2021;7:CD013307.

80. Ely EW, Inouye SK, Bernard GR, et al. Delirium in mechanically ventilated patients: validity and reliability of the confusion assessment method for the intensive care unit (CAM-ICU). *JAMA.* 2001;286(21):2703–10.

81. Bergeron N, Dubois MJ, Dumont M, Dial S, Skrobik Y. Intensive Care Delirium Screening Checklist: evaluation of a new screening tool. *Intensive Care Med.* 2001;27(5):859–64.

82. Gusmao-Flores D, Salluh JI, Chalhub RA, Quarantini LC. The confusion assessment method for the intensive care unit (CAM-ICU) and intensive care delirium screening checklist (ICDSC) for the diagnosis of delirium: a systematic review and meta-analysis of clinical studies. *Crit Care.* 2012;16(4):R115.

83. Reznik ME, Drake J, Margolis SA, et al. Deconstructing poststroke delirium in a prospective cohort of patients with intracerebral hemorrhage. *Crit Care Med.* 2020;48(1):111–8.

84. O'Regan NA, Ryan DJ, Boland E, et al. Attention! A good bedside test for delirium? *J Neurol Neurosurg Psychiatry.* 2014;85(10):1122–31.

85. Pandharipande PP, Ely EW, Arora RC, et al. The intensive care delirium research agenda: a multinational, interprofessional perspective. *Intensive Care Med.* 2017;43(9):1329–39.

86. Luetz A, Weiss B, Boettcher S, at al. Routine delirium monitoring is independently associated with a reduction of hospital mortality in critically ill surgical patients: a prospective, observational cohort study. *J Crit Care.* 2016;35:168–73.

87. Jackson JC, Pandharipande PP, Girard TD, et al. Depression, post-traumatic stress disorder, and

functional disability in survivors of critical illness in the BRAIN-ICU study: a longitudinal cohort study. *Lancet Respir Med.* 2014;**2**(5):369–79.

88. Shi Q, Presutti R, Selchen D, Saposnik G. Delirium in acute stroke: a systematic review and meta-analysis. *Stroke.* 2012;**43**(3):645–9.

89. Riker RR, Fraser GL, Simmons LE, Wilkins ML. Validating the Sedation-Agitation Scale with the Bispectral Index and Visual Analog Scale in adult ICU patients after cardiac surgery. *Intensive Care Med.* 2001;**27**(5):853–8.

90. Sessler CN, Gosnell MS, Grap MJ, et al. The Richmond Agitation-Sedation Scale: validity and reliability in adult intensive care unit patients. *Am J Respir Crit Care Med.* 2002;**166**(10):1338–44.

91. Khan BA, Guzman O, Campbell NL, et al. Comparison and agreement between the Richmond Agitation-Sedation Scale and the Riker Sedation-Agitation Scale in evaluating patients' eligibility for delirium assessment in the ICU. *Chest.* 2012;**142**(1):48–54.

92. Riker RR, Shehabi Y, Bokesch PM, et al. Dexmedetomidine vs midazolam for sedation of critically ill patients: a randomized trial. *JAMA.* 2009;**301**(5):489–99.

93. Hughes CG, Mailloux PT, Devlin JW, et al. Dexmedetomidine or propofol for sedation in mechanically ventilated adults with sepsis. *N Engl J Med.* 2021;**384**(15):1424–36.

94. Shehabi Y, Howe BD, Bellomo R, et al. Early sedation with dexmedetomidine in critically ill patients. *N Engl J Med.* 2019;**380**(26):2506–17.

95. Chanques G, Sebbane M, Barbotte E, et al. A prospective study of pain at rest: incidence and characteristics of an unrecognized symptom in surgical and trauma versus medical intensive care unit patients. *Anesthesiology.* 2007;**107**(5):858–60.

96. Puntillo KA, Max A, Timsit JF, et al. Determinants of procedural pain intensity in the intensive care unit. The Europain(R) study. *Am J Respir Crit Care Med.* 2014;**189**(1):39–47.

97. Desbiens NA, Wu AW, Broste SK, et al. Pain and satisfaction with pain control in seriously ill hospitalized adults: findings from the SUPPORT research investigations. For the SUPPORT investigators. Study to Understand Prognoses and Preferences for Outcomes and Risks of Treatment. *Crit Care Med.* 1996;**24**(12):1953–61.

98. Navarro-Garcia MA, Marin-Fernandez B, de Carlos-Alegre V et al. [Preoperative mood disorders in patients undergoing cardiac surgery: risk factors and postoperative morbidity in the intensive care unit]. *Rev Esp Cardiol.* 2011;**64**(11):1005–10.

99. Karahan A. Comparison of three rating scales for assessing pain intensity in an intensive care unit. *Turk J Thorac Cardiovasc Surg.* 2012;**20**(1).

100. Echegaray-Benites C, Kapoustina O, Gelinas C. Validation of the use of the Critical-Care Pain Observation Tool (CPOT) with brain surgery patients in the neurosurgical intensive care unit. *Intensive Crit Care Nurs.* 2014;**30**(5):257–65.

101. Joffe AM, McNulty B, Boitor M, Marsh R, Gelinas C. Validation of the Critical-Care Pain Observation Tool in brain-injured critically ill adults. *J Crit Care.* 2016;**36**:76–80.

102. Dehghani H, Tavangar H, Ghandehari A. Validity and reliability of behavioral pain scale in patients with low level of consciousness due to head trauma hospitalized in intensive care unit. *Arch Trauma Res.* 2014;**3**(1):e18608.

103. Yu A, Teitelbaum J, Scott J, et al. Evaluating pain, sedation, and delirium in the neurologically critically ill-feasibility and reliability of standardized tools: a multi-institutional study. *Crit Care Med.* 2013;**41**(8):2002–7.

104. Arbour C, Choiniere M, Topolovec-Vranic J, et al. Detecting pain in traumatic brain-injured patients with different levels of consciousness during common procedures in the ICU: typical or atypical behaviors? *Clin J Pain.* 2014;**30**(11):960–9.

105. Stotts NA, Puntillo K, Bonham Morris A, et al. Wound care pain in hospitalized adult patients. *Heart Lung.* 2004;**33**(5):321–32.

106. Arroyo-Novoa CM, Figueroa-Ramos MI, Puntillo KA, et al. Pain related to tracheal suctioning in awake acutely and critically ill adults: a descriptive study. *Intensive Crit Care Nurs.* 2008;**24**(1):20–7.

107. Aissaoui Y, Zeggwagh AA, Zekraoui A, Abidi K, Abouqal R. Validation of a behavioral pain scale in critically ill, sedated, and mechanically ventilated patients. *Anesth Analg.* 2005;**101**(5):1470–6.

108. Denehy L, Lanphere J, Needham DM. Ten reasons why ICU patients should be mobilized early. *Intensive Care Med.* 2017;**43**(1):86–90.

109. Fan E, Dowdy DW, Colantuoni E, et al. Physical complications in acute lung injury survivors: a two-year longitudinal prospective study. *Crit Care Med.* 2014;**42**(4):849–59.

110. Dinglas VD, Aronson Friedman L, Colantuoni E, et al. Muscle weakness and 5-year survival in acute respiratory distress syndrome survivors. *Crit Care Med.* 2017;**45**(3):446–53.

111. Needham DM, Wozniak AW, Hough CL, et al. Risk factors for physical impairment after acute lung injury in a national, multicenter study. *Am J Respir Crit Care Med.* 2014;**189**(10):1214–24.

112. Kamdar BB, Combs MP, Colantuoni E, et al. The association of sleep quality, delirium, and sedation status with daily participation in physical therapy in the ICU. *Crit Care*. 2016;**19**:261.

113. Nydahl P, Sricharoenchai T, Chandra S, et al. Safety of patient mobilization and rehabilitation in the intensive care unit. Systematic review with meta-analysis. *Ann Am Thorac Soc*. 2017;**14** (5):766–77.

114. Kumar MA, Romero FG, Dharaneeswaran K. Early mobilization in neurocritical care patients. *Curr Opin Crit Care*. 2020;**26**(2):147–54.

115. Stickgold R. Neuroscience: a memory boost while you sleep. *Nature*. 2006;**444**(7119):559–60.

116. Fuller PM, Gooley JJ, Saper CB. Neurobiology of the sleep-wake cycle: sleep architecture, circadian regulation, and regulatory feedback. *J Biol Rhythms*. 2006;**21**(6):482–93.

117. Altman MT, Knauert MP, Pisani MA. Sleep disturbance after hospitalization and critical illness: a systematic review. *Ann Am Thorac Soc*. 2017;**14**(9):1457–68.

118. Cooper AB, Thornley KS, Young GB, et al. Sleep in critically ill patients requiring mechanical ventilation. *Chest*. 2000;**117**(3):809–18.

119. Cordoba-Izquierdo A, Drouot X, Thille AW, et al. Sleep in hypercapnic critical care patients under noninvasive ventilation: conventional versus dedicated ventilators. *Crit Care Med*. 2013;**41** (1):60–8.

120. Gabor JY, Cooper AB, Crombach SA et al. Contribution of the intensive care unit environment to sleep disruption in mechanically ventilated patients and healthy subjects. *Am J Respir Crit Care Med*. 2003;**167**(5):708–15.

121. Roche-Campo F, Thille AW, Drouot X, et al. Comparison of sleep quality with mechanical versus spontaneous ventilation during weaning of critically III tracheostomized patients. *Crit Care Med*. 2013;**41**(7):1637–44.

122. Patel SB, Poston JT, Pohlman A, Hall JB, Kress JP. Rapidly reversible, sedation-related delirium versus persistent delirium in the intensive care unit. *Am J Respir Crit Care Med*. 2014;**189**(6): 658–65.

123. Ely EW, Shintani A, Truman B, et al. Delirium as a predictor of mortality in mechanically ventilated patients in the intensive care unit. *JAMA*. 2004;**291**(14):1753–62.

124. Thomason JW, Shintani A, Peterson JF, et al. Intensive care unit delirium is an independent predictor of longer hospital stay: a prospective analysis of 261 non-ventilated patients. *Crit Care*. 2005;**9**(4):R375–81.

125. Girard TD, Jackson JC, Pandharipande PP, et al. Delirium as a predictor of long-term cognitive impairment in survivors of critical illness. *Crit Care Med*. 2010;**38**(7):1513–20.

126. Van Rompaey B, Elseviers MM, Van Drom W, Fromont V, Jorens PG. The effect of earplugs during the night on the onset of delirium and sleep perception: a randomized controlled trial in intensive care patients. *Crit Care*. 2012;**16**(3):R73.

127. Le Guen M, Nicolas-Robin A, Lebard C, Arnulf I, Langeron O. Earplugs and eye masks vs routine care prevent sleep impairment in post-anaesthesia care unit: a randomized study. *Br J Anaesth*. 2014;**112**(1):89–95.

128. Alexopoulou C, Kondili E, Diamantaki E, et al. Effects of dexmedetomidine on sleep quality in critically ill patients: a pilot study. *Anesthesiology*. 2014;**121**(4):801–7.

129. Nishikimi M, Numaguchi A, Takahashi K, et al. Effect of administration of ramelteon, a melatonin receptor agonist, on the duration of stay in the ICU: a single-center randomized placebo-controlled trial. *Crit Care Med*. 2018;**46** (7):1099–105.

130. Sun Y, Jiang M, Ji Y, et al. Impact of postoperative dexmedetomidine infusion on incidence of delirium in elderly patients undergoing major elective noncardiac surgery: a randomized clinical trial. *Drug Des Devel Ther*. 2019;**13**:2911–22.

131. Paul T, Lemmer B. Disturbance of circadian rhythms in analgosedated intensive care unit patients with and without craniocerebral injury. *Chronobiol Int*. 2007;**24**(1):45–61.

132. Foreman B, Westwood AJ, Claassen J, Bazil CW. Sleep in the neurological intensive care unit: feasibility of quantifying sleep after melatonin supplementation with environmental light and noise reduction. *J Clin Neurophysiol*. 2015;**32** (1):66–74.

133. Duclos C, Dumont M, Blais H, et al. Rest-activity cycle disturbances in the acute phase of moderate to severe traumatic brain injury. *Neurorehabil Neural Repair*. 2014;**28**(5):472–82.

134. Kishore K, Cusimano MD. The fundamental need for sleep in neurocritical care units: time for a paradigm shift. *Front Neurol*. 2021;**12**:637250.

135. Swoboda SM, Lipsett PA. Impact of a prolonged surgical critical illness on patients' families. *Am J Crit Care*. 2002;**11**(5):459–66.

136. Alfheim HB, Rosseland LA, Hofso K, Smastuen MC, Rustoen T. Multiple symptoms in family caregivers of intensive care unit patients. *J Pain Symptom Manage*. 2018;**55**(2):387–94.

137. Siegel MD, Hayes E, Vanderwerker LC, Loseth DB, Prigerson HG. Psychiatric illness in the next of kin of patients who die in the intensive care unit. *Crit Care Med.* 2008;**36**(6):1722–8.

138. Gries CJ, Engelberg RA, Kross EK, et al. Predictors of symptoms of posttraumatic stress and depression in family members after patient death in the ICU. *Chest.* 2010;**137**(2):280–7.

139. Hickman RL Jr, Douglas SL. Impact of chronic critical illness on the psychological outcomes of family members. *AACN Adv Crit Care.* 2010;**21**(1):80–91.

140. Rodriguez AM, Gregorio MA, Rodriguez AG. Psychological repercussions in family members of hospitalised critical condition patients. *J Psychosom Res.* 2005;**58**(5):447–51.

141. Scott LD, Arslanian-Engoren C. Caring for survivors of prolonged mechanical ventilation. *Home Health Care Manage Pract.* 2002;**14**(2):122–8.

142. Bastawrous M. Caregiver burden – a critical discussion. *Int J Nurs Stud.* 2013;**50**(3):431–41.

143. Anderson WG, Arnold RM, Angus DC, Bryce CL. Posttraumatic stress and complicated grief in family members of patients in the intensive care unit. *J Gen Intern Med.* 2008;**23**(11):1871–6.

144. Pankrath AL, Weissflog G, Mehnert A, et al. The relation between dyadic coping and relationship satisfaction in couples dealing with haematological cancer. *Eur J Cancer Care (Engl).* 2018;**27**(1).

145. Berg CA, Upchurch R. A developmental-contextual model of couples coping with chronic illness across the adult life span. *Psychol Bull.* 2007;**133**(6):920–54.

146. Haines KJ, Denehy L, Skinner EH, Warrillow S, Berney S. Psychosocial outcomes in informal caregivers of the critically ill: a systematic review. *Crit Care Med.* 2015;**43**(5):1112–20.

147. Moore CD, Bernardini GL, Hinerman R, et al. The effect of a family support intervention on physician, nurse, and family perceptions of care in the surgical, neurological, and medical intensive care units. *Crit Care Nurs Q.* 2012;**35**(4):378–87.

148. Arslanian-Engoren C, Scott LD. The lived experience of survivors of prolonged mechanical ventilation: a phenomenological study. Heart Lung. 2003;**32**(5):328–34.

149. Bergbom I, Askwall A. The nearest and dearest: a lifeline for ICU patients. *Intensive Crit Care Nurs.* 2000;**16**(6):384–95.

150. Lyons KS, Lee CS. The Theory Of Dyadic Illness Management. *J Fam Nurs.* 2018;**24**(1):8–28.

151. Vranceanu AM, Bannon S, Mace R, et al. Feasibility and efficacy of a resiliency intervention for the prevention of chronic emotional distress among survivor-caregiver dyads admitted to the neuroscience intensive care unit: a randomized clinical trial. *JAMA Netw Open.* 2020;**3**(10):e2020807.

152. van Beusekom I, Bakhshi-Raiez F, de Keizer NF, Dongelmans DA, van der Schaaf M. Reported burden on informal caregivers of ICU survivors: a literature review. *Crit Care.* 2016;**20**:16.

153. LaBuzetta JN, Rosand J, Vranceanu AM. Review: Post-Intensive Care Syndrome: Unique Challenges in the Neurointensive Care Unit. Neurocrit Care. 2019;**31**(3):534–45.

154. Bautista CA, Nydahl P, Bader MK, et al. Executive summary: post-intensive care syndrome in the neurocritical intensive care unit. *J Neurosci Nurs.* 2019;**51**(4):158–61.

155. Society of Critical Care Medicine. ICU Liberation Bundle (A-F). Available from: www.sccm.org/Clinical-Resources/ICULiberation-Home/ABCDEF-Bundles.

156. Rosa RG, Ferreira GE, Viola TW, et al. Effects of post-ICU follow-up on subject outcomes: a systematic review and meta-analysis. *J Crit Care.* 2019;**52**:115–25.

157. McPeake J, Iwashyna TJ, Boehm LM, et al. Benefits of peer support for intensive care unit survivors: sharing experiences, care debriefing, and altruism. *Am J Crit Care.* 2021;**30**(2):145–9.

Prognostication in Sepsis-Associated Encephalopathy

William Roth, Marie-Carmelle Elie-Turenne, and Carolina B. Maciel

Sepsis: Introduction

Sepsis, a life-threatening dysregulated host response to infection, represents the leading cause of death among adults in US hospitals and remains one of the most prevalent causes of death in children worldwide.[1,2] Every year in the United States, 1 in 1,000 people will become septic, and over half of these will require intensive care.[3,4] The estimated 5-year mortality related to sepsis approaches 80%.[5] Following the widespread implementation of sepsis guidelines, 3-year absolute mortality has significantly decreased by 20%.[6] The increased survivorship of sepsis patients has prompted the investigation of long-term outcomes including cognitive, psychiatric, functional, and quality-of-life sequelae.

Sepsis-Associated Encephalopathy: Introduction

Sepsis-associated encephalopathy (SAE), broadly defined as a rapid decline in cognitive function in the setting of sepsis,[7] occurs in an estimated 8–70% of septic patients.[8,9] The presentation of SAE may be described as malaise, impaired attention, agitation, disorientation, hypersomnolence, delirium, or coma.[10] Despite advances in the recognition of this syndrome, and in the absence of a standard diagnostic tool, SAE remains a diagnosis of exclusion once other causes of altered mentation in a febrile patient with infection have been investigated.

While the pathophysiology of SAE remains poorly defined, it is generally understood to occur as a consequence of a maladaptive inflammatory response to a systemic infection.[11–13] The increased release of cytokines and inflammatory markers impairs the integrity of the blood–brain barrier (BBB), potentiates the production of neurotoxic factors such as reactive oxygen and nitrogen species, development of cerebral edema, and alterations in neurotransmission.[14] Additionally, a loss of endothelial integrity and dysregulation of brain perfusion lead to ischemia and microhemorrhages.[15–18] Further, translocation of bacteria to the brain leading to direct promotion of neuroinflammatory mediators and alterations in the cerebrovasculature has also been demonstrated.[19,20] The consequence of this constellation of processes is neuronal degeneration and cell death.[21]

SAE and Outcomes

Mortality

Clinical studies of sepsis patients have consistently demonstrated that SAE is an independent predictor of mortality. One early estimate from a prospective observational study of 1,333 septic patients with acutely altered mental status secondary to sepsis demonstrated a 49% versus 26% mortality for those with versus without mental status change, respectively.[22] The degree or magnitude of encephalopathy may also impact survival. In one prospective cohort of 50 septic patients, mortality worsened with lower scores on the Glasgow Coma Scale (GCS). Mortality ranged from 16% in those with a GCS of 15 to 63% in those with a GCS of 3–8.[23] Other retrospective reviews of septic and intensive care unit (ICU) patients describe similar mortality estimates.[24–26]

Neurocognitive Sequelae

Clinical Data

Long-term follow-up data collected in sepsis survivors illustrate the persistence of neurocognitive sequelae following hospitalization. The prevalence of long-term cognitive impairment is 20–50% following severe sepsis. Several prospective cohort studies characterize a wide range of cognitive impairments in multiple domains, including working memory, attention, task-switching, verbal memory, and verbal fluency, following the discharge of the index hospitalization for sepsis. [27,28]

Comorbidities

Dementia

Survivors of sepsis also appear to have a higher risk of subsequent dementia. In one large prospective cohort study of 623 survivors of severe sepsis, patients had a 10.6% higher prevalence of moderate or severe cognitive impairment at 3 years after hospital discharge, and a high rate of functional limitation up to 8 years after discharge. Compared to other hospitalized patients, sepsis survivors were three times as likely to develop cognitive impairment.[5] A retrospective cohort analysis of Medicare data reinforced these findings, showing a high burden of functional disability and cognitive impairment following sepsis hospitalization. [3] Another retrospective analysis of Medicare billing data showed an increased incidence of cognitive decline in patients with infection or severe sepsis.[29] In a subset analysis of the Cardiovascular Health Study, 399 patients with severe sepsis, 639 patients with pneumonia, and 1,932 patients with infection but without sepsis underwent cognitive evaluation with the Mini-Mental Status Exam (MMSE). All groups showed similar cognitive decline following hospitalization and were twice as likely as controls to develop dementia in 5–10 years.[30] Further work is needed to elucidate confounding conditions that may lead to further cognitive decline including sedatives, non-SAE delirium, acute respiratory distress syndrome (ARDS), or preexisting neurodegenerative conditions, which themselves may render septic patients more susceptible to the development of SAE.[31]

ARDS

Acute respiratory distress syndrome (ARDS) is a serious complication of sepsis, defined by profound hypoxia, bilateral lung infiltrate, and non-cardiogenic pulmonary edema, necessitating prolonged ventilatory support. The mortality rate from ARDS ranges from 20–80% and is associated with both short- and long-term morbidity. Prospective studies in patients with sepsis and ARDS provide additional insight into cognitive impairments in septic patients. The duration of delirium during ARDS correlates with worse

global cognitive function up to 1 year after discharge. Nearly 100% of ARDS survivors demonstrate some degree of cognitive impairment 2 years following discharge.[32–34]

Understanding of neurological and functional outcomes in ARDS may provide insight and guide the prognostication in the many patients afflicted by COVID-19 (infection by SARS-CoV2 virus). While data continue to evolve, the high prevalence of acute lung injury and severe hypoxic respiratory failure that resembles ARDS among novel SARS-CoV-2 infected patients or COVID-19 cannot be underemphasized. The incidence of COVID-19 related acute lung injury is high, up to 88% in hospitalized patients, with limited longitudinal data on outcomes.[35] Postmortem examinations of patients who died of COVID-19 demonstrate a variety of neuropathological findings including microglial nodule formation with neuronophagia with surprisingly sparse infiltration of circulating immune cells or viral mRNA detected, hemorrhagic leukoencephalopathy, and microvascular thrombosis. These patients show more significant injury attributable to hypoxia and ischemia in typically vulnerable areas of the brain.[36,37] COVID-related hypercoagulability also increases risk of ischemic stroke which likely contributes largely to functional outcomes.[38] ARDS severity and disorders of consciousness have emerged as prognostic markers for increased risk of mortality. [39] Survivors of COVID have reported persistent neuropsychological symptoms such as lethargy, cognitive difficulties, anxiety, depression, dysautonomia, and pain, a constellation of symptoms referred to as "long-haul COVID."[40] The pathophysiological correlates, prognostic markers, and long-term consequences of this syndrome remain to be fully elucidated.

Preclinical Data

Translational researchers have performed numerous studies to replicate the cognitive dysfunction observed in patients with SAE. They have employed various methods, primarily in mouse and rat models, including cecal ligation puncture (CLP), induced endotoxemia and others to mimic sepsis and its sequelae. Barichello and colleagues provide a comprehensive review of translational research involving SAE and cognitive outcomes. [41] The most commonly observed cognitive deficits in preclinical models include impaired short- and long-term memory, learning, locomotor and exploratory activities, and depressive and anxious behaviors.[42,43] Investigators have postulated based on preclinical models that memory deficits are associated with sepsis-induced neuronal loss in the hippocampus and prefrontal cortex, as well as lower cholinergic innervation of the parietal cortices.[44]

Psychiatric Sequelae

Depression

Psychiatric symptoms are common after critical illness and sepsis. Estimates of prevalence range from 10–58%.[45] One subset analysis of 439 severe sepsis patients in the Health and Retirement Study showed that pre-sepsis depression and functional impairment after sepsis best predicted subsequent development of depression.[46] Depressive behavior is also noted in CLP models of SAE; one such study demonstrated reversal of depressive symptoms after treatment with the antidepressant imipramine. [43,47]

Post-Traumatic Stress Disorder

Up to one in four ICU patients will suffer from post-traumatic stress disorder (PTSD) symptoms. [48] Among survivors of septic shock, those who received stress-dose steroids developed fewer PTSD symptoms than those who did not receive steroids.[49] Further work is needed to understand the role that SAE may play in the development of post-traumatic symptoms after hospitalization, and whether this can be prevented by specific measures.

Quality-of-Life and Functional Outcomes

The current understanding of the impact of SAE on quality-of-life and functional outcomes is limited. Sepsis, however, is known to significantly impact quality of life and functionality after hospitalization. Secondary analyses of 580 septic patients in two large clinical trials – PROWESS-SHOCK and ACCESS – reported that 41.6% of patients could not live independently 6 months after hospitalization. Over 45% of these patients reported limitations with mobility and self-care. [50] All survivors of sepsis in another small study scored significantly lower on physical functioning, general health, and social function domains when compared to established norms for the general US population.[51]

Outcomes in Children

Mortality

The impact of sepsis and SAE in children may be similar to that in adults. In a meta-analysis of 12 studies evaluating outcomes in patients with neonatal sepsis, infants who suffered neonatal sepsis had higher rates of mortality and developmental delay compared to other neonates.[52]

Neurocognitive Sequelae

Children who survive sepsis with SAE more often develop cognitive deficits than healthy controls. Fifty children with SAE underwent neuropsychiatric evaluation at short-term follow-up following hospitalization. They had significantly worse mean verbal IQ, general development, physical, adaptive, social-emotional, and communication subscale performance. Moreover, these children had lower intelligence, worse school performance, and more disobedience and irritability than healthy controls. [53] A retrospective cohort of 50 children who survived septic shock demonstrated similar findings, with 44% of children scoring less than the 25th percentile in cognitive testing and 14% requiring special education. In this study, younger age at admission was associated with worse cognitive outcomes.[54]

SAE Biomarkers

Plasma Biomarkers

Plasma biomarkers for diagnosis and prognosis in brain injury and critical illness have been broadly studied in SAE (see Zenaide and Gusmao-Flores, 2013, for a detailed systematic review).[55] Despite many promising biomarkers, including S100 calcium-binding protein beta (S100B) and neuron-specific enolase (NSE), none is sufficiently sensitive or specific for routine clinical use given variable results.[56–58] The calcium-binding protein S100B is found primarily in glia (though also found in other extracranial sources) that has been used in many disease models as a marker of brain injury.[59] NSE is a cytoplasmic neuronal protein, also present red blood cells, platelets, and neuroendocrine cells, which is used as a surrogate for neuronal injury in patients who suffer cardiac arrest and traumatic brain injury.[60]

In one cohort of 170 patients with sepsis, 42% demonstrated increased S100B levels, and 53% had elevated NSE levels within the first 72 hours of diagnosis.[61] In another study of 112 patients, of whom 48 patients had SAE, higher S100B and NSE levels were seen in those with SAE compared to controls. A threshold of 0.131 µg/L for diagnosing SAE had 67.2% specificity and 85.4% sensitivity (area under the curve [AUC] 0.824; 95% confidence interval [CI]: 0.750–0.898), whereas NSE levels above 24.15 ng/mL for diagnosing SAE had 82.8% specificity and 54.2% sensitivity (AUC 0.664; 95% CI: 0.561–0.767).[62] S100B was also highly associated with both low GCS score and hospital mortality.[62]

Other novel biomarkers under investigation in the diagnosis and prognosis of SAE are calcium-binding protein A8, tumor necrosis factor receptor-associated factor 6, glial fibrillary acidic protein (GFAP), neurofilament light/heavy chain, and ubiquitin C-terminal hydrolase; however, further work is needed before their implementation in clinical practice.[63–65] Importantly, there are numerous brain injury and neurodegenerative biomarkers under investigation that may expose parallel pathways and be applicable in SAE, including UCH-L1, tau protein, Copeptin, SBDP 145, SBDP150, spectrum N-terminal fragment (SNTF), neurofilament, myelin basic protein (MBP), and secretoneurin. Other biomarkers identified in sepsis and delirium, such as amyloid-beta, interleukin-6, -8, -10, procalcitonin, C4d, and tumor necrosis factor-alpha, show reasonable accuracy in prediction of shock, coma, mortality, and cognitive dysfunction, but have not undergone extensive evaluation in patients with SAE.[66–68] Many studies among older adults are limited by a lack of harmonization of behavioral batteries for neurocognitive assessments, or lack sufficient data on baseline cognitive status.

Biomarker studies in children yield similar results. In a prospective cohort study of 48 children diagnosed with septic shock, S100B, NSE, and GFAP were significantly elevated compared to controls, and most highly elevated in non-survivors.[69] Cerebrospinal fluid analysis in a cohort of pediatric patients revealed significantly higher intrathecal synthesis of nitric oxide, S100B, and lipid peroxides in children with SAE compared with those with sepsis alone.[70] While a clinical diagnosis of SAE in neonates is challenging, numerous biomarkers have been identified in neonatal sepsis. The most extensively studied include C-reactive protein,

procalcitonin, mannose-binding lectin, serum amyloid A, interleukin-6 and -8, adrenomedullin, lipopolysaccharide-binding protein, soluble triggering receptor expressed on myeloid cells, and soluble urokinase plasminogen activator. Despite this extensive work, clinicians have not reached a consensus on their routine use. Bersani and colleagues provide a comprehensive systematic review of biomarkers in neonatal sepsis.[71]

Neurophysiology

Electroencephalography (EEG)

Clinicians and researchers have utilized neurophysiological studies in patients with sepsis and SAE for diagnostic and prognostic purposes. Not surprisingly, nearly all patients with SAE have abnormalities on electroencephalography (EEG); these are summarized in Table 13.1. Some have posited that the high sensitivity of EEG in SAE patients makes it more sensitive than clinical criteria for diagnosis.[72] In a systematic review of 17 studies, background abnormalities were seen in 12–100% of septic patients.[73] Both background slowing and suppression were independently associated with increased mortality. In a retrospective study of 201 medical ICU patients who underwent EEG, sepsis was the only independent predictor of nonconvulsive seizures, which were associated with higher mortality and worse functional outcomes.[74] Several prospective observational studies have demonstrated characteristic EEG features during SAE, which are nonspecific. The most common findings include absence of reactivity, theta- or delta-predominant slowing, background suppression, triphasic waves, epileptiform discharges, and nonconvulsive seizures. Seizures and lack of EEG reactivity are often associated with increased hospital mortality and rates of re-admission within 30-days post-discharge.[75] In survivors, background slowing can persist up to 2 years after hospital discharge.[76–78] EEG abnormalities may also help predict outcome in children. One prospective study of 108 premature neonates showed a significant increase in the prevalence of a burst-suppression background in septic (57%) compared to non-septic (22%) patients.[79] The prevalence of status epilepticus in adults admitted with sepsis has doubled (from 0.1% to 0.2%) in a cross-sectional study of nearly 8 million admissions of sepsis identified through the Nationwide Inpatient Sample database from 1988 to 2008.[80]

Table 13.1 Summary of electroencephalography (EEG) findings in SAE

Study	Patient characteristics	EEG findings
Lavy et al., 1970 [114]	Case series of 3 adults with generalized convulsions receiving intravenous penicillin	Disorganized background slowing and paroxysmal sharp and spike activity, which were transient
Young et al., 1992 [72]	Retrospective cohort of 62 adults with bacteremia and varying degrees of encephalopathy	Normal, excessive theta, predominantly delta, triphasic waves, and suppression/burst suppression, loss of reactivity
Hsu et al., 2008 [69]	Prospective cohort of 24 children with septic shock	Increase in beta and delta activity, decreased or increased voltages, burst suppression, loss of or impaired reactivity
Oddo et al., 2009 [74]	Retrospective cohort of 120 adults admitted to Medical ICU with sepsis (from 201 total)	9% electrographic seizures, 16% with periodic discharges, 7% with seizures and periodic discharges
Ter Horst et al., 2010 [115]	Retrospective cohort 22 neonates with sepsis/meningitis monitored with amplitude EEG	40.9% decreased voltages: 22% burst suppression, 13.5% with "flat trace" (< 5 µV), 4.5% continuous but low voltage 54.5% continuous or discontinuous with normal voltages 22.7% electrographic seizure activity: 9.1% status epilepticus and 13.6% repeated seizure
Helderman et al., 2010 [79]	Retrospective cohort of 42 premature neonates with sepsis monitored with repeated amplitude EEG (from 108 infants that completed study)	57% burst suppression transiently (vs. 22% burst suppression in nonseptic infants)
Semmler et al., 2013 [27]	Prospective follow up cohort of 25 adults with sepsis that survived ICU hospitalization (from 44 total)	Increased theta and gamma power than healthy controls
Azabou et al., 2015 [116]	Prospective cohort 110 adults with sepsis admitted to ICU	25% absent reactivity, 19% periodic discharges, 15% electrographic seizures
Gilmore et al., 2015 [78]	Prospective cohort of 98 patients with severe sepsis (100 episodes of sepsis) admitted to Medical ICU	28% absent reactivity, 25% periodic discharges, 11% electrographic seizures
Berisavac et al., 2016 [77]	Prospective cohort of 39 adult patients with SAE	100% abnormal EEG: 15.4% increased theta, 48.7% increased delta, 23% triphasic waves, 12.8% suppression, 17.9% epileptiform discharges, 43.6% seizures
Velissaris et al., 2018 [117]	Retrospective cohort of 17 adults with sepsis presenting to Emergency Room	64.7% normal EEG, 35.3% abnormal EEG: 23.5% increased theta, 11.7% increased delta
Nielsen et al., 2019 [118]	Prospective cohort of 102 adults with sepsis and septic shock admitted to Medical ICU	14.7% periodic discharges (87% of which were delirious) In those *without* delirium, preserved beta activity and reactivity were more frequently seen

While the mortality from sepsis decreased modestly during the study period (from 20% to 18%), the mortality in status epilepticus during sepsis demonstrated a sharp decrease from 43% to 28%, which may reflect improved diagnostic evaluation with early detection and prompt treatment of status epilepticus.[80]

Somatosensory Evoked Potentials (SSEPs)

Several studies have investigated somatosensory evoked potentials (SSEPs) to prognosticate following a diagnosis of sepsis or SAE. Preclinical models of SAE demonstrate deterioration in latencies and amplitudes of SSEP peaks.[81] In a study in which 68 patients with SAE underwent SSEP testing, 34% demonstrated subcortical pathway impairment, 84% involving the cortical pathways.[82] Whether preexisting pathway impairment renders patients more susceptible to SAE, or SAE is causative of these impairments, remains uncertain.

Neuroimaging and Neuropathology

A variety of abnormal neuroimaging findings have been described in patients with SAE and sepsis and are summarized in Table 13.2. Many of the reported studies are retrospective, limiting the interpretation of the findings in the absence of prior imaging. In one prospective cohort of patients with SAE, the presence of abnormal neuroimaging findings were associated with more severe illness and altered biomarkers.[68] The most common findings in patients with SAE include ischemic stroke, frontal and periventricular white matter hyperintensities, vasogenic edema, and global cerebral atrophy.[83,84] Stubbs and colleagues[85] have compiled a number of case series and case reports describing imaging findings in patients with SAE. Akin to findings in animal models, septic patients have atrophic left hippocampi and increased global atrophy compared to non-septic ICU survivors. [27,28] While the mechanism of lateralized atrophy remains unclear, it has been proposed that asymmetric density of protective neurotransmitters (such as norepinephrine) on the right hemisphere or a general susceptibility of the left hemisphere to neurodegenerative disease may play a role. Postmortem histopathological evaluation confirms many of the findings seen on neuroimaging. One study of 23 patients with septic shock who died of non-neurological causes was compared to controls which comprised deceased ICU patients without septic shock and patients who died suddenly from extra-cranial injury. All of the septic patients showed evidence of ischemic changes, with neuronal apoptosis particularly in autonomical centers including the amygdala, supraoptic and paraventricular hypothalamic nuclei, locus ceruleus, and vegetative nuclei of the anterior fourth ventricle. Less common findings included hemorrhage, thrombosis, micro-abscesses, and necrotizing leukoencephalopathy.[18] A cohort of 12 patients with SAE demonstrated a high prevalence of microabscesses, infarcts, astrocyte

Table 13.2 Summary of neuroimaging findings in SAE

Study	Imaging and patient characteristics	Findings
Bartynski et al. 2006 [119]	Magnetic resonance imaging (MRI), magnetic resonance angiography (MRA), computed tomography (CT) in 106 patients with posterior reversible encephalopathy syndrome (PRES)	23.6% of patients with infection, sepsis, or shock
Sharshar et al., 2007 [83]	MRI in 9 patients with septic shock sand brain dysfunction	22% normal, 22% multiple ischemic strokes, 56% white matter lesions
Piazza et al., 2009 [84]	MRI in 4 patients with severe sepsis or septic shock	50% normal, 50% white matter lesions
Morandi et al., 2010 [120]	MRI in 4 patients with septic shock and delirium	100% white matter lesions
Fugate et al. 2010 [121]	MRI in 109 patients with PRES	17% of patients with sepsis, predominantly parieto-occipital involvement
Gunther et al. 2012 [28]	MRI in 47 patients with ICU delirium, 57% with sepsis	Longer duration of delirium associated with larger ventricle-to-brain ratio, smaller superior frontal and hippocampal volumes
Polito et al., 2013 [15]	MRI in 71 patients with septic shock who developed focal neurological deficit, seizure, coma, or delirium	52% normal, 29% ischemic stroke, 21% leukoencephalopathy, 8% mixed lesions
Semmler et al., 2013 [27]	MRI in 25 septic and 19 non-septic ICU survivors	Septic survivors with less left hippocampal volume
Sutter et al., 2015 [122]	MRI in 23 patients with sepsis and mental status change	48% with abnormality; 70% with white matter hyperintensities; 43% with ischemic infarcts
Ehler et al., 2017 [123]	MRI in 13 sepsis patients in ICU	69% with white matter hyperintensities
Orhun et al., 2019 [124]	MRI and voxel-based morphometric (VBM) analysis of 93 patients with sepsis-induced brain dysfunction	29% normal, 54.9% brain lesions, 16.1% atrophy; VBM with atrophy in insula, cingulate cortex, frontal lobe, precuneus, thalamus

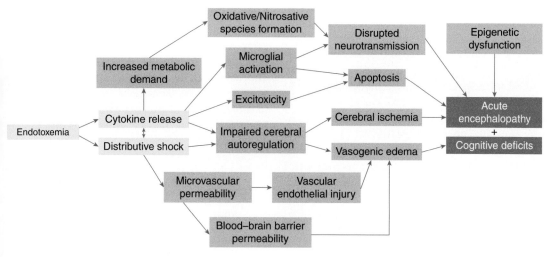

Figure 13.1 Simplified model of SAE pathophysiology.

and microglial proliferation, white matter microhemorrhages, and pontine myelinolysis.[86] Neuroimaging may greatly benefit clinicians with prognostication in patients with SAE, but further work is needed to establish consistent findings and associated outcomes.

SAE Pathophysiology

Greater understanding of these mechanisms is necessary for the characterization of risk factors for poor outcomes and, by extension, the identification of relevant biomarkers for prognostication. For an extensive systematic review of the pathophysiology of SAE, see Papadopolous et al.[11] The mechanisms implicated in the SAE development are summarized in Figure 13.1.

Cerebral Blood Flow

Sepsis and its accompanying inflammatory cascade are known to cause macrovascular and microvascular damage. Cytokines disrupt the protective mechanisms in the cerebral vasculature, rendering patients susceptible to hypoperfusion and hypoxic–ischemic injury. Specifically, vasomotor reactivity and loss of integrity of cerebral autoregulation may play a role in sepsis.[87–91] One study utilizing near infrared spectroscopy in SAE patients showed disturbed autoregulation was associated with worse neurological status, though the impact on outcomes is unclear.[92] In the setting of hypotension and shock, there is likely a multifactorial pathway thought to impact

cognition and induce SAE, including signaling of apoptotic pathways, intracellular calcium accumulation, glutamatergic excitation, reactive oxygen species, and microvascular permeability inducing vascular endothelial injury, vasodilation, and increased metabolic demand.[93] Preclinical studies largely suggest that microvascular perfusion and activation-flow coupling is impaired in animal models of sepsis.[94,95]

Blood–Brain Barrier (BBB)

The BBB becomes altered in experimental sepsis, with increased permeability and diffuse perivascular edema (especially in the CA1 region of the hippocampus) associated with systemic and brain-derived increase in inflammatory mediators as the cardinal manifestations.[96] The detachment of pericytes – multifunctional and polymorphic cells located in the basal lamina of microvessels – results in disorganization of the basal lamina unit and an increase in cerebrovascular permeability; these findings are also associated with increased microglial activation and demonstrate the complexity of the pathophysiology of BBB disruption.[96]

Inflammation

The dysregulated inflammatory response of sepsis induces or potentiates other known pathogenic mechanisms in SAE. Microglial activation appears to be particularly important, as activated microglia are a primary pathological finding in postmortem studies of patients who died of sepsis.[97]

Investigators hypothesize the vagal and circumventricular organ activation or cytokine-induced inhibition of cholinergic neurons may mediate microglial activation in sepsis.[98] Indeed, microglial regulators mitigated memory, coordination and motor deficits in a mouse model of SAE.[99] Several preclinical studies have elucidated the role of cytokines in the brain and the associated regulatory anti-inflammatory cascade.[100] The cytokine IL-1 beta, for example, has been shown to depress long-term potentiation.[101] Tumor necrosis factor knock-out mice had less lipopolysaccharide-induced apoptosis, neutrophil infiltration, cerebral edema, and inducible nitric oxide synthase (iNOS) mRNA expression than wild-type mice.[102]

Oxidative and Nitrosative Stress

Nitric oxide and free oxygen species appear to have a deleterious effect on the brain and cognitive function based on animal models of SAE and some postmortem pathological data. Postmortem histopathological findings demonstrate increased iNOS expression in association with neuronal apoptosis in septic patients.[18,103] Animal models of sepsis and SAE demonstrate induction of iNOS in association with cognitive deficits. Inhibition or knockdown of iNOS is sufficient to mitigate these deficits.[104–106] Other preclinical models demonstrate mitochondrial dysfunction and associated oxidative stress are relevant in the pathogenesis of SAE. In fact, memory deficits in a mouse model of sepsis were mitigated by administration of the antioxidants N-acetylcysteine and deferoxamine.[107–110]

Other

Dysregulation of amino acids, disrupted neurotransmission, and epigenetic dysfunction all are posited to play a role in the pathogenesis of SAE as well.[111–113] Disruption of tryptophan catabolism, the kynurenine pathway, was demonstrated to mediate cognitive impairment via indoleamine 2,3-dioxygenase activation in a mouse model of sepsis using cecal ligation and perforation.[111] In a similar rat model of sepsis, inhibition of acetylated histones 3 and 4 (AcH3 and AcH4), cytoplasmic histone deacetylase 4, and Bcl-XL deacetylases in hippocampi was noted and associated with apoptosis; these cells were rescued with histone deacetylases inhibitor, demonstrating that epigenetic modulation is at least in part implicated in the cognitive dysfunction in sepsis.[113]

Conclusion

Patients with sepsis-associated encephalopathy carry a significant risk of mortality, cognitive impairment, progressive decline, and psychiatric disorders such as depression and PTSD. While several promising biomarkers may influence efforts to prognosticate in patients with SAE, none is yet ready for clinical practice. Advancing the understanding of the mechanisms underlying SAE can enable future efforts at improving prognostication.

References

1. Kutko MC, Calarco MP, Flaherty MB, et al. Mortality rates in pediatric septic shock with and without multiple organ system failure. *Pediatr Crit Care Med.* 2003;4:333–7.

2. Lagu T, Rothberg MB, Shieh MS, et al. Hospitalizations, costs, and outcomes of severe sepsis in the United States 2003 to 2007. *Crit Care Med.* 2012;40:754–61.

3. Iwashyna TJ, Cooke CR, Wunsch H, Kahn JM. Population burden of long-term survivorship after severe sepsis in older Americans. *J Am Geriatr Soc.* 2012;60:1070–7.

4. Stevenson EK, Rubenstein AR, Radin GT, Wiener RS, Walkey AJ. Two decades of mortality trends among patients with severe sepsis: a comparative meta-analysis. *Crit Care Med.* 2014;42:625–31.

5. Iwashyna TJ, Ely EW, Smith DM, Langa KM. Long-term cognitive impairment and functional disability among survivors of severe sepsis. *JAMA.* 2010;304:1787–94.

6. Castellanos-Ortega A, Suberviola B, Garcia-Astudillo LA, et al. Impact of the Surviving Sepsis Campaign protocols on hospital length of stay and mortality in septic shock patients: results of a three-year follow-up quasi-experimental study. *Crit Care Med.* 2010;38:1036–43.

7. Widmann CN, Heneka MT. Long-term cerebral consequences of sepsis. *Lancet Neurol.* 2014;13:630–6.

8. Gofton TE, Young GB. Sepsis-associated encephalopathy. *Nat Rev Neurol.* 2012;8:557–66.

9. Lamar CD, Hurley RA, Taber KH. Sepsis-associated encephalopathy: review of the neuropsychiatric manifestations and cognitive outcome. *J Neuropsychiatry Clin Neurosci.* 2011;23:237–41.

10. Chaudhry N, Duggal AK. Sepsis associated encephalopathy. *Adv Med.* 2014;2014:762320.

11. Papadopoulos MC, Davies DC, Moss RF, Tighe D, Bennett ED. Pathophysiology of septic

encephalopathy: a review. *Crit Care Med.* 2000;**28**:3019–24.

12. Consales G, De Gaudio AR. Sepsis associated encephalopathy. *Minerva Anestesiol.* 2005;**71**:39–52.

13. Jacob A, Brorson JR, Alexander JJ. Septic encephalopathy: inflammation in man and mouse. *Neurochem Int.* 2011;**58**:472–6.

14. Davies DC. Blood-brain barrier breakdown in septic encephalopathy and brain tumours. *J Anat.* 2002;**200**:639–46.

15. Polito A, Eischwald F, Maho AL, et al. Pattern of brain injury in the acute setting of human septic shock. *Crit Care.* 2013;**17**:R204.

16. Zhang QH, Sheng ZY, Yao YM. Septic encephalopathy: when cytokines interact with acetylcholine in the brain. *Mil Med Res.* 2014;**1**:20.

17. Szatmári S, Végh T, Csomós Á, et al. Impaired cerebrovascular reactivity in sepsis-associated encephalopathy studied by acetazolamide test. *Crit Care.* 2010;**14**:R50.

18. Sharshar T, Annane D, de la Grandmaison GL, et al. The neuropathology of septic shock. *Brain Pathol.* 2004;**14**:21–33.

19. Tang AT, Choi JP, Kotzin JJ, et al. Endothelial TLR4 and the microbiome drive cerebral cavernous malformations. *Nature.* 2017;**545**:305–10.

20. Singer BH, Dickson RP, Denstaedt SJ, et al. Bacterial dissemination to the brain in sepsis. *Am J Respir Crit Care Med.* 2018;**197**:747–56.

21. Bozza FA, D'Avila JC, Ritter C, Sonneville R, Sharshar T, Dal-Pizzol F. Bioenergetics, mitochondrial dysfunction, and oxidative stress in the pathophysiology of septic encephalopathy. *Shock (Augusta, Ga).* 2013;**39** Suppl 1:10–16.

22. Sprung CL, Peduzzi PN, Shatney CH, et al. Impact of encephalopathy on mortality in the sepsis syndrome. The Veterans Administration Systemic Sepsis Cooperative Study Group. *Crit Care Med.* 1990;**18**:801–6.

23. Eidelman LA, Putterman D, Putterman C, Sprung CL. The spectrum of septic encephalopathy. Definitions, etiologies, and mortalities. *JAMA.* 1996;**275**:470–3.

24. Zhang LN, Wang XT, Ai YH, et al. Epidemiological features and risk factors of sepsis-associated encephalopathy in intensive care unit patients: 2008–2011. *Chin Med J (Engl).* 2012;**125**:828–31.

25. Suchyta MR, Jephson A, Hopkins RO. Neurologic changes during critical illness: brain imaging findings and neurobehavioral outcomes. *Brain Imaging Behav.* 2010;**4**:22–34.

26. Raicevic R, Jovicic A, Dimitrijevic R, Surbatovic M, Marenovic T. [Septic encephalopathy–prognostic value of the intensity of consciousness disorder to the outcome of sepsis]. *Vojnosanit Pregl.* 2001;**58**:151–6.

27. Semmler A, Widmann CN, Okulla T, et al. Persistent cognitive impairment, hippocampal atrophy and EEG changes in sepsis survivors. *J Neurol Neurosurg Psychiatry.* 2013;**84**:62–9.

28. Gunther ML, Morandi A, Krauskopf E, et al. The association between brain volumes, delirium duration, and cognitive outcomes in intensive care unit survivors: the VISIONS cohort magnetic resonance imaging study. *Crit Care Med.* 2012;**40**:2022–32.

29. Guerra C, Hua M, Wunsch H. Risk of a diagnosis of dementia for elderly medicare beneficiaries after intensive care. *Anesthesiology.* 2015;**123**:1105–12.

30. Shah FA, Pike F, Alvarez K, et al. Bidirectional relationship between cognitive function and pneumonia. *Am J Respir Crit Care Med.* 2013;**188**:586–92.

31. Jackson JC, Gordon SM, Ely EW, Burger C, Hopkins RO. Research issues in the evaluation of cognitive impairment in intensive care unit survivors. *Intensive Care Med.* 2004;**30**:2009–16.

32. Girard TD, Jackson JC, Pandharipande PP, et al. Delirium as a predictor of long-term cognitive impairment in survivors of critical illness. *Crit Care Med.* 2010;**38**:1513–20.

33. Hopkins RO, Weaver LK, Pope D, et al. Neuropsychological sequelae and impaired health status in survivors of severe acute respiratory distress syndrome. *Am J Respir Crit Care Med.* 1999;**160**:50–6.

34. Hopkins RO, Weaver LK, Collingridge D, et al. Two-year cognitive, emotional, and quality-of-life outcomes in acute respiratory distress syndrome. *Am J Respir Crit Care Med.* 2005;**171**:340–7.

35. Grasselli G, Zangrillo A, Zanella A, et al. Baseline characteristics and outcomes of 1591 patients infected with SARS-CoV-2 admitted to ICUs of the Lombardy region, Italy. *JAMA.* 2020;**323** (16):1574–81.

36. Al-Dalahmah O, Thakur KT, Nordvig AS, et al. Neuronophagia and microglial nodules in a SARS-CoV-2 patient with cerebellar hemorrhage. *Acta Neuropathol Commun.* 2020;**8**:1–7.

37. Thakur KT, Miller EH, Glendinning MD, et al. COVID-19 neuropathology at Columbia University Irving Medical center/New York Presbyterian Hospital. *Brain.* 2021;**144** (9):2696–2708.

38. Tan Y-K, Goh C, Leow AS, et al. COVID-19 and ischemic stroke: a systematic review and meta-summary of the literature. *J Thromb Thrombolysis*. 2020;**50**:587–95.

39. Boehme AK, Doyle K, Thakur KT, et al. Disorders of consciousness in hospitalized patients with COVID-19: the role of the systemic inflammatory response syndrome. *Neurocrit Care*. 2022;**36** (1):89–96.

40. Huang C, Huang L, Wang Y, et al. 6-month consequences of COVID-19 in patients discharged from hospital: a cohort study. *Lancet*. 2021;**397**:220–32.

41. Barichello T, Sayana P, Giridharan VV, et al. Long-term cognitive outcomes after sepsis: a translational systematic review. *Mol Neurobiol*. 2019;**56**:186–251.

42. Barichello T, Martins MR, Reinke A, et al. Cognitive impairment in sepsis survivors from cecal ligation and perforation. *Crit Care Med*. 2005;**33**:221–3; discussion 262–223.

43. Barichello T, Martins MR, Reinke A, et al. Long-term cognitive impairment in sepsis survivors. *Crit Care Med*. 2005;**33**:1671.

44. Semmler A, Frisch C, Debeir T, et al. Long-term cognitive impairment, neuronal loss and reduced cortical cholinergic innervation after recovery from sepsis in a rodent model. *Exp Neurol*. 2007;**204**:733–70.

45. Streck EL, Comim CM, Barichello T, Quevedo J. The septic brain. *Neurochem Res*. 2008;**33**:2171–7.

46. Davydow DS, Hough CL, Langa KM, Iwashyna TJ. Symptoms of depression in survivors of severe sepsis: a prospective cohort study of older Americans. *Am J Geriatr Psychiatry*. 2013;**21**:887–97.

47. Tuon L, Comim CM, Antunes MM, et al. Imipramine reverses the depressive symptoms in sepsis survivor rats. *Intensive Care Med*. 2007;**33**:2165–7.

48. Myhren H, Ekeberg O, Toien K, Karlsson S, Stokland O. Posttraumatic stress, anxiety and depression symptoms in patients during the first year post intensive care unit discharge. *Crit Care*. 2010;**14**:R14.

49. Schelling G, Stoll C, Kapfhammer HP, et al. The effect of stress doses of hydrocortisone during septic shock on posttraumatic stress disorder and health-related quality of life in survivors. *Crit Care Med*. 1999;**27**:2678–83.

50. Yende S, Austin S, Rhodes A, et al. Long-term quality of life among survivors of severe sepsis: analyses of two international trials. *Crit Care Med*. 2016;**44**:1461–7.

51. Heyland DK, Hopman W, Coo H, Tranmer J, McColl MA. Long-term health-related quality of life in survivors of sepsis. Short Form 36: a valid and reliable measure of health-related quality of life. *Crit Care Med*. 2000;**28**:3599–3605.

52. Bakhuizen SE, de Haan TR, Teune MJ, et al. Meta-analysis shows that infants who have suffered neonatal sepsis face an increased risk of mortality and severe complications. *Acta Paediatr*. 2014;**103**:1211–18.

53. Kaur J, Singhi P, Singhi S, Malhi P, Saini AG. Neurodevelopmental and behavioral outcomes in children with sepsis-associated encephalopathy admitted to pediatric intensive care unit: a prospective case control study. *J Child Neurol*. 2016;**31**:683–90.

54. Bronner MB, Knoester H, Sol JJ, et al. An explorative study on quality of life and psychological and cognitive function in pediatric survivors of septic shock. *Pediatr Crit Care Med*. 2009;**10**:636–42.

55. Zenaide PV, Gusmao-Flores D. Biomarkers in septic encephalopathy: a systematic review of clinical studies. *Rev Bras Ter Intensiva*. 2013;**25**:56–62.

56. Iacobone E, Bailly-Salin J, Polito A, et al. Sepsis-associated encephalopathy and its differential diagnosis. *Crit Care Med*. 2009;**37**:S331–6.

57. Pierrakos C, Vincent JL. Sepsis biomarkers: a review. *Crit Care*. 2010;**14**:R15.

58. Piazza O, Russo E, Cotena S, Esposito G, Tufano R. Elevated S100B levels do not correlate with the severity of encephalopathy during sepsis. *Br J Anaesth*. 2007;**99**:518–21.

59. Berger RP, Adelson PD, Pierce MC, et al. Serum neuron-specific enolase, S100B, and myelin basic protein concentrations after inflicted and noninflicted traumatic brain injury in children. *J Neurosurg*. 2005;**103**:61–8.

60. Isgro MA, Bottoni P, Scatena R. Neuron-specific enolase as a biomarker: biochemical and clinical aspects. *Adv Exp Med Biol*. 2015;**867**:125–43.

61. Nguyen DN, Spapen H, Su F, et al. Elevated serum levels of S-100beta protein and neuron-specific enolase are associated with brain injury in patients with severe sepsis and septic shock. *Crit Care Med*. 2006;**34**:1967–74.

62. Yao B, Zhang LN, Ai YH, Liu ZY, Huang L. Serum S100beta is a better biomarker than neuron-specific enolase for sepsis-associated encephalopathy and determining its prognosis: a prospective and observational study. *Neurochem Res*. 2014;**39**:1263–9.

63. Zhang LN, Wang XH, Wu L, et al. Diagnostic and predictive levels of calcium-binding protein A8 and tumor necrosis factor receptor-associated factor 6 in sepsis-associated encephalopathy: a prospective observational study. *Chin Med J (Engl)*. 2016;**129**:1674–81.

64. Wu L, Ai ML, Feng Q, et al. Serum glial fibrillary acidic protein and ubiquitin C-terminal hydrolase-L1 for diagnosis of sepsis-associated encephalopathy and outcome prognostication. *J Crit Care*. 2019;**52**:172–9.

65. Ehler J, Petzold A, Wittstock M, et al. The prognostic value of neurofilament levels in patients with sepsis-associated encephalopathy – a prospective, pilot observational study. *PLoS One*. 2019;**14**:e0211184.

66. van den Boogaard M, Kox M, Quinn KL, et al. Biomarkers associated with delirium in critically ill patients and their relation with long-term subjective cognitive dysfunction; indications for different pathways governing delirium in inflamed and noninflamed patients. *Crit Care*. 2011;**15**:R297.

67. Fioretto JR, Martin JG, Kurokawa CS, et al. Interleukin-6 and procalcitonin in children with sepsis and septic shock. *Cytokine*. 2008;**43**:160–4.

68. Orhun G, Tuzun E, Ozcan PE, et al. Association between inflammatory markers and cognitive outcome in patients with acute brain dysfunction due to sepsis. *Noro Psikiyatr Ars*. 2019;**56**:63–70.

69. Hsu AA, Fenton K, Weinstein S, et al. Neurological injury markers in children with septic shock. *Pediatr Crit Care Med*. 2008;**9**:245–51.

70. Hamed SA, Hamed EA, Abdella MM. Septic encephalopathy: relationship to serum and cerebrospinal fluid levels of adhesion molecules, lipid peroxides and S-100B protein. *Neuropediatrics*. 2009;**40**:66–72.

71. Bersani I, Auriti C, Ronchetti MP, et al. Use of early biomarkers in neonatal brain damage and sepsis: state of the art and future perspectives. *Biomed Res Int*. 2015;**2015**:253520.

72. Young GB, Bolton CF, Archibald YM, Austin TW, Wells GA. The electroencephalogram in sepsis-associated encephalopathy. *J Clin Neurophysiol*. 1992;**9**:145–52.

73. Hosokawa K, Gaspard N, Su F, et al. Clinical neurophysiological assessment of sepsis-associated brain dysfunction: a systematic review. *Crit Care*. 2014;**18**:674.

74. Oddo M, Carrera E, Claassen J, Mayer SA, Hirsch LJ. Continuous electroencephalography in the medical intensive care unit. *Crit Care Med*. 2009;**37**:2051–6.

75. Fox J, Lekoubou A, Bishu KG, Ovbiagele B. Seizure comorbidity boosts odds of 30-day readmission after an index hospitalization for sepsis. *Epilepsy Behav*. 2019;**95**:148–53.

76. Azabou E, Magalhaes E, Braconnier A, et al. Early standard electroencephalogram abnormalities predict mortality in septic intensive care unit patients. *PLoS One*. 2015;**10**:e0139969.

77. Berisavac, II, Padjen VV, Ercegovac MD, et al. Focal epileptic seizures, electroencephalography and outcome of sepsis associated encephalopathy-A pilot study. *Clin Neurol Neurosurg*. 2016;**148**:60–6.

78. Gilmore EJ, Gaspard N, Choi HA, et al. Acute brain failure in severe sepsis: a prospective study in the medical intensive care unit utilizing continuous EEG monitoring. *Intensive Care Med*. 2015;**41**:686–94.

79. Helderman JB, Welch CD, Leng X, O'Shea TM. Sepsis-associated electroencephalographic changes in extremely low gestational age neonates. *Early Hum Dev*. 2010;**86**:509–13.

80. Urtecho J, Snapp M, Sperling M, et al. Hospital mortality in primary admissions of septic patients with status epilepticus in the United States. *Crit Care Med*. 2013;**41**:1853–62.

81. Kafa IM, Bakirci S, Uysal M, Kurt MA. Alterations in the brain electrical activity in a rat model of sepsis-associated encephalopathy. *Brain Res*. 2010;**1354**:217–26.

82. Zauner C, Gendo A, Kramer L, et al. Impaired subcortical and cortical sensory evoked potential pathways in septic patients. *Crit Care Med*. 2002;**30**:1136–9.

83. Sharshar T, Carlier R, Bernard F, et al. Brain lesions in septic shock: a magnetic resonance imaging study. *Intensive Care Med*. 2007;**33**:798–806.

84. Piazza O, Cotena S, De Robertis E, Caranci F, Tufano R. Sepsis associated encephalopathy studied by MRI and cerebral spinal fluid S100B measurement. *Neurochem Res*. 2009;**34**:1289–92.

85. Stubbs DJ, Yamamoto AK, Menon DK. Imaging in sepsis-associated encephalopathy–insights and opportunities. *Nat Rev Neurol*. 2013;**9**:551–61.

86. Jackson AC, Gilbert JJ, Young GB, Bolton CF. The encephalopathy of sepsis. *Can J Neurol Sci*. 1985;**12**:303–7.

87. Szatmari S, Vegh T, Csomos A, et al. Impaired cerebrovascular reactivity in sepsis-associated encephalopathy studied by acetazolamide test. *Crit Care*. 2010;**14**:R50.

88. Fulesdi B, Szatmari S, Antek C, et al. Cerebral vasoreactivity to acetazolamide is not impaired in

203

patients with severe sepsis. *J Crit Care.* 2012;**27**:337–43.

89. Matta BF, Stow PJ. Sepsis-induced vasoparalysis does not involve the cerebral vasculature: indirect evidence from autoregulation and carbon dioxide reactivity studies. *Br J Anaesth.* 1996;**76**:790–4.

90. Terborg C, Schummer W, Albrecht M, et al. Dysfunction of vasomotor reactivity in severe sepsis and septic shock. *Intensive Care Med.* 2001;**27**:1231–4.

91. Taccone FS, Castanares-Zapatero D, Peres-Bota D, et al. Cerebral autoregulation is influenced by carbon dioxide levels in patients with septic shock. *Neurocrit Care.* 2010;**12**:35–42.

92. Rosenblatt K, Walker KA, Goodson C, et al. Cerebral autoregulation-guided optimal blood pressure in sepsis-associated encephalopathy: a case series. *J Intensive Care Med.* 2020;**35**(12):1453–64.

93. Reis C, Akyol O, Araujo C, et al. Pathophysiology and the monitoring methods for cardiac arrest associated brain injury. *Int J Mol Sci.* 2017;**18**(1):129.

94. Taccone FS, Su F, Pierrakos C, et al. Cerebral microcirculation is impaired during sepsis: an experimental study. *Crit Care.* 2010;**14**:R140.

95. Rosengarten B, Hecht M, Auch D, et al. Microcirculatory dysfunction in the brain precedes changes in evoked potentials in endotoxin-induced sepsis syndrome in rats. *Cerebrovasc Dis.* 2007;**23**:140–7.

96. Nishioku T, Dohgu S, Takata F, et al. Detachment of brain pericytes from the basal lamina is involved in disruption of the blood–brain barrier caused by lipopolysaccharide-induced sepsis in mice. *Cell Mol Neurobiol.* 2009;**29**:309–16.

97. Lemstra AW, Groen in't Woud JC, Hoozemans JJ, et al. Microglia activation in sepsis: a case–control study. *J Neuroinflammation.* 2007;**4**:4.

98. van Gool WA, van de Beek D, Eikelenboom P. Systemic infection and delirium: when cytokines and acetylcholine collide. *Lancet.* 2010;**375**:773–5.

99. Gamal M, Moawad J, Rashed L, et al. Evaluation of the effects of Eserine and JWH-133 on brain dysfunction associated with experimental endotoxemia. *J Neuroimmunol.* 2015;**281**:9–16.

100. Abramova AY, Pertsov SS, Kozlov AY, et al. Cytokine levels in rat blood and brain structures after administration of lipopolysaccharide. *Bull Exp Biol Med.* 2013;**155**:417–20.

101. Imamura Y, Wang H, Matsumoto N, et al. Interleukin-1beta causes long-term potentiation deficiency in a mouse model of septic encephalopathy. *Neuroscience.* 2011;**187**:63–9.

102. Alexander JJ, Jacob A, Cunningham P, Hensley L, Quigg RJ. TNF is a key mediator of septic encephalopathy acting through its receptor, TNF receptor-1. *Neurochem Int.* 2008;**52**:447–56.

103. Sharshar T, Gray F, Lorin de la Grandmaison G, et al. Apoptosis of neurons in cardiovascular autonomic centres triggered by inducible nitric oxide synthase after death from septic shock. *Lancet.* 2003;**362**:1799–1805.

104. Satta MA, Jacobs RA, Kaltsas GA, Grossman AB. Endotoxin induces interleukin-1beta and nitric oxide synthase mRNA in rat hypothalamus and pituitary. *Neuroendocrinology.* 1998;**67**:109–16.

105. Eckel B, Ohl F, Bogdanski R, Kochs EF, Blobner M. Cognitive deficits after systemic induction of inducible nitric oxide synthase: a randomised trial in rats. *Eur J Anaesthesiol.* 2011;**28**:655–63.

106. Weberpals M, Hermes M, Hermann S, et al. NOS2 gene deficiency protects from sepsis-induced long-term cognitive deficits. *J Neurosci.* 2009;**29**:14177–84.

107. Cepinskas G, Wilson JX. Inflammatory response in microvascular endothelium in sepsis: role of oxidants. *J Clin Biochem Nutr.* 2008;**42**:175–84.

108. Brealey D, Karyampudi S, Jacques TS, et al. Mitochondrial dysfunction in a long-term rodent model of sepsis and organ failure. *Am J Physiol Regul Integr Comp Physiol.* 2004;**286**:R491–7.

109. Crouser ED, Julian MW, Blaho DV, Pfeiffer DR. Endotoxin-induced mitochondrial damage correlates with impaired respiratory activity. *Crit Care Med.* 2002;**30**:276–84.

110. Barichello T, Machado RA, Constantino L, et al. Antioxidant treatment prevented late memory impairment in an animal model of sepsis. *Crit Care Med.* 2007;**35**:2186–90.

111. Gao R, Kan MQ, Wang SG, Yang RH, Zhang SG. Disrupted tryptophan metabolism induced cognitive impairment in a mouse model of sepsis-associated encephalopathy. *Inflammation.* 2016;**39**:550–60.

112. Cassol OJ Jr, Comim CM, Constantino LS, et al. Acute low dose of MK-801 prevents memory deficits without altering hippocampal DARPP-32 expression and BDNF levels in sepsis survivor rats. *J Neuroimmunol.* 2011;**230**:48–51.

113. Fang J, Lian Y, Xie K, Cai S, Wen P. Epigenetic modulation of neuronal apoptosis and cognitive functions in sepsis-associated encephalopathy. *Neurol Sci.* 2014;**35**:283–8.

114. Lavy S, Stein H. Convulsions in septicemic patients treated by penicillin. The value of

electroencephalograph examination. *Arch Surg.* 1970;**100**:225–8.

115. Ter Horst HJ, van Olffen M, Remmelts HJ, de Vries H, Bos AF. The prognostic value of amplitude integrated EEG in neonatal sepsis and/or meningitis. *Acta Paediatr.* 2010;**99**:194–200.

116. Azabou E, Magalhaes E, Braconnier A, et al. Early standard electroencephalogram abnormalities predict mortality in septic intensive care unit patients. *PLoS One.* 2015;**10**:e0139969.

117. Velissaris D, Pantzaris ND, Skroumpelou A, et al. Electroencephalographic abnormalities in sepsis patients in correlation to the calculated prognostic scores: a case series. *J Transl Int Med.* 2018;**6**:176–80.

118. Nielsen RM, Urdanibia-Centelles O, Vedel-Larsen E, et al. Continuous EEG monitoring in a consecutive patient cohort with sepsis and delirium. *Neurocrit Care.* 2020;**32**(1):121–30.

119. Bartynski WS, Boardman JF, Zeigler ZR, Shadduck RK, Lister J. Posterior reversible encephalopathy syndrome in infection, sepsis, and shock. *AJNR Am J Neuroradiol.* 2006;**27**:2179–90.

120. Morandi A, Gunther ML, Vasilevskis EE, et al. Neuroimaging in delirious intensive care unit patients: a preliminary case series report. *Psychiatry (Edgmont).* 2010;**7**:28–33.

121. Shankar J, Banfield J. Posterior reversible encephalopathy syndrome: a review. *Can Assoc Radiol J.* 2017;**68**:147–53.

122. Sutter R, Chalela JA, Leigh R, et al. Significance of parenchymal brain damage in patients with critical illness. *Neurocrit Care.* 2015;**23**:243–52.

123. Ehler J, Barrett LK, Taylor V, et al. Translational evidence for two distinct patterns of neuroaxonal injury in sepsis: a longitudinal, prospective translational study. *Crit Care.* 2017;**21**:262.

124. Orhun G, Esen F, Ozcan PE, et al. neuroimaging findings in sepsis-induced brain dysfunction: association with clinical and laboratory findings. *Neurocrit Care.* 2019;**30**:106–17.

Prognostication in Delirium

Eyal Y. Kimchi and Sophia L. Ryan

Background, Epidemiology, and Public Health importance

Background

Delirium is an acute disturbance of attention and awareness that can be associated with poor prognosis, including dependence and death.[1,2] Delirium is exceedingly common in critically ill patients across many different contexts, and can be considered a state of acute organ dysfunction or failure. Neuroprognostication in the setting of delirium is challenging due to the multifactorial nature of the syndrome and requires careful consideration of the various ways in which delirium manifests.

Epidemiology

Delirium is common in hospitalized adults, particularly as clinical acuity increases.[3] Unsurprisingly, delirium incidence is highest in the critical care population, afflicting 32–84% of intensive care unit (ICU) patients.[4–6] Delirium also tends to be common in patients with neurological diseases,[7] for example, with a prevalence between 13 and 48% in patients with stroke.[8] Even in the general medical population, where the prevalence of delirium ranges from 10 to 25%, delirium remains more likely to afflict neurologically vulnerable patients, such as those with dementia.[9]

Assessing Delirium in Critically Ill Patients

The bedrock of delirium management is recognition of its presence, which can be challenging in the ICU setting. Delirium is formally defined in the *Diagnostic and Statistical Manual of Mental Disorders* (DSM-5) as an acute change or fluctuation in attention and awareness that is associated with additional disturbances in cognition, such as

disorientation.[1] Formal diagnosis of delirium requires an evaluation by a clinical expert with experience diagnosing delirium. The assessment of mental status and delirium typically depends upon verbal responses, which may be difficult for patients who are intubated.

Specialized delirium screening tools have been developed to identify delirium in critically ill patients unable to respond verbally, such as the Confusion Assessment Method for the Intensive Care Unit (CAM-ICU) [10,11] and the Intensive Care Delirium Screening Checklist (ICDSC) [12]. These tools can be integrated into routine clinical care in the ICU and can be performed by trained nurses or research staff. Without such tools, it is estimated that the majority of delirium is missed by healthcare teams.[13,14] Therefore, clinical practice guidelines recommend that "critically ill adults should be regularly assessed for delirium using a valid tool."[15]

The CAM-ICU, based on the Confusion Assessment Method (CAM) algorithm.[16] operationalizes the four components of the CAM with adaptations for patients who are unable to speak. For example, examiners can test sustained attention by asking patients to squeeze the examiner's hand when they hear the letter "A," but not other letters. The CAM-ICU has been validated for use specifically in ventilated patients, with a sensitivity of 81% (95% confidence interval [CI]: 57%–93%) and specificity of 98% (95% CI: 86%–100%) in a meta-analysis.[10,17] The CAM-ICU has also been studied in neurocritically ill patients [18] and nonmechanically ventilated stroke patients, [19] but it still depends on verbal comprehension, and studies often do not clarify how they account for aphasia or distinguish between delirium related to overt cerebral pathology versus a systemic process.

Delirium can present with a range of phenotypes, from a hyperactive subtype, characterized by increased activity, hypervigilance, and agitation, to a hypoactive phenotype, characterized by decreased activity, lethargy, and even coma. While past neurological literature often distinguished these two subtypes, it is increasingly clear that the two are related, and delirium often presents as a mixed subtype with both hyperactive and hypoactive components. Patients with delirium in the ICU may have more hypoactive and mixed presentations, rather than the more conspicuous hyperactive presentation, potentially accounting for some of the underrecognition of delirium.[20]

Confusion regarding the terminology of delirium relative to other causes of altered mental status also suggests that its impact may not always be fully appreciated. Delirium in the ICU is sometimes referred to as encephalopathy or ICU psychosis. However, a recent expert panel has recommended that encephalopathy be used to refer to pathobiological processes in the brain, and delirium used to refer to the clinical state characterized by the aforementioned features, as affirmed by multiple societies.[21]

Multifactorial Nature of Delirium

By definition, delirium is a direct physiological consequence of another medical condition,[1] such as infection or intoxication. More commonly, however, delirium is thought to result from a multifactorial combination of predisposing and precipitating factors.[9] Predisposing factors, such as neurodegenerative disease, make patients vulnerable to delirium. Delirium may only emerge, however, in the presence of additional precipitating factors, for example, a new infection. For patients with severe predisposing factors, even a simple trigger may suffice to induce delirium, for example, a urinary tract infection in a patient with advanced Alzheimer's disease. In contrast, severe precipitants may induce delirium even in otherwise cognitively healthy patients, for example, severe burns in an adolescent. Patients with delirium and critical illness in the ICU may therefore be younger and less likely to have dementia than patients who more typically have delirium on the wards.[22]

Predisposing and precipitating factors are sometimes inferred before they can be diagnosed, but even when such factors are clearly identified it can be hard to predict the quality, severity, and prognosis of the ensuing delirium. Because of the multifactorial nature of delirium, acute and long-term prognostication depends upon the implications, modifiability, and interactions of three sets of factors:

1. Predisposing factors: Some predisposing factors for delirium may be modifiable, such as decreased hearing, for which hearing aids may help. Other predisposing factors, however, may lack meaningful disease modifying treatments and portend poorer long-term outcomes, for example, Alzheimer's disease.

2. Precipitating factors: Some precipitating factors for delirium may be more easily modifiable with a good prognosis, for example, dehydration, while other precipitating factors may be hard to treat and have a poor prognosis, for example, sepsis due to multi-drug resistant organisms.

3. Complications of delirium: Some delirium may remit quickly when appropriate multimodal behavioral interventions are initiated early. However, more severe delirium may cause more serious complications, for example, causing the patient to fall, or even prompting care providers to use off-label medications such as anti-psychotics, which in turn can cause iatrogenic adverse effects such as cardiac arrhythmias.

Public Health Importance

While different factors and complications interact to influence prognosis in unique ways for individual patients, from a public health perspective the importance of delirium crosses many clinical boundaries and is magnified by its scale. When delirium occurs in the ICU, its impact frequently extends into the rest of the hospitalization as well as into ensuing post-acute care. Due to its widespread nature, the annual healthcare costs associated with delirium have been estimated to be $38–152 billion in the United States alone.[23] In the ICU, delirium is associated with higher costs even after adjusting for factors such as age, comorbidities, and illness severity.[24,25] Preventing the personal, social, and financial costs of delirium requires proactive evaluation and management of delirium on a systems level. Because the course of individual patient's delirium can vary so widely but occurs in the context of such a large population, even modest improvements in delirium prediction and prognostication could have tremendous public health impact.

Neuroprognostication in Acute Settings

Clinical

Predicting Who Will Get Delirium

Predicting outcomes in delirium is rooted first in predicting who is at risk for developing delirium. Given the heterogeneous presentation and multifactorial pathophysiology, this has proven to be challenging. Several predisposing factors have been described in cohort studies, specifically age and clinically recognized cognitive impairment [9,26]. Subclinical or more specific cognitive impairments may also increase the risk of delirium and can be assessed before its onset, such as in the case of elective surgery, where delirium may develop during postoperative ICU care. For example, delirium following cardiac surgery is associated with impairments in delayed recall and working memory.[27]

The range of precipitants associated with delirium are broad, and their impact depends upon severity and context, complicating delirium prediction in general populations. In general, markers of critical illness severity, such as the Acute Physiology and Chronic Health Evaluation (APACHE) score, Sequential Organ Failure Assessment (SOFA), and the need for mechanical ventilation, are strongly associated with delirium.[5,26] Additionally, delirium is associated with emergent or invasive procedures and trauma.[26,28]

Several groups have developed multivariable models to predict ICU delirium, such as the PRE-DELIRIC model, whose factors include age, APACHE-II score, coma type, admission type, infection, metabolic acidosis, morphine dose, sedatives, urea concentration, and urgent admission.[29] With a sensitivity of 0.70 and a specificity of 0.73 in a multisite validation study, the PRE-DELIRIC score, like other predictive scores,[30] currently has moderate utility for predicting delirium. Similar models have been developed to try to predict delirium earlier in the patient's ICU course [31] or more dynamically throughout,[32] including machine learning methods.[33] Another risk model has even tried to predict daily changes in a wider number of brain states in ICU patients, including either coma or delirium.[34] Some reviewers, however, have raised concerns that the predictive

capabilities of most models to date may not be robust enough to be useful clinically.[35]

Predicting Delirium Severity and Course

The severity and course of delirium have been described in several ways.[36] Various severity scores for delirium assessment, duration of delirium across assessments, and even combinations of severity and duration to describe the trajectory or cumulative burden of delirium have been described.[37] As expected for a heterogeneous process, such predictions about the severity and course of delirium are conflicting. One study has found that patients with dementia tend to have higher peak delirium severity than those without, [38] whereas another has found that patients with cognitive decline have a higher likelihood of a mild but accelerated course of delirium.[37] Regarding duration, older ICU patients [39] or those with hypoactive delirium [40] tend to have a longer course, independent of sedation. In a randomized controlled trial, the dose and duration of sedative medications was found to be associated with a higher likelihood of both delirium and a prolonged course of delirium.[41]

Sociodemographic factors are additionally important, as patients who identify as African American are more likely to have a more severe trajectory of delirium.[37] The severity and duration of delirium are highly correlated. Patients with more severe delirium at the time of presentation tend to have a more prolonged course as well. [42] Surprisingly, the PRE-DELIRIC score, which can predict delirium modestly, predicts the duration of delirium poorly.[43] Several patient-, disease-, and treatment-related characteristics can determine the duration and severity of delirium. Outcomes in patients with delirium depend on whether the precipitating causes for delirium are potentially reversible or not.

Imaging

Multiple imaging modalities have been used in patients with delirium to study predisposing risk factors, precipitating pathologies, and long-term prognosis. Although relatively few studies have been prospective and large or unbiased evaluations of ICU patients. As expected, given that the most important risk factors for delirium are older age and dementia, neuroimaging markers associated with an increased risk for delirium include atrophy and white matter hyperintensities.[44,45] When trying to identify acute precipitants in heterogeneous patients, neuroimaging tends to have a low yield,[46] although acute ischemic lesions may be associated with delirium after cardiothoracic surgery.[44] In patients with stroke, right hemispheric and total anterior circulation strokes may be associated with delirium.[44] Measures of anatomical connectivity may also be promising predictors of delirium, including reductions in fractional anisotropy on diffusion tensor imaging.[44]

Functional imaging has also been performed in patients with delirium using a variety of modalities. Increased correlation between dorsolateral prefrontal cortex and posterior cingulate cortex on functional magnetic resonance imaging (fMRI) appears to be associated with delirium. Additionally, greater precuneus connectivity with the posterior cingulate cortex predicted less severe and shorter duration delirium. Low regional cerebral oxygenation on near infrared spectroscopy (NIRS) has been associated with delirium in the ICU.[47] Other vascular findings have been demonstrated intraoperatively during cardiac surgery to predict subsequent delirium.[48] A few longitudinal studies have suggested that some of the structural findings are unsurprisingly persistent. For example, brain atrophy is associated with a longer duration of delirium, and longer duration of delirium is correlated with increased brain atrophy at 3 months after the index hospitalization.[49] In contrast, some functional findings associated with delirium may improve with its clinical resolution.[50]

Biomarkers

There is great interest in identifying biomarkers of delirium both to aid in the diagnosis and to improve our understanding of pathophysiology. Targeted studies have primarily focused on markers of inflammation, blood brain barrier dysfunction, and neural injury. Most biomarker studies have been performed on serum, with fewer studies of cerebrospinal fluid (CSF) or brain tissue. In serum, C-reactive protein (CRP) is commonly elevated in patients with delirium in the ICU, and higher elevations are associated with prolonged delirium.[51] Other inflammatory markers collected early in an ICU stay, such as interleukins IL-6, IL-7, IL-10 and tumor necrosis factor alpha (TNFα), are also associated with both the severity and duration of coma.[52]

Findings from studies assessing the relationship between delirium and markers of neural injury have been less consistent. Neuron-specific enolase (NSE) may correlate with post-cardiac surgery delirium.[53] In critically ill coronavirus disease 2019 (COVID-19) patients, delirium was associated with higher levels of neurofilament-light chain (NfL) and glial fibrillary acidic protein (GFAP).[54] NfL is also higher in patients with other types of sepsis-associated encephalopathy and correlates with delirium severity.[55] Other markers such as brain-derived neurotrophic factor (BDNF) have not been as consistently associated with delirium. [56] Some markers, such as S100B, are increased not only in patients with delirium but also those with sepsis.[57] Protein S100B in the CSF has not been consistently associated with delirium; [58] however, higher CSF levels of dopamine metabolites are associated with delirium in hospitalized neurological patients.[59]

Electrophysiology

Electroencephalography (EEG) may be a particularly reliable biomarker of delirium.[60] Even early EEG studies recognized that generalized EEG slowing can be associated with delirium.[61] EEG findings can correlate with delirium severity [62,63] and can predict outcomes such as length of stay and mortality. [63–65] EEG studies have been performed at various timepoints in relationship to delirium.[66] For example, intraoperative suppression on EEG can predict subsequent delirium in the ICU.[67] This may reflect vulnerability rather than a causal effect, as titrating anesthesia to EEG does not appear to decrease the risk of delirium.[68]

Researchers have also looked at whether other types of physiological data may help predict delirium. Heart rate variability appears increased in some studies of patients with delirium in the ICU.[69] Limb actigraphy does not appear predictive of who has or will develop delirium. Eye movements, however, may distinguish cardiac ICU patients with delirium from those without.[70,71] Additionally, decreases in the percentage and speed of pupillary constriction have also been associated with an increased risk of delirium in the ICU, possibly even preceding clinical diagnosis.[72] The relationship of these findings to longer-term prognosis remains undetermined.

Neuroprognostication Over Time

Delirium is not only common but also associated with worse long-term outcomes. While traditionally thought of as a transient condition, delirium can persist for extended periods, through the hospitalization and even following discharge. In a 2009 systemic review, Cole and colleagues reported that 45% of delirious patients remained delirious upon discharge, and 33% was still delirious 1 month after discharge.[73] Delirium is associated with numerous sequelae, including longer mechanical ventilation, longer ICU and hospital stays, increased dependence after discharge, and death.[6] While it remains unclear how much of this association is due to risk factors versus delirium itself, delirium worsens outcomes in already vulnerable patients.

Mortality

Delirium has been consistently associated with an approximately 2- to 3-fold increased risk of mortality across many patients over several decades, particularly for patients who experience delirium in the ICU.[6,74] Mortality is increased both in the ICU and in the hospital, even when accounting for acute physiology scores or organ failure.[5] Mortality tends to be increased most in patients with hypoactive [75] or refractory [57] delirium. An increasing duration of delirium is associated with increased 30-day mortality in multivariable analysis, with even a single day of delirium associated with a hazard ratio for mortality of 1.70.[76] Delirious patients are at increased risk of complications such as self-extubation.[78] The attributable mortality of delirium, however, is often more challenging to determine.[77]

Cognitive

The strongest long-term association of delirium is with worsened cognition. A longer duration of delirium is associated with worse cognition at 3 months and 1 year, even after controlling for various factors such as age and preexisting cognitive impairment in a multivariable analysis.[79] Other studies have shown more specifically that a longer duration of hypoactive delirium is associated with worse long-term cognition.[40] Specific cognitive deficits that have been noted include global cognition and executive function,[79] as well as memory and naming.[80] Some of the factors associated

with the development of delirium in the ICU, such as sedation, seem less associated with long-term cognitive outcomes in randomized trials.[41]

Traditionally, the association between delirium and worsened long-term cognition has been explained by potentially unrecognized neurodegenerative disease in such patients, even in patients who had been previously cognitively intact. While this may be the case for some patients, an autopsy study of almost 1,000 patients demonstrated that the cognitive decline observed in patients with delirium superimposed on neurodegenerative disease outpaces that seen with delirium alone or neurodegeneration alone, suggesting an additional, as yet unrecognized, neuropathological processes in delirium.[81]

Functional

Many patients suffer functional impairments after ICU care, which has been increasingly recognized with the term "post-intensive case syndrome" (PICS), which includes functional, cognitive, and mental health features. While delirium is clearly associated with the cognitive features of PICS, the relationship between delirium and functional measures has not been as fully studied. One study has demonstrated that the duration of delirium is associated with worse functional outcomes over 1 year compared to those who did not experience delirium, as assessed by basic activities of daily living (ADLs), though not instrumental ADLs.[82] The same study also found lower motor-sensory function in patients who had experienced delirium in the ICU, though not overall worse physical health.[82] However, expert review across a wider range of studies has not found that delirium is consistently associated with worse long-term functional outcomes.[15]

Some efforts being tried to prevent PICS are similar to those advocated to prevent delirium, for example bundled care.[83] An ICU intervention that was targeted to improve functional status, early physical and occupational therapy, additionally decreased the duration of delirium during the ICU. [84] Therefore, even if delirium is not independently associated with PICS, the two may continue to be related based on shared precipitating and predisposing factors and attempted interventions.

Behavioral

The experience of delirium for the patient, family, and care team is often distressing.[85] Delirium in the ICU is highly associated with patient reports of distress in follow-up, including delusional memories.[86] Survivors of delirium often have memories of torture and fearing for their lives, and approximately 20% of patients experience post-traumatic stress disorder (PTSD) symptoms following ICU care.[87] While sometimes necessary for safety, restraining a confused and frightened patient can foment even more confusion and fear. Due to this, there has been significant concern that patients who experience delirium in the ICU may be at higher risk of developing PTSD. However, while some studies have demonstrated that delirium is associated with subsequent PTSD symptoms,[88] larger studies [89] and expert panels [15] have found no clear evidence yet that delirium in critically ill adults is consistently associated with an increased risk of PTSD. Similarly, larger studies [89] and expert panels [15] have found no clear evidence that delirium in critically ill adults is consistently associated with subsequent depression. In contrast, preoperative depression may be associated with an increased risk of post-cardiac surgery delirium.[90]

Gaps in Current Knowledge

Prognosis of Family and Caregivers

The experience of delirium for the patient, family, and care team is often a tragic one. Families can be devastated to witness their loved ones behaving erratically or even violently. And even staff suffer not only because of the stress and all-consuming nature of the care but also when confused patients mistakenly see attempts to provide care as a threat. Under these circumstances, delirious patients can unintentionally injure their care providers if proper behavioral measures are not taken.[91]

Although much research has focused on the long-term impact of delirium on patients, relatively less is known about its impact on family and caregivers. Increasingly, family members are encouraged to be an active part of delirium screening [92,93] and management, which can have significant benefit. However, if family is involved without enough support, this can unintentionally shift care responsibilities from the medical system to the family, potentially burdening them and exacerbating inequities for those without the flexibility or means to attend to the patient's bedside.

Delirium Assessment in Special Patient Contexts

Despite the availability of several validated tools for assessing delirium, there remain several ICU populations in whom it is particularly challenging to diagnose delirium. Under- or misdiagnosing delirium also presents unique challenges to the understanding of neuroprognostication in these contexts.

One major controversy has been whether delirium can be diagnosed in the context of reduced arousal. The DSM-5 criteria for delirium have been changed to state that inattention should not be assessed "in the context of [a] severely reduced level of arousal such as coma,"[1] given the difficulty of obtaining responses from these patients. In contrast, European Delirium Association and American Delirium Society statements have recommended that reduced arousal, with the exception of coma, is a valid context within which to diagnose delirium, even in the absence of patient responses to cognitive testing.[94] Delirium can sometimes even be a stage of improvement after coma, for example, in the context of post-traumatic confusional state.[95]

Related to considerations regarding arousal are concerns regarding sedation. Acute sedation causes altered mental status in otherwise healthy people, both hypoactive lethargy and even hyperactivity at the time of emergence, but it is not clear that this necessarily represents delirium in terms of typical long-term prognostic associations. Certain aspects of delirium may remain sensitive even in the setting of sedation, such as inattention, but other aspects may become much less specific, such as the level of arousal.[96] The influence of sedation may also depend on the delirium instrument used.[97] At least one study has demonstrated that only delirium that persists despite weaning of sedation has a worse prognosis.[98] While low-level sedation is expected and recommended practice, sedation is often deeper than targeted,[99] and the correct amount of time to lift sedation for reliable mental status assessments may not be achievable depending on other factors, such as ventilator dyssynchrony, nor may it be clear when a sufficient amount of time has passed, particularly after long sedation or in the setting of renal or hepatic insufficiency/dysfunction.

Nearly all delirium and mental status assessments currently depend on verbal communication, and therefore language barriers and potentially cultural ones may also impact assessments. Aphasic patients pose a particular challenge; however, that is not often explicitly addressed in some studies. It is possible that delirium assessment in an aphasic patient may require increased cut-off values.[100] Other brain lesions may also complicate delirium assessment,[101] for example, in intracerebral hemorrhage.[102]

Lastly, there is increasing knowledge about and recognition of delirium in pediatric ICU patients, but relatively less information compared to adults regarding its long-term prognostic impact. [103,104]

Subsyndromal Delirium

It remains unclear whether delirium is best thought of as a binary state: present or absent, or as a spectrum: from mild to severe. Mild delirium symptoms that do not fully meet delirium criteria have been termed subsyndromal delirium, which may be more common than delirium itself.[105] The risk factors of subsyndromal delirium and delirium are similar in many ways, and patients may progress from subsyndromal delirium to delirium.[106] Although effects are varied across studies and definitions, in general subsyndromal delirium is likely associated with lower effects on clinical outcomes than delirium.[107] The majority of patients will recover fully, but in at least one study ~ 29% may have a protracted course.[108] This suggests that the severity of delirium on a spectrum may be a more important prognostic marker than the result of a binary delirium screen.

Determining Causality

While there is a clear association between delirium and poor clinical outcomes, the question of causality is complex. Patients who suffer from delirium are often older and have higher rates of underlying dementia than those who do not develop delirium. Some of the poor outcomes are likely related to patients being sicker at baseline. However, several studies have demonstrated increased rates of death in patients who suffer from delirium, even when controlling for demographic and clinical factors such as age and comorbidities.[109–111]

Patients with delirium also suffer additional consequences related to the behavioral syndrome and iatrogenic responses. For example, patients with delirium are more likely to fall, leading to worse outcomes via resultant fractures, surgeries, and head injuries. Approximately 10% of the association of delirium with death may be mediated through use of restraining devices, hospital-acquired complications, and additional noxious insults acquired during hospitalization (such as sleep disturbance and dehydration). Each of these factors is three times more likely in delirious patients and increases mortality in a graded manner.[112]

Patients with delirium are also (1) more likely to receive sedating medications including those associated with cardiorespiratory compromise, [113,114] (2) more likely to be subjected to restrictive equipment including catheters associated with infection risk,[115] and (3) less likely to undergo potentially beneficial treatments, all of which can worsen outcomes. For example, if a patient with cancer becomes acutely delirious during a hospitalization and is unable to receive chemotherapy, that patient may be more likely to die than a similar patient who did not become delirious. Similarly, a patient with delirium may require a brain magnetic resonance imaging (MRI) procedure as part of a workup for altered mental status, but in order to safely undergo the MRI might receive sedation that can increase the risk of aspiration or prolong the delirium. Additionally, the antipsychotics given in an off-label capacity to manage symptoms of delirium [116,117] are associated with increased mortality in elderly patients, [118] imparting a 2.4-fold increased risk of sudden cardiac death [119,113] and a 40–50% increased risk of aspiration pneumonia.[119] Thus, while some of the poor outcomes observed in delirious patients may be related to baseline vulnerability and precipitating factors, some are also likely directly related to the delirium and its consequences.

Ongoing Research

Although delirium is thought to be both multifactorial and heterogeneous, these features may belie more complex underlying etiological and pathophysiological diversity.[120] Despite delirium being very common in ICU patients, it is unclear what portion of delirium risk in the ICU is due to each of many correlated factors: the critical illness itself, extended multiorgan failure, possible patient predispositions, standard clinical interventions in the ICU such as sedation, or environmental influences in the ICU, for example, intensive 24-hour care that disrupts sleep and circadian rhythms. Each factor may have a different impact on prognosis and potential modifiability and may be measured using different sets of biomarkers.

Only recently have contributing precipitants to delirium been reported more comprehensively in a larger ICU cohort.[121] Most ICU patients in this cohort had more than one delirium precipitant, with sedation being the most common. Among the different types of delirium-precipitating factors, most were associated with worse long-term cognitive function, except for metabolic contributors.

Sometimes precipitating factors are at times challenging to identify for given patients, even when the presence of delirium is clear. Sometimes, predisposing factors such as a neurodegenerative disease become evident or assumed in retrospect. Delirium biomarker research, particularly research that studies their trajectories, will continue to be an important feature of delirium research, both to understand pathophysiology and to predict long-term prognosis. This process may be greatly facilitated by international consortia and biobanks.[120]

Additionally, while delirium can be multifactorial, there is a great temptation to assume that every lab abnormality may be contributing to it. At times it may also be difficult to distinguish the effects of precipitating factors on delirium, such as pain, with their treatments, such as narcotics. It may therefore be challenging to know how to translate risks into interventions, particularly when balancing other important quality-of-life priorities in a given individual. Such research may ultimately require novel and adaptive trial designs.[120] The most effective delirium prevention programs tend to be multimodal and bundled,[122] but therefore hard to study mechanistically. It remains to be seen whether approaches utilizing artificial intelligence will help us overcome the complexity of delirium.

References

1. American Psychiatric Association. *Diagnostic and Statistical Manual of Mental Disorders, DSM-5*. 5th ed. Washington, DC: APA, 2013.

2. World Health Organization. The ICD-10 Classification of Mental and Behavioural Disorders: Clinical Descriptions and Diagnostic Guidelines [online]. World Health Organization, 1992. Accessed at: https://apps.who.int/iris/handle/10665/37958.

3. Vasilevskis EE, Han JH, Hughes CG, Ely EW. Epidemiology and risk factors for delirium across hospital settings. *Best Pract Res Clin Anaesthesiol.* 2012;**26**:277–87.

4. Boettger S, Zipser CM, Bode L, et al. The prevalence rates and adversities of delirium: Too common and disadvantageous. *Palliat Support Care.* 2020 Aug 3:1–9.

5. Salluh JI, Soares M, Teles JM, et al. Delirium epidemiology in critical care (DECCA): an international study. *Crit Care Lond Engl.* 2010;**14**: R210.

6. Salluh JIF, Wang H, Schneider EB, et al. Outcome of delirium in critically ill patients: systematic review and meta-analysis. *BMJ.* 2015;**350**:h2538.

7. Zipser CM, Deuel J, Ernst J, et al. Predisposing and precipitating factors for delirium in neurology: a prospective cohort study of 1487 patients. *J Neurol.* 2019;**266**(12):3065–75.

8. Shi Q, Presutti R, Selchen D, Saposnik G. Delirium in acute stroke: a systematic review and meta-analysis. *Stroke.* 2012;**43**:645–9.

9. Inouye SK, Westendorp RGJ, Saczynski JS. Delirium in elderly people. *Lancet Lond Engl.* 2014;**383**:911–22.

10. Ely EW, Margolin R, Francis J, et al. Evaluation of delirium in critically ill patients: validation of the Confusion Assessment Method for the Intensive Care Unit (CAM-ICU). *Crit Care Med.* 2001;**29**:1370–9.

11. Ely EW, Inouye SK, Bernard GR, et al. Delirium in mechanically ventilated patients: validity and reliability of the confusion assessment method for the intensive care unit (CAM-ICU). *JAMA.* 2001;**286**:2703–10.

12. Bergeron N, Dubois MJ, Dumont M, Dial S, Skrobik Y. Intensive Care Delirium Screening Checklist: evaluation of a new screening tool. *Intensive Care Med.* 2001;**27**:859–64.

13. Rockwood K, Cosway S, Stolee P, et al. Increasing the recognition of delirium in elderly patients. *J Am Geriatr Soc.* 1994;**42**:252–6.

14. Kales HC, Kamholz BA, Visnic SG, Blow FC. Recorded delirium in a national sample of elderly inpatients: potential implications for recognition. *J Geriatr Psychiatry Neurol.* 2003;**16**:32–38.

15. Devlin JW, Skrobik Y, Gélinas C, et al. Clinical practice guidelines for the prevention and management of pain, agitation/sedation, delirium, immobility, and sleep disruption in adult patients in the ICU. *Crit Care Med.* 2018;**46**:e825.

16. Inouye SK, van Dyck CH, Alessi CA, et al. Clarifying confusion: the confusion assessment

213

method. A new method for detection of delirium. *Ann Intern Med.* 1990;**113**:941–8.

17. Shi Q, Warren L, Saposnik G, Macdermid JC. Confusion assessment method: a systematic review and meta-analysis of diagnostic accuracy. Neuropsychiatr Dis Treat. 2013;**9**:1359–70.

18. Patel MB, Bednarik J, Lee P, et al. Delirium monitoring in neurocritically ill patients: a systematic review. *Crit Care Med.* 2018;**46**:1832–41.

19. Mitasova A, Kostalova M, Bednarik J, et al. Poststroke delirium incidence and outcomes: validation of the Confusion Assessment Method for the Intensive Care Unit (CAM-ICU). *Crit Care Med.* 2012;**40**:484–90.

20. Krewulak KD, Stelfox HT, Leigh JP, Ely EW, Fiest KM. Incidence and prevalence of delirium subtypes in an adult ICU: a systematic review and meta-analysis. *Crit Care Med.* 2018;**46**:2029–35.

21. Slooter AJC, Otte WM, Devlin JW, et al. Updated nomenclature of delirium and acute encephalopathy: statement of ten Societies. *Intensive Care Med.* 2020;**46**:1020–2.

22. Canet E, Amjad S, Robbins R, et al. Differential clinical characteristics, management and outcome of delirium among ward compared with intensive care unit patients. *Intern Med J.* 2019;**49**:1496–1504.

23. Leslie DL, Marcantonio ER, Zhang Y, Leo-Summers L, Inouye SK. One-year health care costs associated with delirium in the elderly population. *Arch Intern Med.* 2008;**168**:27–32.

24. Milbrandt EB, Deppen S, Harrison PL, et al. Costs associated with delirium in mechanically ventilated patients. *Crit Care Med.* 2004;**32**:955–62.

25. Vasilevskis EE, Chandrasekhar R, Holtze CH, et al. The cost of ICU delirium and coma in the intensive care unit patient. *Med Care.* 2018;**56**:890–7.

26. Zaal IJ, Devlin JW, Peelen LM, Slooter AJC. A systematic review of risk factors for delirium in the ICU. *Crit Care Med.* 2015;**43**:40–7.

27. Price CC, Garvan C, Hizel LP, Lopez MG, Billings FT. Delayed recall and working memory MMSE domains predict delirium following cardiac surgery. *J Alzheimers Dis.* 2017;**59**:1027–35.

28. Mossello E, Baroncini C, Pecorella L, et al. Predictors and prognosis of delirium among older subjects in cardiac intensive care unit: focus on potentially preventable forms. *Eur Heart J Acute Cardiovasc Care.* 2020;**9**(7):771–8.

29. van den Boogaard M, Schoonhoven L, Maseda E, et al. Recalibration of the delirium prediction model for ICU patients (PRE-DELIRIC): a multinational observational study. *Intensive Care Med.* 2014;**40**:361–9.

30. Cherak SJ, Soo A, Brown KN, et al. Development and validation of delirium prediction model for critically ill adults parameterized to ICU admission acuity. *PLoS One.* 2020;**15**:e0237639.

31. Wassenaar A, Schoonhoven L, Devlin JW, et al. Delirium prediction in the intensive care unit: comparison of two delirium prediction models. *Crit Care Lond Engl.* 2018;**22**:114.

32. Fan H, Ji M, Huang J, et al. Development and validation of a dynamic delirium prediction rule in patients admitted to the Intensive Care Units (DYNAMIC-ICU): A prospective cohort study. *Int J Nurs Stud.* 2019;**93**:64–73.

33. Lucini FR, Fiest KM, Stelfox HT, Lee J. Delirium prediction in the intensive care unit: a temporal approach. *Annu Int Conf IEEE Eng Med Biol Soc.* 2020;**2020**:5527–30.

34. Marra A, Pandharipande PP, Shotwell MS, et al. Acute brain dysfunction: development and validation of a daily prediction model. *Chest.* 2018;**154**:293–301.

35. Lindroth H, Bratzke L, Purvis S, et al. Systematic review of prediction models for delirium in the older adult inpatient. *BMJ Open.* 2018;**8**:e019223.

36. Jones RN, Cizginer S, Pavlech L, et al. Assessment of instruments for measurement of delirium severity: a systematic review. *JAMA Intern Med.* 2019;**179**:231–9.

37. Lindroth H, Khan BA, Carpenter JS, et al. Delirium severity trajectories and outcomes in ICU patients: defining a dynamic symptom phenotype. *Ann Am Thorac Soc.* 2020;**17**(9):1094–103.

38. Hshieh TT, Fong TG, Schmitt EM, et al. Does Alzheimer's disease and related dementias modify delirium severity and hospital outcomes? *J Am Geriatr Soc.* 2020;**68**:1722–30.

39. Pisani MA, Murphy TE, Araujo KLB, Van Ness PH. Factors associated with persistent delirium after intensive care unit admission in an older medical patient population. J Crit Care. 2010;**25**:540.e1–7.

40. Hayhurst CJ, Marra A, Han JH, et al. Association of hypoactive and hyperactive delirium with cognitive function after critical illness. *Crit Care Med.* 2020;**48**:e480–e488.

41. Nedergaard HK, Jensen HI, Stylsvig M, et al. Effect of nonsedation on cognitive function in

survivors of critical illness. *Crit Care Med.* 2020;**48** (12):1790–8.

42. Rudberg MA, Pompei P, Foreman MD, Ross RE, Cassel CK. The natural history of delirium in older hospitalized patients: a syndrome of heterogeneity. *Age Ageing.* 1997;**26**:169–74.

43. Heesakkers H, Devlin JW, Slooter AJC, van den Boogaard M. Association between delirium prediction scores and days spent with delirium. *J Crit Care.* 2020;**58**:6–9.

44. Nitchingham A, Kumar V, Shenkin S, Ferguson KJ, Caplan GA. A systematic review of neuroimaging in delirium: predictors, correlates and consequences. *Int J Geriatr Psychiatry.* 2018;**33**:1458–78.

45. Soiza RL, Sharma V, Ferguson K, et al. Neuroimaging studies of delirium: a systematic review. *J Psychosom Res.* 2008;**65**:239–48.

46. Hijazi Z, Lange P, Watson R, Maier AB. The use of cerebral imaging for investigating delirium aetiology. *Eur J Intern Med.* 2018;**52**:35–9.

47. Bendahan N, Neal O, Ross-White A, Muscedere J, Boyd JG. relationship between near-infrared spectroscopy-derived cerebral oxygenation and delirium in critically ill patients: a systematic review. *J Intensive Care Med.* 2019;**34**:514–20.

48. Bernardi MH, Wahrmann M, Dworschak M, et al. Carotid artery blood flow velocities during open-heart surgery and its association with delirium: A prospective, observational pilot study. *Medicine (Baltimore).* 2019;**98**:e18234.

49. Gunther ML, Morandi A, Krauskopf E, et al. The association between brain volumes, delirium duration, and cognitive outcomes in intensive care unit survivors: the VISIONS cohort magnetic resonance imaging study. *Crit Care Med.* 2012;**40**:2022–32.

50. Choi S-H, Lee H, Chung T-S, et al. Neural network functional connectivity during and after an episode of delirium. *Am J Psychiatry.* 2012;**169**:498–507.

51. Souza-Dantas VC, Dal-Pizzol F, Tomasi CD, et al. Identification of distinct clinical phenotypes in mechanically ventilated patients with acute brain dysfunction using cluster analysis. *Medicine (Baltimore).* 2020;**99**:e20041.

52. Khan BA, Perkins AJ, Prasad NK, et al. Biomarkers of delirium duration and delirium severity in the ICU. *Crit Care Med.* 2020;**48**:353–61.

53. Gailiušas M, Andrejaitienė J, Širvinskas E, et al. Association between serum biomarkers and postoperative delirium after cardiac surgery. *Acta Medica Litu.* 2019;**26**:8–10.

54. Cooper J, Stukas S, Hoiland RL, et al. Quantification of neurological blood-based biomarkers in critically ill patients with coronavirus disease 2019. *Crit Care Explor.* 2020;**2**:e0238.

55. Ehler J, Petzold A, Wittstock M, et al. The prognostic value of neurofilament levels in patients with sepsis-associated encephalopathy – a prospective, pilot observational study. *PLoS One.* 2019;**14**:e0211184.

56. Hayhurst CJ, Patel MB, McNeil JB, et al. Association of neuronal repair biomarkers with delirium among survivors of critical illness. *J Crit Care.* 2020;**56**:94–9.

57. Jorge-Ripper C, Alemán M-R, Ros R, et al. Prognostic value of acute delirium recovery in older adults. *Geriatr Gerontol Int.* 2017;**17**:1161–7.

58. Ayob F, Lam E, Ho G, Chung F, El-Beheiry H, Wong J. Pre-operative biomarkers and imaging tests as predictors of post-operative delirium in non-cardiac surgical patients: a systematic review. *BMC Anesthesiol.* 2019;**19**:25.

59. Ramírez-Bermúdez J, Perez-Neri I, Montes S, et al. Dopaminergic Hyperactivity in Neurological Patients with Delirium. *Arch Med Res.* 2019;**50**:477–83.

60. van der Kooi AW, Leijten FSS, van der Wekken RJ, Slooter AJC. What are the opportunities for eeg-based monitoring of delirium in the ICU? *J Neuropsychiatry Clin Neurosci.* 2012;**24**:472–7.

61. Romano J, Engel GL. Delirium I. Electroencephalographic data. *Arch Neurol Psychiatry.* 1944;**51**:356–77.

62. Numan T, van den Boogaard M, Kamper AM, et al. Recognition of delirium in postoperative elderly patients: a multicenter study. *J Am Geriatr Soc.* 2017;**65**(9):1932–8.

63. Kimchi EY, Neelagiri A, Whitt W, et al. Clinical EEG slowing correlates with delirium severity and predicts poor clinical outcomes. *Neurology.* 2019;**93**:e1260–e1271.

64. Shinozaki G, Bormann NL, Chan AC, et al. Identification of patients with high mortality risk and prediction of outcomes in delirium by bispectral EEG. *J Clin Psychiatry.* 2019;**80** (5):19m12749.

65. Azabou E, Magalhaes E, Braconnier A, et al. Early standard electroencephalogram abnormalities predict mortality in septic intensive care unit patients. *PLoS One.* 2015;**10**(10):e1039969.

66. Boord MS, Moezzi B, Davis D, et al. Investigating how electroencephalogram measures associate

with delirium: a systematic review. *Clin Neurophysiol.* 2020;**132**(1):246–57.

67. Fritz BA, Maybrier HR, Avidan MS. Intraoperative electroencephalogram suppression at lower volatile anaesthetic concentrations predicts postoperative delirium occurring in the intensive care unit. *Br J Anaesth.* 2018;**121**:241–8.

68. Wildes TS, Mickle AM, Ben Abdallah A, et al. effect of electroencephalography-guided anesthetic administration on postoperative delirium among older adults undergoing major surgery: the ENGAGES randomized clinical trial. *JAMA.* 2019;**321**:473–83.

69. Oh J, Cho D, Kim J, et al. Changes in heart rate variability of patients with delirium in intensive care unit. *Annu Int Conf IEEE Eng Med Biol Soc.* 2017;**2017**:3118–21.

70. Matsushima E, Nakajima K, Moriya H, et al. A psychophysiological study of the development of delirium in coronary care units. *Biol Psychiatry.* 1997;**41**:1211–17.

71. van der Kooi AW, Rots ML, Huiskamp G, et al. Delirium detection based on monitoring of blinks and eye movements. *Am J Geriatr Psychiatry.* 2014;**22**:1575–82.

72. Favre E, Bernini A, Morelli P, et al. Neuromonitoring of delirium with quantitative pupillometry in sedated mechanically ventilated critically ill patients. *Crit Care Lond Engl.* 2020;**24**:66.

73. Cole MG, Ciampi A, Belzile E, Zhong L. Persistent delirium in older hospital patients: a systematic review of frequency and prognosis. *Age Ageing.* 2008;**38**:19–26.

74. Aung Thein MZ, Pereira JV, Nitchingham A, Caplan GA. A call to action for delirium research: meta-analysis and regression of delirium associated mortality. *BMC Geriatr.* 2020;**20**:325.

75. Krewulak KD, Stelfox HT, Ely EW, Fiest KM. Risk factors and outcomes among delirium subtypes in adult ICUs: a systematic review. *J Crit Care.* 2020;**56**:257–64.

76. Shehabi Y, Riker RR, Bokesch PM, et al. Delirium duration and mortality in lightly sedated, mechanically ventilated intensive care patients. *Crit Care Med.* 2010;**38**:2311–18.

77. Klein Klouwenberg PMC, Zaal IJ, Spitoni C, et al. The attributable mortality of delirium in critically ill patients: prospective cohort study. *BMJ.* 2014;**349**:g6652.

78. Dubois MJ, Bergeron N, Dumont M, Dial S, Skrobik Y. Delirium in an intensive care unit: a study of risk factors. *Intensive Care Med.* 2001;**27**:1297–1304.

79. Pandharipande PP, Girard TD, Jackson JC, et al. Long-term cognitive impairment after critical illness. *N Engl J Med.* 2013;**369**:1306–16.

80. van den Boogaard M, Schoonhoven L, Evers AWM, et al. Delirium in critically ill patients: impact on long-term health-related quality of life and cognitive functioning. *Crit Care Med.* 2012;**40**:112–18.

81. Davis DHJ, Muniz-Terrera G, Keage HAD, et al. Association of delirium with cognitive decline in late life: a neuropathologic study of 3 population-based cohort studies. *JAMA Psychiatry.* 2017;**74**:244–51.

82. Brummel NE, Jackson JC, Pandharipande PP, et al. Delirium in the ICU and subsequent long-term disability among survivors of mechanical ventilation. *Crit Care Med.* 2014;**42**:369–77.

83. Inoue S, Hatakeyama J, Kondo Y, et al. Post-intensive care syndrome: its pathophysiology, prevention, and future directions. *Acute Med Surg.* 2019;**6**:233–46.

84. Schweickert WD, Pohlman MC, Pohlman AS, et al. Early physical and occupational therapy in mechanically ventilated, critically ill patients: a randomised controlled trial. *Lancet Lond Engl.* 2009;**373**:1874–82.

85. Partridge JSL, Martin FC, Harari D, Dhesi JK. The delirium experience: what is the effect on patients, relatives and staff and what can be done to modify this? *Int J Geriatr Psychiatry.* 2013;**28**:804–12.

86. Svenningsen H, Tønnesen EK, Videbech P, et al. Intensive care delirium – effect on memories and health-related quality of life – a follow-up study. *J Clin Nurs.* 2014;**23**:634–44.

87. Righy C, Rosa RG, da Silva RTA, et al. Prevalence of post-traumatic stress disorder symptoms in adult critical care survivors: a systematic review and meta-analysis. *Crit Care.* 2019;**23**(1):213.

88. Bulic D, Bennett M, Georgousopoulou EN, et al. Cognitive and psychosocial outcomes of mechanically ventilated intensive care patients with and without delirium. *Ann Intensive Care.* 2020;**10**:104.

89. Brown KN, Soo A, Faris P, Patten SB, Fiest KM, Stelfox HT. Association between delirium in the intensive care unit and subsequent neuropsychiatric disorders. *Crit Care Lond Engl.* 2020;**24**:476.

90. Eshmawey M, Arlt S, Ledschbor-Frahnert C, Guenther U, Popp J. Preoperative depression and plasma cortisol levels as predictors of delirium after cardiac surgery. *Dement Geriatr Cogn Disord.* 2019;**48**:207–14.

91. The Joint Commission. Sentinel Event Alert 59: Physical and verbal violence against health care workers. 2018; revised June 2021.

92. Steis MR, Evans L, Hirschman KB, et al. Screening for delirium via family caregivers: convergent validity of the Family Confusion Assessment Method (FAM-CAM) and Interviewer-Rated CAM. *J Am Geriatr Soc.* 2012;**60**:2121–6.

93. Inouye SK, Puelle M, Saczynski J, Steis M. *The Family Confusion Assessment Method (FAM-CAM): Instrument and Training Manual.* Boston: Hospital Elder Life Program, 2012. Available at: www.hospitalelderlifeprogram.org.

94. European Delirium Association, American Delirium Society. The DSM-5 criteria, level of arousal and delirium diagnosis: inclusiveness is safer. *BMC Med.* 2014;**12**:141.

95. Sherer M, Katz DI, Bodien YG, et al. Post-traumatic confusional state: a case definition and diagnostic criteria. *Arch Phys Med Rehabil.* 2020;**101**(11):2041–50.

96. Boettger S, Meyer R, Richter A, et al. Screening for delirium with the Intensive Care Delirium Screening Checklist (ICDSC): Symptom profile and utility of individual items in the identification of delirium dependent on the level of sedation. *Palliat Support Care.* 2019;**17**:74–81.

97. van den Boogaard M, Wassenaar A, van Haren FMP, et al. Influence of sedation on delirium recognition in critically ill patients: a multinational cohort study. *Aust Crit Care.* 2020;**33**(5):420–5.

98. Patel SB, Poston JT, Pohlman A, Hall JB, Kress JP. Rapidly reversible, sedation-related delirium versus persistent delirium in the intensive care unit. *Am J Respir Crit Care Med.* 2014;**189**:658–65.

99. Nassar AP, Zampieri FG, Salluh JI, et al. Organizational factors associated with target sedation on the first 48 h of mechanical ventilation: an analysis of checklist-ICU database. *Crit Care Lond Engl.* 2019;**23**:34.

100. Boßelmann C, Zurloh J, Stefanou M-I, et al. delirium screening in aphasic patients with the Intensive Care Delirium Screening Checklist (ICDSC): a prospective cohort study. *Front Neurol.* 2019;**10**:1198.

101. von Hofen-Hohloch J, Awissus C, Fischer MM, et al. Delirium Screening in neurocritical care and stroke unit patients: a pilot study on the influence of neurological deficits on CAM-ICU and ICDSC outcome. *Neurocrit Care.* 2020;**33**(3):708–17.

102. Reznik ME, Drake J, Margolis SA, et al. Deconstructing poststroke delirium in a prospective cohort of patients with intracerebral hemorrhage. *Crit Care Med.* 2020;**48**:111–18.

103. Janssen NJJF, Tan EYL, Staal M, et al. On the utility of diagnostic instruments for pediatric delirium in critical illness: an evaluation of the Pediatric Anesthesia Emergence Delirium Scale, the Delirium Rating Scale 88, and the Delirium Rating Scale-Revised R-98. *Intensive Care Med.* 2011;**37**:1331–7.

104. Alvarez RV, Palmer C, Czaja AS, et al. Delirium is a common and early finding in patients in the pediatric cardiac intensive care unit. J Pediatr. 2018;**195**:206–12.

105. Bastos AS, Beccaria LM, da Silva DC, Barbosa TP. Identification of delirium and subsyndromal delirium in intensive care patients. *Rev Bras Enferm.* 2019;**72**:463–7.

106. Yamada C, Iwawaki Y, Harada K, et al. Frequency and risk factors for subsyndromal delirium in an intensive care unit. *Intensive Crit Care Nurs.* 2018;**47**:15–22.

107. Serafim RB, Soares M, Bozza FA, et al. Outcomes of subsyndromal delirium in ICU: a systematic review and meta-analysis. *Crit Care Lond Engl.* 2017;**21**:179.

108. Cole MG, Bailey R, Bonnycastle M, et al. Frequency of full, partial and no recovery from subsyndromal deliriumin older hospital inpatients. *Int J Geriatr Psychiatry.* 2016;**31**:544–50.

109. Leslie DL, Zhang Y, Holford TR, et al. Premature death associated with delirium at 1-year follow-up. *Arch Intern Med.* 2005;**165**:1657–62.

110. Kiely DK, Marcantonio ER, Inouye SK, et al. Persistent delirium predicts increased mortality. *J Am Geriatr Soc.* 2009;**57**:55–61.

111. McCusker J, Cole M, Abrahamowicz M, Primeau F, Belzile E. Delirium predicts 12-month mortality. *Arch Intern Med.* 2002;**162**:457–63.

112. Dharmarajan K, Swami S, Gou RY, Jones RN, Inouye SK. Pathway from delirium to death: potential in-hospital mediators of excess mortality. *J Am Geriatr Soc.* 2017;**65**:1026–33.

113. Inouye SK, Marcantonio ER, Metzger ED. Doing Damage in Delirium: The Hazards of Antipsychotic Treatment in Elderly Persons. Lancet Psychiatry. 2014;**1**:312–315.

114. Herzig SJ, Rothberg MB, Guess JR, et al. Antipsychotic Use in Hospitalized Patients: Rates, Indications, and Predictors. *J Am Geriatr Soc.* 2016;**64**:299–305.

115. Pendlebury ST, Lovett NG, Smith SC, et al. Observational, longitudinal study of delirium in consecutive unselected acute medical admissions: age-specific rates and associated factors, mortality and re-admission. *BMJ Open.* 2015;**5**:e007808.

116. Nikooie R, Neufeld KJ, Oh ES, et al. Antipsychotics for treating delirium in hospitalized adults: a systematic review. *Ann Intern Med.* 2019;**171**:485.

117. Oh ES, Needham DM, Nikooie R, et al. Antipsychotics for preventing delirium in hospitalized adults: a systematic review. *Ann Intern Med.* 2019;**171**:474.

118. Kuehn BM. FDA warns antipsychotic drugs may be risky for elderly. *JAMA.* 2005;**293**:2462.

119. Herzig SJ, LaSalvia MT, Naidus E, et al. Antipsychotics and the risk of aspiration pneumonia in individuals hospitalized for nonpsychiatric conditions: a cohort study. *J Am Geriatr Soc.* 2017;**65**:2580–6.

120. Oh ES, Akeju O, Avidan MS, et al. A roadmap to advance delirium research: recommendations from the NIDUS Scientific Think Tank. *Alzheimers Dement J.* 2020;**16**:726–33.

121. Girard TD, Thompson JL, Pandharipande PP, et al. Clinical phenotypes of delirium during critical illness and severity of subsequent long-term cognitive impairment: a prospective cohort study. *Lancet Respir Med.* 2018;**6**:213–22.

122. Inouye SK, Bogardus ST, Baker DI, Leo-Summers L, Cooney LM. The Hospital Elder Life Program: a model of care to prevent cognitive and functional decline in older hospitalized patients. Hospital Elder Life Program. *J Am Geriatr Soc.* 2000;**48**:1697–1706.

Chapter 15

Prognostication in Neuro-Oncology and Neurological Complications of Hemato/Oncological Diseases

Anuj Patel and E. Alton Sartor

Background, Epidemiology, and Public Health Importance

Metastatic brain tumors, which include both primary metastatic disease that initiated within the central nervous system (CNS) and secondary metastatic disease that started systemically and metastasized to the CNS, are collectively the most prevalent types of intracranial tumor.[1] Standardized treatment including surgery followed by either focal or whole-brain radiation have allowed for excellent local control rates.[2,3] In the setting of neurological complications related to these tumors, much work has been done to understand the key markers of prognostic and predictive significance. In addition, improved mortality rates in cancer patients have come at the cost of increasingly complicated treatment regimens including cytotoxic, immunological, surgical, and radiation-based therapies. Underlying heterogeneity across different types of metastatic brain disease is a contributing factor to this challenging decision-making process. In addition, only the presence or absence of brain metastasis at the time of initial diagnosis is noted in many historical studies, decreasing the overall detection of metastatic brain disease that develops later in the disease course. As a result, the decision-making process in the critical care setting has become increasingly complicated.

Approximately 20% of patients with a systemic cancer diagnosis will have secondary metastatic brain disease.[4] This may be an underestimate of the actual burden of metastatic brain disease, as patients live longer, thus granting additional time for metastatic brain disease to develop. Autopsy studies have suggested an incidence of metastatic brain disease of up to 40%.[5] Though any cancer may metastasize to the brain, breast (5–20%), lung (20–56%), and melanoma (7–16%) are the most common.[6] The underlying risk from metastatic

brain disease will also be influenced by the molecular subtype of the underlying disease. For example, anaplastic lymphoma kinase gene (*ALK*)-rearranged non-small-cell lung cancer (NSCLC) has a higher chance of metastasis to the brain compared to other subtypes of NSCLC.

In addition to secondary metastatic brain disease, primary brain cancer such as glioma of varying grades, primary CNS lymphoma (P-CNSL), and other primary metastatic brain diseases present additional challenges for prognostication. Primary brain tumors account for 2% of all malignant neoplasms in adults. Glioblastoma accounts for more than half of gliomas and represents a significant portion of the primary brain cancer population. The median survival of glioblastoma, the most common type of primary brain tumor, ranges from 12 to 18 months depending on underlying prognostic factors.[7] Other common primary

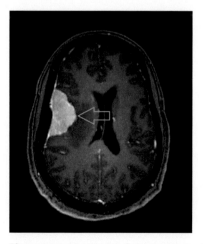

Figure 15.1 Meningioma. Patient presents with no prior metastatic history and recent seizure. Magnetic resonance imaging (MRI) brain T1 post-contrast shows a right homogeneously enhancing tumor with dural tail concerning for meningioma. Recommended for maximal surgical resection for diagnosis and seizure management.

tumors include meningiomas (Figure 15.1), pituitary tumors, and lower-grade gliomas and CNS lymphoma, though the vast majority of meningiomas and pituitary tumors are considered nonmalignant. Overall, there is a very low chance for primary metastatic tumors to metastasize outside of the brain, though the increased seizure risk and the challenge of treating exclusively across the blood–brain barrier and the lack of treatment efficacy across the spectrum of high-grade glioma creates its own set of challenges.

Theory of Decision Making in Neuro-Oncology in the Intensive Care Unit

There are a variety of neurological indications for neurocritical care for patients with CNS metastatic disease. These include close neurological monitoring in the setting of elevated intracranial pressure, seizures, pre- and post-surgical monitoring, and need for or presence of external cerebral spinal fluid (CSF) diversion. Further considerations such as palliative care setting and end-of-life care further complicate the decision-making milieu. These considerations can have a significant impact on assessment of prognostication because each set of problems may imply a different location in the patient treatment life cycle. Initial management for newly diagnosed metastatic disease typically involves early treatment with corticosteroids such as dexamethasone for management of elevated intracranial pressure and associated neurological symptoms such as weakness. When there is a solitary lesion, surgical intervention is always the best, first option, though many tumors can present in surgically inaccessible or eloquent locations or with multifocal disease, which may prevent surgical management. For other admission scenarios, an understanding of the underlying oncological decision making is helpful to assess the best course of action.

Metastatic brain disease, both primary and secondary, is generally resistant to cytotoxic chemotherapy, with a few specific exceptions such as temozolomide and capecitabine.[8] This effect has been associated with the blood–brain barrier and more recently with the blood–tumor barrier in CNS metastatic disease. This barrier has been demonstrated as one of the primary rate-limiting factors for treatment with cytotoxic chemotherapy.[9]

More recently, a variety of inhibitors targeting specific molecular or functional pathways have demonstrated significant efficacy when used to target disease involving the CNS. In NSCLC, epidermal growth factor receptor (EGFR) mutations have shown significant response to agents such as osimertinib, which has been shown to be effective for management of intracranial metastatic disease.[10] Additional treatments that have demonstrated efficacy for CNS disease include dabrafenib and trametinib for *BRAF* V600E mutations in melanoma and crizotinib and *ALK*-rearranged NSCLC.[11,12] Thus, if a cancer demonstrates a functional mutation that may be targetable with a small molecule inhibitor, additional investigation is warranted to understand the likelihood of effective treatment across the blood–brain barrier. If targeted treatment is available, this may substantially change the prognosis for a variety of conditions involving secondary metastatic spread to the brain.

Additional considerations involve management of elevated intracranial pressure related to metastatic brain disease. In the preoperative setting, several studies have demonstrated clinical benefit for 3% hypertonic saline over mannitol. [13–15] To date, there have not been extensive studies comparing the effectiveness of these two agents for urgent reduction of intracranial pressure for brain tumors specifically in the nonsurgical setting, though an extensive review of the available data suggests that both mannitol and hypertonic saline have similar overall efficacy, supporting the use of both options when nonsurgical planning is considered.[16] If there are indications for management with hyperosmolar therapy and no associated plan for surgical intervention, both mannitol and hypertonic saline are reasonable considerations.

Corticosteroids for management of neurological symptoms associated with malignancy of the CNS have been standard for several decades. In addition, treatment with steroids is often included as part of the perioperative surgical plan. The primary mechanism of efficacy of glucocorticoids is reduction of vasogenic edema, which results from increased peritumoral capillary permeability and can be associated with both mass effect and neurological symptoms. Dexamethasone is usually chosen due to its low mineralocorticoid effects and long half-life. Maximal efficacy usually occurs 12–72 hours after administration and should generally be considered for any patients with significant neurological symptoms or associated mass effect. In cases where lymphoma is considered highly likely but the diagnosis is uncertain, steroid management is often held to improve diagnostic yield unless the edema is severe or surgical biopsy is planned within 24–48 hours.

Obstructive and nonobstructive hydrocephalus can play an important role in decision-making for intensive care unit (ICU) patients with cerebral metastatic disease. When a patient presents with symptoms concerning for hydrocephalus such as headache, papilledema, altered mental status, or urinary incontinence, the most important step is to determine whether the patient has an obstructive process, typically determined with high-resolution brain imaging such as magnetic resonance imaging (MRI) with and without contrast. If there is an obstructive process, surgical intervention to alleviate the lesion is the next best step.

Seizures occur in up to 70% of patients with brain tumors. They are most common in patients with low-grade glioma and less common in metastatic brain disease and CNS lymphoma.[17] Pre- and perioperative management with prophylactic anti-seizure medications is common, though postoperative cessation within 4 weeks is recommended for patients who have not demonstrated seizures. In patients with persistent seizures, continued management with an appropriate anti-seizure regimen is recommended, with a preference toward non-enzyme-inducing medications such as levetiracetam, lacosamide, valproate, and zonisamide.[18]

Palliative care begins with early, honest discussions regarding the diagnosis and overall prognosis and attention to symptom management. Re-discussion of goals of care in the event of complications or progression of underlying disease is often indicated.

Metastatic Disease

Metastasis to the central nervous system is a complication of a variety of systemic cancers. It can occur at any point in a cancer's course, including both as the presenting sign of a cancer as well as a late manifestation of advanced disease. Though the true incidence of CNS metastasis is not clearly known, prior studies have estimated 9.6% of all systemic metastatic disease cases will be diagnosed with CNS metastatic disease.[19] Nevertheless, as systemic treatment improves, it is likely that the incidence of CNS metastatic disease will increase with time. Our ability to detect metastatic brain disease has also notably improved with the introduction of MRI as a routine screening tool for patients with metastatic disease. Lung cancer is the most commonly found metastatic cancer in the CNS, representing 45% of intracranial metastatic disease, followed by breast (15%), melanoma (10%), and colorectal (5%).[20]

A number of different systems have been proposed and validated for estimating the prognosis of patients with brain metastases, each with a different methodology and set of variables, with the notable common thread of performance status, age, comorbid medical condition, underlying diagnosis/systemic disease status, and surgical resectability.[21] For example, the recursive partitioning analysis model (RPA) analyzed patients from a collection of clinical trials on numerous potential prognostic factors; the analysis separated into three classes of patients, with the best prognosis in patients under 65 years of age with Karnofsky Performance Status (KPS) ? 70, a controlled primary as well as no extracranial metastases; and the worst in those with a KPS < 70 and a mixed prognosis in the remainder.[22] While there is not one single scoring system that is necessarily superior, these tools can help draw attention to prognostic factors that are easily assessed in the individual patient.

In addition to considering metastatic lesions, assessment of the underlying primary cancer as well as systemic control can also provide important context in the evaluation of a patient with brain or spinal cord metastases. Well-controlled systemic disease with isolated CNS metastatic lesions can present a very different picture from the same lesions in a patient with multisystem metastatic disease. However, given the evolution of treatments with time, it remains important to consider an individual patient's treatment options.

The treatment of brain metastases has long included a role for surgery, with or without radiation. Historically, resection of a solitary brain mass was studied with subsequent whole-brain radiation.[23] In patients with multiple metastases, surgical resection has been less clearly established and continues to be reevaluated. Nevertheless, surgery can play a role in some patients with multiple metastases; in a single center's retrospective analysis, median survival time was no different between patients who underwent surgery for single versus

221

multiple metastatic lesions (with survival instead better predicted by KPS and RPA class).[24]

Radiation, with or without surgery, has an important role in the treatment of brain metastases. It has typically been utilized in two broad forms: whole-brain radiation therapy (WBRT), targeting the entire brain to treat both the lesion as well as the entire brain at risk for undetected metastatic disease, or local treatment in the form of stereotactic radiosurgery (SRS). SRS has been established as an option, in combination with surgery, both alone as well as an adjunct to WBRT; SRS alone is a reasonable option in patients with solitary or oligometastatic lesions.[25] This choice also plays an important role in assessing the neurocognitive prognosis of patients, as WBRT is associated with increased risk of cognitive decline.[26] WBRT continues to play a role in some histologies, such as small cell lung cancer, as well as in patients with a high number of metastases. The combination of surgical resection and focal radiation has resulted in local control rate of > 90%.

Leptomeningeal Disease

Leptomeningeal disease is a relatively common neurological complication, occurring in up to 8% of patients with both primary and secondary metastatic lesions (Figure 15.2).[27,28] Traditionally, the development of this diagnosis is a devastating harbinger and often results in a transition to end-of-life care, and thus deserves special consideration in prognostic assessment. More recently, targeted therapies such as osimertinib have been demonstrated to be very effective for treatment of this disease in cases where there is a suitable target mutation such as EGFR for osimertinib.[29] Initial management should thus be focused on understanding whether the underlying neurological symptoms can be managed with a combination of steroids and CSF diversion. If the patient has a targetable mutation and they have a chance for clinically acceptable response to treatment from radiation and targeted treatments, then aggressive management is reasonable.

Diagnosis of leptomeningeal disease can sometimes pose a challenge, and initial presenting symptoms are sometimes subtle or vague, including cranial neuropathies, headache, or change in mental status. The identification of malignant cells on cerebrospinal fluid cytology is confirmatory,

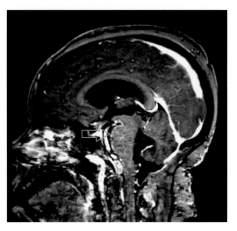

Figure 15.2 Leptomeningeal disease. Patient presents with known diagnosis of breast cancer and new-onset headaches. MRI brain T1 post-contrast shows thin enhancement of the anterior aspect of the mid-brain and pons concerning for leptomeningeal disease. Recommended for lumbar puncture to establish diagnosis and improve symptoms.

though other abnormalities on CSF analysis including both tumor-specific markers as well as elevated protein can also be helpful in making the diagnosis. Suspicion is also raised with characteristic imaging findings, most notably MRI finding of leptomeningeal enhancement as well as nodular appearance of cranial nerves or, in the spinal cord, of the cauda equina. Prompt identification is crucial in suspected cases given the propensity for rapid decline, particularly secondary to hydrocephalus and elevated intracranial pressure.

Elevated intracranial pressure should be treated promptly; as in other CNS metastatic lesions, corticosteroids (e.g., dexamethasone) are utilized.[30] While neurosurgical intervention does not play a large role in the direct treatment of leptomeningeal disease, it can serve a vital role in CSF diversion in cases of symptomatic hydrocephalus or increased intracranial pressure (ICP) not controlled with steroids, which can otherwise lead to significant neurological decline.[31] In cases where intrathecal chemotherapy is being utilized, an Ommaya reservoir may be placed. While the role of shunting in overall survival remains controversial, the benefits include improving symptoms and functional status, and "buying time" for the implementation of chemotherapy or other directed treatment.[32]

Radiation therapy should also be considered, particularly with an aim toward symptom improvement. Treatment can be targeted toward sites of bulky disease, as well as WBRT or craniospinal directed. While WBRT can sometimes be utilized for symptom control, it has not been shown to improve survival overall.[33] There may in addition be a role for radiation as a directed treatment to CSF flow abnormalities as identified by flow studies, particularly to facilitate the use of intrathecal chemotherapy and avoid both protected sites as well as focal toxicities.[34] Particularly as the modern management of metastatic disease evolves, consideration of radiation therapy remains a part of a multimodal approach to treatment and palliation in patients with leptomeningeal disease.

The overall prognosis of leptomeningeal disease has been classically regarded as quite poor. The patient's underlying performance status should be taken into consideration when evaluating prognosis; in one series, patients with a poor performance status (KPS < 70) had median survival of 5 weeks, compared with 15.5 weeks in those with a better level of functioning. In addition, the underlying primary pathology and candidacy for systemic treatments remain considerations. For example, in leptomeningeal carcinomatosis from breast cancer, hormonal receptor and HER2 status can guide both the expected clinical course as well as treatment options.[35] In other histologies, targeted treatment regimens have produced both improvement in neurological symptoms as well as complete response for over 1 year.[36]

In all cases, the patient's response to initial treatment should be monitored and reassessed, particularly considering the gravity of the underlying disease. If elevated ICP and symptoms can be managed, aggressive ongoing treatment can be considered, taking into account candidacy for further treatment options. The approach to decision-making involves addressing both the patient's goals of care and their current level of functioning, in conjunction with their individual pathology and availability of efficacious targeted therapies with adequate CNS penetration.

Novel approaches continue to be pursued, and developments in oncological treatment are being investigated in leptomeningeal disease. In addition to targeted treatments, the use of immunotherapy is being investigated in solid tumor leptomeningeal disease with potentially promising responses.[37]

Primary Brain Tumors

Among primary brain tumors, gliomas make up the largest share in adult patients. The classification of primary brain tumors was historically based upon histological appearance and assigned a grade (I to IV) by criteria; these classifications were revised in 2016 to incorporate new knowledge based on signature molecular genetic features.[38] Within these new features lies the ability to more precisely determine both treatment as well as prognosis; whenever available, this information should be taken into account when considering the prognosis and potential for future treatment of a critically ill neuro-oncology patient.

Among the diffuse gliomas, mutations in isocitrate dehydrogenase (IDH1 and IDH2) are commonly found in lower grade gliomas as well as secondary glioblastomas, that is, those arising from a lower-grade glioma. IDH mutant tumors appear to be distinct both genetically and clinically and are associated with a better prognosis in comparison to tumors that are IDH wild-type.[39] Within these, the methylation status of DNA-repair gene *MGMT* carries both a prognostic and predictive role, and predicts response to alkylating chemotherapies such as temozolomide.[40] Similarly, the presence of a co-deletion of 1p/19q is now defined to be the molecular signature of an oligodendroglioma; moreover, the presence of this codeletion carries a significantly different prognosis, with a much improved overall survival compared with other high-grade gliomas.[41] This is particularly important as tumors carrying this signature codeletion may have previously been histologically classified as grade IV glioblastomas (Figure 15.3), but would instead now be classified as oligodendrogliomas, with a vastly different prognosis.

Initial treatment of glioblastoma typically consists of surgical resection followed by chemoradiation. The extent of resection appears to be associated with survival, and in general a maximal-safe resection strategy is undertaken, taking into account individual patient characteristics.[42] Following surgery, patients generally receive a treatment protocol consisting of fractionated radiotherapy with temozolomide, with subsequent cycles of further temozolomide; in the study establishing this approach, median survival was 14.6 months, compared with 12.1 months in patients receiving radiotherapy alone.[43]

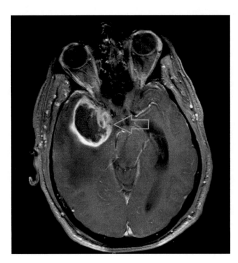

Figure 15.3 Glioblastoma. Patient presents with no prior metastatic history and recent seizure. MRI brain T1 post-contrast shows a right medial temporal rim enhancing lesion with necrotic core. Recommended for surgical resection.

In general, recurrent high-grade glioma carries limited treatment options and portends a worse prognosis. Effective treatment options are generally limited though re-operation, and further medical treatment, including possible experimental trials, can be considered. In one study, patients had a median overall survival of approximately 9 months from the time of progression, either with lomustine monotherapy or in combination with the anti-vascular endothelial growth factor (VEGF) treatment bevacizumab.[44] In patients with additional poor prognostic factors, including poor functional status, large tumor volume, and tumor location in eloquent cortex (pre-specified as motor or speech areas, or directly adjacent to proximal segments of the middle cerebral artery), survival can be as poor as fewer than 2 months.[45] Particularly for patients lacking these poor prognostic factors, which are relatively simple to identify, enrollment in a clinical trial for recurrent glioblastoma should be considered if available and in line with the patient's goals of care.

Though there is relatively limited data on the long-term prognosis in the case of neuro-oncological patients specifically admitted to the ICU, general principles regarding baseline performance status are still useful. In one series of high-grade glioma patients discharged from ICU admissions, 1-year mortality was about 3 in 4; in addition to performance status, the ability to continue oncological treatment was associated with 1-year survival.[46] Therefore, aggressive treatment including intensive care can still be considered in the appropriate patient, even in the face of a comorbid glioma diagnosis.

Lymphoma

Primary central nervous system lymphoma (PCNSL) is a form of non-Hodgkin lymphoma that affects the central nervous system (brain parenchyma, eyes, spinal cord, and the cerebrospinal fluid) without evidence of extra-CNS involvement. The disease is relatively rare, with an annual incidence of about 0.4 per 100,000 patients per year. In immunocompetent hosts, it typically affects patients in the fifth or sixth decade of life. Treatment regimens for this relatively uncommon disease have evolved over recent years, with notable improvement in the overall survival of patients noted, with the notable exception of elderly patients, who have largely been excluded from the trend toward improvement.[47]

There have been two scoring systems that can aid in prognostication of outcome in P-CNSL: the International Extranodal Lymphoma Study Group (IELSG) and the Memorial Sloan Kettering Cancer Center score (MSKCC). The IELSG score takes into account patient age, performance status (measured using Eastern Cooperative Oncology Group score), lactate dehydrogenase (LDH) serum levels, CSF protein concentration, and the presence of involvement of deep structures of the brain and assigns each of these to either favorable or unfavorable factors. Unfavorable values of zero to one were associated with a 2-year overall survival rate of approximately 80%, compared to only 15% in patients with four or five unfavorable factors.[48] The MSKCC score uses a combination of age and KPS to estimate survival of newly diagnosed P-CNSL, with patients age < 50 having an overall survival of 8.5 years, compared with patients > 50 with good performance status (KPS > 70) at 3.2 years and those with worse performance status at 1.1 years.[49]

In contrast to many other brain tumors, the role for neurosurgical intervention is less clearly established in CNS lymphoma. While there are multiple approaches to specific treatment regimens, they are primarily based on medical and radiation treatments. High-dose methotrexate forms the backbone of modern induction therapy regimens, though it may not be tolerated in more frail elderly patients or those with renal failure.[50]

While response to initial treatment is overall improving with time, relapse remains common; in one series, the relapse rate was 36% at a median follow-up of just over 22 months.[51] Treatment remains challenging for recurrent disease, and the prognosis for recurrent P-CNSL remains overall poor. In particular, disease refractory to initial treatment, or with early (< 1 year) recurrence has a particularly poor overall prognosis, with overall survival of about 2 months in refractory patients and about 3 months in early relapsing patients.[52] On the other hand, the course of patients with a relapse remote to their initial treatment is less clear. As a relatively rare disease with ongoing study of novel treatments, including those utilizing Bruton tyrosine kinase inhibitors, the management and expected outcomes of both initial treatment as well as that of refractory or relapsed disease continue to evolve rapidly.

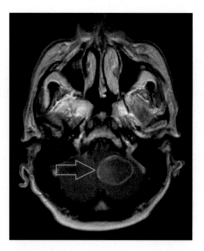

Figure 15.4 Cerebellar metastatic lesion. Patient presents with headaches and known history of lung adenocarcinoma suspicious for new metastatic lesion compressing the fourth ventricle. MRI brain T1 post-contrast shows cystic lesion of the left cerebellum with rim enhancement and compression of the fourth ventricle. Recommended for surgical resection.

Neuroprognostication in the Acute and Chronic Setting

There are few consolidated approaches to evaluating a patient with intracranial metastatic disease in the acute setting (Figure 15.4). Most prognostic approaches rely on the underlying diagnosis, which results in ICU admission in combination with clinical assessments of overall prognosis. Often the decision-making process for patients involves weighing the likelihood of recovery from the underlying acute insult with the long-term prognosis of the patient. If there is a low likelihood for recovery of the acute insult within the likely survival of the patient, then the case is often made to the primary decision maker for a transition to end-of-life care, often with the involvement of palliative medicine. Within this framework, understanding the overall prognosis of the patient, disregarding any acute insult, often becomes critically important. The Palliative Performance Scale (PPS) has been demonstrated to be a valid and reliable tool in the tertiary care setting to help assess short-term prognosis and has been validated for cancer patients.[53,54]

Clinician intuition is often inaccurate, and prognostic uncertainty can cause significant impediments to communication to the primary decision makers.[55] Key prognostic factors that have been identified that can act as reliable assessments for prognosis include changes in dyspnea, performance status, delirium, and cancer anorexia-cachexia syndrome.[56,57] In addition, for patients with advanced cancer a variety of biomarkers including C-reactive protein, low albumin, and leukocytosis have demonstrated independent prognostic value in predicting prognosis in the cancer population.[58] The current standard of care includes incorporating both a well-validated rating scale such as the PPS and understanding of the underlying cancer, treatment options, biomarkers, and active medical issues to determine overall prognosis.

Conclusion

More work remains to be done to improve prognostic models for neuro-oncological disease. As we learn more about CNS metastatic disease and refine our treatments, we will continue to improve our ability to both treat the underlying disease and predict outcomes. Next generation approaches incorporating large quantities of electronic health data with machine learning promise to further increase the accuracy of our predictive models. A recent approach using deep learning, a type of artificial neural network in combination with extensive clinical data, was able to generate accurate prognostic evaluation across 20 different cancer types.[59] Refinements like this promise to significantly improve state-of-the-art determination of prognosis, though potentially at the cost of increased complexity.

Further work remains in a variety of key areas, including prognostic terminology standardization, communication with decision makers, and increasing complexity of medical decision making. Tools such as www.predictsurvival.com can go a long way toward helping providers cope with increasing information available to help make meaningful decisions in terms of prognosis. In addition, much work remains to be done in order to help translate physician understanding of available data to the patients and families in a way that allows for expression of their values when making decisions.

References

1. Ostrom QT, Patil N, Cioffi G, et al. CBTRUS statistical report: primary brain and other central nervous system tumors diagnosed in the United States in 2013–2017. *Neuro Oncol.* 2020;**22**(12 Suppl 2):iv1–iv96.

2. Andrews DW, Scott CB, Sperduto PW, et al. Whole brain radiation therapy with or without stereotactic radiosurgery boost for patients with one to three brain metastases: phase III results of the RTOG 9508 randomised trial. *Lancet.* 2004;**363** (9422):1665–72.

3. Brennan C, Yang TJ, Hilden P, et al. A phase 2 trial of stereotactic radiosurgery boost after surgical resection for brain metastases. *Int J Radiat Oncol Biol Phys.* 2014;**88**(1):130–136.

4. Nayak L, Lee EQ, We PY. Epidemiology of brain metastases. *Curr Oncol Rep.* 2012;**14**:48–54.

5. Tsukada Y, Fouad A, Pickren, JW. Lane, WW. Central nervous system metastasis from breast carcinoma. Autopsy study. *Cancer.* 1983;**52**:2349–54.

6. Barnholtz-Sloan JS, Sloan AE, Davis FG, et al. Incidence proportions of brain metastases in patients diagnosed (1973 to 2001) in the Metropolitan Detroit Cancer Surveillance System. *J Clin Oncol.* 2004;**22**(14):2865–2872.

7. Chinot OL, Wick W, Mason W, et al. Bevacizumab plus radiotherapy–temozolomide for newly diagnosed glioblastoma. *N Engl J Med.* 2014;**370** (8):709–22.

8. Peak S, Abrey LE. Chemotherapy and the treatment of brain metastases. *Hematol Oncol Clin.* 2006;**20**(6):1287–95.

9. Arvanitis CD, Ferraro GB, Jain RK. The blood–brain barrier and blood–tumour barrier in brain tumours and metastases. *Nat Rev Cancer.* 2020;**20** (1):26–41.

10. Soria JC, Ohe Y, Vansteenkiste J, et al. Osimertinib in untreated EGFR-mutated advanced non–small-cell lung cancer. *N Engl J Med.* 2018;**378**(2):113–25.

11. Davies MA, Saiag P, Robert C, et al. Dabrafenib plus trametinib in patients with BRAFV600-mutant melanoma brain metastases (COMBI-MB): a multicentre, multicohort, open-label, phase 2 trial. *Lancet Oncol.* 2017;**18** (7):863–73.

12. Costa DB, Shaw AT, Ou SH, et al. Clinical experience with crizotinib in patients with advanced ALK-rearranged non–small-cell lung cancer and brain metastases. *J Clin Oncol.* 2015;**33** (17):1881.

13. Wu CT, Chen LC, Kuo CP, et al. A comparison of 3% hypertonic saline and mannitol for brain relaxation during elective supratentorial brain tumor surgery. *Anesth Analg.* 2010;**110**(3):903–7.

14. Malik ZA, Mir SA, Naqash IA, Sofi KP, Wani AA. A prospective, randomized, double blind study to compare the effects of equiosmolar solutions of 3% hypertonic saline and 20% mannitol on reduction of brain-bulk during elective craniotomy for supratentorial brain tumor resection. *Anesthesia.* 2014;**8**(3):388.

15. Ali A, Tetik A, Sabanci PA, et al. Comparison of 3% hypertonic saline and 20% mannitol for reducing intracranial pressure in patients undergoing supratentorial brain tumor surgery: a randomized, double-blind clinical trial. *J Neurosurg Anesthesiol.* 2018;**30**(2):171–8.

16. Sokhal N, Rath GP, Chaturvedi A, Singh M, Dash HH. Comparison of 20% mannitol and 3% hypertonic saline on intracranial pressure and systemic hemodynamics. *J Clin Neurosci.* 2017;**42**:148–54.

17. Vecht CJ, Kerkhof M, Duran-Pena A. Seizure prognosis in brain tumors: new insights and evidence-based management. *Oncologist.* 2014;**19** (7):751–9.

18. Pruitt AA. Medical management of patients with brain tumors. *Continuum.* 2015;**21**(2):314–31.

19. Barnholtz-Sloan JS, Sloan AE, Davis FG, et al. Incidence proportions of brain metastases in patients diagnosed (1973 to 2001) in the Metropolitan Detroit Cancer Surveillance System. *J Clin Oncol.* 2004;**22**(14):2865–72.

20. Johnson JD, Young B. Demographics of brain metastasis. *Neurosurg Clin North Am.* 1996;**7** (3):337–44.

21. Stelzer KJ. Epidemiology and prognosis of brain metastases. *Surg Neurol Int.* 2013;**4**(Suppl 4):S192.

22. Gaspar L, Scott C, Rotman M, et al. Recursive partitioning analysis (RPA) of prognostic factors in

three Radiation Therapy Oncology Group (RTOG) brain metastases trials. *Int J Radiat Oncol Biol Phys.* 1997;**37**(4):745–51.

23. Patchell RA, Tibbs PA, Walsh JW, et al. A randomized trial of surgery in the treatment of single metastases to the brain. *N Engl J Med.* 1990;**322**(8):494–500.

24. Paek SH, Audu PB, Sperling MR, Cho J, Andrews DW. Reevaluation of surgery for the treatment of brain metastases: review of 208 patients with single or multiple brain metastases treated at one institution with modern neurosurgical techniques. *Neurosurgery.* 2005;**56**(5):1021–34.

25. Linskey ME, Andrews DW, Asher AL, et al. The role of stereotactic radiosurgery in the management of patients with newly diagnosed brain metastases: a systematic review and evidence-based clinical practice guideline. *J Neurooncol.* 2010;**96**(1):45–68.

26. Chang EL, Wefel JS, Hess KR, et al. in patients with brain metastases treated with radiosurgery or radiosurgery plus whole-brain irradiation: a randomised controlled trial. *Lancet Oncol.* 2009;**10**(11):1037–44.

27. Nayar G, Ejikeme T, Chongsathidkiet P, et al. Leptomeningeal disease: current diagnostic and therapeutic strategies. *Oncotarget.* 2017;**8**(42):73312.

28. Groves MD. Leptomeningeal disease. *Neurosurg Clin.* 2011;**22**(1):67–78.

29. Lamba N, Fick T, Tewarie RN, Broekman ML. Management of hydrocephalus in patients with leptomeningeal metastases: an ethical approach to decision-making. *J Neurooncol.* 2018;**140**(1):5–13.

30. Esquenazi Y, Lo VP, Lee K. Critical care management of cerebral edema in brain tumors. *J Intensive Care Med.* 2017;**32**(1):15–24.

31. Volkov AA, Filis AK, Vrionis FD. Surgical treatment for leptomeningeal disease. *Cancer Control.* 2017;**24**(1):47–53.

32. Lin N, Dunn IF, Glantz M, et al. Benefit of ventriculoperitoneal cerebrospinal fluid shunting and intrathecal chemotherapy in neoplastic meningitis: a retrospective, case–controlled study. *J Neurosurg.* 2011;**115**(4):730–6.

33. Morris PG, Reiner AS, Szenberg OR, et al. Leptomeningeal metastasis from non-small cell lung cancer: survival and the impact of whole brain radiotherapy. *J Thorac Oncol.* 2012;**7**(2):382–5.

34. Glantz MJ, Hall WA, Cole BF, et al. Diagnosis, management, and survival of patients with leptomeningeal cancer based on cerebrospinal fluid-flow status. *Cancer.* 1995;**75**(12):2919–31.

35. Franzoi MA, Hortobagyi GN. Leptomeningeal carcinomatosis in patients with breast cancer. *Crit Rev Oncol Hematol.* 2019;**135**:85–94.

36. Ricciardi GR, Russo A, Franchina T, et al. Efficacy of T-DM1 for leptomeningeal and brain metastases in a HER2 positive metastatic breast cancer patient: new directions for systemic therapy-a case report and literature review. *BMC Cancer.* 2018;**18**(1):1–8.

37. Brastianos PK, Lee EQ, Cohen JV, et al. Single-arm, open-label phase 2 trial of pembrolizumab in patients with leptomeningeal carcinomatosis. *Nat Med.* 2020;**1**:1–5.

38. Louis DN, Perry A, Reifenberger G, et al. The 2016 World Health Organization classification of tumors of the central nervous system: a summary. *Acta Neuropathol.* 2016;**131**(6):803–20.

39. Yan H, Parsons DW, Jin G, et al. IDH1 and IDH2 mutations in gliomas. *N Engl J Med.* 2009;**360**(8):765–73.

40. Hegi ME, Diserens AC, Gorlia T, et al. MGMT gene silencing and benefit from temozolomide in glioblastoma. *N Engl J Med.* 2005;**352**(10):997–1003.

41. Cairncross JG, Wang M, Shaw EG, et al. Phase III trial of chemoradiotherapy for anaplastic oligodendroglioma: long-term results of RTOG 9402. *J Clin Oncol.* 2013;**31**(3):337–43.

42. Marko NF, Weil RJ, Schroeder JL, et al. Extent of resection of glioblastoma revisited: personalized survival modeling facilitates more accurate survival prediction and supports a maximum-safe-resection approach to surgery. *J Clin Oncol.* 2014;**32**(8):774.

43. Stupp R, Mason WP, Van Den Bent MJ, et al. Radiotherapy plus concomitant and adjuvant temozolomide for glioblastoma. *N Engl J Med.* 2005;**352**(10):987–96.

44. Wick W, Gorlia T, Bendszus M, et al. Lomustine and bevacizumab in progressive glioblastoma. *N Engl J Med.* 2017;**377**(20):1954–63.

45. Park JK, Hodges T, Arko L, et alScale to predict survival after surgery for recurrent glioblastoma multiforme. *J Clin Oncol.* 2010;**28**(24):3838.

46. Decavèle M, Gatulle N, Weiss N, et al. One-year survival of patients with high-grade glioma discharged alive from the intensive care unit. *J Neurol.* 2020;**29**:1–10.

47. Mendez JS, Ostrom QT, Gittleman H, et al. The elderly left behind – changes in survival trends of primary central nervous system lymphoma over the past 4 decades. *Neuro Oncol.* 2018;**20**(5):687–94.

48. Ferreri AJ, Blay JY, Reni M, et al. Prognostic scoring system for primary CNS lymphomas: the International Extranodal Lymphoma Study Group experience. *J Clin Oncol.* 2003;**21**(2):266–72.

49. Abrey LE, Ben-Porat L, Panageas KS, et al. Primary central nervous system lymphoma: the Memorial Sloan-Kettering Cancer Center prognostic model. *J Clin Oncol.* 2006;**24**(36):5711–15.

50. Grommes C, Rubenstein JL, DeAngelis LM, Ferreri AJ, Batchelor TT. Comprehensive approach to diagnosis and treatment of newly diagnosed primary CNS lymphoma. *Neuro Oncol.* 2019;**21**(3):296–305.

51. Jahnke K, Thiel E, Martus P, et al. Relapse of primary central nervous system lymphoma: clinical features, outcome and prognostic factors. *J Neurooncol.* 2006;**80**(2):159–65.

52. Langner-Lemercier S, Houillier C, Soussain C, et al. Primary CNS lymphoma at first relapse/progression: characteristics, management, and outcome of 256 patients from the French LOC network. *Neuro Oncol.* 2016 ;**18**(9):1297–303.

53. Anderson F, Downing GM, Hill J, Casorso L, Lerch N. Palliative Performance Scale (PPS): a new tool. *J Palliat Care.* 1996;**12**(1):5–11.

54. Mei AH, Jin WL, Hwang MK, et al. Value of the Palliative Performance Scale in the prognostication of advanced cancer patients in a tertiary care setting. *J Palliat Med.* 2013;**16**(8):887–93.

55. Han PK, Dieckmann NF, Holt C, Gutheil C, Peters E Factors affecting physicians' intentions to communicate personalized prognostic information to cancer patients at the end of life: an experimental vignette study. *Med Decis Making.* 2016;**36**(6):703–13.

56. Trajkovic-Vidakovic M, de Graeff A, Voest EE, Teunissen SC. Symptoms tell it all: a systematic review of the value of symptom assessment to predict survival in advanced cancer patients. *Crit Rev Oncol Hematol.* 2012;**84**(1):130–48.

57. Maltoni M, Caraceni A, Brunelli C, et al. Prognostic factors in advanced cancer patients: evidence-based clinical recommendations–a study by the Steering Committee of the European Association for Palliative Care. *J Clin Oncol.* 2005;**23**(25):6240–8.

58. Dolan RD, McSorley ST, Horgan PG, Laird B, McMillan DC. The role of the systemic inflammatory response in predicting outcomes in patients with advanced inoperable cancer: systematic review and meta-analysis. *Crit Rev Oncol Hematol.* 2017;**116**:134–46.

59. Coudray N, Tsirigos A. Deep learning links histology, molecular signatures and prognosis in cancer. *Nat Cancer.* 2020;**1**(8):755–7.

Chapter 16

Prognostication in the Complications of Neurosurgical Procedures

Zachary L. Hickman and Salazar A. Jones

Introduction

There are many central nervous system (CNS) pathologies that are managed in the neurointensive care unit. Neurocritical patients are a diverse group with vastly different presentations, management, expected duration of their clinical course, and disease-related long-term outcomes. Clinical entities include traumatic brain injury (TBI), ischemic stroke, aneurysmal subarachnoid hemorrhage (aSAH), intraparenchymal hemorrhages (ICH), spinal cord injury (SCI), brain tumors, postoperative craniotomy patients, and nonsurgical diseases, such as myasthenia gravis, Guillain–Barré syndrome, and CNS infections (meningitis and encephalitis).

There are a variety of bedside neurosurgical and neurocritical care procedures that may be required to provide care and mitigate the effects of primary neurologic pathology and to improve outcomes. Despite the many advances in neurosurgical and neurocritical care in that last several decades, complications from these procedures, while generally rare, still can occur (Table 16.1). On the whole, the majority of these complications are minor, and significant complications that negatively impact a patient's prognosis and long-term outcome are even rarer still. One particular challenge in the neurocritical patient is precisely determining the downstream effects of an adverse event related to such a procedure. This challenge exists because the expected hospital course, disposition, and likelihood of recovery are more often significantly related to the patient's underlying neurological insult that required performing the bedside procedure to begin with. For example, in a TBI patient with severe TBI presenting in coma who experiences a complication related to procedure, it is difficult to ascertain and quantify the precise impact of the complication on the patient's prognosis and long-term outcome. A moderate-sized tract hemorrhage

Table 16.1 Complications associated with bedside neurosurgical procedures

Procedure	Complications
External ventricular drain (EVD)/ ventriculostomy	Malposition, hemorrhage, ventriculostomy-associated infection (VAI), shunt dependency, traumatic pseudoaneurysm
Intraparenchymal ICP monitor (IPM)	Malposition, hemorrhage, infection, traumatic pseudoaneurysm
Jugular bulb catheterization	Malposition, carotid puncture, venous hematoma
Subdural drain/ SEPS™	Malposition (brain parenchyma injury), hemorrhage
Lumbar drain	Intracranial hypotension, post-dural puncture headache (PDPH), nausea, nerve root irritation, cerebellar tonsil herniation, intracranial hemorrhage, retained catheter, infection
Lumbar puncture	Intracranial hypotension, post-dural puncture headache (PDPH), nausea

SEPS™ = Subdural Evacuating Port System (Medtronic, Minneapolis, MN, USA).

around a ventriculostomy catheter in such a patient may not result in any appreciable change in the patient's outcome, but certainly could in a good-grade aneurysmal SAH patient with hydrocephalus.

This chapter concerns itself with prognostication in the complications of bedside neurosurgical procedures, including ventriculostomy / external ventricular drain (EVD) placement, invasive intracranial pressure monitor (e.g., brain tissue oxygen monitors, multimodal monitors) placement, jugular bulb catheterization, bedside twist drill placement of subdural drains or use of the subdural evacuating port system (SEPS) for chronic subdural hematoma (CSDH) evacuation, lumbar puncture, and lumbar drain placement. The following discussion is limited to these common neurosurgical procedures, as discussion of complications and outcomes from general intensive care unit (ICU) procedures, such as arterial lines, central venous lines, is outside the scope of this chapter.

For most neurosurgical procedures, there is a paucity of high-quality studies and evidence related to complications, particularly for relatively newer technologies, such as fiberoptic or mini strain-gauge intracranial pressure monitoring devices, or for SEPS. For EVDs, there are significantly more low- and moderate-quality retrospective and observational studies available, given the increased length of time that ventriculostomy catheters have been used in routine clinical practice for emergency cerebrospinal fluid (CSF) diversion and intracranial pressure (ICP) monitoring, their more ubiquitous use (compared to more expensive, newer technologies), and potentially, also related to their relatively higher overall associated risks of malposition, hemorrhage, and infection, compared to other bedside neurosurgical procedures. Despite this, there remains few randomized or prospective trials that report or address complications rates for most bedside neurosurgical procedures. This, combined with the difficulty in ascertaining the clinical impact of a complication of a severely brain-injured patient, makes prognostication related to these complications difficult, except when the complication is severe enough to result in need for additional neurosurgical interventions (e.g., craniotomy for hematoma evacuation) or death.

External Ventricular Drains (EVDs)

A ventriculostomy catheter or EVD is a drain placed within the ventricular system, most commonly the frontal horn of the lateral ventricle, that drains CSF to an external collection system. This is often performed as an emergency procedure for CSF diversion to treat hydrocephalus, to monitor ICP, or both, in a variety of CNS pathologies, including severe TBI, aneurysmal SAH, spontaneous ICH and IVH, as well as cerebral and cerebellar strokes with malignant edema, obstructive hydrocephalus related to tumors, and for patients with infected ventricular shunt systems. ICP is measured through use of a fluid-coupled transducer. According to data from the American

Association of Neurological Surgeons (AANS), there were 42,466 ICP monitoring procedures performed in the United States in 2006.[1] An EVD is still considered the gold standard for ICP monitoring following severe TBI, partly because it is not merely a monitoring device, but also affords the ability to treat elevated ICP via CSF diversion. EVD placement is recommended by the Brain Trauma Foundation in their most recent fourth edition "Guidelines for the Management of Severe Traumatic Brain Injury" for severe TBI patients in coma (Glasgow Coma Scale score ≤ 8) to monitor ICP and decrease 2-week mortality.[2] Evidence suggests that continuous CSF drainage with an EVD following severe TBI results in a reduced elevated ICP burden compared to intermittent CSF drainage.[3] Current American Heart Association (AHA)/American Stroke Association (ASA) guidelines for the management of aneurysmal SAH recommend the use of EVDs for CSF diversion in patients presenting in coma or with acute obstructive hydrocephalus.[4]

External ventricular drains are commonly placed in a several different settings, including the emergency department (ED) and ICU via bedside twist drill craniostomy, or in the operating room (OR) via either twist drill craniostomy or burr hole placement, or through an existing craniotomy/craniectomy defect at the time of surgery. Major complications related to ventriculostomy include catheter malpositioning during placement, hemorrhagic complications, and ventriculostomy-associated infection (VAI). In general, rates of these complications are higher for EVDs compared to intraparenchymal ICP monitors (Table 16.2).[5–7]

Malposition

There is no one standard technique for placement of a ventriculostomy catheter. The most commonly used bedside method is the freehand technique with the entry point and trajectory determined based on external landmarks. The frontal horn of the lateral ventricle is typically canuled, most often the nondominant side, with the target being the foramen of Monro. The most frequent entry point for a frontal EVD is Kocher's point, roughly 2.5–3 cm lateral to the midline (roughly mid-pupillary line) and 1–2 cm anterior to the coronal suture. However, specific pathology or considerations may dictate

Table 16.2 Complication rates for external ventricular drains (EVDs) compared to intraparenchymal ICP monitors (IPMs)

Complication	EVD	IPM
Malposition	2–43% (most 10–15%)	14–17%
Hemorrhage	5–20% (0.5–2% clinically significant)	0–5% (< 1% clinically significant; < 1–2.5% for multimodality monitoring bolts)
Infection	2–26% (most 2–11%)	0–3.7%
Device malfunction	~ 5%	4.5–8.8% (single catheter); 43–58% (multiple catheters)

(a) 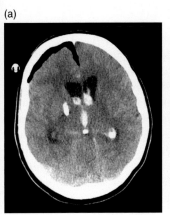 (b)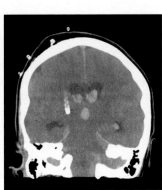

Figure 16.1 Malpositioned right frontal external ventricular drain (EVD) with tip in the basal ganglia. (a) Axial and (b) coronal noncontrast head CT scans following right frontal EVD placement in a 53-year-old female who presented in coma with a Hunt–Hess 5 aneurysmal subarachnoid hemorrhage, intraventricular hemorrhage, and obstructive hydrocephalus from a ruptured left posterior inferior cerebellar artery (PICA) aneurysm. The catheter was misplaced laterally with the tip in the right basal ganglia; the catheter was nonfunctional and was immediately replaced with a new EVD with successful cannulation of the frontal horn of the right lateral ventricle. There was no observable neurological sequela from this misplacement.

placement on the dominant site or via a different trajectory (e.g., significant midline shift, large extra-axial or intraparenchymal hematoma along planned EVD trajectory, lack of an ipsilateral bone flap or a plan for surgery on that side). Alternative entry points include Frazier's point for occipital EVDs (typically performed in the OR) and Keen's point. ED/ICU placement of EVDs is more common for neurosurgical emergencies (severe TBI, aSAH, ICH, and IVH), while OR EVD placement is more common when performed in conjunction with other neurosurgical procedures (hematoma evacuation in head trauma, aneurysm clipping in aSAH, tumor resection, etc.).

The rate of malposition or suboptimal placement of EVD catheters ranges in the literature from 2 to 43%, though the rate in the largest studies specifically investigating this complication is in the 10–15% range; furthermore, the definition of suboptimal placement varies. [5,8–12]. Malposition with the freehand technique is more common in TBI patients, due to smaller ventricles and the presence of cerebral edema and cerebral compression from intracranial hematomas, resulting in midline shift and distorted anatomy.[8,11,12] In

addition, scalp lacerations and scalp swelling may alter the location of the desired entry point. In a retrospective comparison of EVD and intraparenchymal ICP monitor (IPM) placement in 156 consecutive patients with multiple diagnoses, malposition occurred with EVDs at a rate of 20.1%.[5] Kakarla et al. conducted a respective review of 346 consecutive patients who underwent bedside ventriculostomy by neurosurgical trainees.[8] The authors proposed a new grading system, which has been adopted in many subsequent studies: Grade 1, optimal placement in the ipsilateral frontal horn or third ventricle; Grade 2, functional placement in the contralateral ventricle or noneloquent cortex; and Grade 3, suboptimal placement in the eloquent cortex or nontarget cerebrospinal fluid space, with or without functional drainage (Figure 16.1).[8]. Grade I catheter placement occurred in 77% (266/346) of patients, while 10% (34/346) had Grade II and 13% (46/346) had Grade III placement.[8] Suboptimal placement was most common in patients with midline shift and trauma.[8] Another large retrospective study by Saladino et al. of ventriculostomy procedures (both EVDs and shunts) reported an overall malposition rate of 12.3% (26 of 212 procedures), five (2.4%) of which required adjustment.[9] A more recent retrospective cohort study of 308 patients undergoing EVD placement in the ED or ICU by senior neurosurgeons and midlevel practitioners (MLPs) at a level 1 trauma center reported satisfactory placement (in the frontal horn or proximal third ventricle) in 87.4% of cases performed by MLPs and 90.0% of those performed by senior neurosurgeons ($P = 0.5557$).[13] MLPs had an average of 1.2 passes per procedure, with 18 subjects requiring multiple EVD passes. MLP experience did not influence the accuracy of EVD placement. There were a total of 24 EVD-related complications with no difference in the rate of complication between MLPs and neurosurgeons, as well as no notable increase in complications due to multiple pass attempts.[13]

Several adjuncts exist to help improve the accuracy of EVD placement, most commonly the Ghajar guide, which orients the correct trajectory of EVD perpendicular to the skull surface, and image-guided frameless stereotaxy.[12,14,15]. O'Leary et al. demonstrated in a prospective, randomized study comparing freehand EVD placement with Ghajar guide–assisted placement, that use of the Ghajar guide resulted in fewer passes (1.1 ± 0.3 vs. 1.5 ± 0.9 passes, $p = 0.07$) and more accurate placement of the catheter tip in relation to the foramens of Monro (3.7 ± 5.7 mm vs. 9.7 ± 6.3 mm, $p = 0.001$).[16] There was a 4 % complication rate due to malpositioning, with 2 of 49 catheters in the freehand group that were nonfunctional and needed to be replaced.[16] It should be noted that the Ghajar guide is most useful when there is minimal midline shift and the intracranial anatomy is not distorted. Use of bedside electromagnetic (EM) stereotactic navigation has more recently been reported as an adjunct to significantly improve EVD placement accuracy over the freehand technique, with a modest increase in time from determined need to successful placement. [12,15] In a single-center study at a Level 1 trauma center, an overall suboptimal placement rate of 5.3% with navigation versus 42.9% using the freehand technique was reported.[12]

Hemorrhage

A typical EVD catheter has an outer diameter of 2.7–3.5 mm, and a catheter placed via a frontal trajectory traverses approximately 4–5 cm of brain parenchyma prior to entering the ventricle. This distance may be more if there is significant contralateral midline shift. Structures at risk during EVD placement include the corpus callosum, caudate nucleus, internal capsule, and thalamus, as well as vascular structures, such as cortical arteries, veins, and the distal ACA and MCA branches (see "Other Complications" below). Some degree of parenchymal hemorrhage following routine EVD placement is common, with reported incidence rates as high as 40%.[7,17] Most of these are insignificant, punctate intraparenchymal or trace subarachnoid hemorrhage.[17] The average hemorrhage risk appears to be around 5–20%, with more recent, larger retrospective and prospective studies closer to the 20% mark; however, the majority of these are of small volume.[6,9,18–22] A meta-analysis published in 2009 included 13 studies from 1970 to 2008 and reported an overall hemorrhage risk of 5.7% (102/1,790 subjects) and a significant hemorrhage rate of 0.61% (11/1,790 subjects) (Figure 16.2).[18] This was a simple nonweighted average, however, and the meta-analysis was updated by Bauer et al. in 2011 to include 16 studies with 2,428 patients.[23]. The authors reported a cumulative overall hemorrhage rate of 7.0% (95% confidence interval [CI]: 4.5–9.4%; $P < 0.05$) and a cumulative significant hemorrhage rate

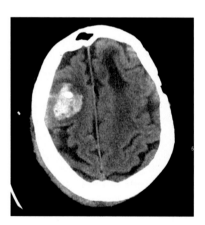

Figure 16.2 Significant tract hemorrhage associated with external ventricular (EVD) drain placement. Noncontrast axial head CT scan following placement of a right frontal EVD in an 81-year-old man who presented with a left thalamic intracerebral hemorrhage with intraventricular extension and obstructive hydrocephalus. The patient was thrombocytopenic with a platelet level of 85,000. He was given a platelet transfusion immediately prior to EVD placement. Post-placement CT demonstrated a large (20 cm³) tract hemorrhage. The hemorrhage was managed conservatively and did not expand further or require surgical intervention. The EVD continued to function properly and was removed on post-bleed day 10.

of 0.8% (95% CI: 0.2–1.4%; $P < 0.05$).[23] As expected, in both meta-analyses, studies that routinely performed post-procedural computed tomography (CT) imaging reported significantly higher hemorrhage rates (10.1–12.1%) compared to those that did not (1.4–1.5%).[18,23] More recently, a retrospective study of 370 EVDs placed in 276 patients at a single center in South Korea reported an overall hemorrhage rate of 20.5% (76 of 370 cases); only 1.4% (5 of 370 cases) were symptomatic.[20] Miller et al. retrospectively reviewed 482 EVDs placed at a single center between 2008 and 2014 and reported an overall hemorrhage rate of 21.6%.[21] Mean hemorrhage volume was small (1.96 ± 6.48 cm^3) with two hemorrhages requiring additional interventions (one surgical evacuation, one contralateral EVD placement). Large (> 30 cm^3) hemorrhage was seen in 2 patients (0.46%).[21] A prospective observational analysis of 1,000 CT scans from all 500 patients (563 EVD catheters) included in the CLEAR III Trial resulted in detection of EVD-related hemorrhage on 14% and 21% of first and last CT scans, respectively.[22] Hemorrhage following EVD removal has also been retrospectively assessed. Miller et al. reported an incidence of 22% with a mean volume of 8.25 ± 20.34 cm^3, with 5 patients (2.0%) having large hemorrhage greater than 30 cm^3 volume.[21] Factors reported to be associated with ventriculostomy-related hemorrhage include preadmission use of antiplatelet medications, thrombocytopenia, multiple placement attempts, accuracy of catheter placement, and bedside (non-OR) catheter placement.[21,22] In a small retrospective series of 69 patients, post-ventriculostomy hemorrhage was not significantly associated with mortality or neurological outcome at discharge or at 3 months post-procedure.[24]

Data on EVD hemorrhage rates in coagulopathic patients or those requiring anticoagulation, dual antiplatelet therapy, or venous thromboembolic prophylaxis are sparse. A small retrospective study of 71 TBI patients requiring 81 ventriculostomies reported no increase in hemorrhage rate in patients with an international normalized ratio (INR) of 1.2–1.6 compared to an INR < 1.2 [19] There were too few patients to accurately assess hemorrhage rate in patients with an INR 1.6–2.0. The overall hemorrhage rate was 6.2% (5 of 81 catheters), with four deemed insignificant and one (1.2%) significant that required surgical inter-

vention. The authors concluded that placement with an INR of 1.6 or less was likely safe.[19] A few studies have reported on hemorrhage rates in patients who underwent heparinization for endovascular ruptured aneurysm repair in close temporal proximity to EVD placement.[25–27] Two of these reported on 119 and 93 patients, respectively, who underwent EVD placement within 24 hours of endovascular coiling and heparinization, with neither study demonstrating an increase in hemorrhage rate compared to patients who did not undergo heparinizaton. [25,26] Conversely, a recent small retrospective study by Gard et al. of 46 patients reported a significantly higher rate of tract hemorrhage in patients undergoing heparinization within 4 hours of EVD placement, compared to those heparinized between 4 and 24 hours after placement (58.8% versus 6.9%, odds ratio [OR] 19.3, 95% CI: 3.4–109; $P < 0.005$).[27] Tract hemorrhages in the early heparinization group were also larger. Three patients had symptomatic hemorrhages, which were all in the early heparinization group; while this group also had a higher prevalence of prehospital aspirin use (41.2% vs. 6.9%), platelet transfusions were administered to these patients prior to, and during, EVD placement. [27] There is also a significantly increased risk of EVD-related hemorrhage in patients receiving dual-antiplatelet therapy (DAPT) compared to those not on DAPT, along with increased size of the hemorrhage for those on DAPT.[28,29] With respect to venous thromboembolic (VTE) prophylaxis, the optimal timing to initiate VTE prophylaxis following EVD or IPM placement is as yet unclear.[7] However, a small study demonstrated that patients who received VTE prophylaxis with unfractionated heparin (UFH) started within 24 hours of EVD placement had no increase in hemorrhagic complications compared to those who had UFH started later than 24 hours (24.4% vs. 19.6%; $P = 0.731$).[30]

Infection

The external portion of the EVD and the CSF drainage system poses a risk for ventriculostomy-associated infections (VAI). Reported VAI rates in the literature vary widely, partly due to the significant variation in the definition as to what constitutes a VAI, as there is no standard, accepted definition.[31,32] Overall, the VAI rate in the

233

literature is generally in the 2–11% range, however, some reports are as high as 22–26%. [7,9,33–45] A meta-analysis of 35 studies with 752 infections from 66,706 catheter-days of observation resulted in a pooled VAI incidence rate of 11.4 per 1,000 catheter days (95% CI: 9.3–13.5).[36] Reported significant factors associated with development of VAI include intraventricular hemorrhage, neurosurgical operations, duration of CSF drainage, need for multiple catheters, manipulation (irrigation or CSF sampling) of the EVD system, CSF leak, longer ICU stays, and concurrent non-CNS infections, particularly pneumonia and urinary tract infections.[7,33,34,46,47]

A retrospective cohort study of VAI in ICH patients using the National Inpatient Sample (NIS) identified 1934 patients (5.6%) diagnosed with VAI between 2002 and 2011.[38] Patients with VAI had a greater than 10% (41.2% vs. 36.5%) relative increase in inpatient mortality and a 43% (50% vs. 35%) relative increase in unfavorable discharge disposition compared to those without an EVD-related infection.[38] In another small retrospective study, mortality in patients with VAI was 48.9%.[43] When all types of intracranial hemorrhage patients are grouped together, patients with a nosocomial infection of the CSF space are nearly three times as likely to have an unfavorable Glasgow Outcome Scale score (83% vs. 30%).[48] There are data to suggest young adults fare just as poorly as older adults.[49] VAI is also significantly associated with increased hospital length of stay and total hospital charges in multiple studies.[35,38] Additionally, in a prospective, randomized trial of silver-impregnated ventricular catheters, patients who developed VAI were significantly more likely to require placement of a permanent CSF shunt than those without an infection (45.7% vs. 19.7%, $P = 0.0002$).[50] The most common causative organism for VAI is coagulase-negative *Staphylococcus* species, followed by *Staphylococcus aureus*.[31,42] Infections with gram-negative bacteria and *Acinetobacter baumannii* have been associated with higher mortality, reaching 64% in some studies.[40,43]

Due to the apparent increase in VAI rate during the first week of CSF drainage, some had previously recommend routine removal and replacement of an EVD catheter at a different site if a duration of use > 5 days was required.[33] However, this practice has since been refuted and more recent studies provide no evidence that routine prophylactic catheter exchange reduces the risk of VAI.[31,51] Furthermore, there does not appear to be a significant advantage to bolt over tunneled EVDs with respect to infection (VAI incidence of 10.0% vs. 14.2%, respectively; $P = 0.2$).[45] Likewise, routine administration of systemic broad-spectrum antibiotic prophylaxis for EVD placement has not been shown to be beneficial compared to those receiving narrow-spectrum or no prophylaxis.[52] In fact, patients who received broad-spectrum prophylaxis had gram-negative infections with significantly greater antibiotic resistance.[52] There is good evidence that the use of antibiotic-impregnated catheters (AIC) and silver-coated catheters (SCC) are associated with significantly reduced rates of VAI.[50,53–56] The number of AICs needed to prevent one infection was 19.[56] The use of AICs has also been demonstrated to be cost-effective, with an estimated net savings of $254,069 per 100 patients treated with AICs. [56,57] However, similar to administration of systemic broad-spectrum antibiotic prophylaxis, there is concern that both AIC and SCCs may select against gram-positive organisms and select for infections with methicillin-resistant *Staphylococcus aureus* (MRSA) and gram-negative bacteria.[54,55]

Malfunction

Compared to data on malposition, hemorrhage, and infection rates following EVD placement, there is a paucity of documented literature regarding the frequency of EVD malfunction from obstruction or dislodgement, or the effect of malfunction and need for replacement on patient prognosis and outcomes. EVD malfunction, however, is not uncommon, and is primarily caused by either malpositioning or migration of the catheter into the brain parenchyma or obstruction of the catheter holes or lumen by blood or cellular debris. [58] Higher rates of occlusion are reported for EVDs with small internal diameters.[58,59] In a study using the NIS from 1998 to 2010, Rosenbaum et al. found that 5.7% of admissions with reported ventriculostomies were followed by at least one additional ventriculostomy.[60] Pooled results from 8 studies with 1,995 EVDs placed in 1,581 patients demonstrated an average of

1.26 EVDs per patient (range 1.09–1.48).[58] Patients requiring EVD catheter replacement were at significantly higher risk of infection (29%) compared to those not requiring replacement (6%) (OR 6.1, 95% CI: 4.2–9.1).[58] Attempts to relieve an EVD obstruction may involve careful aspiration or irrigation with sterile saline, or use of fibrinolytics, such as tissue plasminogen activator (tPA). If the blockage is persistent and the patient continues to require CSF drainage, replacement of the EVD catheter is then undertaken. The need for EVD replacement is, of course, associated with all the risks of initial EVD placement, including malpositoning and hemorrhage. Additionally, in the interim there is the added risk of CSF underdrainage with potential for worsening hydrocephalus, elevated ICP, and neurological compromise. Of note, Jensen et al. found a significantly higher rate of complications in tunneled (40%) versus bolted (6.5%) EVDs in 271 patients, mainly related to inadvertent catheter removal, catheter obstruction, and CSF leak ($P < 0.001$). [61]

Shunt Dependency

While not a complication *per se*, the likelihood of the need for permanent CSF diversion via ventricular shunt placement is an important consideration in assessing the prognosis and eventual outcome of a given patient. The rates of shunt placement following a need for emergency CSF diversion vary with the diagnosis for which CSF drainage was initially required, with the highest rates for aneurysmal SAH and IVH patients (27–63%), followed by TBI (22.5%) and ICH (7–20%) patients.[62–66] Rapid weaning of EVDs has been previously recommended, as no difference in shunt dependency but a shorter ICU and hospital length of stay were reported in comparison to a gradual-weaning protocol in a small randomized control trial of aSAH patients.[62] However, a recent large retrospective trial of 1,171 consecutive aSAH patients treated in a similar fashion, except for the EVD weaning protocol, at two different German university hospitals demonstrated that patients who underwent gradual weaning were significantly less likely to develop shunt dependency (27.5% vs. 34.7%; $P = 0.018$) without an increase in infection rate.[63] The majority (78%) of neurosurgeons and neu-

rointensivists in the United States who responded to a survey on this topic preferred a gradual weaning approach.[67] Predictors of shunt-dependency in a retrospective analysis of a prospective database of nontraumatic ICH patients requiring emergency CSF diversion were only thalamic hemorrhage and elevated ICP.[65]

Other Complications

Iatrogenic Pseudoaneurysms

Delayed intracranial hemorrhage resulting from the formation of traumatic pseudoaneurysms as a result of EVD or intraparenchymal monitors has been reported, though it is extremely rare. [68–73] Most present in a delayed fashion 14–21 days or more after the initial vessel insult with SAH or IVH or a focal intraparenchymal hemorrhage in the region of the prior EVD or intracranial monitor.[68] The cause of the pseudoaneurysm is direct trauma to the vessel either during twist drill craniostomy (when the dura and cortical surface cannot be directly visualized) or by the catheter/probe itself. The most common vessels are the distal anterior cerebral (pericallosal, callosomarginal, A3 segments) or middle cerebral (M4 segment) arteries, though involvement of the middle meningeal and superficial temporal arteries have also been reported. [68,72–74] Suspicion for a traumatic pseudoaneurysm should be high when a delayed hemorrhage occurs in a previously uninjured region of the brain in proximity to a prior ventriculostomy or intracranial monitor placement. Medial trajectories are more likely to result in injury to the anterior cerebral arteries. Delayed hemorrhage rates from traumatic pseudoaneurysms can reach 80% with mortality of up to 50% following rupture.[68] Given this, conservative management is not recommended when a pseudoaneurysm is identified, and prompt treatment should be undertaken via craniotomy with surgical clipping, coagulation, or ligation, or via endovascular embolization with coils or glue.

Diabetes Insipidus

While diabetes insipidus (DI) is a known complication of aSAH, the development of DI immediately following replacement of an EVD (2 weeks after aSAH) where the catheter tip went into the sella has been reported.[75] The DI resolved when the EVD was removed.

Invasive Intracranial Monitoring Devices (Intraparenchymal ICP Monitors, Brain Tissue Oxygen Monitors, Cerebral Blood Flow Monitors, Electroencephalography Depth Electrodes, Cerebral Microdialysis Catheters)

There is significantly less literature on complication rates and prognosis related to complications following the placement of invasive intracranial monitoring devices – such as intraparenchymal ICP monitors (IPM), Pb_tO_2 monitors, cerebral microdialysis (CMD) catheters, and electroencephalography (EEG) depth electrodes – compared to external ventricular drains, largely due to the former's more recent and less ubiquitous incorporation into routine clinical practice. In general, complication rates, particularly for malposition and device-related hemorrhage or infection, are significantly lower for intraparenchymal ICP monitors (IPM) compared to EVDs.[5–7] This is likely related to the smaller diameter of the devices, short depth needed for placement (generally 1.5–3 cm), lack of direct communication between CSF in the ventricular system and the catheter and external system, and reduced need for manipulations.

Malposition

There is a paucity of data on malposition rates for intraparenchymal monitoring devices. Khan et al. reported in a retrospective analysis of 156 patients who had either an EVD or IPM placed that all malpositions occurred in the EVD group (20.1%).[5] In a retrospective review of 61 patients undergoing multimodal intracranial monitoring, 26 (43%) patients had diffuse injury and 35 (57%) had focal injury; of those with focal injuries, 6 (17%) catheters were misplaced within a lesion (infarct or clot), while 16 (46%) were in perilesional tissue (within 2 cm of focal injury).[76] Radiographic malpositioning was noted in 13.9% of patients undergoing multimodal monitoring (MMM) with invasive intracranial monitors.[77] Mean depth of placement has also been shown to vary widely.[78]

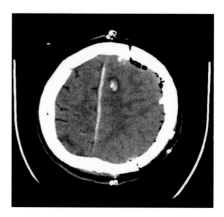

Figure 16.3 Small tract hemorrhage associated with intraparenchymal ICP monitor (IPM) placement. Postoperative noncontrast axial head CT scan following a left craniotomy for evacuation of a traumatic acute subdural hematoma evacuation in a 33-year-old man who had a fall from standing. A bolted left frontal IPM was placed through a small twist drill craniostomy just medial to the craniotomy edge in the operating room at the completion of the case. The patient was mildly thrombocytopenic and there was a small tract hemorrhage that developed around the IPM tip. The hemorrhage remained clinically insignificant and did not expand further, and the probe remained functional.

Hemorrhage

Reported overall hemorrhage rates for IPM range from 0–5%.[6,7,37,78–82,] Most of these are small (< 1 cm³) and asymptomatic, with clinically relevant hemorrhages occurring in less than 1% of patients (Figure 16.3).[78,80] Hemorrhage rates are increased to 7% in patients with acute liver failure and 8.7–15.3% in patients with coagulopathy, with an corresponding increase in clinically significant hemorrhages.[79,80,83] Clinically significant hemorrhage rates in patients undergoing MMM using a triple or quad-lumen bolt are slightly higher, at < 1–2.5%.[76,77,84] In a retrospective review of all patients admitted to a Level 1 trauma center over a 3 year period who had intraparenchymal ICP monitors placed and were stratified by initial INR, 10 patients had a borderline INR (1.2–1.6) and 12 a high INR (≥ 1.7) despite administration of component therapy.[85] Three patients had clinically insignificant, petechial hemorrhages, one in each group with INRs of 1.2, 1.3, and 2.5, respectively. The authors' conclusion was that hemorrhagic complications of IPM placement in patients with INR ≤ 1.6 were infrequent and use of blood products to correct INR below this threshold is unnecessary.[85] In another retrospective review of 155 adult severe TBI patients with invasive intracranial monitors, no new hemorrhages were associated with IPM placement in patients started on VTE prophylaxis at a median time of 3.6 days following injury.[81]

Infection

Clinical infection rates are similarly lower for IPM than for EVDs and range from 0 to 3.7%. [6,7,34,52,78–80,] Culture positivity of removed probe tips has been found in up to 8.5–13.2%, with the most common organism being *Staphylococcus epidermidis*; however, most of these had no clinical evidence of infection.[79,80] Prophylactic administration of antibiotics prior to IPM placement has not been shown to reduce infections and instead may be associated with more infectious complications and infections secondary to multi-drug resistant (MDR) organisms.[86]

Malfunction

Technical complications, including device breakage, dislodgement, or malfunction, are the most common complications associated with IPM placement. Reported rates of these minor complications range from 4.5 to 8.8% when only a single monitor is placed, though when multiple intracranial monitors are placed for MMM, device malfunction or dislodgement rates of up to 43–58% have been documented.[6,76–80,87] No significant difference in complication rates for monitors placed by neurosurgeons (10%), residents (8%), or midlevel providers (7%) has been suggested ($p = 0.09$).[87]

Other Complications

Similarly to EVDs, iatrogenic traumatic pseudoaneurysm formation with resultant delayed hemorrhage has been rarely reported. Two case reports involve injury to a distal cortical branch of the MCA or ACA near the site of IPM insertion, presenting with delayed intraparenchymal hemorrhage 17 and 25 days, respectively, following TBI. [72,73] One case was treated with craniotomy and surgical excision of the pseudoaneurysm, while the other was treated endovascularly with *n*-butyl cyanoacrylate (NBCA) embolization. A more recent case report details the delayed formation of an iatrogenic pseudoaneurysm from the superficial temporal artery (STA) following placement of an intracranial pressure monitor (combined ICP/Pb$_t$ O$_2$ monitor).[74] The patient presented in a delayed fashion with development of a pulsatile

mass with skin breakdown at the apex near the site of the prior monitor placement. This was managed successfully with surgical resection to prevent further wound breakdown and to achieve a good cosmetic result.

Jugular Bulb Catheters

Jugular bulb catheterization (JBC) is occasionally employed in brain-injured patients to monitor jugular venous saturation and, indirectly, cerebral blood flow (CBF) and cerebral metabolism. Jugular venous desaturation and anaerobic metabolism are associated with worse neurological outcomes.[88] In JBC, a small catheter is inserted using the modified Seldinger technique into the internal jugular vein (IJV) and directed in a cephalad fashion to a location approximating the jugular bulb, in order to minimize the contribution by extracerebral venous blood. Significant complications from JBC are rare. The most common complications in two retrospective studies with 123 and 44 patients, respectively, were inadvertent carotid artery puncture (3–4.5%) without adverse effect, venous hematoma (2%), and malpositioning of the catheter (3%).[88,89] In the latter study, of 20 patients who were evaluated by ultrasound, 8 (40%) had asymptomatic nonobstructive IJV thrombi (95% CI: 19–61%).[88] Venous hematomas were easily controlled with mild application of pressure, and most malpositioned catheters were successfully repositioned over a guidewire.[89] No significant complications occurred in either study. Furthermore, contrary to the fears of most physicians reticent to employ JBC, in a prospective study of 37 consecutive pediatric patients with both JBC and ICP monitoring, there was no evidence of jugular venous obstruction in the catheterized vessel or increase in ICP related to jugular bulb catheterization.[90]

Subdural Drains and the Subdural Evacuating Port System (SEPS™)

Chronic subdural hematoma (CSDH) is a diagnosis encountered frequently by many neurosurgeons. The incidence of CSDH increases greatly with age from approximately 3.4 per 100,000 in patients less than 65 years of age to 8–58 per 100,000 in those older than 65 years.[91] Given the increase in the elderly population in the United States, the incidence of CSDH is expected to double in approximately 25 years.[91] CSDH may be asymptomatic, or patients may present with headaches, depressed mental status, or focal neurological deficits. These symptoms are typically reversible and improve with evacuation or resolution of the hematoma.

Several techniques for evacuation of CSDH have been described, including bedside twist drill craniostomy (TDC) and placement of a subdural drain (SDD) or use of the Subdural Evacuating Port System™ (Medtronic, Minneapolis, MN, USA), burr hole craniostomy (BHC) with or without a surgical drain, and craniotomy. The former two techniques are most commonly performed at the bedside in the ED or ICU and will be the focus of this section. They are generally utilized for hypo- or isodense hematomas of chronic or subacute age without significant septations. A thorough discussion of BHC and craniotomy for CSDH evacuation (with or without placement of a surgical drain) is beyond the scope of this chapter; however, the 2012 review by Ducruet et al. provides a useful starting point for the interested reader.[91]

Subdural drain (SDD) misplacement following bedside TDC is not widely reported and limited by small case numbers. One retrospective series of bedside SDD placement reported that 1 out of 39 catheters (2.6%) penetrated the brain parenchyma.[92] Singh et al. reported two parenchymal injuries in 48 patients (4.2%) with bedside SDD placement.[93] When a subdural drain is placed after BHC, typically in the OR, malposition was reported to be 15.7%, with 7% and 12.5% of the misplaced drains causing a hemorrhage and neurological symptoms, respectively.[94] Patients with misplaced subdural drains had longer hospital stays and a nonsignificant trend toward poorer functional outcome and discharge disposition.[94] Acute subdural hematomas occurred in 6% of 79 patients treated with bedside TDC with SDD placement.[95] In another series of 38 patients, one patient (2.6%) had an acute epidural hematoma after SDD placement.[96] Singh et al. reported poor outcome in 2 of 48 patients (4.2%) in the TDC arm compared to 0 of 52 (0%) in the BHC arm; one case involved development of an acute epidural hematoma after TDC and the other case involved two recurrences, followed by BHC, and eventual formation of a brain abscess.[93]

The SEPS™ system consists of a small, hollow cranial bolt that is anchored in the skull at the site of a small bedside TDC with dural opening. The bolt is connected to a suction bulb for the evacuation of a chronic or subacute subdural hematoma. The main advantage of the system is that there is no drain or parts of the system that are intracranial, thereby theoretically minimizing the risk of damage to the brain parenchyma by an malpositioned SDD. Complications of both SDD and SEPS™ placement include parenchymal hemorrhage, infection or subdural empyema, conversion of a chronic or subacute subdural hematoma to an acute subdural hematoma, epidural hematoma, and tension pneumocephalus.

In a large series of 371 SEPS™ cases, the incidence of acute subdural hematoma or parenchymal hemorrhage was < 2%.[97] In another series of 126 SEPS™ cases, a parenchymal hemorrhage occurred in one patient and that hemorrhage did not require any additional procedures.[98] In a large series of 233 patients with 397 TDCs and SDD placement, an acute subdural hematoma in one patient was the only complication, which was treated with immediate craniotomy for evacuation.[99] A total of 260 (67%) of primary or secondary TDC in this study were effective in treating CSDH in 133 (57%) of patients, with the remainder requiring open surgical evacuation. In a retrospective comparison of 41 TDC with SDD placement to 25 SEPS™ procedures, SEPS™ was associated with a significant risk of requiring a second bedside procedure (OR 3.24, 95% CI: 1.03–10.14) relative to SDD placement, as well as longer ICU and hospital lengths of stay.[100] Complication rates did not differ significantly between SDD (2.4%) and SEPS™ (12%) ($P = 0.148$). Adverse events included nonfatal acute hemorrhage, including one in the SEPS™ group that required a craniotomy for evacuation, and four nonfunctioning drains, two in each group (4.9% SDD vs. 8% SEPS; $p = 0.6302$). The two nonfunctioning drains in the SDD group were due to inadvertent placement into the brain parenchyma in one case and into the ventricle in the other, both without neurological deficit. There were no reported infectious complications.[100]

Based upon its low complication profile and reduced risk of brain parenchyma injury, our favored paradigm is to initially attempt SEPS™ evacuation in patients with hypo- or isodense chronic or subacute subdural hematomas without significant subdural membranes. Adjuvant therapies that we commonly use are several weeks of atorvastatin administration and middle meningeal embolization in select patients. Less commonly, systemic corticosteroids may be administered as well. For patients with significant subdural membranes or that fail initial SEPS™ placement, BHC or craniotomy with placement of a surgical drain is performed.

Lumbar Drains

Lumbar drains consist of a small, intrathecal catheter inserted into the lumbar CSF cistern below the L2–L3 level that connects to a closed external collection system. The indications for placement are broad and include management of communicating hydrocephalus, normal pressure hydrocephalus, meningitis, cranial or spinal CSF leak, and during open and endovascular thoracic/thoracoabdominal aortic aneurysm (T/TL-AAA) repair to reduce the risk of spinal cord injury (SCI) resulting from thoracic spinal cord hypoperfusion. Approximately half of all patients with a lumbar drain will experience some complication.[101,102] Fortunately, the most common complications (intracranial hypotension, headaches, nausea, nerve root irritation, cerebellar tonsil herniation) are generally minor and mostly reversible when treated expeditiously. The rates of major complications – meningitis, retained catheter, and intracranial hemorrhage – are not widely reported, but are considered uncommon. The incidence of meningitis is 0.8–8% and resolves with treatment.[101–104]. Symptomatic acute intracranial hemorrhages were noted in 1.2% of patients in one series of 233 patients.[101] In a retrospective review of 230 patients who underwent TAAA repair with prophylactic lumbar drain placement, 8 (3.5%) patients developed an acute subdural hematoma, with a 50% mortality.[105] Of the four patients with acute subdural hematomas who survived, all responded well to neurosurgical intervention and recovered.

Other complications, such as cerebral herniation, posterior cerebral artery (PCA) infarction, temporary or permanent abducens nerve palsy, and sinus thrombosis, are rare, but have been described.[106,107] Neuroprognostication in the setting of these complications should be based on the clinical picture at the time of the complication. Fractured or retained lumbar catheters are also a known complication. Different management strategies have been proposed, including open surgical removal versus leaving the catheter in place so long as it is not causing symptoms or resulting in infection. Neither strategy is expected to routinely change patient outcomes.

Lumbar Puncture

Lumbar puncture is a common procedure performed by internists, intensivists, neurologists, and neurosurgeons, both inside and outside of an ICU setting. The most common complication associated with lumbar puncture by far is development of post-dural puncture headache (PDPH). Significant hemorrhagic complications are exceedingly rare. For the medical treatment of PDPH, caffeine has demonstrated effectiveness compared to placebo, and gabapentin, hydrocortisone, and theophylline have been shown to decrease pain severity.[108] Conversely, there is no evidence that bedrest is beneficial in preventing the development of PDPH, and may in fact increase the probability of it occurring (relative risk [RR] 1.24; 95% CI: 1.04–1.48), compared to immediate mobilization.[109] The role of supplemental intravenous fluids to help prevent PDPH is unclear.[109] One of the most effective methods to prevent PDPH is the use of atraumatic spinal needles. This is borne out in two recent meta-analyses including dozens of studies with up to 31,412 participants in the larger analysis, with the pooled incidence of PDPH significantly reduced from 11.0% (95% CI: 9.1–13.3) in the conventional needle group to 4.2% (3.3–5.2%) in the atraumatic group (RR 0.40, 95% CI: 0.34–0.47, $p < 0.0001$) without a reduction in efficacy.[110,111] Need for adjuvant therapies to treat PDPH, such as intravenous fluids, controlled analgesia, or epidural blood patch, were also reduced.[111] Lastly, two Cochrane reviews found no relevant studies to address the question of whether plasma or platelet transfusions should be given to patients with abnormal anticoagulation or platelet levels, respectively, prior to lumbar puncture.[112,113] In both cases, prospective studies designed with approximately 47,000–50,000 subjects would be needed to answer these questions.

Conclusion

Neurosurgical procedures, including those performed at the bedside, incur some inherent risk. The specific risk is dependent on the procedure type. For bedside ventriculostomy and intracranial pressure monitoring placement, the most feared and studied complications include hemorrhage and infection. However, for both procedures, the overall rate of clinically significant bleeding complications is low. The main key to understanding the significance of a given complication is whether there has a been a neurological change in exam due to the complication. Of all the complications discussed in this chapter, ventriculostomy-associated infection (VAI) is most consistently associated with poor patient outcomes. There exist opportunities to further develop and incorporate into clinical practice noninvasive methods of monitoring ICP and other physiological parameters, as well as improving the accuracy of EVD and monitor placement, infection prevention, and reducing the length of time that invasive intracranial monitors are needed.

References

1. National Neurosurgical Procedural Statistics: American Association of Neurological Surgeons (AANS) Survey, 2006.

2. Carney N, Totten AM, O'Reilly C, et al. Guidelines for the Management of Severe Traumatic Brain Injury, Fourth Edition. *Neurosurgery.* 2017;**80**(1):6–15.

3. Nwachuku EL, Puccio AM, Fetzick A, et al. Intermittent versus continuous cerebrospinal fluid drainage management in adult severe traumatic brain injury: assessment of intracranial pressure burden. *Neurocrit Care.* 2014;**20**(1):49–53.

4. Connolly ES Jr, Rabinstein AA, Carhuapoma JR, et al. Guidelines for the management of aneurysmal subarachnoid hemorrhage: a guideline for healthcare professionals from the American Heart Association/American Stroke Association. *Stroke.* 2012;**43**(6):1711–37.

5. Khan SH, Kureshi IU, Mulgrew T, Ho SY, Onyiuke HC. Comparison of percutaneous ventriculostomies and intraparenchymal monitor: a retrospective evaluation of 156 patients. *Acta Neurochir Suppl.* 1998;**71**:50–2.

6. Liu H, Wang W, Cheng F, et al. External ventricular drains versus intraparenchymal intracranial pressure monitors in traumatic brain injury: a prospective observational study. *World Neurosurg.* 2015;**83**(5):794–800.

7. Tavakoli S, Peitz G, Ares W, Hafeez S, Grandhi R. Complications of invasive intracranial pressure monitoring devices in neurocritical care. *Neurosurg Focus.* 2017;**43**(5):E6.

8. Kakarla UK, Kim LJ, Chang SW, Theodore N, Spetzler RF. Safety and accuracy of bedside external ventricular drain placement. *Neurosurgery.* 2008;**63**(1 suppl_1):ONS162–ONS167.

9. Saladino A, White JB, Wijdicks EF, Lanzino G. Malplacement of ventricular catheters by neurosurgeons: a single institution experience. *Neurocrit Care.* 2009;**10**(2):248–52.

10. Woernle CM, Burkhardt JK, Bellut D, Krayenbuehl N, Bertalanffy H. Do iatrogenic factors bias the placement of external ventricular catheters? – a single institute experience and review of the literature. *Neurol Med Chir (Tokyo).* 2011;**51**(3):180–6.

11. Patil V, Lacson R, Vosburgh KG, et al. Factors associated with external ventricular drain placement accuracy: data from an electronic health record repository. *Acta Neurochir (Wien).* 2013;**155**(9):1773–9.

12. AlAzri A, Mok K, Chankowsky J, Mullah M, Marcoux J. Placement accuracy of external ventricular drain when comparing freehand insertion to neuronavigation guidance in severe traumatic brain injury. *Acta Neurochir (Wien).* 2017;**159**(8):1399–1411.

13. Ellens NR, Fischer DL, Meldau JE, Schroeder BA, Patra SE. external ventricular drain placement accuracy and safety when done by midlevel practitioners. *Neurosurgery.* 2019;**84**(1):235–41.

14. Ghajar JB. A guide for ventricular catheter placement. Technical note. *J Neurosurg.* 1985;**63**(6):985–6.

15. Mahan M, Spetzler RF, Nakaji P. Electromagnetic stereotactic navigation for external ventricular drain placement in the intensive care unit. *J Clin Neurosci.* 2013;**20**(12):1718–22.

16. O'Leary ST, Kole MK, Hoover DA, et al. Efficacy of the Ghajar Guide revisited: a prospective study. *J Neurosurg.* 2000;**92**(5):801–3.

17. Gardner PA, Engh J, Atteberry D, Moossy JJ. Hemorrhage rates after external ventricular drain placement. *J Neurosurg.* 2009;**110**(5):1021–5.

18. Binz DD, Toussaint LG 3rd, Friedman JA. Hemorrhagic complications of ventriculostomy placement: a meta-analysis. *Neurocrit Care.* 2009;**10**(2):253–6.

19. Bauer DF, McGwin G Jr, Melton SM, George RL, Markert JM. The relationship between INR and development of hemorrhage with placement of ventriculostomy. *J Trauma.* 2011a;**70**(5):1112–17.

20. Ko JK, Cha SH, Choi BK, et al. Hemorrhage rates associated with two methods of ventriculostomy: external ventricular drainage vs.

ventriculoperitoneal shunt procedure. *Neurol Med Chir (Tokyo)*. 2014;**54**(7):545–51.

21. Miller C, Tummala RP. Risk factors for hemorrhage associated with external ventricular drain placement and removal. *J Neurosurg*. 2017;**126**(1):289–97.

22. Muller A, Mould WA, Freeman WD, et al. The incidence of catheter tract hemorrhage and catheter placement accuracy in the CLEAR III trial. *Neurocrit Care*. 2018;**29**(1):23–32.

23. Bauer DF, Razdan SN, Bartolucci AA, Markert JM. Meta-analysis of hemorrhagic complications from ventriculostomy placement by neurosurgeons. *Neurosurgery*. 2011c;**69**(2):255–60.

24. Sussman ES, Kellner CP, Nelson E, et al. Hemorrhagic complications of ventriculostomy: incidence and predictors in patients with intracerebral hemorrhage. *J Neurosurg*. 2014;**120**(4):931–6.

25. Hoh BL, Nogueira RG, Ledezma CJ, Pryor JC, Ogilvy CS. Safety of heparinization for cerebral aneurysm coiling soon after external ventriculostomy drain placement. *Neurosurgery*. 2005;**57**(5):845–9; discussion 845–9.

26. Leschke JM, Lozen A, Kaushal M, et al. Hemorrhagic complications associated with ventriculostomy in patients undergoing endovascular treatment for intracranial aneurysms: a single-center experience. *Neurocrit Care*. 2017;**27**(1):11–16.

27. Gard AP, Sayles BD, Robbins JW, Thorell WE, Surdell DL. Hemorrhage rate after external ventricular drain placement in subarachnoid hemorrhage: time to heparin administration. *Neurocrit Care*. 2017;**27**(3):350–5.

28. Kung DK, Policeni BA, Capuano AW, et al. Risk of ventriculostomy-related hemorrhage in patients with acutely ruptured aneurysms treated using stent-assisted coiling. *J Neurosurg*. 2011;**114**(4):1021–7.

29. Hudson JS, Prout BS, Nagahama Y, et al. External ventricular drain and hemorrhage in aneurysmal subarachnoid hemorrhage patients on dual antiplatelet therapy: a retrospective cohort study. *Neurosurgery*. 2019;**84**(2):479–84.

30. Tanweer O, Boah A, Huang PP. Risks for hemorrhagic complications after placement of external ventricular drains with early chemical prophylaxis against venous thromboembolisms. *J Neurosurg*. 2013;**119**(5):1309–13.

31. Lozier AP, Sciacca RR, Romagnoli MF, Connolly ES Jr. Ventriculostomy-related infections: a critical review of the literature. *Neurosurgery*. 2002;**51**(1):170–81.

32. Gozal YM, Farley CW, Hanseman DJ, et al. Ventriculostomy-associated infection: a new, standardized reporting definition and institutional experience. *Neurocrit Care*. 2014;**21**(1):147–51.

33. Mayhall CG, Archer NH, Lamb VA, et al. Ventriculostomy-related infections. A prospective epidemiologic study. *N Engl J Med*. 1984;**310**(9):553–9.

34. Rebuck JA, Murry KR, Rhoney DH, Michael DB, Coplin WM. Infection related to intracranial pressure monitors in adults: analysis of risk factors and antibiotic prophylaxis. *J Neurol Neurosurg Psychiatry*. 2000;**69**(3):381–4.

35. Lyke KE, Obasanjo OO, Williams MA, et al. Ventriculitis complicating use of intraventricular catheters in adult neurosurgical patients. *Clin Infect Dis*. 2001;**33**(12):2028–33.

36. Ramanan M, Lipman J, Shorr A, Shankar A. A meta-analysis of ventriculostomy-associated cerebrospinal fluid infections. *BMC Infect Dis*. 2015;**15**:3.

37. Dimitriou J, Levivier M, Gugliotta M. Comparison of complications in patients receiving different types of intracranial pressure monitoring: a retrospective study in a single center in Switzerland. *World Neurosurg*. 2016;**89**:641–6.

38. Murthy SB, Moradiya Y, Shah J, Hanley DF, Ziai WC. Incidence, predictors, and outcomes of ventriculostomy-associated infections in spontaneous intracerebral hemorrhage. *Neurocrit Care*. 2016;**24**(3):389–96.

39. Poblete R, Zheng L, Raghavan R, et al. Trends in ventriculostomy-associated infections and mortality in aneurysmal subarachnoid hemorrhage: data from the nationwide inpatient sample. *World Neurosurg*. 2017;**99**:599–604.

40. Bari ME, Haider G, Malik K, et al. Outcomes of post-neurosurgical ventriculostomy-associated infections. *Surg Neurol Int*. 2017;**8**:124.

41. Jamjoom AAB, Joannides AJ, Poon MT, et al. Prospective, multicentre study of external ventricular drainage-related infections in the UK and Ireland. *J Neurol Neurosurg Psychiatry*. 2018;**89**(2):120–6.

42. Kohli G, Singh R, Herschman Y, Mammis A. Infection incidence associated with external ventriculostomy placement: a comparison of outcomes in the emergency department, intensive care unit, and operating room. *World Neurosurg*. 2018;**110**:e135–e140.

43. Sam JE, Lim CL, Sharda P, Wahab NA. The organisms and factors affecting outcomes of external ventricular drainage catheter-related

ventriculitis: a penang experience. *Asian J Neurosurg.* 2018;**13**(2):250–7.

44. Hoffman H, Jalal MS, Chin LS. The incidence of meningitis in patients with traumatic brain injury undergoing external ventricular drain placement: a nationwide inpatient sample analysis. *Neurocrit Care.* 2019;**30**(3):666–74.

45. Roach J, Gaastra B, Bulters D, Shtaya A. Safety, accuracy, and cost effectiveness of bedside bolt external ventricular drains (EVDs) in comparison with tunneled EVDs inserted in theaters. *World Neurosurg.* 2019;**125**:e473–e478.

46. Chi H, Chang KY, Chang HC, Chiu NC, Huang FY. Infections associated with indwelling ventriculostomy catheters in a teaching hospital. *Int J Infect Dis.* 2010;**14**(3):e216–19.

47. Sorinola A, Buki A, Sandor J, Czeiter E. Risk factors of external ventricular drain infection: proposing a model for future studies. *Front Neurol.* 2019;**10**:226.

48. Habib OB, Srihawan C, Salazar L, Hasbun R. Prognostic impact of health care-associated meningitis in adults with intracranial hemorrhage. *World Neurosurg.* 2017;**107**:772–7.

49. Srihawan C, Castelblanco RL, Salazar L, et al. Clinical characteristics and predictors of adverse outcome in adult and pediatric patients with healthcare-associated ventriculitis and meningitis. *Open Forum Infect Dis.* 2016;**3**(2): ofw077.

50. Keong NC, Bulters DO, Richards HK, et al. The SILVER (Silver Impregnated Line Versus EVD Randomized trial): a double-blind, prospective, randomized, controlled trial of an intervention to reduce the rate of external ventricular drain infection. *Neurosurgery.* 2012;**71**(2):394–403.

51. Wong GK, Poon WS, Wai S, et al. Failure of regular external ventricular drain exchange to reduce cerebrospinal fluid infection: result of a randomised controlled trial. *J Neurol Neurosurg Psychiatry.* 2002;**73**(6):759–61.

52. May AK, Fleming SB, Carpenter RO, et al. Influence of broad-spectrum antibiotic prophylaxis on intracranial pressure monitor infections and subsequent infectious complications in head-injured patients. *Surg Infect (Larchmt).* 2006;**7**(5):409–17.

53. Sonabend AM, Korenfeld Y, Crisman C, et al. Prevention of ventriculostomy-related infections with prophylactic antibiotics and antibiotic-coated external ventricular drains: a systematic review. *Neurosurgery.* 2011;**68**(4):996–1005.

54. Atkinson RA, Fikrey L, Vail A, Patel HC. Silver-impregnated external-ventricular-drain-related

55. Konstantelias AA, Vardakas KZ, Polyzos KA, Tansarli GS, Falagas ME. Antimicrobial-impregnated and -coated shunt catheters for prevention of infections in patients with hydrocephalus: a systematic review and meta-analysis. *J Neurosurg.* 2015;**122** (5):1096–1112.

56. Root BK, Barrena BG, Mackenzie TA, Bauer DF. Antibiotic impregnated external ventricular drains: meta and cost analysis. *World Neurosurg.* 2016;**86**:306–15.

57. Edwards NC, Engelhart L, Casamento EM, McGirt MJ. Cost-consequence analysis of antibiotic-impregnated shunts and external ventricular drains in hydrocephalus. *J Neurosurg.* 2015;**122**(1):139–47.

58. Aten Q, Killeffer J, Seaver C, Reier L. Causes, complications, and costs associated with external ventricular drainage catheter obstruction. *World Neurosurg.* 2020;**134**:501–6.

59. Gilard V, Djoubairou BO, Lepetit A, et al. Small versus large catheters for ventriculostomy in the management of intraventricular hemorrhage. *World Neurosurg.* 2017;**97**:117–22.

60. Rosenbaum BP, Vadera S, Kelly ML, Kshettry VR, Weil RJ. Ventriculostomy: frequency, length of stay and in-hospital mortality in the United States of America, 1988–2010. *J Clin Neurosci.* 2014;**21**(4):623–32.

61. Jensen TS, Carlsen JG, Sorensen JC, Poulsen FR. Fewer complications with bolt-connected than tunneled external ventricular drainage. *Acta Neurochir (Wien).* 2016;**158**(8):1491–4.

62. Klopfenstein JD, Kim LJ, Feiz-Erfan I, et al. Comparison of rapid and gradual weaning from external ventricular drainage in patients with aneurysmal subarachnoid hemorrhage: a prospective randomized trial. *J Neurosurg.* 2004;**100**(2):225–9.

63. Jabbarli R, Pierscianek D, R RO, et al. Gradual external ventricular drainage weaning reduces the risk of shunt dependency after aneurysmal subarachnoid hemorrhage: a pooled analysis. *Oper Neurosurg (Hagerstown).* 2018;**15** (5):498–504.

64. Bauer DF, McGwin G, Jr, Melton SM, George RL, Markert JM. Risk factors for conversion to permanent ventricular shunt in patients receiving therapeutic ventriculostomy for traumatic brain injury. *Neurosurgery.* 2011b;**68**(1):85–8.

65. Zacharia BE, Vaughan KA, Hickman ZL, et al. Predictors of long-term shunt-dependent hydrocephalus in patients with intracerebral

hemorrhage requiring emergency cerebrospinal fluid diversion. *Neurosurg Focus.* 2012;**32**(4):E5.

66. Peters SR, Tirschwell D. Timing of permanent ventricular shunt placement following external ventricular drain placement in primary intracerebral hemorrhage. *J Stroke Cerebrovasc Dis.* 2017;**26**(10):2120–7.

67. Chung DY, Leslie-Mazwi TM, Patel AB, Rordorf GA. Management of external ventricular drains after subarachnoid hemorrhage: a multi-institutional survey. *Neurocrit Care.* 2017;**26**(3):356–61.

68. Chalil A, Staudt MD, Lownie SP. Iatrogenic pseudoaneurysms associated with cerebrospinal fluid diversion procedures. *Surg Neurol Int.* 2019;**10**:31.

69. Schuette AJ, Blackburn SL, Barrow DL, Cawley CM. Pial arteriovenous fistula resulting from ventriculostomy. *World Neurosurg.* 2012;77 (5–6):785.e1–2.

70. Kosty J, Pukenas B, Smith M, et al. Iatrogenic vascular complications associated with external ventricular drain placement: a report of 8 cases and review of the literature. *Neurosurgery.* 2013;**72**(2 Suppl Operative):ons208–13; discussion ons213.

71. Raygor KP, Mooney MA, Snyder LA, et al. Pseudoaneurysm of distal anterior cerebral artery branch following external ventricular drain placement. Oper Neurosurg (Hagerstown). 2016;**12**(1):77–82.

72. Le H, Munshi I, Macdonald RL, Wollmann R, Frank J. Traumatic aneurysm resulting from insertion of an intracranial pressure monitor. Case illustration.*J Neurosurg.* 2001;**95**(4):720.

73. Shah KJ, Jones AM, Arnold PM, Ebersole K. Intracranial pseudoaneurysm after intracranial pressure monitor placement. *BMJ Case Rep.* 2014;**2014**:bcr2014011410.

74. Pan J, Barros G, Greil ME, et al. pseudoaneurysm of the superficial temporal artery after intracranial pressure monitoring device placement: case report of a rare complication. *Oper Neurosurg (Hagerstown).* 2020;**19**(3):288–91.

75. Kawsar KA, Inam MB, Watts C. Diabetes insipidus-an extremely rare complication from replacement of an external ventricular drain. *Acta Neurochir (Wien).* 2019;**161**(7):1377–80.

76. Stuart RM, Schmidt M, Kurtz P, et al. Intracranial multimodal monitoring for acute brain injury: a single institution review of current practices. *Neurocrit Care.* 2010;**12**(2):188–98.

77. Foreman B, Ngwenya LB, Stoddard E, et al. Safety and reliability of bedside, single burr hole technique for intracranial multimodality monitoring in severe traumatic brain injury. *Neurocrit Care.* 2018;**29**(3):469–80.

78. Koskinen LO, Grayson D, Olivecrona M. The complications and the position of the Codman MicroSensor ICP device: an analysis of 549 patients and 650 Sensors. *Acta Neurochir (Wien).* 2013;**155**(11):2141–8; discussion 2148.

79. Martinez-Manas RM, Santamarta D, de Campos JM, Ferrer E. Camino intracranial pressure monitor: prospective study of accuracy and complications. *J Neurol Neurosurg Psychiatry.* 2000;**69**(1):82–6.

80. Gelabert-Gonzalez M, Ginesta-Galan V, Sernamito-Garcia R, et al. The Camino intracranial pressure device in clinical practice. Assessment in a 1000 cases. *Acta Neurochir (Wien).* 2006;**148**(4):435–41.

81. Dengler BA, Mendez-Gomez P, Chavez A, et al. Safety of chemical DVT prophylaxis in severe traumatic brain injury with invasive monitoring devices. *Neurocrit Care.* 2016;**25**(2):215–23.

82. Okonkwo DO, Shutter LA, Moore C, et al. Brain oxygen optimization in severe traumatic brain injury Phase-II: a phase II randomized trial. *Crit Care Med.* 2017;**45**(11):1907–14.

83. Karvellas CJ, Fix OK, Battenhouse H, et al. Outcomes and complications of intracranial pressure monitoring in acute liver failure: a retrospective cohort study. *Crit Care Med.* 2014;**42**(5):1157–67.

84. Bailey RL, Quattrone F, Curtin C, et al. The safety of multimodality monitoring using a triple-lumen bolt in severe acute brain injury. *World Neurosurg.* 2019;**130**:e62–e67.

85. Davis JW, Davis IC, Bennink LD, et al. Placement of intracranial pressure monitors: are "normal" coagulation parameters necessary? *J Trauma.* 2004;**57**(6):1173–7.

86. Stoikes NF, Magnotti LJ, Hodges TM, et al. Impact of intracranial pressure monitor prophylaxis on central nervous system infections and bacterial multi-drug resistance. *Surg Infect (Larchmt).* 2008;**9**(5):503–8.

87. Kaups KL, Parks SN, Morris CL. Intracranial pressure monitor placement by midlevel practitioners. *J Trauma.* 1998;**45** (5):884–6.

88. Coplin WM, O'Keefe GE, Grady MS, et al. Thrombotic, infectious, and procedural complications of the jugular bulb catheter in the intensive care unit. *Neurosurgery.* 1997;**41**(1):101–7; discussion 107–9.

89. Goetting MG, Preston G. Jugular bulb catheterization: experience with 123 patients. *Crit Care Med.* 1990;**18**(11):1220–3.

90. Goetting MG, Preston G. Jugular bulb catheterization does not increase intracranial pressure. *Intensive Care Med.* 1991;**17**(4):195–8.

91. Ducruet AF, Grobelny BT, Zacharia BE, et al. The surgical management of chronic subdural hematoma. *Neurosurg Rev.* 2012;**35**(2):155–69; discussion 169.

92. Sucu HK, Gokmen M, Ergin A, Bezircioglu H, Gokmen A. Is there a way to avoid surgical complications of twist drill craniostomy for evacuation of a chronic subdural hematoma? *Acta Neurochir (Wien).* 2007;**149**(6):597–9.

93. Singh SK, Sinha M, Singh VK, et al. A randomized study of twist drill versus burr hole craniostomy for treatment of chronic subdural hematoma in 100 patients. *Indian J Neurotrauma.* 2011;**8**(2):83–8.

94. Kamenova M, Wanderer S, Lipps P, et al. When the drain hits the brain. *World Neurosurg.* 2020;**138**:e426–e436.

95. Horn EM, Feiz-Erfan I, Bristol RE, Spetzler RF, Harrington TR. Bedside twist drill craniostomy for chronic subdural hematoma: a comparative study. *Surg Neurol.* 2006;**65**(2):150–3; discussion 153–4.

96. Gokmen M, Sucu HK, Ergin A, Gokmen A, Bezircio Lu H. Randomized comparative study of burr-hole craniostomy versus twist drill craniostomy; surgical management of unilateral hemispheric chronic subdural hematomas. *Zentralbl Neurochir.* 2008;**69**(3):129–33.

97. Flint AC, Chan SL, Rao VA, et al. Treatment of chronic subdural hematomas with subdural evacuating port system placement in the intensive care unit: evolution of practice and comparison with bur hole evacuation in the operating room. *J Neurosurg.* 2017;**127**(6):1443–8.

98. Hoffman H, Ziechmann R, Beutler T, Verhave B, Chin LS. First-line management of chronic subdural hematoma with the subdural evacuating port system: Institutional experience and predictors of outcomes. *J Clin Neurosci.* 2018;**50**:221–5.

99. Jablawi F, Kweider H, Nikoubashman O, Clusmann H, Schubert GA. Twist drill procedure for chronic subdural hematoma evacuation: an analysis of predictors for treatment success. *World Neurosurg.* 2017;**100**:480–6.

100. Ortiz M, Belton P, Burton M, Litofsky NS. Subdural drain versus subdural evacuating port system for the treatment of nonacute subdural hematomas: a single-center retrospective cohort study. *World Neurosurg.* 2020;**139**:e355–e362.

101. Governale LS, Fein N, Logsdon J, Black PM. Techniques and complications of external lumbar drainage for normal pressure hydrocephalus. *Neurosurgery.* 2008;**63**(4 Suppl 2):379–84; discussion 384.

102. Acikbas SC, Akyuz M, Kazan S, Tuncer R. Complications of closed continuous lumbar drainage of cerebrospinal fluid. *Acta Neurochir (Wien).* 2002;**144**(5):475–80.

103. Roland PS, Marple BF, Meyerhoff WL, Mickey B. Complications of lumbar spinal fluid drainage. *Otolaryngol Head Neck Surg.* 1992;**107**(4):564–9.

104. Greenberg BM, Williams MA. Infectious complications of temporary spinal catheter insertion for diagnosis of adult hydrocephalus and idiopathic intracranial hypertension. *Neurosurgery.* 2008;**62**(2):431–5; discussion 435–6.

105. Dardik A, Perler BA, Roseborough GS, Williams GM. Subdural hematoma after thoracoabdominal aortic aneurysm repair: an underreported complication of spinal fluid drainage? *J Vasc Surg.* 2002;**36**(1):47–50.

106. Miglis MG, Levine DN. Intracranial venous thrombosis after placement of a lumbar drain. *Neurocrit Care.* 2010;**12**(1):83–7.

107. Cain RB, Patel NP, Hoxworth JM, Lal D. Abducens palsy after lumbar drain placement: a rare complication in endoscopic skull base surgery. *Laryngoscope.* 2013;**123**(11):2633–8.

108. Basurto Ona X, Osorio D, Bonfill Cosp X. Drug therapy for treating post-dural puncture headache. *Cochrane Database Syst Rev.* 2015;**7**:CD007887.

109. Arevalo-Rodriguez I, Ciapponi A, Roque i Figuls M, Munoz L, Bonfill Cosp X. Posture and fluids for preventing post-dural puncture headache. *Cochrane Database Syst Rev.* 2016;**3**:CD009199.

110. Arevalo-Rodriguez I, Munoz L, Godoy-Casasbuenas N, et al. Needle gauge and tip designs for preventing post-dural puncture headache (PDPH). *Cochrane Database Syst Rev.* 2017;**4**:CD010807.

111. Nath S, Koziarz A, Badhiwala JH, et al. Atraumatic versus conventional lumbar puncture needles: a systematic review and meta-analysis. *Lancet.* 2018;**391**(10126):1197–1204.

112. Estcourt LJ, Desborough MJ, Doree C, Hopewell S, Stanworth SJ. Plasma transfusions prior to lumbar punctures and epidural catheters for people with abnormal coagulation. *Cochrane Database Syst Rev.* 2017;**9**:CD012497.

113. Estcourt LJ, Malouf R, Hopewell S, Doree C, Van Veen J. Use of platelet transfusions prior to lumbar punctures or epidural anaesthesia for the prevention of complications in people with thrombocytopenia. *Cochrane Database Syst Rev.* 2018;4:CD011980.

Chapter 17

Prognostication in Pediatric Neurocritical Care

Kerri L. LaRovere, Matthew Kirschen, Alexis Topjian, Mark S. Wainwright, and Robert C. Tasker

Introduction

Mortality rates for children in the pediatric intensive care unit (PICU) have decreased 5-fold from 1-in-5 [1] to 1-in-25 [2] cases over the past few decades. Despite improvements in rates of survival after critical illness, 1-in-5 children who require life support in the PICU for an acute illness has a new morbidity up to 3 years after discharge.[2,3] That translates to new functional, cognitive, and/or neurological morbidity in 5–10% of PICU survivors.[2,3] Also, for the parents of these children, the child's critical illness may become a chronic condition that leads to ongoing emotional stress for the whole family with significant psychological and social impact.[4]

There are several important distinctions between children and adults in regard to making a prognosis as a result of acute neurological injury – henceforth called *neuroprognostication*. Foremost, during the initial presentation of acute neurological illness, event, or trauma, there is a partnership between clinicians and parents, and the communication of likelihood of possible death versus survival. Then, parents and caregivers want to know what their child's developmental trajectory will be after the critical illness, and whether their child will have the capacity to return to his/her premorbid developmental baseline or better. From the clinician's perspective, however, there is usually no way of knowing what the response of the developing brain after acute injury will be over time, particularly when the child's developmental baseline and trajectory may be unknown. Second, neurological injury in the PICU may be the result of a largely heterogeneous group of acute and chronic neurological and neurosurgical diseases, general medical/surgical conditions, and iatrogenic insults.[5] Third, in regard to prognostication about future neurological function, it is important to remember that some cognitive

functions, such as executive function, do not develop fully until late adolescence. Hence, prognosticating about long-term outcomes in a 5-year-old with new lesions to the frontal lobes, even if we had data, is fraught with challenges.

During the acute phase after neurological injury, the domains of brain function that are impaired likely depend on the extent of injury and its treatment, as well as the presence of pre-existing neurological abnormalities, and individual physiological, genetic, and environmental vulnerabilities that render some domains at risk more than others. Regardless of the cause, the developmental impact of critical illness on the child's physical, cognitive, psychological, and social health is important and, collectively, is now termed "Post-Intensive Care Syndrome – Pediatrics (PICS–p)."[6–10] Therefore, clinical decision making based on important prognostic variables depends upon understanding all of the above factors in combination with the trajectory of recovery.[10]

There are two main perspectives to understanding the effects of acute neurological injury on the development and the trajectory of recovery in children: (1) the child and family and the impact of illness on their life and function; and (2) the clinician's incorporation and understanding of evidence about treatment and interventions and how they impact outcome. This chapter will focus on the latter, but knowledge about the former informs us about which morbidities are clinically relevant. Here we summarize the clinical evidence from the recent pediatric literature on (1) neuroprognostication tools used in the PICU (e.g., clinical, imaging, scales, biomarkers, electrophysiology, and other); and (2) follow-up studies that have used functional, cognitive, behavioral, or other outcomes measures. Neuroprognostication is discussed in the context of acute brain injury due to acute central nervous system

(CNS) infections, congenital heart disease (CHD), cardiac arrest, extracorporeal life support (ECLS), status epilepticus (SE), and traumatic brain injury (TBI).

Acute CNS Infections

The neurological complications of meningitis occurring during childhood include cognitive and behavioral impairments, hearing loss, motor disabilities (weakness, paralysis), epilepsy, hydrocephalus, brain abscess, and ventriculitis.[11–18] These complications have been associated with significant long-term psychosocial consequences, reduced health-related quality of life (HRQOL), and less economic self-sufficiency in adulthood. [19–22] The long-term neurological complications seen after viral encephalitis in childhood include developmental delay (35%), behavioral problems (18%), motor impairment (17%), seizures (10%), [23] and cognitive and neuropsychiatric impairments, such as depression and anxiety.[24–27]

Neuroprognostication in the PICU and Follow-Up

The are no neuroprognostication tools that can be used during the acute illness in the PICU that reliably predict clinically meaningful developmental outcomes after CNS infection. The literature on this topic reveals three issues. First, it must be determined whether there is a specific microbiological or viral neurotropism that may lead to a specific pathogen-related neurotoxicity (e.g., herpes simplex virus encephalitis and injury to the temporal lobes). There are a vast number of microbiological etiologies of meningitis and encephalitis, and yet, the cause is unknown in about two-thirds of children with an acute encephalitis syndrome.[28] Second, many studies focus on the acute neurological problems related to a particular infection rather than the later neurological consequences (e.g., early cerebral edema and vasculitis vs. later development of hydrocephalus, epilepsy, and deafness). Here, it is apparent that the true burden and range of long-term neurological disabilities are unknown because outcomes data are often inconsistently available and not always validated for the population under study. Also, neurological sequelae of CNS infection may appear many months after the initial infection,[29] and outcomes measures that are assigned too early in the acute setting or during follow-up can potentially underestimate clinically significant late onset morbidities. Last, standardization of assessment of outcomes and disability, and their sensitivity/specificity, is needed. In this regard, some consequences of CNS infections may relate to long-term effects on global functioning, whereas others may involve a potential effect on a specific pathway or neurotransmitter system resulting in neurological complications associated with the acute infection. Each of these issues requires further investigation and must be understood in order to devise a list of outcome measures that may be likely to show some effect of an intervention in the acute and chronic phases of illness.

To date, the outcomes measures used after meningitis have included unstructured symptom questionnaires, formal neuropsychological tests, [30,31] and ordinal, qualitative scales of general functional status like the Pediatric Cerebral Performance Category (PCPC) and Glasgow Outcome Scale (GOS).[32,33] HRQOL research may incorporate friends and family, and focuses on the impact one's health status has on different dimensions of quality of life, such as physical, social, psychological, spiritual, emotional, cognitive function, economic status, and intelligence. In a prospective study in the United Kingdom, HRQOL outcomes were assessed using the Pediatric Quality of Life Inventory (PedsQL Core version) at a mean of 8 years' follow-up in 100 children, 5–16 years of age, who survived bacterial (82%), viral (8%), or unspecified (10%) meningitis. The PedsQL measures physical, emotional, social, and school functioning, and is suggested as a core global outcome measure by the National Institute of Neurological Disorders and Stroke Common Data Elements.[34] The authors found significantly reduced HRQOL on PedsQL measures, regardless of acute disease complications.[22] Different conceptualizations of HRQOL exist, and methodological development of this outcomes research model is ongoing.

For children with acute encephalitis in resource-limited settings, the Liverpool Outcome Score is a cross-cultural, validated assessment of functional impairment that reliably identifies children who will likely be dependent in activities of daily living.[35] The modified Rankin Scale (mRS) is another ordinal functional outcome score that has been used in adult studies of acute infectious encephalitis,[36,37] and was utilized in a recent prospective pediatric study that included 49 children, 0–16 years of age, with acute encephalitis syndrome due to enterovirus 71.[38] In summary, for acute CNS infections, the outcomes scales used are mainly general, nonspecific measures of global functioning. While these measures are easy to obtain, they are not age-validated, do not account for neurobehavioral outcomes or variability in developmental age, and are not validated for long-term outcomes, and the PCPC score, in particular, lacks precision at higher severity of disability, particularly when retrospective data from the electronic health record are used.

Congenital Heart Disease (CHD)

Up to two-thirds of children with CHD have neurodevelopmental impairments (e.g., social cognitive, language, motor, executive functioning, and attention) that significantly affect quality of life and daily functioning.[39–49]

Neuroprognostication in the PICU and Follow-Up

A central issue for neuroprognostication in the acute setting of PICU management of children with CHD is whether it is feasible and reliable. There are two features of CHD pathophysiology that need to be considered.

First, several factors may simultaneously influence the prevalence and severity of adverse developmental outcomes. For example, there are (1) patient-related factors, such as underlying genetic and developmental disorders, comorbid medical conditions, and type of CHD; (2) medical and surgical therapies, including the need for ECLS and corrective cardiac surgery; (3) intraoperative and postoperative complications, such as acute cerebrovascular and hypoxic–ischemic events, seizures, and infections; and (4) environmental factors, such as duration of PICU admission, socioeconomic status, and lack of exposure to normal developmental stimuli during prolonged hospitalizations.[50,51] The relative contribution and clinical importance of each of these individual risk factors on developmental outcomes is unknown and may vary case by case. Ideally, neuroprognostication after an acute event should account for the interaction between all of these factors – preexisting patient-specific biological factors, medical/surgical interventions and their complications, and

any environmental influences [52] – which is likely impossible.

Second, neurodevelopmental outcomes in children with CHD are in large part an unmodifiable consequence of genetics.[53] Up to 50% of children with CHD have an underlying identifiable genetic cause.[54] Neurodevelopmental disabilities are nearly always present in children with CHD, and some genetic syndromes, such as trisomy 21, 22q11 deletion, Noonan syndrome, and Williams syndrome.[42] Indeed, in children with hypoplastic left heart syndrome who participated in the Single Ventricle Reconstruction Trial, underlying genetic syndrome/anomalies was an independent predictor of lower scores on the Mental Development Index (MDI) of the Bayley Scales of Infant Development-II.[55] However, when considering a specific genetic disorder, such as trisomy 21, the relative contribution of the underlying genetic syndrome and surgical risk factors to neurodevelopmental outcomes may not be significant.[56,57] There may be other unmodifiable *post hoc* factors associated with adverse neurodevelopmental outcomes, such as lower birth weight, maternal education, and socioeconomic status. Given these challenges, neuroprognostication in the acute setting typically focuses on the question of survival and diagnosing acute neurological complications that may benefit from early treatment. Death after cardiac surgery in children is due to low cardiac output or circulatory failure in about 50%, with the remainder due to sepsis, cardiac arrest, and procedural complications. [58,59] While circulatory failure triggers the pathophysiological cascade that leads to death, the severity of associated acute brain injury very often influences prognostic discussions and treatment decisions.

Based on the available evidence in the CHD population, clinical information along with electroencephalography (EEG) and imaging studies are combined to assist neuroprognostication. While the neurological examination can detect gross deficits, subtler cognitive, language and motor deficits are difficult to assess in the PICU, and evolve over time. Seizures are often the first symptom of hypoxic ischemic injury or stroke in infants and children after cardiac surgery, cardiac catheterization, or cardiac arrest.[60–62] Electrographic seizures may be detected on continuous bedside EEG in up to 25% of infants after cardiac surgery.[63,64] The presence of seizures and an abnormal EEG background have been associated with adverse neurodevelopmental outcomes.[64] Similarly, an abnormal background pattern and ictal discharges generated from amplitude-integrated EEG (aEEG) are also biomarkers for postoperative brain injury; however, aEEG patterns are highly affected by sedatives.[65,66] Hence, from a practical standpoint, there remains uncertainty in the utility of the clinical examination and EEG in the acute setting for the purpose of neuroprognostication. Is this knowledge going to change the care that is provided at the bedside or impact outcome prediction? If so, then the challenges to making a diagnosis [67] in a patient with suspected acute structural brain injury should be overcome, even if it means transportation for head computerized tomography (CT) [68,69] and/or magnetic resonance imaging (MRI),[70,71] rather than using head ultrasound.[72,73]

Last, standardization of long-term outcomes measures across all types of CHD remains a challenge. The Boston Circulatory Arrest Trial is a notable example of a large trial where standardized outcomes were collected on children with transposition of the great arteries.[74] This facilitated characterizing a pattern of neurodevelopmental disabilities in these patients. Similar multicenter studies are under way and very much needed.

Cardiac Arrest

Survival after pediatric cardiac arrest has improved over the years,[75] but neurological outcomes remain unfavorable for many children. There are many factors that may influence prognosis after cardiac arrest, but similar to prognostication in children undergoing cardiac surgery, there are two main issues. First, there are a number of unmodifiable factors for children pre-arrest, such as preexisting conditions, genetics, and pathophysiological vulnerabilities, intra-arrest, such as duration of cardiopulmonary resuscitation (CPR) and CPR quality, and post-arrest. Second, if death is not imminent, when should we prognosticate and how should that impact when and how we withhold or withdraw technological support?

There are numerous factors associated with poor patient outcomes. Pre-arrest factors are out-of-hospital cardiac arrest (OHCA) location,[76] younger age for OHCA,[77, 78] or causes such as sudden infant death syndrome [79] and blunt trauma.[80] Intra-arrest, factors associated with better patient outcomes from OHCA are witnessed arrest,[77, 78] the provision of bystander CPR,[81] and less frequent doses of epinephrine.[82] At best, these data can be used to risk-stratify high-risk individuals who may benefit from post-arrest therapies, but should not be used for neuroprognostication. One such example utilized decision tree analysis to risk stratify 1-month favorable outcome, defined as PCPC 1 or 2 (normal to mild disability), based on pre-arrest and intra-arrest factors. Incorporating pre-hospital return of spontaneous circulation (ROSC), initial shockable rhythm, and witnessed status via decision tree analysis, the authors were able to classify good, moderately good, moderately poor, and poor outcome strata with an area under the receiver operating characteristic (ROC) curve of 0.88 (95% confidence interval (CI): 0.87–0.90).[83] A similar approach can be used in children who suffer in-hospital cardiac arrest (IHCA), and patient group risk stratification models, useful for randomized controlled trials (RCTs), have also been generated using a variety of data.[84]

Neuroprognostication in the PICU

Most studies in pediatric cardiac arrest have focused on mortality and short-term outcomes at discharge using PCPC, which consists of a 6-point scale that provides ratings of overall neurological functioning.[85,86] There are features of the neurological examination that have been associated with worse outcomes after cardiac arrest, including: Glasgow Coma Scale (GCS) score < 5 at 24 hours after admission,[87] absence of spontaneous respiratory activity at 24 hours after admission,[87] absence of pupillary reflexes at 12 hours [88,89] and 24 hours after ROSC,[87,90] and absence of a motor response between 2 and 9 days after arrest.[90] However, much of these data are historical, and thus do not take into account advances in post-arrest care such as targeted temperature management (TTM). The 2020 American Heart Association (AHA) Advanced Cardiac Life Support (ACLS) guidelines suggest that the earliest time for accurate multimodal prognostication in adults treated with TTM is at a minimum of 72 hours *after return to normothermia*.[91] At present, in pediatric practice, the best data come from the Therapeutic Hypothermia After Pediatric Cardiac Arrest (THAPCA) RCTs of TTM (33°C vs. 36.8°C within 6 hours of ROSC) after pediatric OHCA and IHCA.[92,93] There is no pediatric specific guidance on the timing of neuroprognostication after TTM for pediatric cardiac arrest; however, extrapolating from adult guidance to provide adequate time for medication clearance after hypothermia is reasonable.[94]

In regard to EEG and brain imaging, the two important reasons to consider obtaining these tests are (1) whether the findings will inform ongoing management, and (2) the accuracy of findings for prognostication. The Critical Care Continuous EEG Task Force of the American Clinical Neurophysiology Society suggests using EEG monitoring following pediatric cardiac arrest for prognostication.[95] However, the 2020 AHA Pediatric Advanced Life Support (PALS) guidelines update recommends that EEGs performed within the first 7 days after pediatric cardiac arrest *"can be useful as one factor for prognostication augmented by other information."*[96,97] How and when to accurately prognosticate outcome following pediatric cardiac arrest is an area that needs further evaluation.

Last, the one additional area of neuroprognostication research that is unique to the post-cardiac arrest population is the utility of serum biomarkers, such as systemic lactate,[98] brain glial fibrillary acid protein, ubiquitin carboxy-terminal hydrolase L1, S100B, and neuron-specific enolase. To date, however, biomarkers remain investigational and have no role in current decision making.

Extracorporeal Life Support

Extracorporeal membrane oxygenation (ECMO) utilization has quadrupled in children and increased 10-fold in adults in the past 15 years to greater than 2,500 pediatric and 4,500 adult cases reported to the Extracorporeal Life Support Organization (ELSO) registry in 2016.[99] Acute brain injury (e.g., hypoxic-ischemic injury, arterial ischemic strokes, or intracranial hemorrhage) occurs in up to 30% of pediatric ECMO patients, and mortality increases to 89% if acute neurological injury occurs.[100] Up to 50% of pediatric ECMO survivors have clinically important neurological disabilities that impair normal development, quality of life, and school performance.[100–103] ECMO technology has become so advanced that now avoiding neurological complications is the key to survival and better long-term neurological outcomes.

Neuroprognostication in the PICU and Follow-Up

In an attempt to assist prognostication, risk factors associated with acute brain injury have been the focus of many studies. The data here fall into three groups: (1) the circumstances that led to ECMO (e.g., hypoxia, hypotension, acidosis, CPR, cardiac surgery); (2) patient-related factors (e.g., preexisting genetic, pulmonary, and cardiac diseases); and (3) ECMO-related factors (e.g., cerebral venous hypertension from internal jugular vein cannulation, non-pulsatile flow in veno-arterial ECMO, mode and duration of ECMO, anticoagulation strategies, drug neurotoxicity, and embolic phenomena).[104–114] To date, however, there is no prognostic model to estimate the risk of developing acute brain injury, and we are left to speculate whether one or more of these underlying pathophysiologies, as well as any other unknown factors, may contribute to a particular pattern of brain injury. In many cases there is limited ability to obtain brain imaging or perform a neurological examination without neuromuscular blockade early during the course of ECMO. With no definitive prognostic model available to predict outcome, there are no reliable models to support decisions about early withdrawal of life-sustaining therapies. In such situations, these decisions are often considered on a case-by-case basis.

Clinical recognition of an acute neurological event such as stroke or seizure during ECMO may not be possible at the time of ictus. Current neurological monitoring modalities used during ECMO are limited in their ability to detect acute brain injuries. EEG is used intermittently and other modalities including transcranial Doppler (TCD) or near infrared spectroscopy (NIRS) do not reliably detect vascular insults. Most of the pediatric literature supporting the use of neuroimaging, EEG monitoring, cerebral oximetry, and serum biomarkers during ECMO is observational, and its quality is at the level of grades 3B (case-control) and 4 (case series).[115] Serial neurological examinations with support from neuroimaging are a reliable way to detect brain injury in the acute setting, but examinations are commonly limited by sedation and/or neuromuscular blockade in a patient treated with ECMO, and acute neuroimaging studies may be normal in greater than 50% of patients. Other factors, such as the impact of seizures on outcomes, even in the absence of abnormal neuroimaging, must also be considered. [116,117] Further research is under way using brain-specific and inflammatory serum biomarkers to assist in real-time diagnosis of neurological injury and recovery and may enable early prognostication.[118]

There is some literature on long-term neurodevelopmental outcomes following ECMO, but larger studies are needed. According to a systematic review of 60 papers published between 2000 and 2016, a median of 36 (interquartile range, 18–6) children up to 18 years of age underwent standardized measures to evaluate outcomes after ECMO at a median of 26 (interquartile range 8–61) months. Overall, 10–50% of children scored 2 standard deviations (SD) below normal for age on cognitive testing, behavioral problems occurred in up to 46%, severe motor impairment occurred in 12%, and 31–53% of school age/adolescents scored > 1 SD below population mean on quality-of-life measures.[119] Other studies have shown that added supports/services were needed in some school-age children despite normal cognitive testing.[120] International standardized common outcomes measures and longitudinal follow-up of survivors are needed to increase outcome data and better understand neurodevelopmental outcomes, therapeutic needs, quality of life, and prevalence of end-organ dysfunction. Developmental stage as a potential modifier of outcomes warrants increased focus, since early life stress affects brain maturation through multiple mechanisms, including epigenetic alteration of gene expression and stress-related circuits in the cortex, hippocampus, and limbic system.[121]

Status Epilepticus

Seizures are often a symptom of a primary brain insult, and neurological outcomes are likely influenced by a combination of factors beyond the severity of the primary insult, genetics and environment, including (1) seizure detection rate; (2) approach to seizure management, both short- and long-term; and (3) the degree to which seizures contribute to secondary brain insults.[122] The association between status epilepticus (SE) and outcomes in critically ill children has been confounded by variable detection methods and definitions of electrographic seizures (ES) and electrographic SE (ESE). Accordingly, multiple studies report an incidence between 10 and 40%.

[123,124] Seizure detection rates may become more consistent in the future with consensus regarding the indications for use of EEG in the PICU and definitions of EEG abnormalities,[125] but challenges from a resource standpoint (e.g., availability of EEG machines and personnel to read, interpret, and communicate results in a timely fashion) will have to be overcome.

Neuroprognostication in the PICU and Follow-Up

It remains unclear whether treatment of seizures improves outcomes in critically ill children. [126,127] This problem is, in part, due to the variability in outcomes measures used (e.g., mortality, quality of life, short- or long-term decline in neurological function). For example, a prospective study of 259 children who had continuous EEG (cEEG) monitoring in the PICU or cardiac intensive care unit (CICU) identified seizures and SE in 36% and 9%, respectively.[128] Seizure burden was not associated with mortality. However, after adjustment for diagnosis and illness severity, the odds of neurological decline, defined as a decrease in PCPC score at hospital discharge, were strongly associated with a seizure burden of more than 12 minutes in a given hour. Importantly, the odds of mortality were higher with an unreactive EEG background (odds ratio [OR] 7.40) or longer PICU/CICU stay, and not with SE. In contrast, a retrospective multicenter study of 550 children in the PICU identified ES in 30% and ESE in 11%, and reported an association between ESE and mortality in a multivariate analysis.[129] ES was not associated with worse outcomes, but the odds ratio for in-hospital mortality in multivariable analysis was significantly increased for SE (OR 2.2), as well as abnormal EEG backgrounds including both burst-suppression (OR 28.5) and attenuated/featureless (OR 91.5).[129]

Studies of the effects of SE on survivors of critical illness have also used various durations of follow-up. A prospective study of 200 children (3% of all PICU admissions during the study period) with acute encephalopathy who underwent cEEG according to an institutional protocol identified ES (defined as EEG seizures > 10 seconds or shorter if accompanied by a clinical change) in 20.5%, and ESE (defined as ES > 30 minutes) in 21.5%. Mortality in this cohort was high (18%), and 44% had a short-term poor outcome. ESE, but not ES, was associated with a significantly increased risk of mortality (OR 5.1) and worsening PCPC score at PICU discharge (OR 17.3).[122] A retrospective analysis of long-term outcomes between 0.8 and 12 years after discharge in 127 children with SE found that poor outcome (defined as death, a new neurological deficit and/or development of epilepsy) was associated with ESE, younger age (< 5 years) or longer seizures (> 33.5 minutes).[131] In other long-term follow-up studies, both ES and ESE have been linked with risk for poor outcome. In a study of 137 children with normal neurodevelopment before PICU admission for acute encephalopathy, ESE, but not ES, was associated with increased risk for epilepsy (OR 13.3), unfavorable GOS (OR 6.4), and lower pediatric quality-of-life score at a median follow-up of 2.7 years.[132] In a prospective observational study of 300 children who were admitted to the PICU for acute neurological conditions and altered mental status, 60 survivors were neurodevelopmentally normal prior to PICU admission and had outcome data available. In this cohort, ES and ESE were associated with worse adaptive behavior scores and trends toward worse emotional and executive function scores at a median follow-up of 2.6 years after discharge.[133] In studies of the long-term follow-up of the Boston Circulatory Arrest Study, ES were detected in 11% of this cohort of 178 children with transposition of the great arteries. The occurrence of ES was associated with a decrease in executive function and impaired social interactions, but not with academic achievement at 4 years' follow-up.[134]

Collectively, these studies have attempted to associate ES, ESE, and SE with short- and long-term neurological morbidity and mortality. The burden of ES may contribute in a dose-dependent way to poor outcome but not necessarily to mortality.[128] The EEG background (burst-suppression, attenuation) seems to be strongly associated with risk for mortality in some studies. [128,129] With this knowledge, should background EEG abnormalities change the goals of intensive care? The answer currently is no, but rather this information may serve to risk-stratify patients who may benefit from one treatment approach versus another in RCTs. Assessment of the link between SE, ESE or seizures and long-term neurological function must also acknowledge the potential toxicity of the treatments (e.g., benzodiazepines) on outcome.[135,136]

Traumatic Brain Injury (TBI)

Neuroprognostication in cases of pediatric severe TBI is notoriously difficult, and similar to the other clinical scenarios aforementioned, there is an ethical dimension to consider – for example, how to offer guidance when there are diverging views from families and clinicians on aggressiveness of care during a so-called window of opportunity for limiting or withdrawing life-sustaining therapies. [137] There is, most definitely, a need to identify instances of lethal TBI when ongoing intensive care beyond initial resuscitation attempts is not appropriate. In this regard, the types of brain injury in such children older than 2 years of age is remarkably similar to those seen in adults.[2] Some post-resuscitated children with GCS score 3 and bilateral fixed and dilated pupils may be in this category and progress to brain death (i.e., death by neurological criteria). How the regional and local emergency systems deal with such patients should be decided locally. In some practices, admission to the PICU is offered to all children who have entered the emergency system. The teams based in the PICU with its resources and more time to let patients recover are best equipped to deal with the issues surrounding the diagnosis of brain death. In any child with at least one pupil reacting to light, irrespective of the GCS score, all and full TBI-related interventions are offered. In this clinical scenario, it is impossible and inappropriate to use clinical features at the time of the injury to predict survival. Some of these children may well have sustained a fatal injury that will become apparent over the course of intensive care.

Neuroprognostication in the PICU

The prognostication of potential outcomes after PICU care in children with severe TBI is extremely difficult. The prognosis for recovery may be due to a number of primary cerebral and extra-cerebral insults (e.g., hypotension, hypoxemia, hypercarbia) at the time of the injury, and secondary insults (e.g., seizures, increased intracranial pressure [ICP], cerebral edema, axonal injury). It is not an exact science, since some degree of recovery may continue for years after the inciting event in survivors and is more related to white matter integrity. [138,139] Hence, at presentation, the assumption is that initial shearing injury and uncontrolled intracranial hypertension with inadequate cerebral perfusion results in loss of brain tissue, white matter integrity, brain function, and future neurological potential. The question is how best to assess these pathophysiologies. For example, the degree of raised ICP and low cerebral perfusion pressure (CPP) may reflect the severity of injury and provide surrogate information based on associations with outcome, but should not lead to life-determining decision making in the absence of supportive clinical and imaging findings. Similar to the OHCA and IHCA literature, there are also large pediatric TBI series that repeatedly demonstrate associations between clinical parameters (i.e., ICP, CPP, seizures, pupils responses) and mortality, for example, 25–45% in adults and 10–25% in children, which do, at best, help with risk-stratification for RCTs – but no more.[140,141]

In regard to outcomes in survivors, we have limited ability to prognosticate during the acute phase of illness due to lack of adequate clinical, imaging, or electrophysiological tools to assess the degree and nature of white matter injury resulting from severe TBI. There are some data in children with TBI, and a few authors have reported white matter architecture derangements in small series of children.[142–147] There was also a 2012 US National Institutes of Health initiative for common data elements for outcome measures in pediatric TBI research.[34] To date, however, these have not resulted in more than observational information.

Summary

In this review, we have synthesized the available pediatric literature and our collective experience dealing with issues surrounding neuroprognostication for critically ill children with acute CNS infections, following cardiac surgery, cardiac arrest, ECMO, SE, and severe TBI. Some unifying features across all of these disease states are that outcomes likely depend upon a combination of factors, with some occurring before, during, and long after the acute phase of illness; some are potentially unmodifiable consequences of genetics and environment; and some may be modifiable secondary insults themselves (e.g., related to PICU management, seizure burden). There are two key takeaways to consider in terms of neuroprognostication. First, for the few children with acute brain injury in whom death is imminent, the decision to withdraw life-sustaining therapies may be considered. For the majority of children

with acute brain injury, however, the clinical information, trajectory of illness, and decision making do not fall into this category. In these cases, we continue neuroprotective therapies, and perform serial assessments over time to determine whether there is recovery of brain function. Second, is that neuroprognostication is challenging and should thoughtfully incorporate numerous objective patient level factors in order to guide and optimize critical care management and improve patient and family outcomes.

Gaps in Current Knowledge

Prognostic models and risk-stratification may be useful for enrolling children in RCTs, but these do not deal with diagnostic testing and management of individual patients. An overarching goal of care for critically ill children with acute brain injury is to preserve his/her developmental status and trajectory after the acute event, and maximize function of the child and family. In order to achieve this goal, there must be (1) timely and proper diagnostic evaluations of the acute brain injury and its complications; (2) appropriate management of primary and secondary insults to the brain; (3) prevention of iatrogenic insults; (4) accurate and timely diagnostic assessment of clinically meaningful outcomes; (5) access to effective mental health, rehabilitation, and specialty medical services; (6) family/caregiver support; and (7) successful re-entry into home life (friends, school, sports, hobbies, and organizations). The data also suggest that a multidisciplinary approach, including neuropsychological assessments, screening of parents and families for comorbid conditions, and a clear and effective plan for reintegration into life, may optimize outcomes in addition to medical management of comorbid medical, psychological, social, cognitive, behavioral, and motor conditions.[148] One particular subgroup worthy of mention for whom further research is needed, as long-term prognosis and outcomes remain unclear, are those children with so-called *catastrophic* brain injury, leading to coma and disorders of consciousness. Much work is needed to understand the trajectories of recovery in these children in order to improve prognostication and inform clinical decision making as early as possible after the catastrophic event. Table 17.1 outlines some of the gaps in current knowledge by research category (basic, clinical, and translational). The

Table 17.1 Research agenda (basic, clinical, and translational) to address current gaps in knowledge about neuroprognostication in pediatric neurocritical care

Basic	• What animal models are best for modeling acute brain injury in critically ill children, and long-term morbidities and recovery in different diseases?
	• Is there regional cerebral vulnerability related to secondary insults and iatrogenic insults, such as hypoxia/ischemia, hypotension, hypocapnia, hypoglycemia, seizures, cerebral edema, increased intracranial pressure, vasospasm, and medications (e.g., sedatives/analgesics)?
	• What biological mechanisms mediate recovery, and do they differ by disease?
Clinical	• What disease phenotypes are clinically important, and how should they be defined (e.g., by biology and/or effect on function)?
	• What new therapies and clinical trial designs are likely to target a clinically relevant phenotype?
	• What is the best timing and dose for interventions and overall efficacy of interventions on long-term neurological outcomes?
	• How do we define, measure, and monitor recovery trajectories for each disease?
	• What outcomes measures address the full range of functioning of the child and family for each disease?
	• What clinical collaborations and infrastructure are needed to standardize clinical assessments and assess long-term outcomes?
	• How do we better work with families and caregivers when presenting information about potential outcomes and assess their understanding of prognostic risk?
	• What prognosis, and when, should be used to withdraw intensive care?
Translational	• How does the critical illness trajectory impact morbidity and recovery for each disease?
	• How does the expected developmental trajectory impact morbidity and recovery for each disease?
	• What early neuroprognostication tools reliably predict future morbidities and trajectories of recovery for each disease?
	• How do we apply screening tools to determine children at risk for disabilities, best timing and dose for interventions, and overall efficacy of interventions?

major challenges for neuroprognostication include the need for multicenter studies to overcome small patient numbers at individual centers, clinical heterogeneity, standardization of outcomes assessments, and coexistence of multiple risk factors.

References

1. Pollack MM, Ruttimann UE, Getson PR. Accurate prediction of the outcome of pediatric intensive care. A new quantitative method. *N Engl J Med.* 1987;**316**(3):134–9.

2. Pollack MM, Holubkov R, Funai T, et al. Simultaneous prediction of new morbidity, mortality, and survival without new morbidity from pediatric intensive care: a new paradigm for outcomes assessment. *Crit Care Med.* 2015;**43**(8):1699–1709.

3. Pinto NP, Rhinesmith EW, Kim TY, Ladner PH, Pollack MM. Long-term function after pediatric critical illness: results from the survivor outcomes study. *Pediatr Crit Care Med.* 2017;**18**(3):e122–e130.

4. Williams CN, Eriksson C, Piantino J, et al. Long-term sequelae of pediatric neurocritical care: the parent perspective. *J Pediatr Intensive Care.* 2018;**7**(4):173–181.

5. Tasker RC, Menon DK : Critical care and the brain. *JAMA.* 2016, **315**(8):749–50.

6. Hopkins RO, Choong K, Zebuhr CA, Kudchadkar SR. Transforming PICU culture to facilitate early rehabilitation. *J Pediatr Intensive Care.* 2015;**4**(4):204–11.

7. Ong C, Lee JH, Leow MK, Puthucheary ZA. Functional outcomes and physical impairments in pediatric critical care survivors: a scoping review. *Pediatr Crit Care Med.* 2016;**17**(5):e247–259.

8. Ebrahim S, Singh S, Hutchison JS, et al. Adaptive behavior, functional outcomes, and quality of life outcomes of children requiring urgent ICU admission. *Pediatr Crit Care Med.* 2013;**14**(1):10–18.

9. Cunha F, Mota T, Teixeira-Pinto A, et al. Factors associated with health-related quality of life changes in survivors to pediatric intensive care. *Pediatr Crit Care Med.* 2013;**14**(1):e8–15.

10. Watson RS, Choong K, Colville G, et al. Life after critical illness in children – toward an understanding of pediatric post-intensive care syndrome. *J Pediatr.* 2018;**198**:16–24.

11. Stein-Zamir C, Shoob H, Sokolov I, et al. The clinical features and long-term sequelae of invasive meningococcal disease in children. *Pediatr Infect Dis J.* 2014;**33**(7):777–9.

12. Kohli-Lynch M, Russell NJ, Seale AC, et al, Neurodevelopmental impairment in children after group B streptococcal disease worldwide:

systematic review and meta-analyses. *Clin Infect Dis.* 2017;**65**(suppl_2):S190–S199.

13. Edmond K, Clark A, Korczak VS, et al. Global and regional risk of disabling sequelae from bacterial meningitis: a systematic review and meta-analysis. *Lancet Infect Dis.* 2010;**10**(5):317–28.

14. Hudson LD, Viner RM, Christie D. Long-term sequelae of childhood bacterial meningitis. *Curr Infect Dis Rep.* 2013;**15**(3):236–41.

15. Wee LY, Tanugroho RR, Thoon KC, et al. A 15-year retrospective analysis of prognostic factors in childhood bacterial meningitis. *Acta Paediatr.* 2016;**105**(1):e22–9.

16. Tewabe T, Fenta A, Tegen A, et al. Clinical outcomes and risk factors of meningitis among children in referral hospital, Ethiopia, 2016: a retrospective chart review. *Ethiop J Health Sci.* 2018;**28**(5):563–70.

17. Ouchenir L, Renaud C, Khan S, et al. The epidemiology, management, and outcomes of bacterial meningitis in infants. *Pediatrics.* 2017;**140**(1).

18. Sadarangani M, Scheifele DW, Halperin SA, et al., Investigators of the Canadian Immunization Monitoring Program ACTive (IMPACT). Outcomes of invasive meningococcal disease in adults and children in Canada between 2002 and 2011: a prospective cohort study. *Clin Infect Dis.* 2015;**60**(8):e27–35.

19. Roed C, Omland LH, Skinhoj P, et al. Educational achievement and economic self-sufficiency in adults after childhood bacterial meningitis. *JAMA.* 2013;**309**(16):1714–21.

20. Pickering L, Jennum P, Ibsen R, Kjellberg J. Long-term health and socioeconomic consequences of childhood and adolescent onset of meningococcal meningitis. *Eur J Pediatr.* 2018;**177**(9):1309–15.

21. Borg J, Christie D, Coen PG, Booy R, Viner RM. Outcomes of meningococcal disease in adolescence: prospective, matched-cohort study. *Pediatrics.* 2009;**123**(3):e502–9.

22. Sumpter R, Brunklaus A, McWilliam R, Dorris L : Health-related quality-of-life and behavioural outcome in survivors of childhood meningitis. *Brain Injury.* 2011;**25**(13–14):1288–95.

23. Khandaker G, Jung J, Britton PN, et al. Long-term outcomes of infective encephalitis in children: a systematic review and meta-analysis. *Dev Med Child Neurol.* 2016;**58**(11):1108–15.

24. Rao S, Elkon B, Flett KB, et al, Long-term outcomes and risk factors associated with acute encephalitis in children. *J Pediatric Infect Dis Soc.* 2017;**6**(1):20–7.

25. Ramanuj PP, Granerod J, Davies NW, et al. Quality of life and associated socio-clinical factors after encephalitis in children and adults in England: a population-based, prospective cohort study. *PLoS One.* 2014;**9**(7):e103496.

26. Granerod J, Davies NW, Ramanuj PP, et al. Increased rates of sequelae post-encephalitis in individuals attending primary care practices in the United Kingdom: a population-based retrospective cohort study. *J Neurol.* 2017;**264**(2):407–15.

27. Hokkanen L, Launes J : Neuropsychological sequelae of acute-onset sporadic viral encephalitis. *Neuropsychol Rehabil.* 2007;**17**(4–5):450–77.

28. Glaser CA, Gilliam S, Schnurr D, et al. In search of encephalitis etiologies: diagnostic challenges in the California Encephalitis Project, 1998–2000. *Clin Infect Dis.* 2003;**36**(6):731–42.

29. Ooi MH, Lewthwaite P, Lai BF, et al. The epidemiology, clinical features, and long-term prognosis of Japanese encephalitis in Central Sarawak, Malaysia, 1997–2005. *Clin Infect Dis.* 2008;**47**(4):458–68.

30. Bozzola E, Bergonzini P, Bozzola M, et al. Neuropsychological and internalizing problems in acute central nervous system infections: a 1 year follow-up. *Ital J Pediatr.* 2017;**43**(1):96.

31. Martis JMS, Bok LA, Halbertsma FJJ, et al. Brain imaging can predict neurodevelopmental outcome of Group B streptococcal meningitis in neonates. *Acta Paediatr.* 2019;**108**(5):855–64.

32. Rohlwink UK, Mauff K, Wilkinson KA, et al. Biomarkers of cerebral injury and inflammation in pediatric tuberculous meningitis. *Clin Infect Dis.* 2017;**65**(8):1298–1307.

33. Faried A, Arief G, Arifin MZ, Nataprawira HM : Correlation of lactate concentration in peripheral plasma and cerebrospinal fluid with Glasgow Outcome Scale for patients with tuberculous meningitis complicated by acute hydrocephalus treated with fluid diversions. *World Neurosurg.* 2018;**111**:e178–e182.

34. McCauley SR, Wilde EA, Anderson VA, et al. Recommendations for the use of common outcome measures in pediatric traumatic brain injury research. *J Neurotrauma.* 2012;**29**(4):678–705.

35. Lewthwaite P, Begum A, Ooi MH, et al. Disability after encephalitis: development and validation of a new outcome score. *Bull World Health Organ.* 2010;**88**(8):584–92.

36. Lenhard T, Ott D, Jakob NJ, et al. Predictors, neuroimaging characteristics and long-term outcome of severe european tick-borne

encephalitis: a prospective cohort study. *PLoS One.* 2016;**11**(4):e0154143.

37. Kalita J, Mani VE, Bhoi SK, Misra UK. Spectrum and outcome of acute infectious encephalitis/encephalopathy in an intensive care unit from India. *QJM.* 2017;**110**(3):141–8.

38. Teoh HL, Mohammad SS, Britton PN, et al. Clinical characteristics and functional motor outcomes of enterovirus 71 neurological disease in children. *JAMA Neurol.* 2016;**73**(3):300–7.

39. Marino BS, Lipkin PH, Newburger JW, et al. Neurodevelopmental outcomes in children with congenital heart disease: evaluation and management: a scientific statement from the American Heart Association. *Circulation.* 2012;**126**(9):1143–72.

40. Mebius MJ, Kooi EMW, Bilardo CM, Bos AF. Brain injury and neurodevelopmental outcome in congenital heart disease: a systematic review. *Pediatrics.* 2017;**140**(11):e20164055.

41. Sterken C, Lemiere J, Vanhorebeek I, Van den Berghe G, Mesotten D. Neurocognition after paediatric heart surgery: a systematic review and meta-analysis. *Open Heart.* 2015;**2**(1):e000255.

42. Wernovsky G. Current insights regarding neurological and developmental abnormalities in children and young adults with complex congenital cardiac disease. *Cardiol Young.* 2006;**16**(Suppl 1):92–104.

43. Bellinger DC, Wypij D, duPlessis AJ, et al. Neurodevelopmental status at eight years in children with dextro-transposition of the great arteries: the Boston Circulatory Arrest Trial. *J Thorac Cardiovascr Surg.* 2003;**126**(5):1385–96.

44. Mussatto KA, Hoffmann RG, Hoffman GM, et al. Risk and prevalence of developmental delay in young children with congenital heart disease. *Pediatrics.* 2014;**133**(3):e570–7.

45. Bellinger DC, Wypij D, Rivkin MJ, et al. Adolescents with d-transposition of the great arteries corrected with the arterial switch procedure: neuropsychological assessment and structural brain imaging. *Circulation.* 2011;**124**(12):1361–9.

46. Schaefer C, von Rhein M, Knirsch W, et al. Neurodevelopmental outcome, psychological adjustment, and quality of life in adolescents with congenital heart disease. *Dev Med Child Neurol.* 2013;**55**(12):1143–9.

47. Shillingford AJ, Glanzman MM, Ittenbach RF, et al. Inattention, hyperactivity, and school performance in a population of school-age children with complex congenital heart disease. *Pediatrics.* 2008;**121**(4):e759–67.

48. Teixeira FM, Coelho RM, Proenca C, et al. Quality of life experienced by adolescents and young adults with congenital heart disease. *Pediatr. Cardiol.* 2011;**32**(8):1132–8.

49. Neal AE, Stopp C, Wypij D, et al. Predictors of health-related quality of life in adolescents with tetralogy of Fallot. *J Pediatr.* 2015;**166**(1):132–8.

50. Wernovsky G, Licht DJ. Neurodevelopmental outcomes in children with congenital heart disease – what can we impact? *Pediatr Crit Care Med.* 2016;**17**(8 Suppl 1):S232–42.

51. Dominguez TE, Wernovsky G, Gaynor JW. Cause and prevention of central nervous system injury in neonates undergoing cardiac surgery. *Semin Thorac Cardiovasc Surg.* 2007;**19**(3):269–77.

52. Bird GL, Jeffries HE, Licht DJ, et al. Neurological complications associated with the treatment of patients with congenital cardiac disease: consensus definitions from the Multi-Societal Database Committee for Pediatric and Congenital Heart Disease. *Cardiol Young.* 2008;**18**(Suppl 2):234–9.

53. Gaynor JW, Stopp C, Wypij D, et al. Neurodevelopmental outcomes after cardiac surgery in infancy. *Pediatrics.* 2015, **135**(5):816–25.

54. Blue GM, Kirk EP, Giannoulatou E, el al. Advances in the genetics of congenital heart disease: a clinician's guide. *J Am Coll Cardiol.* 2017;**69**(7):859–70.

55. Newburger JW, Sleeper LA, Bellinger DC, et al. Early developmental outcome in children with hypoplastic left heart syndrome and related anomalies: the single ventricle reconstruction trial. *Circulation.* 2012;**125**(17):2081–91.

56. Rosser TC, Edgin JO, Capone GT, et al. Associations between medical history, cognition, and behavior in youth with Down syndrome: a report from the Down Syndrome Cognition Project. *Am J Intellect Dev Disabil.* 2018; **123**(6):514–28.

57. Calderon J, Willaime M, Lelong N, et al., EPICARD study group. Population-based study of cognitive outcomes in congenital heart defects. *Arch Dis Child.* 2018;**103**(1):49–56.

58. Ma M, Gauvreau K, Allan CK, Mayer JE Jr, Jenkins KJ. Causes of death after congenital heart surgery. *Ann Thorac Surg.* 2007;**83**(4):1438–45.

59. Gaies M, Pasquali SK, Donohue JE, et al. Seminal postoperative complications and mode of death after pediatric cardiac surgical procedures. *Ann Thorac Surg.* 2016;**102**(2):628–35.

60. Abend NS, Beslow LA, Smith SE, et al. Seizures as a presenting symptom of acute arterial ischemic stroke in childhood. *J Pediatr.* 2011;**159**(3):479–83.

61. Singh RK, Zecavati N, Singh J, et al. Seizures in acute childhood stroke. *J Pediatr.* 2012;**160** (2):291–6.

62. Marino BS, Tabbutt S, MacLaren G, et al. Cardiopulmonary resuscitation in infants and children with cardiac disease: a scientific statement from the American Heart Association. *Circulation.* 2018;**137**(22):e691–e782.

63. Naim MY, Gaynor JW, Chen J, et al. Subclinical seizures identified by postoperative electroencephalographic monitoring are common after neonatal cardiac surgery. *J Thorac Cardiovasc Surg.* 2015;**150**(1):169–78; discussion 178–80.

64. Abend NS, Dlugos DJ, Clancy RR. A review of long-term EEG monitoring in critically ill children with hypoxic-ischemic encephalopathy, congenital heart disease, ECMO, and stroke. *J Clin Neurophysiol.* 2013;**30**(2):134–42.

65. Mebius MJ, Oostdijk NJE, Kuik SJ, et al. Amplitude-integrated electroencephalography during the first 72 h after birth in neonates diagnosed prenatally with congenital heart disease. *Pediatr Res.* 2018;**83**(4):798–803.

66. Claessens NHP, Noorlag L, Weeke LC, et al. Amplitude-integrated electroencephalography for early recognition of brain injury in neonates with critical congenital heart disease. *J Pediatr.* 2018;**202**:199–205 e191.

67. Sinclair AJ, Fox CK, Ichord RN, et al. Stroke in children with cardiac disease: report from the International Pediatric Stroke Study Group Symposium. *Pediatr Neurol.* 2015;**52**(1):5–15.

68. Larovere KL, Brett MS, Tasker RC, Strauss KJ, Burns JP : Head computed tomography scanning during pediatric neurocritical care: diagnostic yield and the utility of portable studies. *Neurocrit Care.* 2011;**16**(2):251–7.

69. Srinivasan J, Miller SP, Phan TG, Mackay MT. Delayed recognition of initial stroke in children: need for increased awareness. *Pediatrics.* 2009;**124** (2):e227–34.

70. Mahle WT, Tavani F, Zimmerman RA, et al. An MRI study of neurological injury before and after congenital heart surgery. *Circulation.* 2002;**106**(12 Suppl 1):109–14.

71. Verrall CE, Walker K, Loughran-Fowlds A, et al. Contemporary incidence of stroke (focal infarct and/or haemorrhage) determined by neuroimaging and neurodevelopmental disability at 12 months of age in neonates undergoing cardiac surgery utilizing cardiopulmonary bypass. *Interact Cardiovasc Thorac Surg.* 2018;**26**(4):644–50.

72. Golomb MR, Dick PT, MacGregor DL, Armstrong DC, DeVeber GA. Cranial ultrasonography has a low sensitivity for detecting arterial ischemic stroke in term neonates. *J Child Neurol.* 2003;**18**(2):98–103.

73. Cowan F, Mercuri E, Groenendaal F, et al. Does cranial ultrasound imaging identify arterial cerebral infarction in term neonates? *Arch Dis Child Fetal Neonatal Ed.* 2005;**90**(3):F252–6.

74. Rappaport LA, Wypij D, Bellinger DC, et al. Relation of seizures after cardiac surgery in early infancy to neurodevelopmental outcome. Boston Circulatory Arrest Study Group. *Circulation.* 1998;**97**(8):773–9.

75. Girotra S, Spertus JA, Li Y, et al., American Heart Association Get With the Guidelines-Resuscitation Investigators, Survival trends in pediatric in-hospital cardiac arrests: an analysis from Get With the Guidelines – Resuscitation. *Circ Cardiovasc Qual Outcomes.* 2013;**6**(1):42–9.

76. de Caen AR, Berg MD, Chameides L, et al. Part 12: pediatric advanced life support: 2015 American Heart Association Guidelines Update for Cardiopulmonary Resuscitation and Emergency Cardiovascular Care. *Circulation.* 2015;**132**(18 suppl 2):S526–S542.

77. Fink EL, Prince DK, Kaltman JR, et al. Unchanged pediatric out-of-hospital cardiac arrest incidence and survival rates with regional variation in North America. *Resuscitation.* 2016;**107**:121–8.

78. Goto Y, Funada A, Goto Y. Duration of prehospital cardiopulmonary resuscitation and favorable neurological outcomes for pediatric out-of-hospital cardiac arrests: a nationwide, population-based cohort study. *Circulation.* 2016;**134**(25):2046–59.

79. Meert KL, Telford R, Holubkov R, et al. Pediatric out-of-hospital cardiac arrest characteristics and their association with survival and neurobehavioral outcome. *Pediatr Crit Care.* 2016;**17**(12):e543–e550.

80. Matos RI, Watson RS, Nadkarni VM, et al. Duration of cardiopulmonary resuscitation and illness category impact survival and neurologic outcomes for in-hospital pediatric cardiac arrests. *Circulation.* 2013;**127**(4):442–51.

81. Goto Y, Maeda T, Goto Y. Impact of dispatcher-assisted bystander cardiopulmonary resuscitation on neurological outcomes in children with out-of-hospital cardiac arrests: a prospective, nationwide, population-based cohort study. *J Am Heart Assoc.* 2014;**3**(3): e000499.

82. Hoyme DB, Patel SS, Samson RA, et al., American Heart Association Get With the Guidelines-Resuscitation Investigators. Epinephrine dosing interval and survival outcomes during pediatric

in-hospital cardiac arrest. *Resuscitation.* 2017;**117**:18–23.

83. Goto Y, Maeda T, Nakatsu-Goto Y. Decision tree model for predicting long-term outcomes in children with out-of-hospital cardiac arrest: a nationwide, population-based observational study. *Crit Care.* 2014;**18**(3):R133.

84. Holmberg MJ, Moskowitz A, Raymond TT, et al. Derivation and internal validation of a mortality prediction tool for initial survivors of pediatric in-hospital cardiac arrest. *Pediatr Crit Care Med.* 2018;**19**(3):186–95.

85. Fiser DH. Assessing the outcome of pediatric intensive care. *J Pediatr.* 1992;**121**(1):68–74.

86. Fiser DH, Long N, Roberson PK, et al. Relationship of pediatric overall performance category and pediatric cerebral performance category scores at pediatric intensive care unit discharge with outcome measures collected at hospital discharge and 1- and 6-month follow-up assessments. *Crit Care Med.* 2000;**28**(7):2616–20.

87. Mandel R, Martinot A, Delepoulle F, et al. Prediction of outcome after hypoxic-ischemic encephalopathy: a prospective clinical and electrophysiologic study. *J Pediatr.* 2002;**141** (1):45–50.

88. Moler FW, Donaldson AE, Meert K, et al. Multicenter cohort study of out-of-hospital pediatric cardiac arrest. *Crit Care Med.* 2011;**39** (1):141–9.

89. Meert KL, Donaldson A, Nadkarni V, et al. Multicenter cohort study of in-hospital pediatric cardiac arrest. *Pediatr Crit Care Med.* 2009;**10** (5):544–53.

90. Carter BG, Butt W. A prospective study of outcome predictors after severe brain injury in children. *Intensive Care Med.* 2005;**31**(6):840–5.

91. Soar J, Berg KM, Andersen LW, et al., Adult Advanced Life Support Collaborators. Adult Advanced Life Support: 2020 International Consensus on Cardiopulmonary Resuscitation and Emergency Cardiovascular Care Science with Treatment Recommendations. *Resuscitation.* 2020;**156**:A80–A119.

92. Moler FW, Silverstein FS, Holubkov R, et al. Therapeutic hypothermia after out-of-hospital cardiac arrest in children. *N Engl J Med.* 2015;**372** (20):1898–1908.

93. Moler FW, Silverstein FS, Holubkov R, et al. Therapeutic hypothermia after in-hospital cardiac arrest in children. *N Engl J Med.* 2017;**376** (4):318–29.

94. Topjian AA, de Caen A, Wainwright MS, et al. Pediatric post-cardiac arrest care: a scientific statement from the American Heart Association. *Circulation.* 2019;**140**(6):e194–e233.

95. Herman ST, Abend NS, Bleck TP, et al. Consensus statement on continuous eeg in critically ill adults and children, part I: indications. *J Clin Neurophysiol.* 2015;**32**(2):87–95.

96. Topjian AA, Raymond TT, Atkins D, et al., Pediatric Basic and Advanced Life Support Collaborators. Part 4: Pediatric Basic and Advanced Life Support 2020 American Heart Association Guidelines for Cardiopulmonary Resuscitation and Emergency Cardiovascular Care. *Pediatrics.* 2021;**147**(Suppl 1): e2020038505D.

97. Topjian AA, Raymond TT, Atkins D, et al. Pediatric Basic and Advanced Life Support Collaborators. Part 4: Pediatric Basic and Advanced Life Support: 2020 American Heart Association Guidelines for Cardiopulmonary Resuscitation and Emergency Cardiovascular Care. *Circulation.* 2020;**142**(16 Suppl 2):S469–S523.

98. Plog BA, Dashnaw ML, Hitomi E, et al. Biomarkers of traumatic injury are transported from brain to blood via the glymphatic system. *J Neurosci.* 2015;**35**(2):518–26.

99. Thiagarajan RR, Barbaro RP, Rycus PT, et al. Extracorporeal Life Support Organization Registry International Report 2016. *ASAIO J.* 2017;**63**(1):60–7.

100. Barrett CS, Bratton SL, Salvin JW, et al. Neurological injury after extracorporeal membrane oxygenation use to aid pediatric cardiopulmonary resuscitation. *Pediatr Crit Care Med.* 2009;**10**(4):445–51.

101. Waitzer E, Riley SP, Perreault T, Shevell MI. Neurologic outcome at school entry for newborns treated with extracorporeal membrane oxygenation for noncardiac indications. *J Child Neurol.* 2009;**24**(7):801–6.

102. Schiller RM, Madderom MJ, Reuser JJ, et al. Neuropsychological follow-up after neonatal ECMO. *Pediatrics.* 2016;**138**(5).

103. Yu YR, Carpenter JL, DeMello AS, et al. Evaluating quality of life of extracorporeal membrane oxygenation survivors using the pediatric quality of life inventory survey. *J Pediatr Surg.* 2018;**53**(5):1060–4.

104. Nijhuis-van der Sanden MW, van der Cammen-van Zijp MH, Janssen AJ, et al. Motor performance in five-year-old extracorporeal membrane oxygenation survivors: a population-based study. *Crit Care.* 2009;**13**(2):R47.

105. Gupta P, McDonald R, Chipman CW, et al. 20-year experience of prolonged extracorporeal

membrane oxygenation in critically ill children with cardiac or pulmonary failure. *Ann Thorac Surery.* 2012;**93**(5):1584–90.

106. Carpenter JL, Yu YR, Cass DL, et al. Use of venovenous ECMO for neonatal and pediatric ECMO: a decade of experience at a tertiary children's hospital. *Pediatr Surg Int.* 2018;**34** (3):263–8.

107. Teele SA, Salvin JW, Barrett CS, et al. The association of carotid artery cannulation and neurologic injury in pediatric patients supported with venoarterial extracorporeal membrane oxygenation. *Pediatr Crit Care.* 2014;**15**(4):355–61.

108. Golej J, Trittenwein G, Early detection of neurologic injury and issues of rehabilitation after pediatric cardiac extracorporeal membrane oxygenation. *Artif Organs.* 1999;**23**(11):1020–5.

109. Van Heijst A, Liem D, Hopman J, Van Der Staak F, Sengers R. Oxygenation and hemodynamics in left and right cerebral hemispheres during induction of veno-arterial extracorporeal membrane oxygenation. *J Pediatr.* 2004;**144**(2):223–8.

110. Hunter CJ, Blood AB, Bishai JM, et al. Cerebral blood flow and oxygenation during venoarterial and venovenous extracorporeal membrane oxygenation in the newborn lamb. *Pediatr Crit Care.* 2004;**5**(5):475–81.

111. Weber TR, Kountzman B. The effects of venous occlusion on cerebral blood flow characteristics during ECMO. *J Pediatr Surg.* 1996;**31**(8):1124–7.

112. Rodriguez RA, Belway D. Comparison of two different extracorporeal circuits on cerebral embolization during cardiopulmonary bypass in children. *Perfusion.* 2006;**21**(5):247–53.

113. Zanatta P, Forti A, Bosco E, et al. Microembolic signals and strategy to prevent gas embolism during extracorporeal membrane oxygenation. *J Cardiothorac Surg.* 2010;**5**:5.

114. Vogler C, Sotelo-Avila C, Lagunoff D, et al. Aluminum-containing emboli in infants treated with extracorporeal membrane oxygenation. *N Engl J Med.* 1988;**319**(2):75–7.

115. Bembea MM, Felling R, Anton B, Salorio CF, Johnston MV. Neuromonitoring during extracorporeal membrane oxygenation: a systematic review of the literature. *Pediatr Crit Care Med.* 2015;**16**(6):558–64.

116. Schiller RM, Tibboel D. Neurocognitive outcome after treatment with(out) ECMO for neonatal critical respiratory or cardiac failure. *Front Pediatr.* 2019;**7**:494.

117. Bembea MM, Felling RJ, Caprarola SD, et al. Neurologic outcomes in a two-center cohort of

neonatal and pediatric patients supported on extracorporeal membrane oxygenation. *ASAIO J.* 2020;**66**(1):79–88.

118. Bembea MM, Rizkalla N, Freedy J, et al. Plasma biomarkers of brain injury as diagnostic tools and outcome predictors after extracorporeal membrane oxygenation. *Crit Care Med.* 2015;**43** (10):2202–11.

119. Boyle K, Felling R, Yiu A, et al. Neurologic outcomes after extracorporeal membrane oxygenation: a systematic review. *Pediatr Crit Care Med.* 2018;**19**(8):760–6.

120. Madderom MJ, Reuser JJ, Utens EM, et al. Neurodevelopmental, educational and behavioral outcome at 8 years after neonatal ECMO: a nationwide multicenter study. *Intensive Care Med.* 2013;**39**(9):1584–93.

121. Bolton JL, Short AK, Simeone KA, Daglian J, Baram TZ. Programming of stress-sensitive neurons and circuits by early-life experiences. *Front Behav Neurosci.* 2019;**13**:30.

122. Payne ET, Zhao XY, Frndova H, et al. Seizure burden is independently associated with short term outcome in critically ill children. *Brain.* 2014;**137**(Pt 5):1429–38.

123. Lalgudi Ganesan S, Hahn CD : Electrographic seizure burden and outcomes following pediatric status epilepticus. *Epilepsy Behav.* 2019;**101**(Pt B):106409.

124. Abend NS, Gutierrez-Colina AM, Topjian AA, et al. Nonconvulsive seizures are common in critically ill children. *Neurology.* 2011;**76** (12):1071–7.

125. Herman ST, Abend NS, Bleck TP, et al. Consensus statement on continuous eeg in critically ill adults and children, part I: indications. *J Clin Neurophysiol.* 2015;**32**:87–95.

126. Abend NS. Electrographic status epilepticus in children with critical illness: epidemiology and outcome. *Epilepsy Behav.* 2015;**49**:223–7.

127. Pinchefsky EF, Hahn CD. Outcomes following electrographic seizures and electrographic status epilepticus in the pediatric and neonatal ICUs. *Curr Opin Neurol.* 2017;**30**(2):156–64.

128. Payne E, Zhao X, Frndova H, et al. Seizure burden is independently associated with short term outcome in critically ill children. *Brain.* 2014;**137**:1429–38.

129. Abend N, Arndt D, Carpenter J, et al. Electrographic seizures in pediatric ICU patients: cohort study of risk factors and mortality. *Neurology.* 2013;**81**:383–91.

130. Topjian AA, Gutierrez-Colina AM, Sanchez SM, et al. Electrographic status epilepticus is

associated with mortality and worse short-term outcome in critically ill children. *Crit Care Med.* 2013;**41**(1):215–23.

131. Lambrechtsen F, Buchalter J. Aborted and refractory status epilepticus in children: a comparative analysis. *Epilepsia.* 2008;**49**:615–25.

132. Wagenman K, Blake T, Sanchez S, et al. Electrographic status epilepticus and long-term outcome in critically ill children. *Neurology.* 2014;**82**:396–404.

133. Abend NS, Wagenman KL, Blake TP, et al. Electrographic status epilepticus and neurobehavioral outcomes in critically ill children. *Epilepsy Behav.* 2015;**49**:238–44.

134. Gaynor JW, Jarvik GP, Gerdes M, et al. Postoperative electroencephalographic seizures are associated with deficits in executive function and social behaviors at 4 years of age following cardiac surgery in infancy. *J Thorac Cardiovasc. Surg* 2013;**146**(1):132–7.

135. Kachmar AG, Irving SY, Connolly CA, Curley MAQ. A systematic review of risk factors associated with cognitive impairment after pediatric critical illness. *Pediatr Crit Care Med.* 2018;**19**(3):e164–e171.

136. Dervan LA, Di Gennaro JL, Farris RWD, Watson RS. Delirium in a tertiary PICU: risk factors and outcomes. *Pediatr Crit Care Med.* 2020;**21**(1):21–32.

137. Kirschen MP, Walter JK. Ethical issues in neuroprognostication after severe pediatric brain injury. *Semin Pediatr Neurol.* 2015;**22** (3):187–95.

138. Tasker RC, Westland AG, White DK, Williams GB. Corpus callosum and inferior forebrain white matter microstructure are related to functional outcome from raised intracranial pressure in child traumatic brain injury. *Dev Neurosci.* 2010;**32**(5–6):374–84.

139. Tasker RC. Changes in white matter late after severe traumatic brain injury in childhood. *Develop Neurosci.* 2006; **28**(4–5):302–8.

140. Feickert HJ, Drommer S, Heyer R. Severe head injury in children: impact of risk factors on outcome. *J Trauma.* 1999;**47**(1):33–8.

141. Barlow K, Thompson E, Johnson D, Minns RA. The neurological outcome of non-accidental head injury. *Pediatr Rehabil.* 2004;**7**(3):195–203.

142. Tomita H, Ito U, Saito J, Maehara T. Cerebral atrophy after severe head injury. *Adv Neurol.* 1990;**52**:553.

143. Onuma T, Shimosegawa Y, Kameyama M, Arai H, Ishii K. Clinicopathological investigation of gyral high density on computerized tomography following severe head injury in children. *J Neurosurg.* 1995;**82**(6):995–1001.

144. Levin HS, Benavidez DA, Verger-Maestre K, et al. Reduction of corpus callosum growth after severe traumatic brain injury in children. *Neurology.* 2000;**54**(3):647–63.

145. Grados MA, Slomine BS, Gerring JP, et al. Depth of lesion model in children and adolescents with moderate to severe traumatic brain injury: use of SPGR MRI to predict severity and outcome. *J Neurol Neurosurg Psychiatry.* 2001;**70**(3):350–8.

146. Tasker RC, Salmond CH, Westland AG, et al. Head circumference and brain and hippocampal volume after severe traumatic brain injury in childhood. *Pediatr Res.* 2005;**58**(2):302–8.

147. Wilde EA, Hunter JV, Newsome MR, et al. Frontal and temporal morphometric findings on MRI in children after moderate to severe traumatic brain injury. *J Neurotrauma.* 2005;**22**(3):333–44.

148. Wainwright MS, Grimason M, Goldstein J, et al. Building a pediatric neurocritical care program: a multidisciplinary approach to clinical practice and education from the intensive care unit to the outpatient clinic. *Semin Pediatr Neurol.* 2014;**21** (4):248–54.

Chapter 18

Prognostication in Palliative Care and Neurocritical Care

Shannon Hextrum, Viren Patel, and Edward M. Manno

Introduction

Neuroprognostication, the focus of this book, is crucial toward the management of the highly complex patient in the neurological intensive care unit (Neuro ICU). It is of primary importance to understand the nature of the disease and the potential for recovery. Informed prognostication by neurologically trained physicians has been hypothesized to be a significant reason for the improved outcomes of neurological patients managed in a Neuro ICU versus general medical ICUs.[1]

Decisions surrounding withdrawal of life-sustaining therapies (WLST) are highly dependent on prognosis. In a retrospective study of Neuro ICU patients who were terminally extubated, family members surveyed most frequently cited quality of life, prognosis, and the patient's previously known wishes as "very important" in their decision to remove life-sustaining therapy.[2]

Evidence-based prognostication in the Neuro ICU is difficult, and may be biased by the effect of WLST on patient mortality. Rabinstein (2009) argues that studies of prognostic features in this patient population have not adequately factored in the effect of WLST. Physicians may be less aggressive with certain patients deemed to have poor prognosis, leading to early WLST, and those patients' outcomes become further data points to support the notion of poor prognosis, the "self-fulfilling prophecy."[3] Thus. it is important to understand and delineate prognosis as best we can in the Neuro ICU.

This chapter will review the history of grading scales to assess outcomes, the impact of prognostication on both families and ICU personnel, and finally outline suggestions for the process itself.

History of Defining Impaired Neurological States

From the first cardiac defibrillation to ventilatory support and organ transplantation, the twentieth century brought significant progress in medical care. Such advances were seen in tandem with new ethical issues involving the approach to the comatose patient and neuroprognostication.[4,5] In 1968, an ad hoc committee was formed at Harvard Medical School to create a definition of brain death described as irreversible coma, and in part suggested limitation in care based on medical futility.[4,6] The committee defined irreversible coma by the following: unresponsiveness to external stimuli, no spontaneous breathing nor spontaneous muscle movements, and no brainstem reflexes. Electroencephalogram (EEG) was recommended for confirmation testing.[6]

Such clear definitions of brain death did little to address the medical and legal standards for the comatose patient, an issue that would gain significant attention in the following years through landmark cases. In April 1975, Karen Ann Quinlan arrived at the Newton Memorial Hospital after absence of breathing for at least two episodes. She was unresponsive and lacked pupillary activity on arrival. While details of the events leading to her hospitalization are still incomplete, anoxic injury was determined to be the underlying etiology of her coma. Upon transfer to Saint Claire's Hospital, she received a tracheotomy. She subsequently developed sleep-wake cycles, and her level of consciousness was described by physicians as a persistent vegetative state (the more modern term being "unresponsive wakefulness syndrome").[7] When Ms. Quinlan's family requested removal of life-sustaining therapy, their physician refused, a decision supported by the hospital as well as the state of New Jersey. The case entered the New Jersey Supreme Court on appeal, which reversed the initial ruling on the basis that the decision to withdraw life support was protected under the constitutional right of privacy.[8]

The Quinlan case established a legal precedent for withdrawal of life-sustaining therapy, as well

261

as upheld the right of competent, surrogate decision makers to withdraw life support on behalf of an incompetent patient. A remarkable and perhaps unappreciated feature of the Karen Ann Quinlan case was that she survived nearly 10 years after ventilatory support was discontinued. Drs. Siegler and Taylor discussed the importance of acknowledging her prolonged survival, underscoring the outstanding nursing care and support she undoubtedly received.[9]

The Quinlan case set into motion a number of publications concerning the removal of life-sustaining therapy in the ICU.[5] The President's Commission for the Study of Ethical Problems in Medicine and Biomedical and Behavioral Research (1983) established consensus-based ethical guidelines on these issues.[10] With regard to treatment of permanently unconscious patients, the report stressed the importance of respect for the patient's body and appropriate allocation of community resources. The decision to pursue artificial feedings was deemed justified if in line with surrogate goals to sustain the patient for the hope of potential recovery. However, an intervention such as dialysis was described as "very hard to justify" (p. 190) in the permanently unconscious patient. [10]

Further legal precedent was established on the specific question of artificial nutrition in the case of Nancy Cruzan, which was ultimately decided in the US Supreme Court.[11] After suffering the results of an automobile accident, Cruzan was diagnosed as being in a permanent vegetative state, though she did not require ventilatory support. According to Cruzan's parents, a feeding tube was not consistent with her previously stated wishes regarding quality of life. Though a trial judge supported the family's decision, the Missouri Supreme Court reversed this ruling on the grounds that there was not enough evidence that the patient herself would refuse this treatment. In this case, the US Supreme Court ultimately protected the right for patients to refuse life-sustaining therapy; however, the court simultaneously upheld the state's right to require clear evidence of a non-decisional patient's prior wishes for removing life-sustaining interventions. This ruling led to the Patient Self-Determination Act, which promoted widespread use of healthcare advance directives.[5,12]

Contemporary Ethical Issues

The decision to withdraw care in the Neuro ICU is one of the most challenging that families and healthcare providers must face. The right to withhold unwanted treatment is based on a patient's right to autonomy.[3] As the previously discussed court cases highlight, the principle of autonomy may be at odds with the principle of beneficence, or acting in the best interests of the patient.[13] Further, the concept of futility is an ethical challenge in patients with impaired consciousness. Treatments sustaining life in the permanently unconscious patient may be deemed futile by some; however, this concept also implies certainty in the prognosis of future unconsciousness as well as subjective judgments regarding quality of life.[3]

When limits are placed on patient care, there are ethical considerations in how this process should unfold. A consensus statement by the American College of Critical Care Medicine highlights three core ethical principles regarding WLST. First, the act of withholding therapy (not providing it in the first place) and that of withdrawing therapy (removing it once initiated) share equal ethical ground. Second, allowing death is distinct from causing death, a concept explored in the landmark Quinlan case. Third, therapy may be given when intended to relieve pain and suffering, even if such therapy may hasten the dying process.[14]

Decisions regarding limitations on medical therapy in the ICU are complicated by variable approaches in which care is de-escalated.[15] One potentially controversial approach involves not escalating care, which allows for a distinction between withdrawal and withholding treatments. [16] Such an approach may be seen as a compromise between the extremes of comfort measures and full medical therapy, where interventions such as vasopressors, antibiotics, hemodialysis, or mechanical ventilation may be withdrawn or not initiated depending on the patient's or family's preferences.[17] However, this practice has brought up ethical concerns. For one, there may be inherent confusion regarding the true goals of care. When treatment is not aimed strictly on comfort nor strictly on full therapy, it can be seen as ineffective at reaching either goal. Such an approach can be misleading to families, and even prolong suffering and dying. As an alternative, authors Curtis and Rubenfeld advocate the concept of "time limited trial," of full medical therapy prior to formally pursuing comfort-focused measures.[18]

Who, What, When, and Where to Prognosticate

Palliative care decisions may be complicated by the unique trajectories of neurocritical illness, namely the sudden and unanticipated functional decline in the patients' status in contrast to conditions with gradual progression of disease.[19,20] Family members coping with such unexpected events are responsible for crucial end-of-life decision making. Withdrawal of life-sustaining therapies accounts for a majority of deaths in the Neuro ICU, another feature demonstrating the important role of surrogate decision makers in the end-of-life care process.[19,21,22]

The Neurocritical Care Society's (NCS) position statement on devastating brain injury recommends a 72-hour window of observation prior to WLST, as well as multiple examinations over time for the purposes of improved prognostication.[23] Similarly, the American Heart Association (AHA) and American Stroke Association (ASA) guidelines for spontaneous intracerebral hemorrhage recommend waiting until day two of hospitalization prior to placing any new do-not-resuscitate (DNR) orders.[19,24]

Identifying palliative care needs early on is strongly supported by the NCS guidelines.[23] A qualitative study of palliative care consultations within the Neuro ICU at Harborview Medical Center revealed that prognosis was a chief focus of discussion. The authors suggest a distinction between palliative care approaches in medical ICUs, which may focus more attention on symptom management than on prognostication.[25–27]

Available Data: Physician Trends in Withdrawal of Life-Sustaining Treatment

Given the significant role of prognosis in establishing care goals in the Neuro ICU, it is important to examine any variation between how practitioners may prognosticate. A Canadian survey of physicians directly involved in the care of patients with traumatic brain injury (TBI) found significant variation in

scenario-based questions regarding a patient's prognosis. The case involved a 25-year-old male with a Glasgow Coma Scale score of a 6 on admission who remained clinically unchanged after 1 week. Approximately one-third of those surveyed agreed or strongly agreed that the patient's 1-year outcome would be unfavorable. The remaining 41% disagreed or strongly disagreed with such prognosis, and 29% reported feeling neutral. Important variation was observed between specialties, with neurologists most likely to predict unfavorable prognosis (50%).[28]

Variation in physician approach to end-of-life issues may also be affected by religious affiliations, as was demonstrated in a prospective observational study in European ICUs. Cases that involved limitations of care at end of life were analyzed, and such limitations included withholding and withdrawing life-sustaining therapy. Withholding life-sustaining treatment described an approach of not adding or increasing life-sustaining therapy, including withholding cardiopulmonary resuscitation (CPR). By contrast, withdrawing described the active removal of a life-sustaining intervention.[29] Physician religious affiliation showed variation in treatment approach; for instance, physicians identifying as Catholic had a higher frequency of withdrawal of life-sustaining therapy (53%) compared to withholding life-sustaining treatments, while the frequency of withdrawal of life-sustaining therapy was lower for Jewish physicians (19%) and Greek Orthodox physicians (22%).[30]

Research has also been directed at analyzing the content and effectiveness of discussions regarding WLST. One study assessed the perception of physician recommendations using simulated goals-of-care discussion videos between a physician and a surrogate decision maker. The simulated patient was depicted requiring ventilatory support and likely sustaining significant long-term disability. The discussions ended with either the physician providing a recommendation about WLST or no recommendation, and videos were viewed by true surrogate decision makers. Out of 169 participants, 56% indicated their preference for receiving a recommendation directly from the physician, while 42% preferred no recommendation. There was no relationship found between specific preferences and demographic details. Such contrasting views by surrogates underscores the importance of close attention to needs and preference of surrogates in the context of shared decision making.[31,32]

A recent qualitative survey of surrogate decision makers for critically ill patients with TBI assessed communication strategies of practitioners. While the sample size was small (16 surrogates and 20 physicians), striking and important themes were illuminated. For instance, 82% of surrogates indicated preference for precise numerical data in discussions of prognosis, while 75% of physicians reported avoiding the use of specific numbers in outcome predictions. Understandably, surrogates often expressed frustration and difficulty with the uncertainty in prognostication, while physicians tended to cite the importance of communicating issues of uncertainty in prognosis.[33] Greater attention to understanding and validating the concerns of surrogate decision makers may help improve communication and care in the Neuro ICU.

Assessment of Outcomes: Functional Outcome Scales

Since end-of-life decisions are heavily based on prognosis, it is important to understand how we measure long-term functional outcomes. Defining "functional outcome" is somewhat difficult. What may be considered functional for one individual may be totally unacceptable to another. However, in order to assess, codify, and study treatment modalities, functional scores needed to be developed. The most commonly used functional outcome scores, include the Barthel index, modified Rankin Scale, Extended Glasgow Outcome Scale, and Glasgow-Pittsburgh Cerebral Performance Category (Table 18.1). Newer scales are often used in secondary analyses.

The Barthel Index (BI), developed in 1965, is scored from 0 through 100 and is used as a measure of a patient's ability to perform activities of daily living (ADL)[34]. These include, but are not limited to, an evaluation of feeding, bowel and bladder control, grooming, bathing, dressing, and mobility. While the scoring system evaluates a patient's ability to maintain self-care and mobility, there is inconsistent use of the BI in clinical trials within Neurocritical Care. This may be explained by the ambiguity in the definition of a favorable outcome, questioning the clinical relevance of the score.[35] For example, some trials

define favorable outcome as a score greater than 50, whereas others use a cut-off of greater than 95. Achieving a score greater than 60 has been associated with patients moving from assisted dependence to independence, whereas a score of 85 correlates with independence with minimal assistance.[36] Defining a good outcome with the BI remains controversial, and is a limitation of its use in clinical trials.

The modified Rankin Scale (mRS) is one of the most commonly used measures of neurological outcome in clinical trials (see Table 18.1). First introduced in 1957, the mRS was developed to be a gross measure of handicap and impairment after stroke.[37] The original scale developed by Dr. Rankin was a grading system from 1 to 5, with 1 meaning non-disabling stroke. The modification of the scale to its modern form of 0 to 6 was first introduced in the UK-TIA study group through the addition of grade 0 as no symptoms and grade 6 as death. The UK-TIA study group defined mRS grade 0–2 as non-disabling strokes, whereas grades 3–5 were considered disabling. [38,39] There is less variability in the definition of a good outcome on the mRS compared to the BI. [35]

The Glasgow Outcome Scale (GOS), developed in 1975,[40] has historically been used as the primary clinical outcome measure for studies of traumatic brain injury (TBI). A scale of 1 to 5 scale characterized the following outcomes: 1 – death, 2 – vegetative state, 3 – severe disability, 4 – moderate disability, and 5 – good recovery. The Extended Glasgow Outcome Scale (GOS-E) was developed in response to concerns of a relative lack of sensitivity in characterizing and observing improvement in various mental and physical deficits in a TBI patient.[41] The significant difference between the GOS and GOS-E is that severe disability, moderate disability, and good recovery are split into lower and upper categories, resulting in a scale from 1 to 8. This scale expansion allows for more subtle differentiation in clinical outcomes, as well as increased sensitivity to detect changes in clinical trials compared to its predecessor.[42] The GOS-E remains the primary outcome scale used in current studies of TBI.[43]

The Glasgow-Pittsburgh Cerebral Performance Category (CPC) scale is commonly used for neurological prognostication after cardiac arrest (although mRS has recently become the more commonly utilized scale), and is a modification of the

Table 18.1 Primary outcomes used in various landmark trials in neurocritical care

Clinical trial	Primary outcome
Alteplase in Acute Ischemic Stroke – NINDS[80] – ECASS II[81]	– Barthel Index, modified Rankin Scale (mRS), Glasgow Outcomes Scale (GOS), National Institutes of Health Stroke Scale (NIHSS) – Modified Rankin Scale
Delayed Endovascular Thrombectomy in Proximal Large Vessel Occlusion – DAWN[82] – DEFUSE-3[83]	– Modified Rankin Scale – Modified Rankin Scale
Decompressive Hemicraniectomy for Malignant MCA syndrome – DESTINY[84] – DECIMAL[85] – HAMLET[86]	– Modified Rankin Scale – Modified Rankin Scale – Modified Rankin Scale
Blood Pressure Control in Intracranial Hemorrhage (ICH) – INTERACT–2[87] – ATACH–2[88]	– Modified Rankin Scale – Modified Rankin Scale
Surgical Intervention in ICH – STICH II[89] – CLEAR III[90] – MISTIE III[91]	– Extended Glasgow Outcome Scale – Modified Rankin Scale – Modified Rankin Scale
Targeted Temperature Management after Cardiac Arrest – Original TTM study [92] – 33 vs. 36 Degrees TTM[93]	– Discharge Location and Disability – All-cause mortality (Glasgow-Pittsburgh Cerebral Performance Category [CPC] and mRS were secondary)
Select studies in Traumatic Brain Injury: – DECRA[94] – MRC CRASH[95]	– Extended Glasgow Outcomes Scale – Death within 2 weeks, death or dependence at 6 months (based on GOS)

aforementioned Glasgow Outcome Scale. The CPC includes the following scoring system: 1 – conscious and alert with normal function or slight disability, 2 – conscious and alert with moderate disability, 3- conscious with severe disability, 4 – comatose or persistent vegetative state, 5 – brain dead. A good clinical outcome is defined as a CPC grade 1–2.[44] While there is concern about variability in inter- and intra-reviewer agreement, the CPC allows for an efficient evaluation of neurological recovery for landmark clinical trials in patients after cardiac arrest.[45]

Alternative Measures of Outcomes

While the previous outcome scales provided scoring systems for general outcomes, they have been criticized for their limited evaluation of neurocognitive and psychological deficits. In an effort to increase uniformity and improve the evaluation of cognitive function beyond that of disability, a number of outcome assessments have been developed.

The EuroQoL group was formed in 1987, and was composed of a multidisciplinary team of experts from Sweden, Finland, Norway, the Netherlands, and the UK, with an ultimate aim to standardize health-related quality-of-life measures in order to determine the effectiveness of various medical interventions.[46] The EQ-5D was thus developed. The EQ-5D contains a state of health description and a self-evaluation of health. The state of health domains examined include mobility, self-care, conduct of activities, pain/discomfort, and anxiety/depression.[47] The self-evaluation of health involves the patient providing a numeric valuation of his or her health on a visual scale (with 0 = worst imaginable and 100 = best imaginable). The EQ-5D has been expanded for use in a variety of health-related studies, including population health studies, health technology assessment, and cost-effectiveness analysis beyond Neurocritical Care.[46,48]

Similar to the aim of EuroQoL, the National Institutes of Health (NIH) Blueprint in 2006 aimed to develop a battery of assessment tools of core neurological and behavioral functions that would allow for standardization of outcomes across population studies and clinical trials.[49] The NIH Toolbox was thus developed and provided a comprehensive evaluation of motor, cognitive, sensory, and emotional function.[50] The assessment tool has been evaluated by multiple expert working groups and is available online. It is designed to be used across one's life span, ranging from ages 3 through 85 years.

Other health-related quality-of-life measures include the Neuro-QOL, which evaluates 13 measures including anxiety, depression, fatigue, motor function, cognition, emotion, and sleep, as well as ability to participate in social activities.[51] Other tools that have been developed include the TBI-QOL for patients with TBI and the SCI-QOL for patients with spinal cord injury. This multitude of outcome measures attempts to address the more subtle, yet perhaps more clinically meaningful data for patients and their families. Understanding these outcome measures is imperative to neuroprognostication and facilitating family discussions.

The Impact of Withdrawal of Life-Sustaining Measures on Families

In a study of critical care physicians, nearly all (96%) had withheld or withdrawn life-sustaining medical treatment based upon their expectation of a patient's death.[52] From a medicolegal perspective in the United States, withholding or withdrawal of life-sustaining medical treatment is legally acceptable if the decision is made by a competent patient or their healthcare surrogate.[53] The healthcare surrogate, if not decided upon prior to the occurrence of a neurological injury, will often be a spouse or surviving adult children. The surrogacy hierarchy is often legally coded in many states and provides guidance to providers in terms of whom to turn to when considering WLST.

Making a decision regarding WLST and initiating comfort measures can have a significant impact on families. Families have reported anxiety and distress, which can be exacerbated by poor communication from medical providers.[54] Poor communication and mistrust in physicians often leads to healthcare surrogates wanting more control over the decision-making process of WLST.[55] Furthermore, post-traumatic stress disorder (PTSD) has been described 90 days after ICU discharge or death in family members who shared in end-of-life care decision making.[56] While there remains a significant need to better understand the prevalence of PTSD in family members of patients in an ICU,[57] the act of WLST itself appears to have a variable impact on PTSD symptomatology.

Clear and consistent communication appears to be a significant component to improving family satisfaction during this arduous time.

Other studies, however, have found that participating in the end-of-life care decision-making process provided families with a sense of control and relief. This was achieved through the perception of providing an end to suffering and being able to follow a loved one's values.[58]

A majority of families are satisfied with their decision, and their loved one's death is often dignified and compassionate after WLST.[55] A Canadian study found that most families perceive their dying family member as being comfortable during the withdrawal of life-sustaining measures.[59] Factors that were associated with greater family satisfaction included a better understanding of the process, the patient appearing comfortable, adequate time for preparing family and friends, and privacy during the end of life.[60] Other factors that also increased family satisfaction include a decision that is consistent with the patient's wishes, consistency with physician recommendations, and a discussion of family spiritual practices.[61] Economically, effective family communication at the end of life is associated with deceased lengths of stay in the ICU and hospital, as well as decreased financial costs.[62,63]

Caregiver Impact of Prolonged Care in the Neurologically Devastated Patient

The impact of maintaining full medical support in patients with significant neurological injuries has a myriad of effects that extend beyond the patient. The true incidence of devastating neurological injury is unknown and depends on the nature of the injury. An estimated 69 million individuals suffer from a prior TBI worldwide,[64] and the prevalence of patients with in a persistent vegetative state (or unresponsive wakefulness) is estimated to be anywhere from 0.5–3.36 patients per 100,000.[65,66] These numbers do not include patients who have neurological injury from other etiologies, including ischemic or hemorrhage stroke, encephalitis, or other neurological insults. Much of the literature regarding the impact of maintaining prolonged medical treatment, including life-sustaining measures, comes from studies on TBI and patients in a persistent vegetative state.

These studies suggest that caring for a patient with severe TBI or persistent vegetative state can have a profound detrimental impact on the caregiver, described as a "miserable" quality of life.[67] Increased rates of caregiver depression, somatization, and alcoholism have been reported, as well as families neglecting other illnesses in the family. [67–69] As the duration of time that a patient exists in a persistent vegetative state increases, so do feelings of isolation and emotional distress in caregivers and their families.[70] Prolonged grief disorder was found to be present in 60% of caregivers of patients with disorders of consciousness. [71] A study of caregivers of patients in a persistent vegetative state found that the entire family can suffer physical, mental, social, and financial setbacks.[72] The impact of the patients' neurological injuries on families is often underappreciated, and should be considered in the context of palliative care.

Similar issues exist for patients with better outcomes and who are able to participate in rehabilitation. In a study of patients at an average of 14 years post-injury, patients with TBI experienced high levels of depression, a sense of burden to their family, and a higher rate of divorce compared to the national average. This finding exists even in patients who remain employed and are living independently.[73,74] In a 20-year follow-up study of patients with TBI, 32% continued to exhibit aggressive or sexual behavior, and a majority (61%) had no social contacts. The significant psychological and social impact of a brain injury, from increased social isolation to changes in behavior and personality, were described to be more disabling than their physical disability.[74,75]

The Process of Changing Goals of Care and Initiating Withdrawal of Aggressive Medical Support

Once the decision has been made to withdraw aggressive medical support, the focus of care changes from treating a specific illness to providing comfort for the patient and their loved ones. [15] This new goal must be clearly defined and discussed with the surrogate decision makers. The process itself should be described in simple but clear terms. Documentation is crucial and should be documented clearly that these decisions are consistent with the patient's previously

Table 18.2 Opioid protocol for palliative extubation and end-of-life care

Medication	Recommended titration
Morphine	New start: – Morphine 5–10 mg IV bolus. Then 2–5 mg/h continuous infusion • With discomfort, consider additional bolus of 50% of the hourly dose. May titrate dose every 10 minutes with increase by 25%–50% as needed Continuation: – Bolus 100% of the hourly dosage and increase the infusion rate by 25% for discomfort

Fentanyl	New start:
	– Fentanyl 50–100 mcg IV. Then 25–100 mcg/h continuous infusion
	  • With discomfort, consider additional bolus of 50% of the hourly dose. May titrate dose every 10 minutes with increase by 25–50% as needed
	   Continuation of previous opioids:
	– Fentanyl: Bolus 25–50% of the hourly dosage and increase the infusion rate by 25%.

*Adapted from Coradazzi et al.[76]

expressed desires, and that the family is providing substituted judgment based on the patient's values (in other words, saying what the patient themselves would say, if they were able to make the decision were they not incapacitated).

Withdrawal of aggressive medical support typically proceeds in a stepwise fashion, with vasopressor support being discontinued prior to extubation. If airway management is an issue, oral or nasal airways can be placed to prevent acute obstruction. Monitors are turned off in the room (but can be maintained at the nursing station), and alarms and distractions should be minimized. Routine blood draws and medication administration, other than for comfort, are discontinued.

Sedation and pain medications are best titrated in a previously developed protocol or algorithm (e.g., see Table 18.2).[76] Titration can occur expeditiously if needed for comfort. Physicians are covered under the precept of "double effect" – permissibility of performing a morally good act (i.e., controlling pain with medication), which may result in an unintended outcome (i.e., hastening of death).[77] Use of neuromuscular blockade should always be avoided, since it may block evidence of distress.

Prediction of the timing of death is very difficult. It is important to counsel families in potential scenarios, and give a range of time, varying from minutes to hours, and sometimes days, depending on the nature and severity of the injury. Many may wish to stay with their loved one. Some patients develop terminal body or limb movements such as flexion

in the arms, shoulder adduction, and hands crossing to the chin.[78] It is prudent for family members to sit in order to avoid any vasovagal syncope that may occur in the setting of this psychosocial stressor. Clergy are particularly helpful during this time. Most family criticisms occur during this time, if this process is not sensitively managed.[79]

Conclusions

Neurological prognosis after devastating neurological injury remains imprecise, but being able to best approximate how patients will do has important implications for patients and families. The effect of end-of-life decisions has significant impact on both prognostic models and family well-being. Palliation for the neurological patient has a storied history, and both withholding and withdrawal of medical treatments have both legal and ethical support. Understanding outcome scales and their limitations helps delineate what would be best for a given patient based on their previously stated value system. The process of end-of-life palliative care in the Neuro ICU needs to be performed appropriately and managed with great sensitivity in order to provide adequate closure for all involved in the care of the patient.

References

1. Diringer MN, Edwards DF. Admission to a neurologic/neurosurgical intensive care unit is associated with reduced mortality rate after intracerebral hemorrhage. *Crit Care Med.* 2001;29:635–40.

2. Mayer SA, Kossoff SB. Withdrawal of life support in the neurological intensive care unit. *Neurology.* 1999;**52**:1602–9.

3. Rabinstein AA. Ethical dilemmas in the neurologic ICU: withdrawing life-support measures after devastating brain injury. *Continuum Lifelong Learning Neurol.* 2009;**15**:13–25.

4. De Georgia MA. History of brain death as death: 1968 to the present. *J Crit Care.* 2014;**29**:673–8.

5. Luce JM, White DB. A history of ethics and law in the intensive care unit. *Crit Care Clin.* 2009;**25**:221–37.

6. [no authors listed] A definition of irreversible coma: report of the Ad Hoc Committee of the Harvard Medical School to examine the definition of brain death. *JAMA.* 1968;**205**:337340.

7. In Re Quinlan, 70 N.J. 10, 355 A.2d 647. 1976.

8. Falck DP. In re Quinlan: one court's answer to the problem of death with dignity. *Wash Lee Law Rev.* 1977;**34**:285–308.

9. Siegler M, Taylor RM. Intimacy and caring: the legacy of Karen Ann Quinlan. *Trends Health Care Law Ethics.* 1993;**8**:28–30, 38.

10. *President's Commission for the Study of Ethical Problems in Medicine and Biomedical and Behavioral Research. Deciding to Forego Life-Sustaining Treatment. A report on the Ethical, Medical, and Legal Issues in Treatment decisions.* Washington, DC: US Government Printing Office, 1983.

11. US Supreme Court. Cruzan v. Director, Missouri Department of Health. *Wests Supreme Court Report.* 1990;**110**:2841–92.

12. Annas GJ. Nancy Cruzan and the right to die. *N Engl J Med.* 1990;**323**:670–3.

13. Schor NF. Comment: autonomy vs beneficence. *Neurology.* 2014;**83**:1370.

14. Truog RD, Campbell M, Curtis, Jr., et al. Recommendations for end-of-life care in the intensive care unit: a consensus statement by the American Academy of Critical Care Medicine. *Crit Care Med.* 2008;**36**:953.

15. Manno EM, Wijdicks EF. The declaration of death and the withdrawal of care in the neurologic patient. *Neurol Clin.* 2006;**24**:159–69.

16. Morgan CK, Varas GM, Pedroza C, Almoosa KF. Defining the practice of "no escalation of care" in the ICU. *Crit Care Med.* 2014;**42**:357–61.

17. Thompson DR. "No escalation of treatment" as a routine strategy for decision-making in the ICU: pro. *Intensive Care Med.* 2014;**40**:1372–3.

18. Curtis JR, Rubenfeld GD. "No escalation of treatment" as a routine strategy for decision-

19. Frontera JA, Curtis JR, Nelson JE, et al. Integrating palliative care into the care of neurocritically ill patients: a report from the improving palliative care in the ICU project advisory board and the center to advance palliative care. *Crit Care Med.* 2015;**43**:1964–77.

20. Murray SA, Kendall M, Boyd K, Sheikh A. Illness trajectories and palliative care. *BMJ.* 2005;**330**:1007–11.

21. Diringer MN, Edwards DF, Aiyagari V, Hollingsworth H. Factors associated with withdrawal of mechanical ventilation in a neurology/neurosurgery intensive care unit. *Crit Care Med.* 2001;**29**:1792–7.

22. Prendergast TJ, Luce JM. Increasing incidence of withholding and withdrawal of life support from the critically ill. *Am J Respir Crit Care Med.* 1997;**155**:15–20.

23. Souter MJ, Blissitt PA, Blosser S, et al. Recommendations for the critical care management of devastating brain injury: prognostication, psychosocial, and ethical management. *Neurocritical Care.* 2015;**23**:4–13.

24. Hemphill JC 3rd, Greenberg SM, Anderson CS, et al. Guidelines for the management of spontaneous intracerebral hemorrhage: a guideline for healthcare professionals from the American Heart Association/American Stroke Association. *Stroke.* 2015;**46**:2032–60.

25. Tran LN, Back AL, Creutzfeldt CJ. Palliative care consultations in the neuro-ICU: a qualitative study. *Neurocrit Care.* 2016;**25**:266–72.

26. Yoong J, Park ER, Greer JA, et al. Early palliative care in advanced lung cancer: a qualitative study. *JAMA Intern Med.* 2013;**173**:283–20.

27. Jacobsen J, Jackson V, Dahlin C, et al. Components of early outpatient palliative care consultation in patients with metastatic nonsmall cell lung cancer. *J Palliat Med.* 2011;**14**:459–64.

28. Turgeon AF, Lauzier F, Burns KE, et al. Determination of neurologic prognosis and clinical decision making in adult patients with severe traumatic brain injury: a survey of Canadian intensivists, neurosurgeons, and neurologists. *Crit Care Med.* 2013;**41**:1086–93.

29. Sprung CL, Cohen SL, Sjokvist P, et al. End-of-life practices in European intensive care units: the Ethicus study. *JAMA.* 2003;**290**:790–7.

30. Sprung CL, Maia P, Bulow HH, et al. The importance of religious affiliation and culture on end-of-life decisions in European intensive care units. *Intensive Care Med.* 2007;**33**:1732–9.

making in the ICU: con. *Intensive Care Med.* 2014;**40**:1374–6.

31. White DB, Evans LR, Bautista CA, Luce JM, Lo B. Are physicians' recommendations to limit life support beneficial or burdensome? Bringing empirical data to the debate. *Am J Respir Crit Care Med.* 2009;**180**:320–5.

32. Charles C, Whelan T, Gafni A. What do we mean by partnership in making decisions about treatment? *BMJ.* 1999;**319**:780–2.

33. Quinn T, Moskowitz J, Khan MW, et al. What families need and physicians deliver: contrasting communication preferences between surrogate decision-makers and physicians during outcome prognostication in critically ill TBI patients. *Neurocrit Care.* 2017;**27**:154–62.

34. Mahoney FI, Barthel DW. Functional evaluation: the Barthel Index. *Md State Med J.* 1965;**14**:61–5.

35. Sulter G, Steen C, De Keyser J. Use of the Barthel Index and modified Rankin Scale in acute stroke trials. *Stroke.* 1999;**30**:1538–41.

36. Granger CV, Dewis LS, Peters NC, Sherwood CC, Barrett JE. Stroke rehabilitation: analysis of repeated Barthel Index measures. *Arch Phys Med Rehabil.* 1979;**60**:14–17.

37. Rankin J. Cerebral vascular accidents in patients over the age of 60. II. Prognosis. *Scott Med J.* 1957;**2**:200–15.

38. Farrell B, Godwin J, Richards S, Warlow C. The United Kingdom Transient Ischaemic Attack (UK-TIA) aspirin trial: final results. *J Neurol Neurosurg Psychiatry.* 1991;**54**:1044–54.

39. van Swieten JC, Koudstaal PJ, Visser MC, Schouten HJ, van Gijn J. Interobserver agreement for the assessment of handicap in stroke patients. *Stroke.* 1988;**19**:604–7.

40. Jennett B, Bond M. Assessment of outcome after severe brain damage. *Lancet.* 1975;**1**:480–4.

41. Jennett B, Snoek J, Bond MR, Brooks N. Disability after severe head injury: observations on the use of the Glasgow Outcome Scale. *J Neurol Neurosurg Psychiatry.* 1981;**44**:285–93.

42. Weir J, Steyerberg EW, Butcher I, et al. Does the extended Glasgow Outcome Scale add value to the conventional Glasgow Outcome Scale? *J Neurotrauma.* 2012;**29**:53–8.

43. Okonkwo DO, Shutter LA, Moore C, et al. Brain oxygen optimization in severe traumatic brain injury phase-II: a phase II randomized trial. *Crit Care Med.* 2017;**45**:1907–14.

44. Brain Resuscitation Clinical Trial IISG. A randomized clinical study of a calcium-entry blocker (lidoflazine) in the treatment of comatose survivors of cardiac arrest. *N Engl J Med.* 1991;**324**:1225–31.

45. Ajam K, Gold LS, Beck SS, et al. Reliability of the cerebral performance category to classify neurological status among survivors of ventricular fibrillation arrest: a cohort study. *Scand J Trauma Resusc Emerg Med.* 2011;**19**:38.

46. Devlin NJ, Brooks R. EQ-5D and the EuroQol Group: past, present and future. *Appl Health Econ Health Policy.* 2017;**15**:127–37.

47. Whynes DK, Group T. Correspondence between EQ-5D health state classifications and EQ VAS scores. *Health Qual Life Outcomes.* 2008;**6**:94.

48. Rabin R, de Charro F. EQ-5D: a measure of health status from the EuroQol Group. *Ann Med.* 2001;**33**:337–43.

49. Hodes RJ, Insel TR, Landis SC, Research NIHBf N. The NIH Toolbox: setting a standard for biomedical research. *Neurology.* 2013;**80**:S1.

50. Gershon RC, Cella D, Fox NA, et al. Assessment of neurological and behavioural function: the NIH Toolbox. *Lancet Neurol.* 2010;**9**:138–9.

51. Cella D, Lai JS, Nowinski CJ, et al. Neuro-QOL: brief measures of health-related quality of life for clinical research in neurology. *Neurology.* 2012;**78**:1860–7.

52. Asch DA, Hansen-Flaschen J, Lanken PN. Decisions to limit or continue life-sustaining treatment by critical care physicians in the United States: conflicts between physicians' practices and patients' wishes. *Am J Respir Crit Care Med.* 1995;**151**:288–92.

53. Luce JM, Alpers A. End-of-life care: what do the American courts say? *Crit Care Med.* 2001;**29**:N40–5.

54. Hanson LC, Danis M, Garrett J. What is wrong with end-of-life care? Opinions of bereaved family members. *J Am Geriatr Soc.* 1997;**45**:1339–44.

55. Johnson SK, Bautista CA, Hong SY, Weissfeld L, White DB. An empirical study of surrogates' preferred level of control over value-laden life support decisions in intensive care units. *Am J Respir Crit Care Med.* 2011;**183**:915–21.

56. Azoulay E, Pochard F, Kentish-Barnes N, et al. Risk of post-traumatic stress symptoms in family members of intensive care unit patients. *Am J Respir Crit Care Med.* 2005;**171**:987–94.

57. Petrinec AB, Daly BJ. Post-traumatic stress symptoms in post-ICU family members: review and methodological challenges. *West J Nurs Res.* 2016;**38**:57–78.

58. Nunez ER, Schenker Y, Joel ID, et al. Acutely bereaved surrogates' stories about the decision to limit life support in the ICU. *Crit Care Med.* 2015;**43**:2387–93.

59. Rocker GM, Heyland DK, Cook DJ, et al. Most critically ill patients are perceived to die in comfort during withdrawal of life support: a Canadian multicentre study. *Can J Anaesth*. 2004;**51**:623–30.

60. Keenan SP, Mawdsley C, Plotkin D, Webster GK, Priestap F. Withdrawal of life support: how the family feels, and why. *J Palliat Care*. 2000;**16** (Suppl):S40–4.

61. Gries CJ, Curtis JR, Wall RJ, Engelberg RA. Family member satisfaction with end-of-life decision making in the ICU. *Chest*. 2008;**133**:704–12.

62. Ahrens T, Yancey V, Kollef M. Improving family communications at the end of life: implications for length of stay in the intensive care unit and resource use. *Am J Crit Care*. 2003;**12**:317–23; discussion 324.

63. Khandelwal N, Curtis JR. Economic implications of end-of-life care in the ICU. *Curr Opin Crit Care*. 2014;**20**:656–61.

64. Dewan MC, Rattani A, Gupta S, et al. Estimating the global incidence of traumatic brain injury. *J Neurosurg*. 2018:**130**:1080–97.

65. van Erp WS, Lavrijsen JC, Vos PE, et al. The vegetative state: prevalence, misdiagnosis, and treatment limitations. *J Am Med Dir Assoc*. 2015;**16**:e89–5 e14.

66. Donis J, Kraftner B. The prevalence of patients in a vegetative state and minimally conscious state in nursing homes in Austria. *Brain Inj*. 2011;**25**:1101–17.

67. Crispi F, Crisci C. Patients in persistent vegetative state . . . and what of their relatives? *Nurs Ethics*. 2000;**7**:533–5.

68. Li YH, Xu ZP. Psychological crisis intervention for the family members of patients in a vegetative state. *Clinics (Sao Paulo)*. 2012;**67**:341–5.

69. Moretta P, Estraneo A, De Lucia L, et al. A study of the psychological distress in family caregivers of patients with prolonged disorders of consciousness during in-hospital rehabilitation. *Clin Rehabil*. 2014;**28**:717–25.

70. Chiambretto P, Rossi Ferrario S, Zotti AM. Patients in a persistent vegetative state: caregiver attitudes and reactions. *Acta Neurol Scand*. 2001;**104**:364–8.

71. Elvira de la Morena MJ, Cruzado JA. Caregivers of patients with disorders of consciousness: coping and prolonged grief. *Acta Neurol Scand*. 2013;**127**:413–18.

72. Goudarzi F, Abedi H, Zarea K, Ahmadi F. Multiple victims: the result of caring patients in vegetative state. *Iran Red Crescent Med J*. 2015;**17**:e23571.

73. Hoofien D, Gilboa A, Vakil E, Donovick PJ. Traumatic brain injury (TBI) 10–20 years later: a comprehensive outcome study of psychiatric symptomatology, cognitive abilities and psychosocial functioning. *Brain Inj*. 2001;**15**:189–209.

74. Humphreys I, Wood RL, Phillips CJ, Macey S. The costs of traumatic brain injury: a literature review. *Clinicoecon Outcomes Res*. 2013;**5**:281–27.

75. Thomsen IV. Late psychosocial outcome in severe traumatic brain injury. Preliminary results of a third follow-up study after 20 years. *Scand J Rehabil Med Suppl*. 1992;**26**:142–52.

76. Coradazzi A, Inhaia C, Santana M, et al. Palliative withdrawal ventilation: why, when and how to do it? *HPMIJ*. 2019;3.

77. Rubenfeld GD. Principles and practice of withdrawing life-sustaining treatments. *Crit Care Clin*. 2004;**20**:435–51, ix.

78. Ropper AH. Unusual spontaneous movements in brain-dead patients. *Neurology*. 1984;**34**:1089–92.

79. Abbott KH, Sago JG, Breen CM, Abernethy AP, Tulsky JA. Families looking back: one year after discussion of withdrawal or withholding of life-sustaining support. *Crit Care Med*. 2001;**29**:197–201.

80. National Institute of Neurological Disorders and Stroke rt-PA SSG. Tissue plasminogen activator for acute ischemic stroke. *N Engl J Med*. 1995;**333**:1581–7.

81. Hacke W, Kaste M, Fieschi C, et al. Randomised double-blind placebo-controlled trial of thrombolytic therapy with intravenous alteplase in acute ischaemic stroke (ECASS II). Second European-Australasian acute Stroke Study Investigators. *Lancet*. 1998;**352**:1245–51.

82. Nogueira RG, Jadhav AP, Haussen DC, et al. Thrombectomy 6 to 24 hours after stroke with a mismatch between deficit and infarct. *N Engl J Med*. 2018;**378**:11–21.

83. Albers GW, Marks MP, Kemp S, et al. Thrombectomy for stroke at 6 to 16 hours with selection by perfusion imaging. *N Engl J Med*. 2018;**378**:708–18.

84. Juttler E, Schwab S, Schmiedek P, et al. Decompressive surgery for the treatment of malignant infarction of the middle cerebral artery (DESTINY): a randomized, controlled trial. *Stroke*. 2007;**38**:2518–25.

85. Vahedi K, Vicaut E, Mateo J, et al. Sequential-design, multicenter, randomized, controlled trial of early decompressive craniectomy in malignant middle cerebral artery infarction (DECIMAL trial). *Stroke*. 2007;**38**:2506–17.

86. Hofmeijer J, Kappelle LJ, Algra A, et al. Surgical decompression for space-occupying cerebral

infarction (the hemicraniectomy after middle cerebral artery infarction with life-threatening edema trial [HAMLET]): A multicentre, open, randomised trial. *Lancet Neurol.* 2009;**8**:326–33.

87. Anderson CS, Heeley E, Huang Y, et al. Rapid blood-pressure lowering in patients with acute intracerebral hemorrhage. *N Engl J Med.* 2013;**368**:2355–65.

88. Qureshi AI, Palesch YY, Barsan WG, et al. Intensive blood-pressure lowering in patients with acute cerebral hemorrhage. *N Engl J Med.* 2016;**375**:1033–43.

89. Mendelow AD, Gregson BA, Rowan EN, et al. Early surgery versus initial conservative treatment in patients with spontaneous supratentorial lobar intracerebral haematomas (STICH II): A randomised trial. *Lancet.* 2013;**382**:397–408.

90. Ziai WC, Tuhrim S, Lane K, et al. A multicenter, randomized, double-blinded, placebo-controlled phase III study of clot lysis evaluation of accelerated resolution of intraventricular hemorrhage (CLEAR III). *Int J Stroke.* 2014;**9**:536–42.

91. Hanley DF, Thompson RE, Rosenblum M, et al. Efficacy and safety of minimally invasive surgery with thrombolysis in intracerebral haemorrhage evacuation (MISTIE III): a randomised, controlled, open-label, blinded endpoint phase 3 trial. *Lancet.* 2019;**393**:1021–32.

92. Bernard SA, Gray TW, Buist MD, et al. Treatment of comatose survivors of out-of-hospital cardiac arrest with induced hypothermia. *N Engl J Med.* 2002;**346**:557–63.

93. Nielsen N, Wetterslev J, Cronberg T, et al. Targeted temperature management at 33 degrees c versus 36 degrees c after cardiac arrest. *N Engl J Med.* 2013;**369**:2197–2206.

94. Cooper DJ, Rosenfeld JV, Murray L, et al. Decompressive craniectomy in diffuse traumatic brain injury. *N Engl J Med.* 2011;**364**:1493–1502.

95. Edwards P, Arango M, Balica L, et al. Final results of MRC CRASH, a randomised placebo-controlled trial of intravenous corticosteroid in adults with head injury-outcomes at 6 months. *Lancet.* 2005;**365**:1957–9.

Chapter 19

Prognostication in Chronic Critical Illness: Frailty, Geriatrics, Prior Severe Neurological Comorbidities

Sanjeev Sivakumar and Kushak Suchdev

Introduction

The advancement of medical science over the past several decades, while increasing the ability to preserve life among patients who are critically ill, has led to a new and increasing problem of patients who fail to recover full function. Hospitalized patients can be intensive care-dependent, such that they are unable to survive without receiving critical care, for more than a few days. Such patients have been described in the literature as having chronic critical illness,[1–6] persistently critically ill,[7,8] chronically medically complex, [9] requiring prolonged mechanical ventilation, [10–13] or long-stay patients.[14–16] The term "chronically critically ill" was introduced by Girard and Raffin in 1985.[17] They studied patients who survived an initial episode of critical illness but remained dependent on intensive care without recovering. Patients with chronic critical illness are an identifiable group of intensive care unit (ICU) patients with definable characteristics, have substantial stress associated with their care, and have poor perceived long-term outcomes.

Frailty, on the other hand, is a complex syndrome characterized by loss of physiological reserves. A significant proportion of patients admitted to ICUs with chronic critical illness often share several traits, such as preexisting functional and cognitive deficits, as well as multiple medical comorbidities, which make them at risk for adverse outcomes. This chapter reviews prognostication in patients with chronic critical illness and the roles of frailty, geriatric, and other neurological comorbidities as predictors of recovery and functional outcomes.

Chronic Critical Illness: Background, Epidemiology, and Clinical Features

The onset of chronic critical illness has been identified as the day during critical illness beyond which the severity of admission diagnosis and physiological illness cease to predict outcomes more accurately than do simple pre-ICU patient characteristics. Up to 10% of patients who require mechanical ventilation can have chronic critical illness. This includes patients from medical, neurological, and surgical ICUs. Chronic critical illness is believed to develop after a median of 10 days of hospitalization in an intensive care unit.[7,18] Such persistently critically ill patients consume resources in terms of bed-days, have a higher mortality, and have a significantly lower chance of returning home upon hospital discharge. [13] The overall population prevalence rates of such patients are up to 35 per 100,000 individuals.[5] The prevalence varies with age, peaking at about 82 per 100,000 individuals among adults aged 75–79 years.[5] The mean age for adult patients at risk for chronic critical illness is 65 years (standard deviation [SD] 15 years),[19] and for patients in specialized weaning facilities and long-term acute care facilities, it is in the eighth decade.[19,20] Patients with trauma, however, are more commonly younger, are more likely male, and have fewer comorbidities. Approximately $26 billion is spent annually for the care of patients with chronic critical illness in the United States.[5]

Respiratory failure requiring prolonged dependence on mechanical ventilation is a hallmark feature of chronic critical illness. Additional characteristics of chronic critical illness includes severe weakness due to myopathy, neuropathy, and alterations of body composition such as loss of lean body mass, increased adiposity, and anasarca;[21] brain dysfunction manifesting as coma or delirium that is prolonged or permanent;[22] neuroendocrine changes like the loss of pulsatile secretion of anterior pituitary hormones, which results in low target organ hormone levels and impaired anabolism; [23,24] increased predisposition to infection, often with multidrug-resistant organisms;[25] and skin breakdown associated with nutritional deficiencies, edema, incontinence, and prolonged immobility. [26] Survivor and patient reports also capture other significant stressors during the phase of chronic critical illness from the inability to communicate during prolonged mechanical ventilation and from symptoms including pain, thirst, dyspnea, depression, and anxiety.

Neuroprognostication in the Acute and Chronic Phase of Neurocritical Illness

In a study of over 1 million critically ill patients, acute characteristics were less predictive of in-hospital mortality than were antecedent characteristics (age, sex, health status) after 7 days of ICU hospitalization among patients with a neurological diagnosis, compared to a median of 11 days (interquartile range [IQR] 9–17) across other subgroups. [18] Diagnosis and severity of illness at admission play no role in the Prolonged mechanical Ventilation Prognostic model (ProVENT Score) for prognostication of outcomes for patients still in the ICU at day 14 or day 21.[10,27,28] Several prognostic scoring systems, such as the Acute Physiology and Chronic Health Evaluation II (APACHE II), the Simplified Acute Physiology Score II (SAPS II), and the Mortality Prediction Model (MPM II), have been extensively validated among large groups of critical care patients with mixed diagnoses and found to correlate well with observed outcomes. The general hypothesis underlying the use of severity-of-illness scoring systems is that clinical variables that can be assessed on ICU admission, and subsequent days of stay in the ICU predict survival and functional outcomes of critically ill patients. Most of these studies, however, were conducted in the general ICU with highly heterogeneous groups of patients.

A modified APACHE II score was evaluated in a study of 653 patients with neurocritical illness by Su and colleagues.[29] Patients with severe neurological diseases reach their worst condition at 3–5 days or later post-hospitalization, from secondary brain injury or subsequent multiple complications. The authors of this study tested the relationship between APACHE II score and outcomes at different timepoints. The 72 hours APACHE II score was found to have the greatest

correlation with functional outcomes in the neuro ICU. A 72-hour APACHE II score cut-off of 17.5 points, taking into account neurological diagnoses such as cerebral infarction, intracerebral hemorrhage, neuroinfectious, and neuromuscular disease, could predict hospital mortality with a sensitivity of 76.7%, a specificity of 80%, and an accuracy of 87% [area under the receiver operating characteristic curve (AU-ROC) 0.869 (0.834, 0.903)]. The cut-off values of APACHE II for cerebral infarction, intracerebral hemorrhage, neurological infection, neuromuscular disease, and other neurological diseases were 17.5, 19.5, 24.5, 14.5, and 10.5, respectively. Analyzing individual diagnoses, discrimination of the APACHE II score was acceptable for cerebral infarction, intracerebral hemorrhage, and neurological infection, with an AU-ROC exceeding 80%. Of note, discrimination and predictive capacity of APACHE II was poor for patients with chronic critical illness from neuromuscular disease. Patients with neuromuscular disease have a lower mortality, which may be attributable to potentially reversible respiratory failure with the use of positive pressure ventilation. To improve the accuracy of the APACHE II scoring system in predicting mortality, investigators then conducted a prospective study by building a module modified APACHE II score.[30] This study further validated the previous findings that the 72-hours APACHE II score predicted hospital mortality, particularly among patients admitted with cerebral infarction, intracerebral hemorrhage and neurological infections.

A study by Navarrete-Navarro et al. found that hospital mortality was related to the type of stroke. [31] In this study, for the same age and APACHE III score, subarachnoid hemorrhage showed a mortality rate 5.7-fold that of ischemic stroke, and intracerebral hemorrhage showed a mortality rate 4.1-fold that of ischemic stroke. Huang et al. proposed that the APACHE II score was desirable as a predictor of 30-day mortality for patients with primary pontine hemorrhage (AU-ROC, 0.919). [32] In this study, in terms of area under the ROC curve, APACHE II (0.919) was more discriminative than SAPS II (0.890) and intracerebral hemorrhage (ICH) score (0.844) in predicting 30-day mortality. Preoperative APACHE II and Glasgow Coma Scale (GCS) scores as predictors of 6-month outcomes in patients with malignant middle cerebral infarction after decompressive hemicraniectomy was studied by Tsai and colleagues.[33] After ROC analysis, cut-off values of preoperative GCS > 8 ($P = 0.003$) and APACHE II < 13 ($P = 0.006$) were sufficiently sensitive and specific to predict favorable outcome (modified Rankin Scale [mRS] 0–3) at 6 months (APACHE II, sensitivity 80.0% and specificity 96.9%; $P = 0.006$; ROC curve [AUC] 93.8%, 95% confidence interval [CI]: 83.5–100.0, $P = 0.002$ and GCS, sensitivity 100.0% and specificity 84.4%; $P = 0.003$; ROC curve [AUC] 96.3%, 95% CI: 90.1-100.0, $P = 0.001$)

Among patients with subarachnoid hemorrhage (SAH), the amount of extravasated blood on computed tomography (CT) scan (Fisher grade) and the level of consciousness at admission (GCS) are still the most important determinants predicting mortality and unfavorable outcomes.[34–37] Fisher grade is not included in the APACHE II or SAPS II scoring systems. A complementary measurement scale is thus required in neuroprognostication of chronic critical illness from subarachnoid hemorrhage. Age and cardiopulmonary parameters such as systolic blood pressure, PaO_2/FiO_2 ratios, are proven independent predictors for mortality in patients with SAH.[38,39] Myocardial stunning and neurogenic pulmonary edema mediated by systemic catecholamine surge are well-known systemic manifestations following SAH, with an effect on outcomes.[38,40] Hypoxemia, metabolic acidosis, hyperglycemia, and cardiovascular instability within 24 hours of admission are independent prognosticators of death or severe disability in SAH patients.[41] APACHE II and SAPS II scores have several of these systemic factors in their automated calculation tables, and have been shown to correlate with mortality in a dose-dependent fashion in patients with SAH.[42] Although these scoring systems provide prognostic information, it is dangerous to make decisions on intensity of treatment and withdrawal of life-sustaining therapy (WLST) using such predictors of outcomes early in the course of neurocritical illness due to the risk of self-fulfilling prophecy. Some studies show that APACHE II and SAPS II scoring systems could not be relied on to provide prognostic information for individual patients with SAH and traumatic brain injury (TBI).[30,42] Predicted mortality were much higher than actual mortality (APACHE II predicted 34.7% and SAPS II predicted 38.3%, vs. observed 21.4%).[30]

Gao and colleagues recently validated a new score for predicting 3-month functional outcome of neurocritically ill in a cohort of 941 Chinese patients with primary neurological diagnosis as etiology for admission to the ICU.[43] The patient population included those admitted with cerebral infarction, intracerebral hemorrhage, neuroinflammation, status epilepticus, TBI, Guillain–Barré syndrome, hypoxic ischemic encephalopathy, poisoning, and other neurological disease. In this study, the median length of hospital stay was 15 days, and the median ICU length of stay was 10 days. The 44-point scoring system named the INCNS score (Inflammation [I], nutrition [N], consciousness [C], neurological function [N] and systemic function [S]) was based on APACHE II and SAPS II. Patients with a higher INCNS score had worse outcomes, with higher mortality rates and lower recovery with functional independence compared to patients with lower INCNS scores. The score included 19 items categorized into 5 parts (Table 19.1). The INCNS score exhibited better discriminative and prognostic performance than APACHE II and SAPS II at both 24 and 72 hours in the neuro ICU. The 24- and 72-hour INCNS scores achieved an AU ROC of 0.788 (95% CI: 0.759–0.817) and 0.828 (95% CI: 0.802–0.854), respectively. The 72-hour INCNS score predicted 3-month unfavorable outcomes with a predictive accuracy of 75.5% (sensitivity: 75.0%, specificity: 76.0%, positive predictive value [PPV]: 82.0%, negative predictive value [NPV]: 67.7%, correlation coefficient [CC]: 75.5%), and the 24-hour INCNS score had a predictive accuracy of 72.9% (sensitivity: 73.8%, specificity: 71.9%, PPV: 79.2%, NPV: 65.4%, CC: 73%).

Neurological Exam and Outcomes Following Neurocritical Illness

For patients with critical illness admitted to the neurointensive care unit, neurological examination at different time points can inform prognosis. The GCS score as an index of consciousness, at 24 and 72 hours, has been shown to correlate with functional outcomes following acute brain injury due to trauma, stroke, intracerebral hemorrhage, and SAH.[36,37,44–47] In patients with primary neurological disease admitted to the ICU, patients with recovery to functional independence had a median GCS score of 14 compared to patients with patients with death or disability, who had a median GCS of 10, both at 24 and 72 hours ($p < 0.001$).[43] A greater proportion of patients with

Table 19.1 The INCNS scoresheet

Variable		0	1	2	3
				Points	
Inflammation	WBC (10⁹/L)	4 ~ 10	2.9 ~ 3.9, 10.1 ~ 25.0	≤ 2.8, ≥ 25.1	–
	Temperature (axillary, °C)	36 ~ 38.4	≤ 35.9, 38.5 ~ 40	≥ 40.1	–
Nutrition	Albumin (g/L)	≥ 35	25 ~ 34.9	≤ 24.9	–
Consciousness	Arousal	Spontaneous eye opening	Eye opening to verbal command	Eye opening to pain	None
	Awareness	Correct response to question or command [a]	confused response to question or command [a]	Non-reflex movements [b]	None
Neurological function	Pupillary light reflex	Bilateral sensitive	–	Unilateral slow/ absent	Bilateral slow/absent
	Corneal reflex	Bilateral sensitive	–	Unilateral slow/ absent	Bilateral slow/absent
	Verbal response [c]	Accurate speech	Confused/inappropriate speech	Incomprehensible speech/none	–
	Motor response [c]	Unilateral/ bilateral muscle strength scores ≥ 4	Unilateral/bilateral muscle strength scores of 2–3	Unilateral muscle strength scores ≤ 1	Bilateral muscle strength scores ≤ 1
		Obeying to command	Localizing to/ withdrawal from pain	Flexing/extending to pain	None
	Swallowing function	Water swallow test I–II	Water swallow test III–IV/unable to assess	–	–
	Respiration	Not intubated, 12 ~ 24	Not intubated, ≤ 11/≥ 25	Breathes above ventilator rate	Breathes at ventilator rate/apnea
Systemic condition	Age (yr)	≤ 44	45 ~ 64	65 ~ 74	≥ 75
	Heart rate	60 ~ 100	40 ~ 59, 101 ~ 149	≤ 39, ≥ 150	–
	SBP (mmHg)	90 ~ 140	70 ~ 89, 141 ~ 199	≤ 69, ≥ 200	–
	Blood glucose (mmol/L)	3.9 ~ 11.1	2.2 ~ 3.8, 11.2 ~ 19.3	≤ 2.1, ≥ 19.4	–
	Serum sodium (mmol/L)	130 ~ 150	120 ~ 129,151 ~ 159	≤ 119, ≥ 160	–
	Serum potassium (mmol/L)	3.5 ~ 5.5	2.5 ~ 3.4, 5.6 ~ 6.9	≤ 2.4, ≥ 7.0	–
	Serum creatinine (μmol/L)	44 ~ 132	≤ 43, 133 ~ 171	≥ 172	–
	Total bilirubin (μmol/L)	≤ 34.1	34.2 ~ 102.5	≥ 102.6	–

Abbreviations: SBP: systolic blood pressure; WBC: white blood cell.
[a] The examiner may ask a question about the patient's name or command the patient to move eyeballs and/or hands, if appropriate. [b] Include evidence of visual pursuit or non-contingent behaviors.
[c] Either the muscle strength test or motor response to painful stimulus is performed in each patient.

Source: Adapted from Quing Gao, Gang Yan et al. Development and validation of a new score for predicting functional outcome of neurocritically ill patients: The INCNS score. *CNS Neurosci Ther.* 2019 Apr 10. doi: 10.1111/cns.13134. ©2019 The authors, with permission from John Wiley & Sons Ltd.

bilaterally preserved pupillary light reflex and corneal reflex recover with good functional outcomes (mRS 0–2) compared to patients with either a unilaterally or bilaterally absent response, with higher rates of mortality or recovery with functional disability (mRS 3–6). Respiratory status of patients, requirement and duration of mechanical ventilation, and respiratory patterns are other predictors of functional outcome.[39,48,49]

Geriatrics and Frailty in Intensive Care

In high-income countries, older adults (aged ≥ 65 years) comprise about half of all intensive care admissions, receive more intensive treatments than in the past, and are more likely to survive a critical illness than ever before.[50] Among patients over the age of 80 years admitted with critical illness, mortality rates approaching 50% have been reported.[51] Routine assessment of baseline physical function and frailty status can help identify those patients most suitable for palliative, rehabilitative, and therapeutic interventions and aid in prognostication and informed decision making for very old critically ill patients.

Frailty is a complex syndrome characterized by a loss of physiological reserve in multiple domains (energy, physical capacity, cognitive ability), which renders individuals susceptible to adverse outcomes.[52,53] Frailty as a syndrome was originally described in a geriatric patient population and has associations with risk of hospitalization, mortality, falls and disability.[54] It is now evident that frailty is not restricted to a geriatric or other specific age group and is prevalent even among young critically ill patients.[55]

In a meta-analysis of 10 observational studies, the pooled prevalence of frailty in the ICU was 30% (95% CI 29–32%).[56] The prevalence of frailty in the older demographic can be as high as 43%.[52] Frail patients admitted to ICUs share several traits, such as preexisting functional and cognitive deficits and multiple medical comorbidities, are more likely to require assisted living, are more susceptible to adverse events, and are more likely to die compared to age-matched non-frail individuals.[57,58] Frailty assessment can lead to individualized treatment plans and contribute to shared decision making regarding goals of care.

Pathophysiology of Frailty

Interplay between pathophysiological mechanisms involved in frailty are shown in Figure 19.1.

Frail patients have increased levels of interleukin (IL-6),[59] tumor necrosis factor (TNF-alpha), and C-reactive protein (CRP).[60–62] Elevated levels of neopterin, a marker for immune activation, has been demonstrated, suggesting potential monocyte/macrophage-mediated immune activation in the frail elderly,[63] with increased counts of CD8 +/CD28– T cells and CCR5+ T cells.[64,65] Detrimental effects of inflammation on the musculoskeletal and endocrine among other systems, as well as nutritional dysregulation, suggest a causal relationship between chronic inflammation and frailty. Other factors such as obesity, genetics, and chronic or persistent cytomegalovirus infection (CMV), have been associated with frailty.[60,65,66]

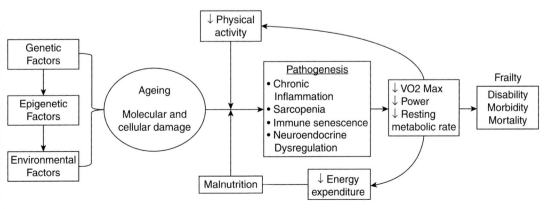

Figure 19.1 Pathogenesis of frailty. Adapted from Walson. *J Am Geriatr Soc.* 2006, *Clegg. Lancet.* 2013, *Lopez-Otin. Cell.* 2013, and Fried. *J Gerontol A Biol Sci Med Sci.* 2001.

Chronic critical illness, due to its characterization with prolonged mechanical ventilation, myopathy, neuropathy, increased susceptibility to infections, and nutritional dysregulation, shares several features with frailty.[67] Both chronic critical illness and frailty are associated with prolonged inflammatory state, sarcopenia, and enhanced catabolism. Thus, unsurprisingly, frailty following an episode of critical illness is independently associated with worse outcomes.[68]

Clinical Assessment and Scoring Systems for Frailty

Commonly used models for frailty include the Fried Frailty Phenotype (FFP), Frailty Index, and the Clinical Frailty Scale (CFS) (Table 19.2). In the rules-based model or the FFP, patients meeting criteria for three out of five symptoms (unintentional > 10 lb weight loss, weak grip strength, slow walking speed based on walking time/15 feet, poor endurance based on self-reported exhaustion, and low activity measured as kcals/week) are categorized as being frail, while those having one or two of five symptoms are categorized as pre-frail.[69] The frailty index takes into account the proportion of cumulative deficits present for a given individual and age based on a structured clinical exam.[70] These deficits represent loss in domains such as functional capacity, sensory impairment, and general medical, health, and behavioral problems. Modifications of frailty index to include comprehensive geriatric assessment (FI-CGA) have been proposed and validated in the acute care setting.[54] Rockwood

et al. demonstrated a moderate correlation between the FFP and the Frailty Index among an elderly population.[71] The CFS uses a judgment-based scale ranging from 1 (robust health) to 9 (terminally ill), can be used readily at bedside, and is thus a feasible alternative tool to measure frailty among elderly.[52] The score correlated well with frailty index (Pearson coefficient 0.80), and showed good criterion validity and dose-response effect for 5-year prediction of death or admission to an institutional facility.[52]

Biomarkers of Frailty

Several blood inflammatory precursors and hormonal biomarkers for frailty have been proposed to increase the predictive capacity of established clinical indices. Serum biomarkers described for frailty include hemoglobin, vitamin D, vitamin B12, albumin, cholesterol, and serum transaminases.[72] Hormonal biomarkers evaluated include testosterone, dehydroepiandrosterone sulphate (DHEA-S),and insulin-like growth factor-1 (IGF-1).[72,73] Sex hormones (estrogen in women and testosterone in men) are lower in frail adults, as is 25-hydroxyvitamin D.[74–77] Frail adults have lower levels of IGF-1, the signaling target of growth hormone and a key anabolic effector of muscle.[73,74] Chronic systemic inflammation is a key pathophysiological process that drives frailty. An elevation in inflammatory markers such as IL-1, IL-6, TNF-alpha, and CRP have been demonstrated in frail individuals. [59,61,74,78,79] Biomarkers, such as IL-6 and TNF-α, directly induce muscle catabolism. The sensitivity and specificity of these biomarkers,

Table 19.2 Clinical assessment of frailty

1. Fried Frailty Phenotype (FFP)	Rules based model Diagnostic criteria: 1. Unintentional weight loss 2. Weak grip strength 3. Slow walking speed 4. Poor endurance 5. Low activity 　　Classified as frail if meeting three of five criteria 　　Pre-frail if one or two of five criteria
2. Frailty Index	Structured exam-based scoring index Frailty defined by proportion of cumulative deficits at a given age
3. Clinical Frailty Scale (CFS)	Clinical judgment–based scale based on presence and extent of control of comorbid illness and level of dependence Classify patients into nine categories ranging from "very fit" to "severely frail"

however, are modest at best and use of clinical tools such as the CFS along with biomarkers can improve diagnostic accuracy.[80]

Prognostication among the Elderly and Frail

Frailty on Admission to an ICU

The association between pre-hospitalization frailty and outcomes, such as mortality, quality of life, and healthcare resource utilization, has been of interest in the past decade. In a meta-analysis of 10 observational studies, frailty was associated with higher hospital mortality (relative risk [RR] 1.71, 95% CI: 1.43–2.05; $p < 0.00001$; heterogeneity (I^2) = 32%) and long-term mortality (RR 1.53; 95% CI: 1.40–1.68; $p < 0.00001$; I^2 = 0%). Frail patients are less likely to get discharged home (RR 0.59; 95% CI: 0.49–0.71; $p < 0.00001$; I^2 = 12%).[56] Frailty and subsequent disability and mortality in critical illness were studied in a combined cohort of 1,040 patients from five centers enrolled in the identical BRAIN-ICU (Bringing to Light the Risk Factors and Incidence of Neuropsychological Dysfunction in ICU Survivors) and MIND-ICU (Delirium and Dementia in Veterans Surviving ICU Care) studies.[81,82] Median age was 62 years, and the median Clinical Frailty Scale (CFS) score on admission was 3. Higher CFS scores were independently associated with death and disability at 12 months. In a large study of frailty in critical illness, investigators measured the CFS at ICU admission in 421 adults aged 50 years or older across six hospitals.[52] Frailty, when defined as a CFS greater than 4, amounted to 33% of patients who were frail on ICU admission.[52] Independent of age, sex, critical illness severity, and comorbidities, frail adults were twice as likely to die in the hospital (32% vs. 16%; adjusted odds ratio [OR], 1.81; 95% CI: 1.09–3.01) and were twice as likely to die within 1 year (48 vs. 25%; adjusted hazard ratio [HR], 1.82; 95% CI: 1.28–2.60). Frail adults are more likely to be functionally dependent at hospital discharge and have lower health-related quality of life in the subsequent year.[83,84]

A multicenter prospective cohort study of 196 intensive care patients aged 65 years or older showed independent associations between pre-hospitalization frailty, measured by CFS, and in-hospital and 6-month mortality.[85] Investigators also measured pre-hospitalization frailty by the FFP. However, measurements of grip strength and walking speed were replaced with self- or proxy reports of mobility before critical illness, which may have compromised its construct validity. The modified frailty phenotype was independently associated with ICU, but not long-term, mortality.

Although advanced age is often associated with frailty, it is not exclusive to the elderly. This was shown in a Canadian study, where 28% of the critically ill patients aged 50–64.9 years met criteria for diagnosis of frailty, and frailty was independently associated with increased 1-year mortality compared to patients who were not frail (33% vs. 20 %; adjusted HR 1.8, 95 % CI: 1.0–3.3; $p = 0.039$) and re-hospitalization nutritional support.[55] However, less than 16% of patients in this study had a primary neurological diagnosis.

Frailty on Admission to an ICU among Adults Aged 80 Years or Older

A large multicenter cohort study of 5,021 patients over the age of 80 years admitted to intensive care units across Europe showed that frailty, as assessed using the Clinical Frailty Score, was associated with higher 30-day mortality (HR 1.54; 95% CI: 1.38–1.73 for frail vs. non-frail).[86] Overall, ICU and 30-day mortality rates were 22.1% and 32.6%, respectively. In an observational study among critically ill elderly patients with a median age of 71 years, pre-ICU frailty was independently associated with mortality.[87] The ICU mortality rates were significantly higher among frail patients, when compared to pre-frail and robust patients during hospital stay, over 3 and 6 months. Length of stay, Sequential Organ Failure Assessment (SOFA) score and APACHE II scores were also significantly higher among frail adults and were independent predictors for mortality among critically ill elderly population.

In a prospective Canadian study that enrolled 610 critically ill patients over the age of 80 years, overall mortality rates were 14% in ICU, 26% in hospital, and 44% at 12-month follow-up.[51] Only one-quarter of patients aged 80 years or older who are admitted to the ICU survived and returned to their baseline levels of physical function at 1 year. In a geriatric population, frailty, measured by the Frailty Index-Comprehensive

Geriatric Assessment (FI-CGA), was independently associated with a higher risk of death and other adverse outcomes in older people admitted to an acute care hospital. The risk of dying increased with each 0.01 increment in the FI-CGA (HR = 1.05, 95% CI: = 1.04–1.07). People discharged home had the lowest admitting mean FI-CGA = 0.38 (±standard deviation 0.11) compared with those who died, FI-CGA = 0.51 (±0.12) or were discharged to a nursing home, FI-CGA = 0.49 (±0.11).

Prior Severe Neurological Comorbidities

The effects of frailty and prior severe neurological diagnoses on functional outcomes, morbidity, and mortality following critical illness have been rarely studied. Hope et al. published data from 47,427 elderly Medicare beneficiaries with frailty admitted to the ICU with critical illness, and examined mortality based on pre-ICU health categories.[88] Patients with ≥ 1 healthcare claim in the preceding 12 months with a diagnosis of stroke, dementia from Alzheimer's disease or senility, other dementias, acute or sub-acute delirium, Parkinson's disease, or functional urinary and fecal incontinence were categorized into the "frailty" group and were compared across other pre-ICU health categories of cancer, chronic organ failure, and robust health. The mean age (SD) of the cohort with neurological diagnosis was 79.4 (±7.3) years, and 57.4% were women. Patients with prior neurological disease as their reason for frailty had higher rates of severe sepsis, acute renal failure, and mechanical ventilation and the lowest probability of discharge home with self-care. There were higher rates of in-hospital mortality (17.3%) when compared with groups with cancer (13.6%) and chronic organ failure (13.4%). Hospital and 3-year mortality (%) of patients with pre-ICU frailty stratified by specific diagnoses were as follows: dementia (15.2% and 54%), dementia diagnoses and skilled nursing facility (SNF) in the year prior (21.6% and 71.1%), dementia and other frailty diagnoses (17.7% and 63.9%), and dementia, other frailty diagnoses, and SNF in the year prior (23.7% and 74.7%), respectively.[88] Patients with pre-ICU neurological diagnoses and frailty had higher in-hospital mortality compared to patients with the same pre-ICU health categories without frailty (adjusted ORs ranged from 1.27 (95% CI: 1.10–1.47) to 1.52 (95% CI: 1.35–1.63)). Pre-ICU frailty conferred a higher

3-year mortality compared to pre-ICU categories without frailty (adjusted HRs ranged from 1.54 (95% CI: 1.45–1.64) to 1.84 (95% CI: 1.70–1.99).

Among patients with intracerebral hemorrhage, the ICH score is the most commonly used clinical grading scale,[47] which was initially validated for 30-day outcomes, and subsequently for 12-month functional outcomes.[89] Older age (≥ 80 years) was an independent predictor of 30-day mortality (p = 0.001) in patients admitted with ICH. Scoring systems, such as the INCNS score for predicting functional outcomes in patients with neurological critical illness, show an association between age > 75 years and worse outcomes, including death and functional disability (mRS 3–6).[43] It is important to note that the literature on frailty and clinical outcomes among critically ill patients is mostly based on heterogeneous groups of patients admitted to general medical ICUs. There is paucity of data on the effect of frailty among neurocritically ill patients, and it is prudent to exercise caution when extrapolating data based on other patient populations to those with neurological disease.

The association between pre-ICU health categories and outcomes has important methodological implications for studies focused on the long-term effects of critical illness in elderly patients. Studies of long-term outcomes have found that older survivors of critical illness have limitations and deficits – muscle weakness, cognitive impairment, muscle wasting – that mirror the frailty syndrome.[90–92]

Frailty in Survivors of Critical illness

Patients admitted to the ICU as "pre-frail" can leave the ICU categorized as frail, as critical illness can hasten processes that contribute to frailty. Undernutrition, weight loss, muscle wasting, and weakness, which are the typical deficits among frail individuals, take years to develop in outpatient geriatric populations. However, these deficits can develop or worsen rapidly in the critically ill, regardless of the diagnosis that led to critical illness.[93] Measuring the Fried Frailty Phenotype domains in the heterogeneous population of survivors of critical illness may help posthospitalization outcome prognostication, as well as identify potential deficits as therapeutic targets for intervention. In a pilot study, a modified Fried's Frailty Index was used in older medical survivors of critical illness after they were moved out of the ICU.[68] Defining frailty as three or more deficits and using Fried's established cut-offs for each component, 81% of older survivors of critical illness were frail. Each 1-point increase in the Fried frailty score was associated with a 3-fold increase in 6-month mortality (RR 3.0; 95% CI: 1.4–6.3), and those with a score of 5 had an 83% 6-month mortality.

Frailty as a Therapeutic Target in Critical Illness

Multidimensional interventions with individualized nutritional, social, psychological and physical interventions targeted at frailty have been evaluated in recent years.[94] Studies in older populations show that frailty may be reversible through targeted exercise and nutrition interventions.[95–97] Muscle wasting, weakness, and malnutrition are common among those with neurological disease and could be responsive to physical exercise training and nutrition optimization, which highlights the importance of rehabilitation. Treating frailty constructs can partially explain why rehabilitation improves exercise capacity, disability, and health-related quality of life. It is unclear whether the pathophysiology causing frailty is universal across different neurological diseases with heterogeneous pathophysiology, or whether it differs by groups based on disease category underlying mechanisms (e.g., sarcopenic or malnourished vs. hyperinflammatory). Clarifying these factors may help identify subgroups at differential risk for poor outcomes and inform interventions to improve outcomes.

In the ICU, minimizing sedation and encouraging early mobilization have been shown to reduce ICU delirium and disability at hospital discharge and can prevent frailty among mechanically ventilated patients.[98] Novel rehabilitative strategies for critically ill patients and survivors of critical illness too weak to ambulate, such as bedside cycle ergometry [99] and neuromuscular electrical stimulation, have being tested.[100,101] The molecular mechanisms of skeletal muscle dysfunction and wasting in aging and critical illness have been elucidated.[102] This has helped identify novel pharmacological targets, such as ubiquitin proteasome system mediators [103] and myostatin agonists [104,105] to prevent muscle wasting and improve recovery of muscle function.

Trials to treat undernutrition during critical illness with supplemental nutrition actually potentiated muscle atrophy and weakness.[102,106,107] A trial of growth hormone replacement in acutely critically ill medical and surgical patients doubled the risk of in-hospital death.[108] Thus, targeting nutritional and hormone replacement therapies following ICU discharge to reverse weight loss and exhaustion in survivors of critical illness has been the subject of interest, with the aim to reverse weight loss and exhaustion in survivors of critical illness.[109,110]

Conclusion

The current literature on chronic critical illness and frailty informs debates regarding the value of intensive care for older adults. Older adults without frailty prior to critical illness tend to benefit most from intensive care, while those who are frail prior to critical illness are more likely to suffer in-hospital mortality and are more likely to develop chronic critical illness or severe disability leading to early death. Future research with a focus on chronic critical illness among patients with neurological illness, biological mechanisms that contribute to frailty with attention to novel targets, pre-ICU and post-ICU frailty scoring systems and their impact on long-term neurological outcomes are needed.

References

1. Nelson, J.E., Cox, C.E., Hope, A.A., Carson, S.S. Chronic critical illness. *Am J Respir Crit Care Med* 2010;**182**(4):446–54.

2. Sjoding, M.W., Cooke, C.R. Chronic critical illness: a growing legacy of successful advances in critical care. *Crit Care Med* 2015; **43**(2):476–7.

3. Kahn, J.M., Werner, R.M., David, G., et al. Effectiveness of long-term acute care hospitalization in elderly patients with chronic critical illness. *Med Care* 2013;**51**(1):4–10.

4. Carson, S.S., Bach, P.B. The epidemiology and costs of chronic critical illness. *Crit Care Clin* 2002;**18**(3):461–76.

5. Kahn, J.M., Le, T., Angus, D.C., et al. The epidemiology of chronic critical illness in the United States. *Crit Care Med* 2015;**43**(2):282–7.

6. Cox, C.E. Persistent systemic inflammation in chronic critical illness. *Respir Care* 2012;**57** (6):859–64; discussion 64–6.

7. Iwashyna, T.J., Hodgson, C.L., Pilcher, D., Bailey, M., Bellomo, R. Persistent critical illness

characterised by Australian and New Zealand ICU clinicians. *Crit Care Resusc* 2015;**17**(3):153–8.

8. Iwashyna, T.J., Hodgson, C.L., Pilcher, D., et al. Towards defining persistent critical illness and other varieties of chronic critical illness. *Crit Care Resusc* 2015;**17**(3):215–18.

9. Kandilov, A., Ingber, I.M., Morley, M, et al. Chronically critically ill population payment recommendations (CCIP-PR): final report. RTI Project No. 0212355.000.010. RTI International. March 2014.

10. Hough, C.L., Caldwell, E.S., Cox, C.E., et al. Development and validation of a mortality prediction model for patients receiving 14 days of mechanical ventilation. *Crit Care Med* 2015;**43**(11):2339–45.

11. Chelluri, L., Mendelsohn, A.B., Belle, S.H., et al. Hospital costs in patients receiving prolonged mechanical ventilation: does age have an impact? *Crit Care Med* 2003;**31**(6):1746–51.

12. Kahn, J.M. Improving outcomes in prolonged mechanical ventilation: a road map. *Lancet Respir Med* 2015;**3**(7):501–2.

13. Damuth, E., Mitchell, J.A., Bartock, J.L., Roberts, B.W., Trzeciak, S. Long-term survival of critically ill patients treated with prolonged mechanical ventilation: a systematic review and meta-analysis. *Lancet Respir Med* 2015;**3**(7):544–53.

14. Hughes, M., MacKirdy, F.N., Norrie, J. Grant, I.S. Outcome of long-stay intensive care patients. *Intensive Care Med* 2001;**27**(4):779–82.

15. Kramer, A.A., Zimmerman, J.E. A predictive model for the early identification of patients at risk for a prolonged intensive care unit length of stay. *BMC Med Inform Decis Mak* 2010;**10**:27.

16. Arabi, Y., Venkatesh, S., Haddad, S., Al Shimemeri, A. Al Malik, S. A prospective study of prolonged stay in the intensive care unit: predictors and impact on resource utilization. *Int J Qual Health Care* 2002;**14**(5):403–10.

17. Girard, K., Raffin, T.A. The chronically critically ill: to save or let die? *Respir Care* 1985;**30**(5):339–47.

18. Iwashyna, T.J., Hodgson, C.L., Pilcher, D., et al. Timing of onset and burden of persistent critical illness in Australia and New Zealand: a retrospective, population-based, observational study. *Lancet Respir Med* 2016;**4**(7):566–73.

19. Cox, C.E., Carson, S.S., Holmes, G.M., Howard, A. Carey, T.S. Increase in tracheostomy for prolonged mechanical ventilation in North Carolina, 1993–2002. *Crit Care Med* 2004;**32**(11):2219–26.

20. Scheinhorn, D.J., Hassenpflug, M.S., Votto, J.J., et al. Ventilator-dependent survivors of catastrophic illness transferred to 23 long-term care hospitals for weaning from prolonged mechanical ventilation. *Chest* 2007;**131**(1):76–84.

21. Hollander, J.M., Mechanick, J.I. Nutrition support and the chronic critical illness syndrome. *Nutr Clin Pract* 2006;**21**(6):587–604.

22. Nelson, J.E., Tandon, N., Mercado, A.F., et al. Brain dysfunction: another burden for the chronically critically ill. *Arch Intern Med* 2006;**166**(18):1993–9.

23. Van den Berghe, G., de Zegher, F., Veldhuis, J.D., et al. The somatotropic axis in critical illness: effect of continuous growth hormone (GH)-releasing hormone and GH-releasing peptide-2 infusion. *J Clin Endocrinol Metab* 1997;**82**(2):590–9.

24. Van den Berghe, G., de Zegher, F., Veldhuis, J.D., et al. Thyrotrophin and prolactin release in prolonged critical illness: dynamics of spontaneous secretion and effects of growth hormone-secretagogues. *Clin Endocrinol (Oxf)* 1997;**47**(5):599–612.

25. Scheinhorn, D.J., Hassenpflug, M.S., Votto, J.J., et al. Post-ICU mechanical ventilation at 23 long-term care hospitals: a multicenter outcomes study. *Chest* 2007;**131**(1):85–93.

26. Carasa, M., Polycarpe, M. Caring for the chronically critically ill patient: establishing a wound- healing program in a respiratory care unit. *Am J Surg* 2004;**188**(1A Suppl):18–21.

27. Carson, S.S., Kahn, J.M., Hough, C.L., et al. A multicenter mortality prediction model for patients receiving prolonged mechanical ventilation. *Crit Care Med* 2012;**40**(4):1171–6.

28. Carson, S.S., Garrett, J., Hanson, L.C., et al. A prognostic model for one-year mortality in patients requiring prolonged mechanical ventilation. *Crit Care Med* 2008;**36**(7):2061–9.

29. Su, Y.Y., Li, X., Li, S.J., et al. Predicting hospital mortality using APACHE II scores in neurocritically ill patients: a prospective study. *J Neurol* 2009;**256**(9):1427–33.

30. Su, Y., Wang, M., Liu, Y., et al. Module modified acute physiology and chronic health evaluation II: predicting the mortality of neuro-critical disease. *Neurol Res* 2014;**36**(12):1099–105.

31. Navarrete-Navarro, P., Rivera-Fernandez, R., Lopez-Mutuberria, M.T., et al. Outcome prediction in terms of functional disability and mortality at 1 year among ICU-admitted severe stroke patients: a prospective epidemiological study in the south of the European Union

(Evascan Project, Andalusia, Spain). *Intensive Care Med* 2003;**29**(8):1237–44.

32. Huang, K.B., Ji, Z., Wu, Y.M., et al. The prediction of 30-day mortality in patients with primary pontine hemorrhage: a scoring system comparison. *Eur J Neurol* 2012;**19**(9):1245–50.

33. Tsai, C.L., Chu, H., Peng, G.S., et al. Preoperative APACHE II and GCS scores as predictors of outcomes in patients with malignant MCA infarction after decompressive hemicraniectomy. *Neurol India* 2012;**60**(6):608–12.

34. Szklener, S., Melges, A., Korchut, A., et al. Predictive model for patients with poor-grade subarachnoid haemorrhage in 30-day observation: a 9-year cohort study. *BMJ Open* 2015;**5**(6):e007795.

35. Claassen, J., Bernardini, G.L., Kreiter, K., et al. Effect of cisternal and ventricular blood on risk of delayed cerebral ischemia after subarachnoid hemorrhage: the Fisher scale revisited. *Stroke* 2001;**32**(9):2012–20.

36. Lantigua, H., Ortega-Gutierrez, S., Schmidt, J.M., et al. Subarachnoid hemorrhage: who dies, and why? *Crit Care* 2015;**19**:309.

37. Teasdale, G.M., Drake, C.G., Hunt, W., et al. A universal subarachnoid hemorrhage scale: report of a committee of the World Federation of Neurosurgical Societies. *J Neurol Neurosurg Psychiatry* 1988;**51**(11):1457.

38. Schuiling, W.J., Dennesen, P.J., Rinkel, G.J. Extracerebral organ dysfunction in the acute stage after aneurysmal subarachnoid hemorrhage. *Neurocrit Care* 2005;**3**(1):1–10.

39. Gruber, A., Reinprecht, A., Gorzer, H., et al. Pulmonary function and radiographic abnormalities related to neurological outcome after aneurysmal subarachnoid hemorrhage. *J Neurosurg* 1998;**88**(1):28–37.

40. Lee, V.H., Oh, J.K., Mulvagh, S.L., Wijdicks, E.F. Mechanisms in neurogenic stress cardiomyopathy after aneurysmal subarachnoid hemorrhage. *Neurocrit Care* 2006;**5**(3):243–9.

41. Claassen, J., Vu, A., Kreiter, K.T., et al. Effect of acute physiologic derangements on outcome after subarachnoid hemorrhage. *Crit Care Med* 2004;**32**(3):832–8.

42. Park, S.K., Chun, H.J., Kim, D.W., et al. Acute Physiology and Chronic Health Evaluation II and Simplified Acute Physiology Score II in predicting hospital mortality of neurosurgical intensive care unit patients. *J Korean Med Sci* 2009;**24**(3):420–6.

43. Gao, Q., Yuan, F., Yang, X.A., et al. Development and validation of a new score for predicting functional outcome of neurocritically ill patients:

44. the INCNS score. *CNS Neurosci Ther* 2020;**26**(1):21–9.

44. Balestreri, M., Czosnyka, M., Chatfield, D.A., et al. Predictive value of Glasgow Coma Scale after brain trauma: change in trend over the past ten years. *J Neurol Neurosurg Psychiatry* 2004;**75**(1):161–2.

45. Marshall, L.F., Gautille, T., Klauber, M.R., et al.: The outcome of severe closed head injury. *J Neurosurg* (Suppl) **75**:28–36, 1991.

46. Tsao, J.W., Hemphill, J.C., 3rd, Johnston, S.C., Smith, W.S., Bonovich, D.C. Initial Glasgow Coma Scale score predicts outcome following thrombolysis for posterior circulation stroke. *Arch Neurol* 2005;**62**(7):1126–9.

47. Hemphill, J.C., 3rd, Bonovich, D.C., Besmertis, L., Manley, G.T., Johnston, S.C. The ICH score: a simple, reliable grading scale for intracerebral hemorrhage. *Stroke* 2001;**32**(4):891–7.

48. Lahiri, S., Mayer, S.A., Fink, M.E., et al. Mechanical ventilation for acute stroke: a multi-state population-based study. *Neurocrit Care* 2015;**23**(1):28–32.

49. Roch, A., Michelet, P., Jullien, A.C., et al. Long-term outcome in intensive care unit survivors after mechanical ventilation for intracerebral hemorrhage. *Crit Care Med* 2003;**31**(11):2651–6.

50. Lerolle, N., Trinquart, L., Bornstain, C., et al. Increased intensity of treatment and decreased mortality in elderly patients in an intensive care unit over a decade. *Crit Care Med* 2010;**38**(1):59–64.

51. Heyland, D.K., Garland, A., Bagshaw, S.M., et al. Recovery after critical illness in patients aged 80 years or older: a multi-center prospective observational cohort study. *Intensive Care Med* 2015;**41**(11):1911–20.

52. Rockwood, K., Song, X., MacKnight, C., et al. A global clinical measure of fitness and frailty in elderly people. *CMAJ* 2005;**173**(5):489–95.

53. Rajabali, N., Rolfson, D., Bagshaw, S.M. Assessment and utility of frailty measures in critical illness, cardiology, and cardiac surgery. *Can J Cardiol* 2016;**32**(9):1157–65.

54. Evans, S.J., Sayers, M., Mitnitski, A., Rockwood, K. The risk of adverse outcomes in hospitalized older patients in relation to a frailty index based on a comprehensive geriatric assessment. *Age Ageing* 2014;**43**(1):127–32.

55. Bagshaw, M., Majumdar, S.R., Rolfson, D.B., et al. A prospective multicenter cohort study of frailty in younger critically ill patients. *Crit Care* 2016;**20**(1):175.

56. Muscedere, J., Waters, B., Varambally, A., et al. The impact of frailty on intensive care unit outcomes: a systematic review and meta-analysis. *Intensive Care Med* 2017;**43**(8):1105–22.

57. Joseph, B., Pandit, V., Zangbar, B., et al. Superiority of frailty over age in predicting outcomes among geriatric trauma patients: a prospective analysis. *JAMA Surg* 2014;**149** (8):766–72.

58. Robinson, T.N., Eiseman, B., Wallace, J.I., et al. Redefining geriatric preoperative assessment using frailty, disability and co-morbidity. *Ann Surg* 2009;**250**(3):449–55.

59. Leng, S., Chaves, P., Koenig, K., Walston, J. Serum interleukin-6 and hemoglobin as physiological correlates in the geriatric syndrome of frailty: a pilot study. *J Am Geriatr Soc* 2002;**50** (7):1268–71.

60. Chen, X., Mao, G., Leng, S.X. Frailty syndrome: an overview. *Clin Interv Aging* 2014;**9**:433–41.

61. Hubbard, R.E., O'Mahony, M.S., Savva, G.M., Calver, B.L., Woodhouse, K.W. Inflammation and frailty measures in older people. *J Cell Mol Med* 2009;**13**(9B):3103–9.

62. Collerton, J., Martin-Ruiz, C., Davies, K., et al. Frailty and the role of inflammation, immunosenescence and cellular ageing in the very old: cross-sectional findings from the Newcastle 85+ Study. *Mech Ageing Dev* 2012;**133**(6):456–66.

63. Leng, S.X., Tian, X., Matteini, A., et al. IL-6-independent association of elevated serum neopterin levels with prevalent frailty in community-dwelling older adults. *Age Ageing* 2011;**40**(4):475–81.

64. De Fanis, U., Wang, G.C., Fedarko, N.S., et al. T-lymphocytes expressing CC chemokine receptor-5 are increased in frail older adults. *J Am Geriatr Soc* 2008;**56**(5):904–8.

65. Qu, T., Yang, H., Walston, J.D., Fedarko, N.S., Leng, S.X. Upregulated monocytic expression of CXC chemokine ligand 10 (CXCL-10) and its relationship with serum interleukin-6 levels in the syndrome of frailty. *Cytokine* 2009;**46**(3):319–24.

66. Schmaltz, H.N., Fried, L.P., Xue, Q.L., et al. Chronic cytomegalovirus infection and inflammation are associated with prevalent frailty in community-dwelling older women. *J Am Geriatr Soc* 2005;**53**(5):747–54.

67. Jeejeebhoy, K.N. Malnutrition, fatigue, frailty, vulnerability, sarcopenia and cachexia: overlap of clinical features. *Curr Opin Clin Nutr Metab Care* 2012;**15**(3):213–19.

68. Baldwin, M.R., Reid, M.C., Westlake, A.A., et al. The feasibility of measuring frailty to predict disability and mortality in older medical intensive care unit survivors. *J Crit Care* 2014;**29**(3):401–8.

69. Fried, L.P., Tangen, C.M., Walston, J., et al. Frailty in older adults: evidence for a phenotype. *J Gerontol A Biol Sci Med Sci* 2001;**56**(3):M146–56.

70. Mitnitski, A.B., Graham, J.E., Mogilner, A.J., Rockwood, K. Frailty, fitness and late-life mortality in relation to chronological and biological age. *BMC Geriatr* 2002;**2**:1.

71. Rockwood, K., Andrew, M., Mitnitski, A. A comparison of two approaches to measuring frailty in elderly people. *J Gerontol A Biol Sci Med Sci* 2007;**62**(7):738–43.

72. Vina, J., Tarazona-Santabalbina, F.J., Perez-Ros, P., et al. Biology of frailty: modulation of ageing genes and its importance to prevent age-associated loss of function. *Mol Aspects Med* 2016;**50**:88–108.

73. Leng, S.X., Cappola, A.R., Andersen, R.E., et al. Serum levels of insulin-like growth factor-I (IGF-I) and dehydroepiandrosterone sulfate (DHEA-S), and their relationships with serum interleukin-6, in the geriatric syndrome of frailty. *Aging Clin Exp Res* 2004;**16**(2):153–7.

74. Puts, M.T., Visser, M., Twisk, J.W., Deeg, D.J., Lips, P. Endocrine and inflammatory markers as predictors of frailty. *Clin Endocrinol (Oxf)* 2005;**63** (4):403–11.

75. Cawthon, P.M., Ensrud, K.E., Laughlin, G.A., et al. Sex hormones and frailty in older men: the osteoporotic fractures in men (MrOS) study. *J Clin Endocrinol Metab* 2009;**94**(10):3806–15.

76. Joseph, C., Kenny, A.M., Taxel, P., et al. Role of endocrine-immune dysregulation in osteoporosis, sarcopenia, frailty and fracture risk. *Mol Aspects Med* 2005;**26**(3):181–201.

77. Travison, T.G., Nguyen, A.H., Naganathan, V., et al. Changes in reproductive hormone concentrations predict the prevalence and progression of the frailty syndrome in older men: the concord health and ageing in men project. *J Clin Endocrinol Metab* 2011;**96**(8):2464–74.

78. Cesari, M., Penninx, B.W., Pahor, M., et al. Inflammatory markers and physical performance in older persons: the InCHIANTI study. *J Gerontol A Biol Sci Med Sci* 2004;**59**(3):242–8.

79. Barzilay, J.I., Blaum, C., Moore, T., et al. Insulin resistance and inflammation as precursors of frailty: the Cardiovascular Health Study. *Arch Intern Med* 2007;**167**(7):635–41.

80. Calvani, R., Marini, F., Cesari, M., et al. Biomarkers for physical frailty and sarcopenia: state of the science and future developments. *J Cachexia Sarcopenia Muscle* 2015;**6**(4):278–86.

81. Brummel, N.E., Bell, S.P., Girard, T.D., et al. Frailty and subsequent disability and mortality among patients with critical illness. *Am J Respir Crit Care Med* 2017;**196**(1):64–72.

82. Jackson, J.C., Pandharipande, P.P., Girard, T.D., et al. Depression, post-traumatic stress disorder, and functional disability in survivors of critical illness in the BRAIN-ICU study: a longitudinal cohort study. *Lancet Respir Med* 2014;**2**(5):369–79.

83. Bagshaw, S.M., Stelfox, H.T., McDermid, R.C., et al. Association between frailty and short- and long-term outcomes among critically ill patients: a multicentre prospective cohort study. *CMAJ* 2014;**186**(2):E95–102.

84. Bagshaw, S.M., Stelfox, H.T., Johnson, J.A., et al. Long-term association between frailty and health-related quality of life among survivors of critical illness: a prospective multicenter cohort study. *Crit Care Med* 2015;**43**(5):973–82.

85. Le Maguet, P., Roquilly, A., Lasocki, S., et al. Prevalence and impact of frailty on mortality in elderly ICU patients: a prospective, multicenter, observational study. *Intensive Care Med* 2014;**40** (5):674–82.

86. Flaatten, H., De Lange, D.W., Morandi, A., et al. The impact of frailty on ICU and 30-day mortality and the level of care in very elderly patients (>/= 80 years). *Intensive Care Med* 2017;**43**(12):1820–8.

87. Kizilarslanoglu, M.C., Civelek, R., Kilic, M.K., et al. Is frailty a prognostic factor for critically ill elderly patients? *Aging Clin Exp Res* 2017;**29** (2):247–55.

88. Hope, A.A., Gong, M.N., Guerra, C., Wunsch, H. Frailty before critical illness and mortality for elderly Medicare beneficiaries. *J Am Geriatr Soc* 2015;**63**(6):1121–8.

89. Hemphill, J.C., 3rd, Farrant, M., Neill, T.A., Jr. Prospective validation of the ICH score for 12-month functional outcome. *Neurology* 2009;**73** (14):1088–94.

90. Herridge, M.S., Cheung, A.M., Tansey, C.M., et al. One-year outcomes in survivors of the acute respiratory distress syndrome. *N Engl J Med* 2003;**348**(8):683–93.

91. Herridge, M.S., Tansey, C.M., Matte, A., et al. Functional disability 5 years after acute respiratory distress syndrome. *N Engl J Med* 2011;**364**(14):1293–304.

92. Ehlenbach, W.J., Hough, C.L., Crane, P.K., et al. Association between acute care and critical illness hospitalization and cognitive function in older adults. *JAMA* 2010;**303**(8):763–70.

93. McDermid, R.C., Stelfox, H.T., Bagshaw, S.M. Frailty in the critically ill: a novel concept. *Crit Care* 2011;**15**(1):301.

94. Dudek, F.E., Tasker, J.G., Wuarin, J.P. Intrinsic and synaptic mechanisms of hypothalamic neurons studied with slice and explant preparations. *J Neurosci Methods* 1989;**28** (1–2):59–69.

95. Latham, N.K., Harris, B.A., Bean, J.F., et al. Effect of a home-based exercise program on functional recovery following rehabilitation after hip fracture: a randomized clinical trial. *JAMA* 2014;**311**(7):700–8.

96. Abizanda, P., Lopez, M.D., Garcia, V.P., et al. Effects of an oral nutritional supplementation plus physical exercise intervention on the physical function, nutritional status, and quality of life in frail institutionalized older adults: the ACTIVNES study. *J Am Med Dir Assoc* 2015;**16**(5):439 e9–e16.

97. Fragala, M.S., Dam, T.T., Barber, V., et al. Strength and function response to clinical interventions of older women categorized by weakness and low lean mass using classifications from the Foundation for the National Institute of Health sarcopenia project. *J Gerontol A Biol Sci Med Sci* 2015;**70** (2):202–9.

98. Schweickert, W.D., Pohlman, M.C., Pohlman, A. S., et al. Early physical and occupational therapy in mechanically ventilated, critically ill patients: a randomised controlled trial. *Lancet* 2009;**373** (9678):1874–82.

99. Burtin, C., Clerckx, B., Robbeets, C., et al. Early exercise in critically ill patients enhances short-term functional recovery. *Crit Care Med* 2009;**37**(9):2499–505.

100. Segers, J., Hermans, G., Bruyninckx, F., et al. Feasibility of neuromuscular electrical stimulation in critically ill patients. *J Crit Care* 2014;**29**(6):1082–8.

101. Kho, M.E., Truong, A.D., Zanni, J.M., et al. Neuromuscular electrical stimulation in mechanically ventilated patients: a randomized, sham-controlled pilot trial with blinded outcome assessment. *J Crit Care* 2015;**30** (1):32–9.

102. Puthucheary, Z.A., Rawal, J., McPhail, M., et al. Acute skeletal muscle wasting in critical illness. *JAMA* 2013;**310**(15):1591–600.

103. Cohen, S., Nathan, J.A., Goldberg, A.L. Muscle wasting in disease: molecular mechanisms and promising therapies. *Nat Rev Drug Discov* 2015;**14** (1):58–74.

104. Leitner, L.M., Wilson, R.J., Yan, Z. Godecke, A. Reactive oxygen species/nitric oxide mediated inter-organ communication in skeletal muscle wasting diseases. *Antioxid Redox Signal* 2017;**26** (13):700–17.

105. Haidet, A.M., Rizo, L., Handy, C., et al. Long-term enhancement of skeletal muscle mass and strength by single gene administration of myostatin inhibitors. *Proc Natl Acad Sci U S A* 2008;**105**(11):4318–22.

106. Doig, G.S., Simpson, F., Sweetman, E.A., et al. Early parenteral nutrition in critically ill patients with short-term relative contraindications to early enteral nutrition: a randomized controlled trial. *JAMA* 2013;**309**(20):2130–8.

107. Hermans, G., Casaer, M.P., Clerckx, B., et al. Effect of tolerating macronutrient deficit on the development of intensive-care unit acquired weakness: a subanalysis of the EPaNIC trial. *Lancet Respir Med* 2013;**1**(8):621–9.

108. Takala, J., Ruokonen, E., Webster, N.R., et al. Increased mortality associated with growth hormone treatment in critically ill adults. *N Engl J Med* 1999;**341**(11):785–92.

109. Schulman, R.C., Mechanick, J.I. Metabolic and nutrition support in the chronic critical illness syndrome. *Respir Care* 2012;**57**(6):958–77; discussion 77–8.

110. Van den Berghe, G. Novel insights into the neuroendocrinology of critical illness. *Eur J Endocrinol* 2000;**143**(1):1–13.

Prognostication in the Transition of Neurocritical Care: Neurorehabilitation and Placement, Role of Post-ICU Recovery Clinics, Insurance, Case Management

Cappi Lay and Sarah Lelin

Introduction

Following hospitalization and treatment for an acute neurological illness, most patients will not immediately regain their previous level of function or be able to return home. As discharge from the hospital becomes imminent, patients must be assessed for what environment and level of services are best suited for them, taking into account their medical needs, appropriateness for therapy, bed availability at different facilities, family preferences, and available financial resources. Clinicians and hospital administrators tend to focus on the clinical resources a discharge facility possesses, and may overlook elements of the discharge plan important to the patient and their family. Discussions about the patient's condition at discharge and needs for a discharge facility can come as a surprise to family members and may engender anger and conflict between the patient's family and the medical team when expectations for a quick recovery are not met. Communication early in the patient's hospitalization between medical providers and family members about the projected course of recovery and need for rehabilitation or a long-term care facility is important to prepare the family for the path ahead. This chapter will describe the different facility options that may be available for patients after hospitalization in the United States and considerations surrounding the appropriateness of different patients for each. Patients with special medical needs are discussed, followed by a discussion of some frequently encountered challenges during discharge planning.

Inpatient Rehabilitation

For patients who are not ready to transition directly back to their homes after hospitalization, inpatient rehabilitation offers a supervised environment that includes speech, physical, and occupational therapists, as well as other rehabilitation specialists who can work with patients to help them recover from an injury, illness, or surgery. Two forms of inpatient rehabilitation – acute and subacute – are commonly encountered and differ in terms of their admission requirements, as well as the intensity of therapy patients typically receive. At both acute and subacute rehabilitation facilities, specialists customize a plan of care for each patient depending on the nature of their disease process and specific disabilities. In order to qualify for either form of inpatient rehabilitation, patients are evaluated during their hospital stay to determine how much therapy, and the intensity, they are anticipated to tolerate during their recovery. Once rehab begins, physical and occupational therapists will work with patients to increase balance and gait steadiness, increase independence in activities of daily living (ADLs), and improve overall safety during ambulation. Insurance coverage plays a key role in determining whether a patient will be admitted to an inpatient rehabilitation facility and is always examined prior to a transfer taking place. The goal of inpatient rehab is to have patients return to their prior level of function and reintegrate them into their home or place of residence.

Differentiating between the subtypes of inpatient rehab, acute rehab is usually integrated

	Acute Care Rehab	Subacute Care Rehab
Focus	Make significant functional gains and medical improvement within a reasonable timeframe	A better choice for patients who are very sick and do not have the energy for longer daily rehabilitation sessions. On the other hand, this is also good for patients who have completed **acute care rehab**
Physician Involvement	Daily face-to-face assessment and treatment plan update	At least once a month (every 30 days)
Treatments Available	Combination of physical, occupational, and speech therapies	Combination of physical, occupational, and speech therapies
Therapy Intensity	3 or more hours of therapy per day up to 5 days a week; one-to-one therapy and group therapy sessions are both provided depending on the patient's needs; additional services may be offered such as respiratory therapy	Generally, patients receive 1 or 2 hours of therapy per day

Figure 20.1 Comparison between acute and subacute care rehab.[3]

within a hospital setting, although the hospital is frequently not the same one where a patient received acute medical care. Patients who are admitted to acute rehab facilities can expect intensive therapy, receiving up to 3 hours of therapy per day, 5 to 6 days per week, depending on the facility protocol. In this setting, therapy can be provided as either a one-to-one session with a therapist, or in a group with other patients, Acute rehab is considered to be short term, with a typical length of stay between 10 to 14 days, the length of which also depends upon the duration approved by the patient's insurance company. Acute rehab is most appropriate for patients who are anticipated to be able to make significant improvements in their level of function over a relatively short amount of time.[1] Another notable difference between inpatient rehabilitation facilities is that admission to an acute rehab facility requires the patient to possess one of several prespecified qualifying diagnoses. This specific set of diagnoses is set by insurance companies, and can include, but is not limited to, stroke, subarachnoid hemorrhage, multiple sclerosis, myasthenia gravis, seizures, traumatic brain injury (TBI), and brain tumors.

Subacute rehabilitation (SAR) also utilizes a combination of physical, occupational, and speech therapy services that are the same as acute rehab, but the number of hours that a patient receives will be lower in this setting. Typically, patients can expect to receive between 1 to 3 hours of therapy per day, depending on the individual facility.[1] Subacute rehab is most frequently provided in a licensed skilled nursing facility (SNF), though there are some hospitals that have their own SAR. In contrast to acute rehab, for which a qualifying diagnosis is a prerequisite for admission, no particular diagnosis is needed in order to qualify for SAR. Admission to SAR is also considered to be short term, but is more commonly longer than that in acute rehab. The length of stay at SAR can vary greatly for each patient, depending on the extent of their improvement, whether an assessment of discharge to their home environment is safe, and of course, on insurance coverage. Based on the aforementioned factors, a length of stay at SAR can be as little as a few days, but up to 100 days.[2] On occasion, while a patient is in acute rehabilitation it may be determined that they would continue to benefit from longer-term rehab, which can also lead to a transfer from an acute rehab facility to a SAR (Figure 20.1).

Home Health Services/Home Care

It is common for patients to need help at home following a hospitalization or inpatient rehab admission. Home health services are provided by a Certified Home Health Agency (CHHA).[4] Home healthcare includes any professional support services that allow a patient to live

SERVICES	HOME HEALTH	HOME CARE
BATHING/DRESSING ASSISTANCE	X	✓
BATHROOM NEEDS	X	✓
CLEANING SERVICES	X	✓
COMPANIONSHIP	X	✓
FORMAL HEALTH MONITORING	✓	X
INJECTIONS	✓	X
MAJOR WOUND CARE	✓	X
MEAL DELIVERY/PREP	X	✓
MEDICAL TESTS	✓	X
ADMINISTER MEDICATIONS	✓	X
MEDICATION REMINDERS	✓	✓
PAIN MANAGEMENT	✓	✓
REHABILITATION THERAPY	✓	X
SKILLED NURSING	✓	X
TRANSPORTATION	X	✓

Figure 20.2 A comparison between the different types of service for home health and home care services. Adapted from [5].

safely in their home. These services strive to help patients with ADLs, such as dressing and bathing, safely ambulating around the home, rehabilitative services, and short-term nursing care for management of an illness or disability. [4] Nursing services at home are prescribed by a physician and provide support in the care of wounds, administering newly prescribed injections, and assessing vital signs.[4] Home health services are approved by and paid for by Medicare, Medicaid, and private insurances.

Home health services are not to be confused with *home care* services. Home health services are medical in nature, whereas home care services include support and assistance in services such as meal preparation, companionship, supervision, chores, housecleaning, and grocery errands.[5] Medicaid is typically the only insurance provider that will cover these services, with coverage varying by state (Figure 20.2).[5]

Long-Term Care

Due to the severity or complexity of illness, many patients will not meet criteria to be safely discharged home or attend an inpatient rehabilitation program. While some families with significant financial resources may be able to secure the personnel and equipment necessary to care for a family member at home, this is out of reach for many families and has the potential to overwhelm family members' other life responsibilities and emotional bandwidth, even if financially feasible. Participation in therapy is a prerequisite for admission to an inpatient rehab facility, often making those destinations inappropriate for patients who remain with a depressed level of consciousness or severe impairment in communication ability. When neither home nor inpatient rehabilitation is an option, two types of facility may be considered: a long-term acute care hospital, or a skilled nursing facility.

Long-Term Acute Care Hospital (LTACH)

Long-term acute care hospitals (LTACHs) serve patients who have complex medical needs, typically those who continue to require ventilator support, but who no longer require a hospital level of care. An LTACH can provide a continuation of sophisticated hospital care for patients who are deemed stable to leave the hospital environment, once they no longer require high level diagnostics or procedures.[6] These facilities provide services including, but not limited to: ventilator weaning, complex wound care, intravenous medications, tube feedings, and the management of comorbid medical conditions.[6] While patients can receive some forms of inpatient rehabilitation during their stay at an LTACH, rehab is not the main focus. LTACHs involve round-the-clock medical care, similar to that of a hospital with a physician on site.[6] In order to qualify for LTACH admission, an intensive care unit (ICU) stay in an acute care hospital of at least 3 days is commonly required. In many cases, patients in a hospital ICU will be directly transferred to an LTACH due to their need for continuous management of mechanical ventilation. Patients' stays at an LTACH frequently last 1 month, but can vary greatly depending on their progress. As with other discharge destinations, prior to transfer to an LTACH, the patient's insurance company should be contacted for authorization.

Skilled Nursing Facility (SNF)

Skilled nursing facilities (SNFs) are appropriate for patients who do not require the intensive level of an acute care hospital or LTACH, but who are not candidates for inpatient rehabilitation and still require medical care that cannot be managed at home. SNFs provide continuing medical care for patients who have suffered from severe illness. They also focus on a patient's custodial needs, and support patients in bathing, dressing, toileting and other ADLs. If patients are able to participate in rehabilitation, SNFs can provide therapy, however, it is not their main priority. Patients may remain at an SNF for as little as a few weeks but may ultimately reside in such a facility for years. While Medicare and private insurance plans may sometimes cover patients for the initial portion of their SNF stay, long-term SNF placement requires that a patient needs to have a nursing facility benefit under a Medicaid plan.

Hospice and Palliative Care

Palliative care is best thought of as an interdisciplinary approach to optimize the quality of life while limiting pain and anxiety associated with a complex medical condition, and may be provided in any clinical care environment, beginning at the time of diagnosis, throughout treatment, until the end of life. The provision of palliative care should not be reserved only for those patients who are imminently dying. A patient with late-stage cancer undergoing curative chemotherapy may therefore receive palliative care, as could another patient who has no further curative options available. Under a palliative care approach, physicians are not required to certify a prognosis, and therapy can begin at any point.[7] Palliative care is typically provided in the hospital, though recently, options for the provision of palliative care at home or at other care facilities have emerged.[7]

When patients, or their caregivers decide to shift the focus of care from actively reversing disease to the pursuit of comfort at the end of life, there are multiple options, depending on the patient's expected prognosis, goals, and complexity of needs. Hospice care and palliative care are both approaches that have the objective of pain and symptom relief, but differ in that hospice care is more appropriate when curative therapy is no longer desired or available.[7] Furthermore, in order for a person to be eligible for hospice services, a physician must certify that the patient has a prognosis anticipating death within 6 months.[7] Hospice care can be covered under Medicare, Medicaid, and private insurances, and requires authorization prior to the initiation. Hospice can be provided at one's home, a hospice-specific residence, an SNF, acute hospitals, LTACHs, and other facilities (Figure 20.3).[7]

Barriers from a Payment Perspective

Both nursing and rehabilitation facilities require insurance authorization prior to accepting patients for transfer. Difficulties in securing these authorizations can be a thorny obstacle to transitioning patients out of the acute care setting. Medicare Part A covers short-term SNF care after a qualifying hospital stay as long as

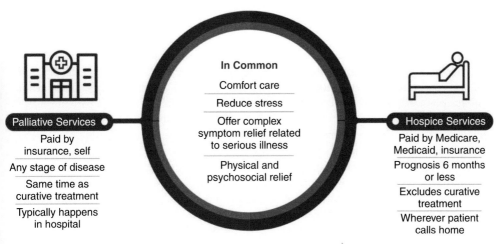

In Common

Comfort care

Reduce stress

Offer complex symptom relief related to serious illness

Physical and psychosocial relief

Palliative Services

Paid by insurance, self

Any stage of disease

Same time as curative treatment

Typically happens in hospital

Hospice Services

Paid by Medicare, Medicaid, insurance

Prognosis 6 months or less

Excludes curative treatment

Wherever patient calls home

Figure 20.3 A comparison of the services offered in hospice and palliative care [7].

medical care is required. For patients over the age of 65, Medicare typically pays for the full cost of the first 20 days of SNF care, paying any fees exceeding $128 per day for days 21 through 100.[8] Long-term custodial care that does not require medical management is not covered by Medicare.

Medicaid is a federal government program jointly administered with the states and provides support for low-income/asset individuals in paying for long- term nursing home care. Unlike Medicare, Medicaid can be used to pay for long-term custodial care even if medical care is not needed. Income cut-offs for individual Medicaid eligibility vary by state but are typically less than $2,300 per month.

Avoiding delays in insurance authorization for long- term care and rehab facilities starts with knowing what form of coverage a patient has. While knowing what kind of insurance a patient has seems like an obvious piece of information that all hospitals would gather, after an acute hospitalization it is not infrequent that the coverage a patient's family member believed them to have either has been changed to a different carrier or has lapsed altogether. Hospital teams should seek to identify and then confirm active insurance coverage as soon as possible after the patient has been admitted. If no insurance coverage is present, the hospital social worker and case management team can start exploring alternative insurance coverage options or begin obtaining the documentation necessary to apply for emergency Medicaid. Knowing what insurance coverage a patient has

will also help the discharge team communicate to the patient's family what facility options they have once the acute hospitalization has occurred.

Lack of insurance and/or lack of legal immigration status create tremendous barriers to safely discharging patients from an acute care hospital who require post-discharge services such as rehab or an SNF. Hospitals struggle to find solutions to these situations because although the patient no longer meets criteria to remain hospitalized, there are limited options to pay for the necessary post-hospitalization services. From the perspective of the hospital administrator, in some situations it may be more cost efficient for the hospital to pay for post-discharge services than to keep the patient hospitalized. Some hospitals, anticipating these types of cases, have responded by earmarking funds to help cover the costs of providing discharge services for these patients.

For uninsured patients who are US citizens, different forms of Medicaid may pay for home care, outpatient physician services, and even nursing home placement. The discharge team can determine whether a patient is eligible for Medicaid and apply. Medicaid programs vary from state to state. Each state has a great deal of flexibility in designing and administering their programs, as the federal guidelines are broad. For instance, in New York State, in order to qualify for nursing home coverage through Medicaid, an evaluation of the patient's financial statements from the previous 5 years is required. Many patients cannot qualify for Medicaid due to excess income or assets. Additional legal assistance, such as an elder law attorney, may be enlisted by the patient or family to assist in navigating Medicaid eligibility.

A special case that deserves mention and can pose extreme challenges to the discharge team is the unauthorized immigrant without health insurance who is hospitalized with a neurological injury. Many undocumented immigrants are especially vulnerable to poor health outcomes due to low rates of health insurance, poor health literacy, [9] high rates of diabetes,[10] and inadequate preventive care. In 2011, only 29% of unauthorized immigrants had some form of private health insurance, leaving the remaining 71% without any form of healthcare coverage.[11] The majority of government-based programs created to support financially struggling patients are prohibited from funding undocumented patients. As of the writing of this chapter, undocumented immigrants are not eligible to apply for Medicaid or Medicare on the Affordable Care Act (ACA) exchanges.

Undocumented immigrants pose a major challenge with respect to discharge planning after critical illness. These patients face extremely limited options and, at this time, there are no feasible solutions to fully meet the needs of this population. In fortunate situations, family members of an undocumented immigrant may be willing to assist in their care during recovery. If the needs of the patient are too great or complex for the patient to return home, some hospitals will assist in providing funds for patients to receive care in a skilled nursing facility, though it should not be assumed that all hospitals have the means or the will to provide this level of financial support. In some instances, hospitals have paid to have the patient flown back to their country of origin to receive care. This process, known as medical repatriation, has been used by hospitals to reduce their costs in the face of a lack of reimbursement. It raises many controversial issues, including those related to consent, social justice, and the fulfillment of international human rights obligations. While a full treatment of this complex and ethically controversial issue is beyond the scope of this chapter, medical repatriation should only be considered when all other options have been exhausted, there is a family member or other party willing to accept responsibility for the patient's care in the destination country, and only if a hospital in the country the patient is being flown back to can accommodate the patient's medical needs.[12] Any

consideration of this option should be discussed with hospital administration and legal and ethics teams before proceeding.

Even those with active insurance coverage can experience barriers if they have needs for skilled services at the time of discharge. For instance, Medicare Part A helps to cover a patient's hospital stay, inpatient rehab, and SNF placement, but will not cover these services indefinitely. Especially after long hospitalizations, patients receiving Medicare may find that they have exhausted the coverage and that additional discharge facility fees cannot be covered. In these cases, if patients don't have supplemental insurance, discharge facilities may not accept the patient, which can lead to long delays to discharge. Discharge teams should try to anticipate limited insurance resources in advance when a prolonged hospitalization seems imminent, and try to apply for additional resources such as Medicaid as soon as possible to limit delays later on.

Facility Delays

Patients who have sustained acute neurological injury often will be left with permanent physical and cognitive disabilities or may require months or sometimes years to slowly recover. There are several commonly encountered obstacles that arise when planning for hospital discharge and the transition to a facility that will continue caring for the patient during this phase of recovery or convalescence. The clinicians at an SNF or rehabilitation center may reject the application of a patient to their facility due to medical instability or inappropriateness. Only medically stable patients should be transferred out of an acute care hospital to one of these destinations, as these facilities seldom have the capacity to take care of unstable or critically ill patients. Hypotension, tachycardia, or tachypnea are obvious reasons why a facility might reject the transfer of a patient, but other medical problems, such as worsening renal failure or a recent change in the patient's mental status, might also be grounds for delay. For the clinicians, social workers and case managers involved in planning post-hospital discharges, it is important to understand what medical requirements different facilities have before applying for admission there, as well as understanding of what type of patients the facility has the capacity care for.

Most facilities will conduct a medical review of the candidate patient's case before they grant acceptance. If a significant change occurs in the patient's clinical status prior to transfer, facilities often elect to repeat the medical review process, inevitably causing delays. When procedures such as tracheostomy, percutaneous feeding tube placement, or ventriculoperitoneal shunting are anticipated, many facilities will refuse to begin an application for transfer until all medically relevant procedures have been completed. In some cases, however, especially when the sending hospital and receiving rehab or long-term care facility have established a trusted relationship working with each other, applications can begin to be processed even before these procedures have been completed, usually contingent on the patient avoiding any procedural complications and remaining stable.

A pause is warranted at this point to restate this important fact: the value of forming relationships between the hospital discharge team and representatives from long-term care facilities and rehab centers pays off tremendously in terms of improved efficiency and a reduction in administrative delays. People naturally work better with those whom they have seen or spoken with in person and who they trust to provide straightforward and honest assessments of patients. Hospital physicians and discharge staff should strongly consider taking the time to visit, in person, facilities they commonly work with, and speak directly with staff there. While this of course does not guarantee that delays won't occur, a facility is much more likely to hold a bed for a patient or go the extra mile to expedite the patient's transition if they have a personal relationship with the hospital's staff.

Keeping the discharge team, including social work and case management, aware of the patient's clinical status with regular updates during their hospitalization helps the team anticipate when a patient may be approaching a discharge date. Regular documentation about changes in the patient's prognosis and discharge planning are another way of conveying information to those team members who will inevitably need this information to decide when it is appropriate to engage a potential discharge facility. As with any team-based task, maintaining clear and open lines of communication is vital and ensures that a social worker does not continue to pursue a discharge plan to a rehab facility when the patient has experienced a clinical deterioration and may now require a nursing home or an extension of their hospital stay that makes transfer timing uncertain.

Staff caring for the patient should anticipate the patient's specific medical needs and will need to convey these to the receiving facility. Most facilities have the capability of continuing intravenous antibiotic therapy, for instance, but many cannot accommodate patients who require dialysis or frequent oral or tracheal suctioning. If the team does not understand a specific facility's limitations, they may waste time planning discharge to a facility that will ultimately reject the patient. Regularly scheduled, daily rounding between clinical providers and the discharge team, including social work and case management, has been shown to improve discharge outcomes and reduce lengths of stay.[13] These daily rounds include an update on the patient's medical status from the clinical team, a description of procedures the patient will require before discharge (e.g., tracheostomy, feeding tube placement), the clinicians' assessment of the patient's functional status (e.g., whether they are able to participate in rehab or not), and the expected date of the patient's readiness for discharge. Sharing information between the clinical and discharge teams on a daily basis helps the latter know when discussions with family and applications to facilities are appropriate and, in our experience, decrease patients' length of stay.

Family Communication

Another important consideration in discharge planning is communication with family members and healthcare surrogates regarding the ultimate disposition of the patient. Acute neurological injuries, such as stroke or TBI, often strike suddenly and unexpectedly. Many family members have difficulty understanding the nature of a brain injury and the possibility that nervous tissue may not heal the way other parts of the body do, leading to permanent deficits. Even after the patient's condition has been explained, family members can have trouble accepting the reality that their loved one has been irrevocably changed, or that they may require an extended duration of care in a long-term facility with an unclear path for recovery. Differences in understanding between clinicians and family members are often a source of tension between the two parties and can lead to antagonism and varying degrees of counter-transference on the part of the physicians or nurses responsible for conveying information to the family.

Communicating the details of a patient's condition to family members should always occur in plain language that includes the most important aspect of the disease process at hand but also lays out a roadmap for what the recovery process will look like. In our experience, in an attempt to remain hopeful and solidify a collaborative rapport with family members, many clinicians speak to families in optimistic terms during the initial phase of hospitalization, sometimes avoiding a discussion about the deficits or difficulties that they foresee the patient having until later in the patient's course when discharge is closer. It is the opinion of the authors that this is a mistake. Clinicians often have enough clinical experience to know early in the patient's course if they are likely to require discharge to a nursing facility or inpatient rehab facility. Conveying a mediocre prognosis, or one that is less hopeful than what family members expect, can create feelings of conflict between family and clinical providers. Family members may interpret realistic prognoses as the medical team "giving up" on the patient. It is essential that clinicians communicate that they are working to do what is best for the patient and help the family through what may be the most difficult time in their lives. Using supportive language, taking the time to listen to families' concerns and desires, and consistently demonstrating presence and compassion to the families of patients is immensely important in building the therapeutic relationship necessary to tackle the patient's transition of care together.

Families naturally prefer discharge to a rehab facility due to the association with active recovery and a better prognosis, but often this is an unrealistic goal. If the need for an SNF or LTACH discharge is foreseen, it is essential to discuss this with family members as early as possible. While often distressing for family members to hear, it allows families time to process this news and begin making plans for life changes that may accompany the patient's illness, as well as giving families time to learn about the different facility options they may have available to them.

Often families wish to visit nursing and rehabilitation facilities in advance, which may delay applications if this is left until later in the patient's course. Family members also frequently reject the idea that their loved ones need to be transferred to a nursing home, and may see the hospital staff's planning around such a discharge as reflecting an abandonment of the patient. It is important to convey early on in the patient's course that the hospital is there to stabilize the patient and carry out any procedures or treatments necessary to set them up for recovery, but that much of the clinical improvement the patient will experience naturally takes place after discharge from the hospital. Discharge planning should be presented as a part of the recovery process.

A second common obstacle related to families of neurologically injured patients comes when there is internal conflict within the family about who is to make medical decisions on behalf of a patient without decision-making capacity. The stress and anxiety induced in individuals after the acute neurological injury in a family member are only exacerbated by discord among the various individuals who almost always want what is best for the patient but differ in opinion about what the best course of action should be. Hospital team members often become the unwitting mediators of conflicts between family members, and are best served by a calm approach, making sure to acknowledge the love every participant shares for the patient, while also listening to and acknowledging the various perspectives that are not universally shared. When discussions about prognosis are first being given, it is often advantageous to include as many individuals in the patient's family as are interested in participating. This establishes a base level of information that everyone can receive simultaneously, and allows for clarifying questions to be asked and answered in front of all concerned. The medical team should avoid having separate conversations with different family members to avoid confusion or the appearance that some information is being withheld from specific individuals. Again, when clinicians feel confident about the patient's future need for skilled nursing facility placement, we advocate introducing this possibility to the family early on. In the event that patients make a more rapid recovery than expected and qualify for inpatient rehab placement instead of an SNF, families tend to accept the change in prognosis better than if their early expectation of a salutary recovery is disappointed and they learn about the need for nursing facility placement later.

Once information about the patient's condition is shared, if there is conflict between family members about medical decisions, the clinician leading the conversation should remind everyone that, ultimately, the goal of discussing medical options is *to do for the patient what they would have wanted for themselves*, a process referred to as "substituted judgment." Reframing medical decision making as an effort to honor the patient's own unspoken desires, rather than a referendum on what individual family members want, often adds a clarity of purpose to the discussion, and creates a common goal among the participants.

In a minority of cases, however, family members may continue to have irreconcilable differences regarding whether a patient would, for example, wish to pursue recovery in a skilled nursing facility after tracheostomy and gastrostomy tube placement, or rather focus on comfort measures in the absence of aggressive medical support. In every case, attempts should be made to achieve unanimity in these decisions, but unfortunately, there are occasions in which agreement will not be reached. In these cases, it is even more important to identify which individual(s) have the legal standing to make medical decisions for the patient. A legally documented healthcare proxy signed by the patient, when present, establishes a healthcare agent to make decisions for the patient that supersedes the authority of all other individuals. In cases where an official healthcare agent has not been designated in writing by the patient, a healthcare surrogate may be established by default on the basis of the individuals' relationship to the patient. In 35 of the US states, a surrogate hierarchy of relatives and partners is established. All of these states grant a spouse highest priority, but only seven allow a partner similar priority, and parents, children, siblings, and friends occupy different rungs of the ladder in different states.[14] Clinicians should familiarize themselves with the provisions that exist in their own state of practice regarding the surrogacy hierarchy that applies to them.

Conclusion

Recovery after neurological injury or disease is a process that commonly requires ongoing medical support and coordinated care at a discharge facility after the acute hospitalization. For those patients whose care needs cannot be delivered in the home, there are several different discharge options that can be considered, including inpatient rehab, an SNF, or an LTACH. Transfer to a discharge facility should be viewed and presented to patients' families as an expected phase in the recovery process. Common challenges in disposition planning include anticipating the patient's medical readiness for discharge, communication with families, and inadequate financial resources. Clear communication about the patient's status between the clinical team caring for the patient and the hospital discharge team can help reduce delays and improve families' satisfaction with the discharge process.

References

1. Burke Rehabilitation. Physical therapy. Available at: www.burke.org/inpatient/admissions/what-is-acute-rehab

2. Columbia University Department of Rehabilitation and Regenerative Medicine. Rehabilitation and regenerative medicine. Available at : www.cumc.columbia.edu/rehab/patient-resources/subacute-inpatient-rehabilitation

3. Vigor Physical Therapy. Comparison between acute and subacute care rehab.

4. New York State Department of Health. NYS Health Profiles. About Certified Home Health Agencies (CHHAs). Available at: https://profiles.health.ny.gov/home_care/pages/chha

5. A Place for Mom. Home care vs. home health care: what's the difference? www.aplaceformom.com/planning-and-advice/articles/home-health-vs-home-care

6. Muldoon SR. Why LTAC hospitals are a choice for critically ill patients. Kindred Hospitals. 2020. Available at: www.kindredhealthcare.com/resources/blog-kindred-continuum/2020/03/19/why-ltac-hospitals-are-often-the-right-choice-for-critically-ill-patients

7. Vitas Health Care. What are the differences and commonalities between hospice and palliative care? Available at: www.vitas.com/hospice-and-palliative-care-basics/about-palliative-care/hospice-vs-palliative-care-whats-the-difference

8. Caring.com. Nursing home costs and ways to pay. Available at: www.caring.com/senior-living/nursing-homes/how-to-pay/

9. Derose KP, Escarce JJ, Lurie N. Immigrants and health care: sources of vulnerability. *Health Aff (Millwood)*. 2007;26(5):258–68.

10. Lee H, Zakhary BL, Firek MA, et al. The prevalence and impact of diabetes mellitus among undocumented immigrants in an indigent care program in Riverside, California. *Diabetes.* 2018;**67**(supplement 1):1625-P.

11. Capps R, Fix M, VanHook J, Bachmeier JD. *A Demographic, Socioeconomic, and Health Coverage Profile of Unauthorized Immigrants in the United States.* Washington, DC; Migration Policy Institute, 2013. Available at: www.migrationpolicy .org/sites/default/files/publications/CIRbrief-Profi le-Unauthorized_1.pdf.

12. Fruth S. Medical repatriation: the intersection of mandated emergency care, immigration consequences, and international obligations. *J Leg Med.* 2015;**36**(1):45–72;.

13. Patel, H, Yirdaw E. Improving early discharge using a team-based structure for discharge multidisciplinary rounds. *Prof Case Manag.* 2019;**24**(2):83–9.

14. DeMartino ES, Dudzinski DM, Doyle CK, et al. Who decides when a patient can't? Statutes on alternate decision makers. *New Engl J Med.* 2017;**376**(15):1478–82.

Chapter 21

Religious and Legal Issues in Neuroprognostication

Aaron Sylvan Lord and Ariane Lewis

Introduction

Of all areas of medicine, the practice of neurological prognostication requires one of the deepest understandings of the humanistic aspects of medicine. Neurological injuries affect the most human aspects of a patient's life – the ability to think, feel, talk, eat, and walk. The impact of neurological injuries must be considered in the context of a patient's and their family's cultural, moral, and religious beliefs. Additionally, a patient's geographical location influences their case from legal and social perspectives. Neurological prognostication for a severely brain-injured patient is practiced in a very different way by a clinician at a major medical center in New York City caring for an Orthodox Jewish patient than it is by a clinician in Bangladesh caring for a Muslim patient. All neurological prognostication requires an intimate understanding of a patient's ethical and religious beliefs and the local laws and customs. Notably, many of the religious, ethical, and legal issues that must be considered when prognosticating after neurological injury have emerged in the past century in the context of the development of advanced ventilators and neurocritical care interventions and are, thus, comparatively new issues to the field of religious studies and bioethics.

In this chapter, we will address religious and legal issues in neurological prognostication. We will start by reviewing religious considerations at the end of life for the six largest religions in the United States and the manner in which these considerations impact the practice of neurological prognostication. With this context in mind, we will then discuss legal issues surrounding neurological prognostication by reviewing some of the most prominent medicolegal cases in the United States and Europe. Many of the conflicts leading to legal action resulted from differences in religious views about the end of life. Lastly, we will discuss the notion of "futility" and review appropriate language and mental constructs to frame discussions around care at the end of life.

Of note, while discussing determination of death by neurological criteria (brain death) is the most concrete, yet the most extreme form of neurological prognostication, this chapter is focused on the broader topic of neurological prognostication. There are a number of papers addressing the ethical, legal, and religious considerations when discussing death by neurological criteria, and we encourage the interested reader to review them.[1,2]

Additionally, we would like to openly acknowledge that neither author is an authority on any of the world's major religions, and neither of us is a lawyer. Lastly, the purpose of this chapter is to aid the clinician in navigating some of the major religious and legal challenges associated with neurological prognostication; it should not be construed as legal advice.

Religious Considerations

Overview

According the 2014 Pew Research Center Religious Landscape Study, the most common religions in the United States are Christianity 70.6% (46.6% Protestant, 20.8% Catholic, 1.6% Mormon, 0.8% Jehovah's Witness), Judaism 1.9%, Islam 0.9%, Buddhism 0.7%, and Hinduism 0.7%.[3] Importantly, 22.8% of the population are so-called religious nones, meaning they are either atheist, or agnostic, or subscribe to no particular religious beliefs.

Viewpoints about end of life, withdrawal of life-sustaining treatment, and euthanasia vary widely within each of the major world religions, as there are a multitude of sects and traditions within each religion. Different denominations of a given religion often have different foundational theologies and beliefs about how to resolve questions about end-of-life decision making. Even within specific religious communities, beliefs and customs might vary from church to church or religious leader to religious leader. With this in mind, we highlight major themes to help the clinician in their daily practice.

As clinicians meet with families to discuss neurological prognostication, it is important not only to ask about a patient's religion, but also to inquire specifically about how their religious views inform the situation at hand. One should never assume certain beliefs, and compassionate inquiry is an essential skill in ensuring a patient's wishes are respected. Notably, just as beliefs vary within certain religions, a patient may have different religious beliefs from other members of their family. Similarly, members of a patient's family may have differing beliefs among themselves. These different beliefs or interpretations can be a source of conflict when determining how to approach neurological prognostication. Open dialogue is crucial, as is consultation with a patient's spiritual leader or local chaplain. Clinicians should consider involving their hospital's chaplain or religious officials in family discussions, as well as inviting a patient's spiritual leader to participate in these discussions.

Specific Religious Considerations

The "Abrahamic" religions, Judaism, Christianity, and Islam, all trace their roots to a single ancestor, Abraham. Abrahamic religions believe that each individual is created at a specific point in time by God and that each individual is unique. Each individual remains themselves throughout their life and then passes into an afterlife. All three traditions rely heavily on sacred, written texts. Many of the laws and customs in the western world derive from a Judeo-Christian understanding of ethics.

Judaism

While there are many branches of Judaism, the three largest are the Orthodox, Conservative, and Reform movements. The Orthodox movement believes in mandatory obedience to Jewish law (Halacha), and adheres to the strictest interpretations of the biblical mandates.[4] Conservative Jews also believe that adherence to Halacha is mandatory, but they believe that the law is under continual evolution. Conservative rabbinical interpretation of the law is often more flexible than that of Orthodox rabbis. The Reform movement has the most liberal interpretation of Jewish law; it places a prominent emphasis on individual autonomy. In Reform Judaism, Halacha is not strictly followed, and the rabbi is often one of many resources Reform Jews seek out in times of need for moral clarity.[5]

Jewish medical ethics relies on a number of principles, but the key one is that life is of the utmost value.[6] There exists not just a permission to heal, but also an obligation to do so because the body belongs to God.[5] In general, it is against Jewish law to hasten death. This mandate, however, is complicated by the additional beliefs that the dying process should not be unnecessarily prolonged and that decisions about treatment should be made to benefit the patient. Therefore, there is considerable disagreement between rabbis as to the correct course of action in many end-of-life decisions. [5] For example, strict interpretations of Halacha do not allow for the withdrawal of artificial nutrition and hydration, but Conservative and Reform rabbis have ruled that that they can be removed at end of life because they are delivered through tubes and look like drugs, not like food or water. Additionally, although most rabbis allow for hospice care, strict interpretations of Halacha do not allow for the use of morphine if it could hasten death; however, Conservative and Reform interpretations allow for the use of morphine as long as the dose is not high enough to cause certain death. A recent survey of rabbis demonstrated that although only 5% of all rabbis believe a person who is brain dead could recover, 22% did not believe brain death is death and 18% believed mechanical ventilation should be continued after brain death.[1] Orthodox rabbis were less likely to accept the concept of brain death than Conservative and Reform rabbis.[1] Conservative and Reform rabbis defend the belief that brain death is death based on eleventh-century Talmudic interpretations that death occurs with cessation of the ability to breathe, and that a decapitated animal should be considered dead, even if the body is still moving.[4] Orthodox rabbis interpret these texts differently.

Christianity

Christianity evolved from Judaism and is based on the belief that Jesus is the son of God and the savior of humankind; his death by crucifixion and eventual resurrection inform many Christian beliefs. With respect to the end of life, Christianity teaches that its members may pursue eternal life through repentance of their sins. Believers in traditional Christianity may seek to use medical technology to postpone death so that they have sufficient time to repent as well as to practice ceremonial last rites.[7] The ability to be conscious to repent may affect end-of-life decisions due to sedation and analgesia, although this may be less of an issue in patients with severe brain injury who may have significant alterations in consciousness due to their injury. Given the importance in Christianity of submitting to God's will, suicide, physician-assisted suicide, and euthanasia are considered murder as they are in conflict with God's will.[7]

However, there are limits to the utility of medicine according to Christian theology. St. Basil the Great argued that while medicine is a "gift from God," it can be harmful to the soul when the use of medicine to stave off death gets so intense that staying alive becomes an all-consuming burden.[7]

Catholicism

The Catholic Church has a distinct hierarchy, with the Pope being its spiritual leader, though different viewpoints exist as a result of varied theological and philosophical methodologies.[8] There is a rich history of bioethical inquiry in the Catholic Church beginning with St. Basil in the fourth century, notions of ordinary versus extraordinary and obligatory versus nonobligatory healthcare in the sixteenth century, and Pope John Paul II's "Evangelium Vitae" in 1995 that reiterated that withdrawal and withholding of therapies is permitted so long as such treatment imposed extreme burden and danger to the patient.[8,9] Euthanasia is not permitted under the 1980 *Declaration on Euthanasia*, and withdrawal of artificial nutrition from those in a vegetative state is forbidden by a 2004 papal decree.[10,11] However, withdrawal of "futile" treatments is permitted under church doctrine.

An important bioethical concept of the "Double Effect" emerged from Catholicism and the writings of St. Thomas Aquinas in the thirteenth century. The principle of Double Effect explains that a harm that alone may be impermissible, such as a hastening of death, may indeed be permissible if it brings about some other good, such as the alleviation of suffering.[12] According to the *New Catholic Encyclopedia*, there are four conditions that need to be met for the Double Effect principle to be applied:[12]

1. The act itself must be morally good or at least indifferent.
2. The agent may not positively will the bad effect, but may permit it. If they could attain the good effect without the bad effect, they should do so.
3. The good effect must flow from the action at least as immediately (in the order of causality, though not necessarily in the order of time) as the bad effect. In other words, the good effect must be produced directly by the action, not by the bad effect. Otherwise, the agent would be using a bad means to a good end, which is never allowed.
4. The good effect must be sufficiently desirable to compensate for the allowing of the bad effect.

Catholics believe that "death ... results from the separation of the life-principle (or soul) from the corporal reality of the person." Given there is no way to determine when this has happened, the Church defers to medical authorities, and all Catholic hospitals in the United States accept death by neurological criteria.[4]

Protestantism

Protestantism emerged in the 1500s in Western Europe. It places particular emphasis on an individual's own interpretation of scripture to determine moral decisions, as opposed to interpretation by authoritative figures in the clergy. Since that time, innumerable sects of Protestantism have emerged and continue to emerge. Beliefs vary widely. Most, but not all, forms of Protestantism recognize death by neurological criteria. Additionally, most forms of Protestantism believe it is moral to withdraw mechanical support as well as artificial nutrition and hydration if it is only prolonging the dying process.[4]

Islam

Islam began in the seventh century. It shares the same monotheistic God as Judaism and Christianity, but it also revolves around the belief that a series of prophets, including Abraham,

Jesus, and the final prophet, Mohammed, have helped lead humanity to God. The foundational sacred Islamic text is the Qur'an. Islamic social and legal customs are described in the Sunnah.[13] There is significant variation in the interpretation of Qur'an and Sunnah as it applies to death and dying, and there is no definitive authority, so beliefs vary widely. There is a deep-rooted respect for science and medicine in Islam, and while there is widespread support for death by neurological criteria within the Muslim medical community, there is significant debate by religious scholars as to its validity.[4] However, less disagreement is seen when it comes to withdrawal of treatment that only prolongs the dying process, as it is believed to be a decision that should be made by the family after they have weighed the benefits and burdens of the options.

Hinduism

Hinduism is a diverse group of beliefs and practices that originated in the Indus Valley (modern-day India). The body is considered a vehicle for this life only and does not represent the true self. Life on earth is considered a continuum from a previous life into the next, through reincarnation into another vessel for another life on earth or becoming one with the highest being, Brahman. Hindus usually accept Western medicine in serious diseases, but if this is not beneficial, they often turn to more traditional practices (healing mantras, gems, dances, fasts, etc.) as a last resort.[14] Great emphasis is placed on a "good death" that occurs at the right time, at the right place, in the correct manner, and in the right state of mind.[15] Given the importance of the process of death, most Hindus in India die at home and thus discontinue medical treatment prior to death. Heroic medical attempts are often considered as interfering with the process of death, and so mechanical support is often quickly removed. Of importance, death with excessive bodily fluids is considered a "bad death," making it harder for the soul to leave the body, so artificial nutrition and hydration are often withheld.[4]

Buddhism

Buddhism was founded in India in the sixth century B.C.E. and quickly spread throughout Asia, where it is at present practiced alongside local traditions. Buddhism shares with Hinduism the belief that life is a cycle of deaths and rebirths,

samsara, with the possibility of eventual liberation, which Buddhism refers to as Nirvana.[4] Buddhism was founded by Siddhartha Gautama, also known as Buddha, and the story of his life is a key source of ethical guidance. There is no central authority in Buddhism, though Buddhists may seek the guidance of monks or spiritual leaders such as the Dalai Lama in Tibetan Buddhism. However, there is no obligation to follow their directives given Buddha's emphasis on finding one's own path through life. The acceptance of withdrawal of treatment or of death by neurological criteria is often heavily informed by local custom, as there are few rigid formalities in modern Buddhism.[16] However, many Buddhists do not accept death by neurological criteria given that death is defined by the absence of vitality, sentience, and heat.[16] Withdrawal of treatment or artificial nutrition and hydration for those suffering from severe neurological injury may be regarded with unease, given the Buddhist belief that all people are deserving of compassion regardless of their physical condition. Deferring treatment of secondary complications, such as pneumonia, is permissible, however, given Buddhist teaching that it is permissible to accept death when one has exhausted medical care.[16] Beliefs and customs around end of life vary widely, however, given the blending of Buddhism into local culture and ancient customs.

Legal Considerations

Medicine remains a mostly self-regulated profession, but it is important to be aware of certain laws and legal cases when managing patients who are severely neurologically impaired. Whenever there is doubt about the legality of an action, it is important to involve the hospital legal and risk management teams. Here, we will review a few legal cases that have brought clarity to the legality of refusing medical interventions by patients and their surrogates in the United States and Europe. We will also review some of the bioethical principles around surrogate decision making at the end of life.

Refusal of Medical Treatment

Two very similar cases form the basis of case law around refusing medical therapies: Karen Ann Quinlan and Nancy Beth Cruzan. Karen Quinlan suffered hypoxic–ischemic brain damage and was in a vegetative state over a year later when her surrogate, her father, asked that she be removed from the ventilator.[17] The hospital initially refused to take her off the ventilator, but the New Jersey Supreme Court ruled in 1976 that the constitutional right to privacy included the right to refuse medical treatments and that this right could be exercised by surrogates for patients who lacked decision-making capacity.[2]

The US Supreme Court weighed in on this issue at a national level when they reviewed the case of Nancy Cruzan, who was in a persistent vegetative state 4 years after suffering a traumatic brain injury. The Supreme Court ruled that, based on the Fourteenth Amendment right to "due process," competent patients have the right to refuse medical care, including withdrawal of artificial nutrition and hydration.[17] However, the court also argued that states could require a higher level of scrutiny of patients' known wishes when the decision to refuse medical treatment was made by a surrogate decision maker.[18]

Additional similar cases have reached national and international prominence. The case of Theresa "Terri" Schiavo, a woman in a persistent vegetative state whose husband wished to discontinue artificial nutrition and hydration, but whose parents did not, was brought to court in Florida. The court ruled that there was "clear and convincing evidence" she would not want to live in a dependent state, and the Supreme Court's refusal to hear the appeal strengthened the right under *Cruzan* of surrogate decision makers to refuse medical treatment.[17]

A more recent and almost identical case in France has reached international prominence. Vincent Lambert is a nurse who has been in a persistent vegetative state since 2008. His wife states that he had clearly indicated he would not want to live in a dependent state, but his parents do not want to remove artificial nutrition and hydration. The case was settled in the French courts and nutrition was stopped, only to be reinstated hours later when a French court issued a stay of the decision so that the UN-affiliated Committee on the Rights of Persons with Disabilities could review his case.[19]

Physician-Assisted Death

While the US Supreme Court has upheld a patient's right to refuse any and all medical treatment for themselves or their surrogate based on the "due process" clause of the Constitution, it has not found that a patient has a fundamental right to euthanasia or physician-assisted suicide. In *Washington* v. *Glucksberg* and *Vacco* v. *Quill*, the court ruled that states are allowed to set their own laws and regulations on physician-assisted suicide, and seven states currently allow the practice.[2] Importantly, palliative sedation is not considered physician-assisted death and is legal in all 50 states, given it is "widely recognized that the provision of pain medication is ethically and professionally acceptable even when the treatment may hasten the patient's death, if the medication is intended to alleviate pain and severe discomfort, not to cause death."[20]

Objections to Death by Neurological Criteria

In the past 50 years, there have been a number of lawsuits objecting to death by neurological criteria. [21] These lawsuits have been issued both prior to completion of an evaluation for determination of death by neurological criteria and prior to discontinuation of organ support.

Two cases in the United States reached conflicting decisions about management of objections to apnea testing. A Montana court ruled that a hospital could not perform an apnea test over a family's objection because Montana law does not mandate that clinicians perform a brain death evaluation, and performance of a medical procedure on a child requires consent by their parents. [22] Contrastingly, in the same year (2016), a Virginia court ruled that a hospital could perform an apnea test over a family's objection.[23]

While some lawsuits on continuation of organ support after declaration of death have resulted in the decision that support should be discontinued, others have resulted in the opposite decision. In a 2015 case in the United Kingdom, the High Court of England and Wales ruled that organ support should be discontinued despite a family's objections that this would violate their Muslim beliefs.[24] Similarly, a court in Toronto ruled that organ support should be discontinued after Taquisha McKitty was declared dead by neurological criteria in 2017, despite her father's religious objection.[25] However, in the highly publicized case of Jahi McMath, a teenager whose family objected to discontinuation of organ support after she suffered hypoxic–ischemic brain injury at a hospital in California in 2013, the court ruled that organ support could be continued and her body could be transferred to her mother's custody, after which she was transferred to New Jersey (where the law requires continuation of organ support until cardiopulmonary arrest if a family voices religious objections to death by neurological criteria).[26]

Requests for "Potentially Inappropriate" Care

In intensive care settings (ICU), clinicians may be asked by surrogates to institute therapies that they feel will not benefit the patient. The etiology for these requests is multifactorial, and it can in part be attributed to poor communication between clinicians and surrogates or misunderstanding by surrogates of prognosis, but it may also be based on differences in religious and ethical beliefs about end-of-life care. Due to these differences, critical care organizations have issued consensus statements on how to deal with such requests. In June 2015, the American Thoracic Society (ATS), American Association of Critical Care Nurses (AACN), American College of Chest Physicians (ACCP), European Society for Intensive Care Medicine, and the Society of Critical Care Medicine issued a Policy Statement with four recommendations on how to respond to requests

for "potentially inappropriate" treatments in the ICU.[27] These recommendations include developing strategies and processes to mitigate treatment conflicts including ample communication and early expert consultation; using the term "potentially inappropriate" in lieu of "futile" for treatments that have at least some chance of accomplishing the effect sought by the patient or surrogate, but clinicians believe that competing ethical considerations justify not providing them; and having medical professionals engage with the public and government officials to advocate for appropriate policies and legislation regarding when life-prolonging technologies should not be used.

Conclusion

The implications of a poor neurological prognosis vary greatly depending on a patient's religious beliefs. Clinicians will benefit from having an understanding of the manner in which the major world religions view end-of-life issues, with the understanding that viewpoints within each religion vary greatly (Table 21.1). Landmark legal cases provide case law defining the rights of patients and their families in the United States who are neurologically devastated or at the end of their life. These cases inform the options we present to patients in similar circumstances, and clinicians should remain up to date on how future cases may impact care in the future (Table 21.2).

Table 21.1 Views on end-of-life issues of major religions in the United States

Religion	% of United States	Basic tenets about end of life	Other considerations
Christianity – Protestant	46.6 %	Individual interpretation of scripture to determine moral decisions is emphasized. Significant variation exists, but many Protestants are comfortable withdrawing treatment if injury is severe or treatments burdensome.	Innumerous denominations exist throughout the United States
Christianity – Catholic	20.8	Repentance of sin and administration of last rights before death is of great importance. Withdrawing and withholding therapies is permitted when treatments impose an extreme burden on a patient. Withdrawal of artificial nutrition for those in a vegetative state is not permitted (2004 Papal Decree).	The Catholic Church has a distinct hierarchy, with the Pope as its leader. Euthanasia is not permitted under the 1980 Papal "Declaration on Euthanasia."

Table 21.1 (cont.)

Religion	% of United States	Basic tenets about end of life	Other considerations
Judaism	1.9	Life is of the utmost value; there is an obligation to heal because the body belongs to God. It is against Jewish law to hasten death and the strictest interpretations do not allow for withdrawal of ongoing treatments including nutrition/ hydration.	Views vary widely between the three major branches in respect to observance of traditional Jewish law. 1. Orthodox: mandatory obedience, strict interpretation; 2. Conservative: mandatory obedience, interpretation evolves; 3. Reform: liberal interpretation; individual autonomy emphasized.
Islam	0.9	Everything should be done to avoid an early death. Withdrawal can be considered if death is certain. Deep rooted respect for medicine and science. There is significant variation in interpretation of the major texts (Qur'an and Sunna).	Withdrawal decisions are left to families who may consult with a spiritual leader (ımam).
Buddhism	0.7	Life is a cycle of deaths and rebirths. The life of Buddha is key to ethical decision-making. Local customs determine most withdrawal decisions. Deferring treatment when death is imminent is permitted, but withdrawal for those with severe neurological injury could be viewed as not being compassionate, which is a central tenant.	No central authority, although many seek spiritual guidance from monks or leaders such as Dalai Lama in Tibetan Buddhism.
Hinduism	0.7	Life is a cycle of deaths and rebirths. Great emphasis is placed on a "good death": the right time, the right place, in the right state of mind. Heroic efforts may be considered to interfere with the process of death. Excessive bodily fluids is considered a "bad death." Artificial nutrition/hydration is often withheld.	There is a preference to die at home. There is general acceptance of western medicine, but emphasis is placed on traditional practices when this has failed.

Table 21.2 Major legal cases affecting neuroprognostication in the United States

Case	Decision year	Jurisdiction	Importance in neuroprognostication
In re Quinlan	1976	New Jersey Supreme Court	Constitutional right to privacy includes right to refuse medical treatments. These rights can be exercised by a surrogate for patients lacking capacity.
Cruzan v. Director, Missouri Dept. of Health	1990	U.S. Supreme Court	Constitutional right to due process includes the right to refuse medical care, or "right to die," but states could require high level of scrutiny when medical care is refused by surrogates.
In Re: Allen Callaway	2016	Montana District Court	Families have the right to refuse testing for determination of death by neurological criteria because (1) the law does not mandate

Table 21.2 (cont.)

Case	Decision year	Jurisdiction	Importance in neuroprognostication
			performance of an assessment for determination of death by neurological criteria, and (2) parents have the right to refuse medical procedures.
In re Mirranda Grace Lawson	2016	Virginia Circuit Court	Families do not have the right to refuse testing for determination of death by neurological criteria.

References

1. Lewis, A. A survey of multidenominational rabbis on death by neurologic criteria. *Neurocrit Care.* 2019;**31**(2):411–18.

2. Gostin, L.O. Deciding life and death in the courtroom. *JAMA.* 1997;**278**(18);1523.

3. Pew Research Center 2014 U.S. religious landscape study. Pew Research Center. 2014.

4. Setta, S.M., S.D. Shemie. An explanation and analysis of how world religions formulate their ethical decisions on withdrawing treatment and determining death. *Philos Ethics Humanit Med.* 2015;**10**:6.

5. Dorff, E.N. End-of-life: Jewish perspectives. *Lancet.* 2005;**366**(9488):862–5.

6. Kassim, P., F. Alias. Religious, ethical, and legal consideration in end-of-life issues: fundamental requisites for medical decision making. *J Relig Health.* 2016;**55**:119–34.

7. Engelhardt, H.T. Jr, A.S. Iltis. End-of-life: the traditional Christian view. *Lancet.* 2005;**366** (9490):1045–9.

8. Markwell, H. End-of-life: a Catholic view. *Lancet,* 2005;366(9491):1132–5.

9. Bulow, H.H., C.L. Sprung, K. Reinhart, et al. The world's major religions' points of view on end-of-life decisions in the intensive care unit. *Intensive Care Med.* 2008;**34**(3):423–30.

10. Sacred Congregation for the Doctrine of the Faith. *Declaration on Euthanasia.* May 5, 1980.

11. Pope John Paul II, Address to the Participants in the International Congress on "Life-Sustaining Treatment and Vegetative State: Scientific Advances and Ethical Dilemmas." March 20, 2004.

12. Carson, T. *The New Catholic Encyclopedia.* 2nd ed. Gale Research, 2002.

13. Sachedina, A. End-of-life: the Islamic view. *Lancet.* 2005;**366**(9487):774–9.

14. Young, K.K. The discourses of Hindu medical ethics. In R.B. Baker, L.B. McCullough, editors. *The Cambridge World History of Medical Ethics.* Cambridge: Cambridge University Press, 2009; 175–84.

15. Firth, S. End-of-life: a Hindu view. *Lancet.* 2005;**366**(9486):682–6.

16. Keown, D. End of life: the Buddhist view. *Lancet.* 2005;**366**(9489):952–5.

17. Pope, T.M. Legal aspects in palliative and end-of-life care in the United States. *UptoDate.* 2019. Last updated September 22, 2023.

18. Schwartz, J.L., A.L. Caplan. Vaccination refusal: ethics, individual rights, and the common good. *Prim Care.* 2011;**38**(4):717–28, ix.

19. Breeden, A. Hours after French patient is taken off life support, a court orders it be restored. *New York Times.* May 20, 2019.

20. Ollove, M. Palliative sedation, an end-of-life practice that is legal everywhere. Stateline, an initiative of the Pew Charitable Trusts, 2018.

21. Lewis, A., O. Scheyer. Legal objections to use of neurologic criteria to declare death in the United States: 1968 to 2017. *Chest.* 2019;**155**(6):1234–45.

22. *In re Callaway, Montana Ninth Judicial District Court, Pondera County, no. DG-16-08.* 2016.

23. *In re Lawson, No. CL16-2358 (City of Richmond Cir. Ct., Va., June 10, 2016) (order).*

24. Choong, K.A., M.Y. Rady. *Re A (A Child)* and the United Kingdom Code of Practice for the Diagnosis and Confirmation of Death: should a secular construct of death override religious values in a pluralistic society? *HEC Forum.* 2018;**30**(1):71–89.

25. *McKitty v. Hayani,* in *ONSC 4015 (CanLII).* 2018.

26. Lewis, A. The legacy of Jahi McMath. *Neurocrit Care.* 2018;**29**(3):519–20.

27. Bosslet, G.T., T.M. Pope, G.D. Rubenfeld, et al. An official ATS/AACN/ACCP/ESICM/SCCM policy statement: responding to requests for potentially inappropriate treatments in intensive care units. *Am J Respir Crit Care Med.* 2015;**191**(11):1318–30.

Chapter 22

New Frontiers in Neuroprognostication: Machine Learning and AI

Charlene Ong and Matthew Miller

Introduction

Artificial intelligence (AI) refers to a wide range of computational methods that approximate human reasoning. Machine learning is a subclass of AI that uses predictive computer models that adjust and improve their performance after exposure to data. [1–3] Machine learning is increasingly used for various purposes, including facial recognition, financial strategy, automated vehicles, and medical applications.[2,3] While objections to AI stem both from skepticism that automation can approach human reasoning and fears of obsolescence, a basic understanding of AI methods, uses, and limitations will be increasingly important as it continues to weave itself into the fabric of our society.

What contribution can machine learning offer the field of neuroprognostication? Certainly, AI approaches hold great promise in advancing our pathophysiological understanding of neurological injury, improving the accuracy of prognostication for patients and families, and streamlining clinical workflows. However, continued progress in this field depends on deliberate consideration of *which* problems machine learning can reasonably solve, rigorous methods for data quality control, and an understanding of how to evaluate the performance of machine learning models. The objective of this chapter is to introduce readers to basic machine learning history, foundational concepts, and examples of how this exciting field has recently been applied to neuroprognostication research.

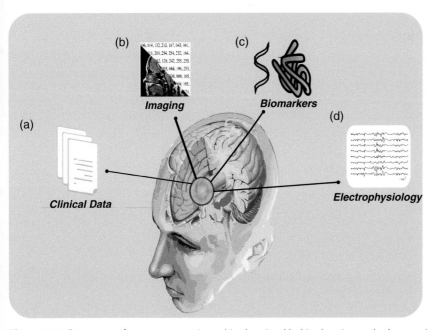

Figure 22.1 Data sources for neuroprognostic machine learning. Machine learning methods can assist investigators and clinicians integrating profoundly heterogeneous datatypes collected on patients over time. Within the next 10 years, clinicians and researchers may benefit from programs that automatically extract relevant data from (a) Structured clinical information, (b) Imaging, (c) Biomarkers, and (d) Continuous data streams like electrophysiology to provide real-time risk stratification metrics for patients during their hospital stay and beyond.

Background

How Do Machines "Learn"?

The anthropomorphic notion of *learning* implies a degree of "human" or sentient agency. However, machine learning algorithms improve their performance over time by simply adjusting their predictions to minimize a *loss function,* or error (Table 22.1).[2,3] This function guides the model in how to adjust its underlying mathematical structure to approximate patterns in a particular data set. The more guidance an algorithm has (through exposure to data), the greater its ability to minimize its loss. Thus, the increasing availability of large data sources (so-called big data) for training is key to machine learning's exploding popularity and its application to the medical field. Data inputs span various types of information. Examples include continuous vital sign measurements, magnetic resonance imaging (MRI) pixel intensities, or genomic data, all of which can effectively train "intelligent" (i.e. high-performing) algorithms (Figure 22.1).

Brief History

Interest in machine learning approaches to clinical problems predates its current use by at least 50 years.[4,5] As early as the 1950s, teams at Cornell University and IBM attempted to automate hematological diagnoses with early punch card–based computing systems, spurring what is now a familiar debate regarding whether computers would replace their human counterparts.[5,6] In the 1970s, Stanford University researchers developed an algorithm designed to automatically propose antimicrobial therapy given user descriptions of infectious symptoms.[7] Several groups in the 1980s experimented with automated computation to generate diagnoses from symptoms and discover interactions between medical variables, including prednisone and cholesterol.[8–10] Even neural networks (Table 22.2), often touted as a cutting-edge machine learning development, were used as early as the 1990s to develop automatic diagnostic systems.[11] These early forays were hampered by both limited training data and laborious manual feature input. They were consequently poorly generalizable to external data sets, and failed to generate mainstream impact.[12] The mid-1990s witnessed a significant research slowdown, as delays in substantive results led to decreased funding and development, often referred to as an "AI Winter."[2,13]

Several factors led to machine learning's resurgence. Increased access to large electronic data sets, exponential improvements in computational capacity, and the democratization of cost-free

Table 22.1 Machine learning nomenclature

Artificial intelligence: A collection of computational methods mimicking human reasoning capabilities.

Machine learning: The study of statistical methodologies whose predictive capacity improves with exposure to exemplary data. This ability to "learn" from data makes machine learning a means to achieve AI.

Model: A consistent framework for predicting an outcome of interest given a set of inputs. It is also referred to as an *algorithm*.

Feature: A relevant data set variable inputted into a machine learning model. All the features in a given data set are referred to as the model's *feature space*.

Loss function: A mathematical measure of a machine learning model's "incorrectness." Algorithms are programmed to minimize their loss function after exposure to training data.

Training set: The set of all observations to which a model is exposed. It is the data set from which the model learns to identify salient patterns as it forms its final model. Often, training sets will be composed of a majority of the full data set, with a portion reserved for testing.

Testing set: The set of observations "unseen" by the model. It is the data set that tests how well the model learned how to perform its task. These data should remain entirely separate from the training set. It is typically derived from either a subset of the original data or a separate data set entirely.

Classification: A machine learning task in which the outcome of interest is a categorical (or binary) value rather than a continuous prediction.

Regression: A machine learning task in which the outcome of interest is a continuous value rather than a categorical prediction.

Interpretability: How well an investigator can identify features leading to a machine learning model's prediction.

Supervised learning: A branch of machine learning in which models "learn" their predictions following exposure to a set of predetermined labeled examples, whose outcome of interest is known *a priori*.

Unsupervised learning: A branch of machine learning in which there are no manual "gold standard" labels. Models infer patterns in data without prior hypotheses. Common applications include clustering of observations for hypothesis generation and reducing the size of large feature spaces (*dimensionality reduction*).

Table 22.2 Selected machine learning methods

- **Tree-based methods**: Several machine learning models use branching logic reminiscent of a tree. These models are often highly interpretable given the ease with which the decision-making process can be followed. We highlight three tree-based methods here:
  - *Classification and Regression Trees (CART):* CARTs are supervised flow charts that predict continuous and categorical outcomes (Figure 22.2A).[22] Branch points (nodes) of the tree are formed by applying binary conditions (yes/no) to datapoints based on their comparison to observed training set features.
  - *Random Forests (RF):* RFs combine many randomly generated decision trees to provide an overall prediction.[23] Each tree in the forest is constructed by randomly sampling a subset of the total features (Figure 22.2A). The ultimate prediction results from majority voting or averaging of all trees in the forest.
  - *Optimal Classification Trees (OCTs):* OCTs optimize every split within the tree simultaneously, rather than considering only the prior feature. This results in improved performance over CART while retaining interpretability through a single tree structure.[24]
- **K-Nearest Neighbors (KNN):** KNN is a supervised algorithm that infers the value of an observation from the *k* closest points in the feature space, where *k* is a number chosen by the researcher (Figure 22.2B).[25] In classification, the category of an unknown observation is evaluated by a majority vote of these *k* neighbors. In regression, this value is inferred from the mean of the neighbors.
- **Support Vector Machines (SVM):** SVMs are a class of supervised learning models that categorize observations by defining boundaries (*margins*) that maximize the separation between observations in a feature space (Figure 22.2C). For more complex data not easily separated by linear functions, a so-called kernel trick allows SVMs to draw nonlinear boundaries.
- **Neural Networks:** Neural networks use successive, codependent mathematical functions (or "layers") to make an ultimate classification/regression. (Figure 22.2D).[26] When many such layers are connected, the network is *deep*, and the study of neural networks is referred to as *deep learning*. Three common types of neural networks include:
- *Multilayer Perceptrons (MLPs)*: These networks consist of **an input layer** of feature values that undergo further functions via **hidden layers** to make a final classification.
- *Convolutional Neural Networks (CNNs):* CNNs use sequential filters that distill data patterns to their most essential properties. This is particularly useful in computer vision, in which these algorithms learn to represent complex images (e.g., tumors or hemorrhages) by combinations of simpler features (e.g., edges and corners).
- *Recurrent Neural Networks (RNNs):* RNNs process sequential data using looped calculations that allow the network to form a "memory" of its previous processing behavior. This is highly useful for time series data such as electroencephalogram *(EEG)*.

Table 22.2 cont.| Essential Machine Learning Algorithms (cont.)

Naïve Bayes: Naïve Bayes combines simple conditional probabilities to make an ultimate prediction of whether a given outcome will occur (Figure 22.2E). It is "naïve" because it assumes equal and independent contributions of all features to the model's decision. In practice, although this condition is frequently violated, its classification performance remains strong.

Linear and Logistic Regression: Linear and logistic regression refers to a broad class of models that predict continuous and categorical outcomes, respectively, as a function of input data. Often considered "traditional" statistics, the ability of regression models to refine their predictions given increasing amounts of data fits the definition of supervised machine learning.[27]

Ensembling: In ensembling, the predictions of several machine learning models are combined to improve classification or regression. When models learn from each other in a successive fashion to improve performance, it is called *boosting*.

programming software [14,15] have created the necessary environment for AI to thrive. As a result, we have witnessed remarkable advances in navigation (e.g., Google Maps), personalized web content (e.g., personalized ads), and computer vision (e.g., facial recognition).[16] While nonmedical machine learning developments currently outpace medical applications,[17] healthcare researchers are increasingly using machine learning methods to identify clinically relevant associations, augment clinician workflow, and predict outcomes. Notable examples include the accurate diagnosis and classification of skin cancer,[18] AI-based detection of diabetic retinopathy,[19] and automated cardiologist-level atrial fibrillation detection from electrocardiograms.[20]

Public Health Importance

Machine learning has enormous potential to impact public health. One can envision a near future in which machine learning models assist in the discovery of new genetic patterns, imaging findings, or combinations of patient characteristics that link disease and outcome. Such findings could provide new targets for therapeutic approaches, help physicians introduce preventive behavioral modifications, or accurately identify which patients are most likely to recover after catastrophic injury. However, in the domain of neuroprognostication, we must be cognizant of machine learning's limitations and intrinsic biases. They are just as likely to reveal practice variations that lead to withdrawal of life-sustaining therapies (the so-called self-fulfilling prophecy),[21] as they are intrinsic patient-related predictors of outcomes. These revelations nevertheless may prove useful by demonstrating opportunities to standardize prognostication across centers.

It would be overly optimistic to presume that machine learning in isolation will be a panacea to all of healthcare's woes. Similar to the implementation of the electronic health record in the past decade, the assimilation of machine learning approaches requires stakeholder buy-in from multiple players, including clinicians, information technologists (IT), hospital administrators, and patients. Its integration will likely encounter obstacles such as overextension of IT services, privacy concerns, and the labor/resources required to adequately validate developed models. Despite these hurdles, machine learning's role in medicine is increasingly apparent, and we would be hard pressed to overstate its potential impact on the healthcare landscape.

Machine Learning Nomenclature and Subtypes

Different machine learning subtypes have their own set of advantages and disadvantages, and the choice of the optimal method depends on (1) the task, (2) available computational processing speed, and (3) the extent to which the investigator wishes to learn the contributing features of the final model (*interpretability*). For instance, neural networks perform very well at computer vision tasks, but they require a significant amount of processing speed to train the classifier. Moreover, it can be difficult to identify *how* the classifier made its ultimate prediction. Linear regression, commonly used and underrecognized as a machine learning subtype, requires less processing speed, and investigators can interrogate input features. Basic machine learning terms and definitions are provided in Table 22.1. Essential machine learning methods and accompanying visuals are included in Table 22.1 and Figure 22.2.

Model Performance Metrics

Investigators use several metrics to evaluate machine learning performance, some of which overlap with traditional epidemiological and statistical terms. *Sensitivity* ($\frac{TP}{TP+FN}$), alternatively known as *Recall*, and *Specificity* ($\frac{TN}{TN+FP}$) forms the basis of

the receiver operator characteristic (ROC) curve, which plots the true positive rate against the false positive rate. The area under the curve of an ROC (commonly denoted **AUC** or **c-statistic**) represents a hybrid assessment of the model's ability to tease out true and false positives in the classification, with AUC > 0.5 suggesting predictive capacity beyond chance. AUCs are commonly used to quickly evaluate and compare machine learning–based model performance.

Depending on the objective and context, clinicians may value different performance criteria. For prediction of potentially reversible conditions, sensitivity may be most important to screen patients, whereas specificity, or even false positives, may be most warranted in the diagnosis of severe, intractable disorders.

Other methods of assessing model performance include positive predictive value PPV ($\frac{TP}{TP + FP}$), otherwise known as **Precision**, negative predictive value NPV ($\frac{TN}{TN + FN}$), **Accuracy** ($\frac{TP}{TN + FN + TP + FP}$), and **F1 score** ($\frac{2 \times Precision \times Recall}{Precision + Recall}$), which represents a type of average (the *harmonic mean*) between precision and recall. Finally, in continuous regression tasks, performance may be evaluated by metrics such as mean squared error (MSE), or R^2, the proportion of variability in the data that is represented within the model.

It is increasingly common to find multiple metrics of model performance, especially as journal reviewers gain better familiarity with machine learning models. We have structured the remainder of this chapter to include examples of recent machine learning approaches to assist in both acute and chronic prognostication within the domains of (1) clinical data, (2) imaging, (3) biomarkers, and (4) electrophysiology.

Neuroprognostication

Clinical

Risk prediction scores are powerful tools for clinical decision making. Well-known examples such as the CHA_2DS_2-VASc score for stroke after atrial fibrillation,[28] or the ABCD score for risk of stroke after transient ischemic attack,[29] are easily implemented and provide meaningful classifications to prognosticate and inform management.[30,31] However, traditional risk scores are often limited by (1) incomplete inclusion of all potential risk factors, and (2) the frequent

A) Tree-Based Methods (CART/RF)

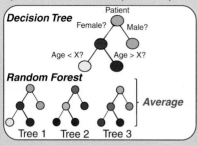

CARTs separate observations by sequentially applying binary conditions to features such as age and sex. **Random Forests (RFs)** aggregate many randomly generated CARTs and averagthe results, improving the model's overall performance.

B) K-Nearest Neighbors (KNN)

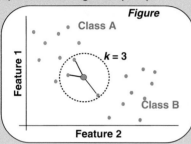

KNN searches for the *k* most similar data points, or "neighbors." In the case that $k = 3$, a datapoint of uncertain class (green) is closest to 2 blue points and 1 orange point. KNN will assign it a "blue" label by a majority vote.

C) Support Vector Machine (SVM)

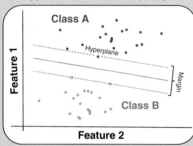

SVMs separate datasets by defining a boundary (hyperplane) that maximally separates the distance (margin) between data classes in a feature space

D) Neural Networks (Deep Learning)

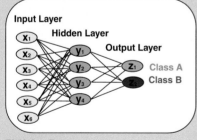

Neural Networks aggregate computational *nodes* (colored circles) into successive layers linked by weighted connections (black lines). The input layer (x_1-x_6) typically consists of input data and is processed via *hidden* nodes (y_1-y_6) resulting in an output layer (z_1,z_2)

E) Naive Bayes

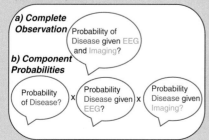

Naive Bayes concludes an ultimate probability that a condition (disease) occurs given numerous features simultaneously by computing the product of simpler conditional probabilities

Figure 22.2 Graphical depiction of selected supervised learning methods (see Table 22.2 for explication).

assumption that risk factors are linearly cumulative, when they may in fact have complex interrelationships that change their collective prognostic value.[32] Machine learning methods and their ability to model nonlinear interactions can therefore potentially greatly improve risk prediction accuracy and precision.

Wong and colleagues used machine learning approaches to improve delirium detection in non–intensive care unit (ICU) patients[33]. They used 796 variables selected by an expert panel and trained five different algorithms on a cohort of 14,227 adults to predict delirium as defined by a commonly used nursing delirium screening scale. Their best-performing model, a gradient boosted random forest (RF) (see Table 22.2) using a subset of 345 variables, yielded an AUC of 0.86 and outperformed a clinically validated delirium score (AWOL: Age ≥ 80 years, unable to spell "World" backward, not fully Oriented to place, and moderate to severe iLlness severity).[34] Heo and colleagues similarly found that a neural network improved prediction of modified Rankin Scale (mRS) scores 3 months after ischemic stroke compared to the 6 variable ASTRAL (Age, Severity of stroke, Time delay between stroke and admission, Range of visual fields, Acute glucose, and Level of consciousness) prognostic scoring system (AUC 0.88 vs. 0.839).[35] However their model's performance depended on the use of 38 clinical variables, and demonstrated no significant performance difference when using only the six variables identified by ASTRAL.[36]

Several groups attempted to forecast outcomes after acute events by developing machine learning models using demographic, procedural, and manually extracted imaging information. In 2014, Asadi and colleagues used neural networks and Support Vector Machines (SVMs, see Table 22.2) to classify good (mRS ≤ 2) and poor outcome in 107 acute stroke patients who underwent mechanical thrombectomy, with an accuracy shy of 70%.[37] Liu and colleagues used a similar approach to combine baseline clinical features and manually identified radiographic variables in their analysis of 1,157 patients with spontaneous intracranial hemorrhage (ICH) to predict hematoma expansion.[38] Their SVM model achieved a mean sensitivity of 81.3%, specificity of 84.8%, overall accuracy of 83.3%, and AUC of 0.89. In 2018, van Os and colleagues used clinical, treatment, and manually derived radiological variables to predict a number of outcomes related to mechanical thrombectomy after stroke. They trained several models including RF, SVM, and neural networks on 1,383 patients. AUCs across all models ranged from 0.88–0.91 predicting 3-month functional independence (as assessed by mRS), but only 0.53–0.57 in predicting good reperfusion after therapy (defined as modified Thrombolysis in Cerebral Infarction Score ≥ 2b).[39]

Investigators are also beginning to use machine learning to quantify and classify clinical signs that historically relied on subjective assessment. Pirlo and Drotár both used various algorithms to classify handwriting kinematics to detect early Alzheimer's and Parkinson's disease, respectively. [40,41] Other groups have analyzed audio recorded speech samples with k-nearest neighbors [42] or ensemble approaches [43] to identify patients with Parkinson's disorders. Tu and colleagues used deep neural networks to automatically distinguish dysarthria subtypes including ataxic, mixed flaccid-spastic, hyper- and hypokinetic speech patterns.[44] While the work in this field has focused mainly on classifying dysarthria subgroups, its potential for prognosticating clinically meaningful outcome metrics like swallowing function, return to work, and disease severity is promising.

Imaging

Because images are composed of potentially millions of pixel values, they are ideally suited to machine learning analytic techniques. The field of computer vision (machine learning image analysis) exploded after Krizhevsky and colleagues used a convolutional neural network (CNN) to accurately classify 1.2 million high-resolution images in 2012 [45]. In subsequent years, research using machine learning approaches to automatically classify and/or analyze medical images has become increasingly popular. In neuroimaging especially, researchers hope to highlight and/or quantify nuanced, clinically relevant radiographic information. In general, machine learning is applied to neuroimaging analysis in one of two ways:

1. Classification: In which either manually interpreted imaging features (e.g., measured midline shift) or raw image inputs (e.g., whole computed tomography [CT] scan) are fed into a model predicting a specified outcome. This approach often makes simultaneous use of other forms of structured or unstructured data (e.g., clinical notes), making multimodal

modeling an increasingly popular strategy in classification problems.

2. Segmentation: In which machine learning methods are used to automatically define the boundaries of structures of interest, such as tumors, brain volume, or cerebrospinal fluid (CSF).

Acute Neurological Emergencies

Machine learning efforts to identify radiological signs of ischemia in the acute setting and their subsequent outcomes span multiple imaging modalities. Several groups have experimented with a variety of methods to automatically identify or segment acute stroke from MRI.[46,47] Additionally, Thornhill and colleagues used unsupervised methods, neural networks, and SVMs to identify free-floating intraluminal thrombi on CT angiograms (CTA) (with accuracy between 65.2 and 76.4%).[48] Dhar and colleagues validated an automated method for intracranial CSF segmentation from an initial cohort of 155 patients by an RF-based method in head CTs performed within 6 and 24 hours of stroke onset to predict cerebral edema development.[49] Other recent work shows the ability of AI models to determine acute ischemic core volume from CTAs [50] and automatically calculate the Alberta Stroke Program early CT score from head CTs.[51] Automated generation of this information by software agents may assist in predicting outcome after mechanical thrombectomy and guiding treatment decisions.

Long-term prediction of post-ischemic outcomes is also a key use in neuroprognostic machine learning, and exciting work has emerged in the literature. Forkert and colleagues hypothesized that precise quantification of infarcted brain volume was an important prognostic indicator of functional outcome. They calculated percentages of infarcted tissue within various overlying anatomical maps to predict an mRS score and obtained a binary accuracy of 85% (mRS > 2 vs. ≤ 2) using SVM.[52] Nielsen and colleagues predicted tissue infarct volume in 29 untreated patients and 35 patients who received IV tissue plasminogen activator (tPA), using mean capillary transit time, cerebral blood volume, and three imaging modalities (diffusion-weighted imaging [DWI], apparent diffusion coefficient [ADC], and T2 fluid attenuated inversion recovery [FLAIR]) as CNN inputs. They found that their model achieved 88% accuracy in predicting final infarct volume, outperforming a simpler regression approach.[53] Functional deficits following ischemia may also be inferred from imaging, and Rehme and colleagues' use of functional MRI (fMRI) as inputs for an SVM model to predict hand-motor impairment stands out as an example.[54]

Several groups have attempted to outperform standardly used risk prediction scales by integrating imaging information and clinical data. Bentley and colleagues used an SVM algorithm to predict symptomatic ICH using head CTs from 116 patients treated with IV tPA, of whom 16 had symptomatic ICH.[55] They found that their algorithm performed better than previously published clinical scales, including SEDAN (**S**ugar (glucose), **E**arly infarct sign, **D**ense cerebral artery sign, **A**ge > 75, **N**IH Stroke Scale > 10),[56] and HAT (**H**emorrhage **A**fter **T**hrombosis).[57] Yu and colleagues also used source perfusion-weighted imaging, DWI, and arterial input function (AIF) to determine the risk of hemorrhagic transformation after ischemic stroke using a variety of machine learning models including SVM, linear regression, decision trees, and neural networks. They ultimately achieved an accuracy of 83.7% in identifying patients who would go on to develop radiographic hemorrhagic transformation.[58]

Other groups have used machine learning to "segment" (i.e. automatically identify) lesions. Hemorrhage is a prime target for study. Takahashi and colleagues' early attempts to automatically identify an MCA "dot sign" using a four-feature SVM also reflect a notable effort in the identification of high-risk hemorrhage, though their method resulted in 54 false positives out of 109 cases.[59] More recently, Lee and colleagues reported a deep convolutional neural network (CNN) strategy that accurately classified hemorrhage into five subtypes (intraparenchymal hemorrhage, intraventricular hemorrhage, subdural hemorrhage, epidural hemorrhage, and subarachnoid hemorrhage [SAH]), demonstrating up to 98% sensitivity and 95% specificity in their validation cohort.[60]

Other examples of machine learning–based neuroprognostication include the work of Gunter and colleagues, who published an automated segmentation method for imaging features of disproportionately enlarged subarachnoid space hydrocephalus. [61] Ramos and colleagues predicted delayed cerebral ischemia from 317 patients with subarachnoid hemorrhage using an RF model composed of clinical and unsupervised feature extraction of baseline CT image data (AUC 0.74).[62] To increase the interpretability of their results, they also computed average clinical feature importance (estimated measures of each feature's contribution to the final model) from their RF and ranked them, finding that total blood volume, presence of intraparenchymal blood, and the time from ictus to CT made important contributions to the model's performance.[63] This type of post-hoc interrogation of machine learning models will likely become a standard practice in the literature, as they can reveal mechanistic contributors to outcome.

Cancer

Oncology is another field in which the quantification of neuroimaging features can improve prediction of recurrence and outcome. Shrot and colleagues used manual tumor segmentation of diffusion tensor and perfusion-weighted MRI to calculate radiographic features in 141 patients with glioblastoma, cerebral metastases, meningioma, or central nervous system lymphoma. The authors used an SVM classifier to differentiate glioblastoma from other tumor types, achieving accuracies of > 90%.[64] Liao and colleagues similarly examined 72 manually derived features from various MRI sequences including intensity, shape, and textural features, as well as selected metagenes on 137 glioblastoma patients to construct various prediction models. Their gradient-boosted decision tree model (see Table 22.2) achieved an accuracy of 81% in classifying patients with greater or less than 1 year survival.[65] Peeken and colleagues developed an RF model using MRI, clinical, and pathological features to predict overall survival and progression-free survival in 189 patients with glioblastoma, achieving an AUC of 0.73.[66] Several groups have also proposed a variety of strategies (SVM, RF, deep learning) to predict isocitrate dehydrogenase (IDH) genotype from tumor imaging features such as shape and texture, given its importance in glioma progression.[64,67–69]

Dementia

Several groups have experimented with how to detect the insidious progression of dementing illnesses. In Alzheimer's disease (AD) in particular, a great deal of attention has been devoted to predicting conversion from the mild cognitive impairment (MCI) prodromal phase of disease to clinical AD. Lu and colleagues used neuroanatomical segmentation

software [70] to delineate 87 regions of interest from both MRI and positron emission tomography (PET), and used average region of interest (ROI) voxel intensities from three levels of resolution to train a neural network with 82.4% accuracy in predicting 3-year conversion to AD.[71] With 626 patients tested, this represented the largest AI-based study of MCI to AD conversion to date, and a substantial increase in accuracy relative to similar published results.[72–77] Notably, however, the authors reported less than 50% accuracy in predicting AD onset in individuals with normal cognition.

Other groups have also used intelligent methods to quantify novel imaging markers of dementia. Kaufmann and colleagues recently used machine learning to identify advanced aging out of proportion to a patient's documented calendar age.[78] Using structural MRI data from over 45,000 individuals aged 3–96 years, they constructed a boosted-RF classifier with 1,118 structural features to predict the so-called brain-age gap. They trained separate models for males and females, and correlated their findings with genetic loci associated with numerous disorders including schizophrenia, multiple sclerosis, and dementia. Such a metric may prove clinically useful both as a marker of chronic decline, as well as an important indicator of recovery potential after acute brain injury.

Biomarkers: Peripheral Indicators, Histopathology, and "Omics"

A "biomarker" has been defined a measurable indicator of the presence or severity of a disease state. [79] While use of the term has expanded to include nonmaterial indicators of pathology (i.e. imaging biomarkers), it has traditionally been used to describe molecular- and cellular-level factors in physical specimens including blood, CSF, or biopsy.

A number of recent studies have used machine learning to study the neuroprognostic significance of serum protein biomarkers. Muller and colleagues used serial readings of neuron-specific enolase (NSE) in order to predict poor outcome (as assessed by Cerebral Performance Category) in patients with anoxic–ischemic disorders of consciousness. They used K-Nearest Neighbors (**KNN**) (see Table 22.2) to impute missing data points and ultimately found that a Naïve Bayes classifier (see Table 22.2) outperformed logistic regression (AUC 0.81).[80] Peacock and colleagues trained an RF classifier on

251 people using peripheral levels of neurogranin, NSE, and metallothionein-3 to predict mild traumatic brain injury (defined as Glasgow Coma Scale ≥ 13) in patients with head trauma with 78% accuracy.[81] Tanioka's group used serum matricellular proteins obtained within the first 3 days of hospitalization in conjunction with clinical variables to predict delayed cerebral ischemia (DCI) following aneurysmal SAH using an RF classifier, achieving 95% accuracy in a cohort of 95 patients.[82]

Machine learning techniques can also be constructively employed to the identification of histopathological biomarkers. In 2015, Olar and colleagues used Classification and Regression Trees (**CARTs**, see Table 22.2) to identify staining characteristics of immunohistochemically treated meningiocytes suggestive of high mitotic index. They then used these indices to derive a novel pathology score for recurrence-free meningioma survival.[83] Chang and colleagues built on their work with a deep learning approach to create a hypercellularity score for gliomas. They examined the relationship between the hypercellularity score and various MRI features, which allowed them to project tissue-level tumor infiltration information directly onto imaging scans.[84] Orringer and colleagues worked with neurosurgeons, chemists, and engineers to develop a portable augmented microscopy system that simulated hematoxylin and eosin staining on site.[85] After validating their virtually stained slides, they piloted the implementation of a neural network to automate "pathologist-free" analysis. They trained their algorithm on 2,919 slides from 101 patients. They identified glial and nonglial tumors with greater than 90% accuracy and achieved specificities and sensitivities greater than 94% in differentiating lesional and nonlesional specimens. Their exciting work combined fundamental engineering and image processing advances with standard deep learning techniques to develop a streamlined pipeline for intraoperative prediction of brain tumor subtype.

Finally, machine learning methods are particularly well suited to investigation of the so-called omics disciplines (including genomics, epigenomics, and proteomics). In 2018, Huang and colleagues used an SVM approach to identify new candidate genes associated with AD.[86] Their team used 355 previously characterized AD-associated loci to train their SVM algorithm, and subsequently screened more than 20,000 candidate genes for possible association with AD dementia.

They validated their classifier on a holdout test-set of known associated genes (AUC 0.94).

Other groups have proposed using deep learning methods to identify relevant signatures of inter-gene regulation to infer interactions between genetic loci in AD,[87] or to discern clinically relevant *epigenetic* biomarker patterns leading to disease phenotypes. Cowgey and colleagues used an unsupervised method [88] to classify methylation patterns in peripheral blood cells from adolescents with clinically diagnosed cerebral palsy, and tested their classifier on a younger set of patients (1–5 years) with an accuracy of 73%.[89] Bahado-Singh and colleagues used deep neural networks to identify cerebral palsy from methylation status in neonates with 95% sensitivity and 94% specificity.[90] Aref-Eshghi and colleagues used SVM to classify 14 different Mendelian-inherited neurodevelopmental disorders, though their panel of conditions was largely limited to rare diseases with highly nonoverlapping methylation signatures.[91]

Electrophysiology

Like imaging, electrophysiological studies like electroencephalography (EEG) are composed of an enormous amount of quantitative data. Similar to how radiographic studies are assessed, trained clinicians subjectively evaluate EEG features and provide interpretations. Using traditional methods, studies have revealed that certain EEG features are associated with clinically relevant outcomes. For instance, lack of background reactivity [92–94] and refractory status epilepticus [95] are both associated with poor prognosis after cardiac arrest. The subjective amount of epileptiform activity, maximum amplitude, or presence of monomorphic bursts during burst suppression are associated with lower likelihood of attaining seizure freedom after weaning sedation.[96] However, it has historically been difficult to definitively determine the clinical significance of many subtler EEG findings due to the subjective nature of how features are defined, and a lack of standardized language for reporting those features until 2013.[97]

Automatic identification of potentially prognostic EEG features is an increasing area of interest. In 2011, Cruse and colleagues conducted a landmark study in which a linear SVM classifier was trained with filtered and artifact-rejected data to classify EEG recordings into either right-hand or toe motor imagery.[98] They used their trained algorithm to assess 16 patients in an Unresponsive Wakefulness State (formerly Persistent Vegetative State, or PVS) to identify those who may have demonstrated subclinical signs of responsiveness to commands. They found 3 of 16 patients consistently modulated their EEG responses to command, leading to the authors' suggestion that EEG could be used to identify patients who may go on to regain consciousness. However, the findings of this study were contested by Goldfine and colleagues, who felt that their statistical model did not sufficiently account for relations between adjacent EEG blocks.[99] When they redid the analysis, they found that none of the 16 patients had significant changes.

Support Vector Machines have been subsequently used to identify potential EEG features indicative of consciousness in various studies, [100–105] but are not the only machine learning method used to classify EEGs. Engemann and colleagues analyzed 327 recordings on patients with disorders of consciousness and 66 healthy controls using a tree-based method,[106] and found that their approach was generalizable to different centers, EEG configurations, and protocols.[107]

Additional groups have also investigated the ability of neural networks to automatically detect EEG features, especially seizures.[108–111] All studies face limitations that include relatively small sample sizes, decreased intra-patient performance, and false alarms. Emami and colleagues used a CNN approach to identify seizures that was found to identify true positives better than commercial seizure detection algorithms such as BESA and Persyst.[108] However, its false alarm rate (misclassification of true negatives) was clinically unacceptable at an alarm every 100 seconds. Similar investigative efforts have found that many algorithms with apparent high performance fail to generalize beyond the patient populations used for model training.[112] Furthermore, the preprocessing required of raw EEG signal into "clean" data inputs ready for analysis requires extensive preparation, including defining when to crop data, whether to use sliding time windows, and artifact removal.[109] The manual labor obviously offsets some of the "automation" of automated EEG classification, and is an important caveat of all machine learning applications.

Despite these challenges, the application of machine learning to detect prognostic EEG patterns has profound prognostic potential. In 2019, Claassen and colleagues used an SVM algorithm to identify Cognitive-Motor Dissociation (CMD) in unresponsive patients with acute neurological injury.[102] They trained their algorithm on a group of 10 healthy volunteers who were instructed to follow particular commands, for example, "open and close your fist." They then applied their algorithm, which had an AUC of 0.86 on the healthy cohort, on unresponsive patients. Forty-four percent of patients who were classified as having CMD had had an Extended Glasgow Outcome Scale (GOS-E) greater or equal to 4, whereas only 14% of patients without CMD achieved this state (odds ratio 4.6; 95% confidence interval [CI]: 1.2–17.1). This seminal work reinforces how machine learning methods may be creatively applied to discern occult patterns that profoundly impact our ability to prognosticate and understand recovery.

Challenges in AI-Based Neuroprognostication

The excitement surrounding machine learning-based neuroprognostication is motivated by our belief that we can optimize the interpretation of complex and heterogeneous streams of patient data. By analyzing patterns that currently escape our notice, we hope to improve the identification of patients with potential for recovery after acute neurological injury, and more accurately define the clinical course of patients with chronic conditions.

Nevertheless, there are numerous challenges to AI-based neuroprognostication. The application of a machine learning algorithm is often the easiest step in the investigative pipeline. It is the acquisition, annotation, standardization, and curation of large data sets that represent the most resource-intensive and significant bottleneck in the research workflow. Furthermore, we must consider how machine learning models are best implemented within the extant clinical workflow. Are they well validated in internal data sets? Are they generalizable? Are models clinically useful, and if so, do they have associated user-friendly platforms within the medical record? Can humans override the model? So-called *human-in-the-loop* strategies, [113] which allow physician confirmation of AI predictions, will be essential to successful clinical integration and application of machine learning algorithms.

Finally, given historical inequalities in the delivery of healthcare, the potential for machine learning systems to deepen disparities in medicine is important to consider and mitigate. Notably, unbalanced training sets may boost the performance of diagnostic software for well-represented groups, while decreasing accuracy for minority patients.[18] While the move toward medical machine learning remains nascent, questions about its adverse potential at the population level must be answered before its widespread clinical implementation.[114]

Future Directions

As we consider whether AI methods will improve our ability to prognosticate outcome, it is natural to question whether they can change outcome too. In 2016, Bouton and colleagues decoded neural signals with an SVM in a machine interface system that enabled forearm movement in a quadriplegic male.[115] Farina and colleagues demonstrated similar results using mechanical prostheses control by amputees.[116] As one considers the frontiers of neuroprognostication, we will undoubtedly gravitate toward approaches that not only accurately predict neurological outcome, but are coupled with neurorehabilitation interventions that reduce morbidity for patients with deficits.

Conclusion

Machine learning is a growing class of advanced numerical methods that promise to generate powerful new insights in clinical medicine. Their application to neuroprognostication has already led to remarkable results, fundamentally challenging clinicians to look beyond the obvious when assessing recovery potential.

However, it is wise to remember that the tools we use to counsel patients and family members are neither omnipresent, nor a substitute for human contact. As Beam and Kohane put it in their 2018 article on the subject, "Machine learning is not a magic device that can spin data into gold."[117] It is instead a natural extension of traditional statistical approaches, and its proper implementation requires a very human touch.

References

1. Michie D, Spiegelhalter DJ, Taylor C. *Machine Learning. Neural and Statistical Classification*, self-published, 1994;13.

2. Goodfellow I, Bengio Y, Courville A. *Deep Learning*. Cambridge, MA: MIT Press, 2016.

3. Mohri M, Rostamizadeh A, Talwalkar A. *Foundations of Machine Learning*: Cambridge, MA: MIT Press, 2018.

4. Schwartz WB. Medicine and the computer: the promise and problems of change. In *Use and Impact of Computers in Clinical Medicine*. New York: Springer, 1970;321–35.

5. Greene JA, Lea AS. Digital futures past – the long arc of big data in medicine. *N Engl J Med* 2019;**381** (5):480–5.

6. Nash F. Differential diagnosis, an apparatus to assist the logical faculties. *Lancet* 1954;**266**:8745.

7. Shortliffe EH. *Computer-Based Medical Consultations: MYCIN*. New York: Elsevier, 1976.

8. Miller RA, McNeil MA, Challinor SM, Masarie Jr FE, Myers JD. The INTERNIST-1/QUICK MEDICAL REFERENCE project – status report. *West J Med* 1986;**145**:816.

9. Shwe MA, Middleton B, Heckerman DE, et al. Probabilistic diagnosis using a reformulation of the INTERNIST-1/QMR knowledge base. *Methods Inf Med* 1991;**30**:241–55.

10. BLUM RL. Computer-assisted design of studies using routine clinical data: analyzing the association of prednisone and cholesterol. *Ann Int Me* 1986;**104**:858–868.

11. Papik K, Molnar B, Schaefer R, et al. Application of neural networks in medicine-a review. *Med Sci Monitor* 1998;4:MT538–MT546.

12. Penny W, Frost D. Neural networks in clinical medicine. *Med Decis Making* 1996;**16**:386–98.

13. Crevier D. *AI: The Tumultuous History of the Search for Artificial Intelligence*. New York: Basic Books, 1993.

14. Pedregosa F, Varoquaux G, Gramfort A, et al. Scikit-learn: machine learning in Python. *J Mach Learn Res*. 2011;**12**:2825–30.

15. Dabbish L, Stuart C, Tsay J, Herbsleb J. Social coding in GitHub: transparency and collaboration in an open software repository. *Proceedings of the ACM 2012 Conference on Computer Supported Cooperative Work*. 2012: ACM: 1277–86.

16. Tegmark M. *Life 3.0: Being Human in the Age of Artificial Intelligence*. New York: Knopf, 2017.

17. Rajkomar A, Dean J, Kohane I. Machine learning in medicine. *N Engl J Med* 2019;**380**:1347–58.

18. Esteva A, Kuprel B, Novoa RA, et al. Dermatologist-level classification of skin cancer with deep neural networks. *Nature* 2017;542:115.

19. De Fauw J, Ledsam JR, Romera-Paredes B, et al. Clinically applicable deep learning for diagnosis and referral in retinal disease. *Nat Med* 2018;**24**:1342–50.

20. Hannun AY, Rajpurkar P, Haghpanahi M, et al. Cardiologist-level arrhythmia detection and classification in ambulatory electrocardiograms using a deep neural network. *Nat Med* 2019;**25**:65–9.

21. Hemphill JC 3rd, White DB. Clinical nihilism in neuroemergencies. *Emerg Med Clin North Am* 2009;**27**:27–37, vii–viii.

22. Breiman L. *Classification and Regression Trees.* New York: Routledge, 2017.

23. Breiman L. Random forests. *Machine Learn* 2001;**45**:5–32.

24. Bertsimas D, Dunn J. Optimal classification trees. *Machine Learn* 2017;**106**:1039–82.

25. Cover T, Hart P. Nearest neighbor pattern classification. *IEEE Trans Inf Theory* 1967;**13**:21–7.

26. Haykin S. *Neural Networks: A Comprehensive Foundation.* Englewood Cliffs: Prentice-Hall, 1994.

27. Hastie T, Tibshirani R, Friedman J, Franklin J. The elements of statistical learning: data mining, inference and prediction. *Math Intell* 2005;**27**:83–5.

28. Lip GY, Nieuwlaat R, Pisters R, Lane DA, Crijns HJ. Refining clinical risk stratification for predicting stroke and thromboembolism in atrial fibrillation using a novel risk factor-based approach: the Euro Heart Survey on Atrial Fibrillation. *Chest* 2010;**137**:263–72.

29. Rothwell P, Giles M, Flossmann E, et al. A simple score (ABCD) to identify individuals at high early risk of stroke after transient ischaemic attack. *Lancet* 2005;**366**:29–36.

30. Koton S, Rothwell P. Performance of the ABCD and ABCD2 scores in TIA patients with carotid stenosis and atrial fibrillation. *Cerebrovasc Dis* 2007;**24**:231–5.

31. Shariff N, Aleem A, Singh M, Li YZ, Smith SJ. AF and venous thromboembolism – pathophysiology, risk assessment and CHADS-VASc score. *J Atr Fibrillation* 2012;**5**:649.

32. Keegan MT, Gajic O, Afessa B. Severity of illness scoring systems in the intensive care unit. *Crit Care Med* 2011;**39**:163–9.

33. Wong A, Young AT, Liang AS, et al. Development and validation of an electronic health record–based machine learning model to estimate delirium risk in newly hospitalized patients without known cognitive impairment. *JAMA Netw Open* 2018;**1**:e181018–e181018.

34. Douglas VC, Hessler CS, Dhaliwal G, et al. The AWOL tool: derivation and validation of a delirium prediction rule. *J Hosp Med* 2013;**8**:493–9.

35. Heo J, Yoon JG, Park H, et al. Machine learning–based model for prediction of outcomes in acute stroke. *Stroke* 2019;**50**:1263–5.

36. Ntaios G, Faouzi M, Ferrari J, et al. An integer-based score to predict functional outcome in acute ischemic stroke: the ASTRAL score. *Neurology* 2012;**78**:1916–22.

37. Asadi H, Dowling R, Yan B, Mitchell P. Machine learning for outcome prediction of acute ischemic stroke post intra-arterial therapy. *PloS One* 2014;**9**:e88225.

38. Liu J, Xu H, Chen Q, et al. Prediction of hematoma expansion in spontaneous intracerebral hemorrhage using support vector machine. *EBioMedicine* 2019;**43**:454–9.

39. Van Os HJ, Ramos LA, Hilbert A, et al. Predicting outcome of endovascular treatment for acute ischemic stroke: potential value of machine learning algorithms. *Front Neurol* 2018;**9**:784.

40. Drotár P, Mekyska J, Rektorová I, et al. Evaluation of handwriting kinematics and pressure for differential diagnosis of Parkinson's disease. *Artif Intell Med* 2016;**67**:39–46.

41. Pirlo G, Diaz M, Ferrer MA, et al. Early diagnosis of neurodegenerative diseases by handwritten signature analysis. In *International Conference on Image Analysis and Processing.* New York: Springer, 2015; 290–7.

42. Zhang H-H, Yang L, Liu Y, et al. Classification of Parkinson's disease utilizing multi-edit nearest-neighbor and ensemble learning algorithms with speech samples. *Biomed Eng Online* 2016;**15**:122.

43. Li Y, Yang L, Wang P, et al. Classification of Parkinson's disease by decision tree based instance selection and ensemble learning algorithms. *J Med Imaging Health Inform* 2017;**7**:444–52.

44. Tu M, Berisha V, Liss J. Interpretable objective assessment of dysarthric speech based on deep neural networks. *Proc Interspeech* 2017:1849–53.

45. Krizhevsky A, Sutskever I, Hinton GE. ImageNet classification with deep convolutional neural networks. *Comm ACM* 2017;**60**:84–90.

46. Griffis JC, Allendorfer JB, Szaflarski JP. Voxel-based Gaussian naïve Bayes classification of ischemic stroke lesions in individual T1-weighted MRI scans. *J Neurosci Methods* 2016;**257**:97–108.

47. Kamnitsas K, Ledig C, Newcombe VF, et al. Efficient multi-scale 3D CNN with fully

connected CRF for accurate brain lesion segmentation. *Med Image Anal* 2017;**36**:61–78.

48. Thornhill RE, Lum C, Jaberi A, et al. Can shape analysis differentiate free-floating internal carotid artery thrombus from atherosclerotic plaque in patients evaluated with CTA for stroke or transient ischemic attack? *Acad Radiol* 2014;**21**:345–54.

49. Dhar R, Chen Y, An H, Lee J-M. Application of machine learning to automated analysis of cerebral edema in large cohorts of ischemic stroke patients. *Front Neurol* 2018;**9**:687.

50. Sheth SA, Lopez-Rivera V, Barman A, et al. Machine learning–enabled automated determination of acute ischemic core from computed tomography angiography. *Stroke* 2019;**50**:3093–3100.

51. Albers GW, Wald MJ, Mlynash M, et al. Automated calculation of Alberta Stroke Program early CT score: validation in patients with large hemispheric infarct. *Stroke* 2019;**50**:3277–9.

52. Forkert ND, Verleger T, Cheng B, et al. Multiclass support vector machine-based lesion mapping predicts functional outcome in ischemic stroke patients. *PLoS One* 2015;**10**:e0129569.

53. Nielsen A, Hansen MB, Tietze A, Mouridsen K. Prediction of tissue outcome and assessment of treatment effect in acute ischemic stroke using deep learning. *Stroke* 2018;**49**:1394–1401.

54. Rehme AK, Volz LJ, Feis D-L, et al. Identifying neuroimaging markers of motor disability in acute stroke by machine learning techniques. *Cereb Cortex* 2014;**25**:3046–56.

55. Bentley P, Ganesalingam J, Jones ALC, et al. Prediction of stroke thrombolysis outcome using CT brain machine learning. *Neuroimage Clin* 2014;**4**:635–40.

56. Strbian D, Engelter S, Michel P, et al. Symptomatic intracranial hemorrhage after stroke thrombolysis: the SEDAN score. *Ann Neurol* 2012;**71**:634–41.

57. Lou M, Safdar A, Mehdiratta M, et al. The HAT score: a simple grading scale for predicting hemorrhage after thrombolysis. *Neurology* 2008;**71**:1417–23.

58. Yu Y, Guo D, Lou M, Liebeskind D, Scalzo F. Prediction of hemorrhagic transformation severity in acute stroke from source perfusion MRI. *IEEE Trans Biomed Eng* 2017;**65**:2058–65.

59. Takahashi N, Lee Y, Tsai D-Y, et al. An automated detection method for the MCA dot sign of acute stroke in unenhanced CT. *Radiol Phys Technol* 2014;**7**:79–88.

60. Lee H, Yune S, Mansouri M, et al. An explainable deep-learning algorithm for the detection of acute intracranial haemorrhage from small datasets. *Nat Biomed Eng* 2019;**3**:173.

61. Gunter NB, Schwarz CG, Graff-Radford J, et al. Automated detection of imaging features of disproportionately enlarged subarachnoid space hydrocephalus using machine learning methods. *Neuroimage Clin* 2019;**21**:101605.

62. Ramos LA, van der Steen WE, Barros RS, et al. Machine learning improves prediction of delayed cerebral ischemia in patients with subarachnoid hemorrhage. *J Neurointerv Surg* 2019;**11**:497–502.

63. Ribeiro MT, Singh S, Guestrin C. "Why should I trust you?": explaining the predictions of any classifier. Proceedings of the 22nd ACM SIGKDD International Conference on Knowledge Discovery and Data Mining; 2016: 1135–44.

64. Shrot S, Salhov M, Dvorski N, et al. Application of MR morphologic, diffusion tensor, and perfusion imaging in the classification of brain tumors using machine learning scheme. *Neuroradiology* 2019;**61**:757–65.

65. Liao X, Cai B, Tian B, et al. Machine-learning based radiogenomics analysis of MRI features and metagenes in glioblastoma multiforme patients with different survival time. *J Cell Mol Med* 2019;**23**:4375–85.

66. Peeken JC, Goldberg T, Pyka T, et al. Combining multimodal imaging and treatment features improves machine learning-based prognostic assessment in patients with glioblastoma multiforme. *Cancer Med* 2019;**8**:128–36.

67. Zhang B, Chang K, Ramkissoon S, et al. Multimodal MRI features predict isocitrate dehydrogenase genotype in high-grade gliomas. *Neurooncol* 2016;**19**:109–17.

68. Akkus Z, Ali I, Sedlář J, et al. Predicting deletion of chromosomal arms 1p/19q in low-grade gliomas from MR images using machine intelligence. *J Digit Imaging* 2017;**30**:469–76.

69. Zhou H, Chang K, Bai HX, et al. Machine learning reveals multimodal MRI patterns predictive of isocitrate dehydrogenase and 1p/19q status in diffuse low-and high-grade gliomas. *J Neurooncol* 2019;**142**:299–307.

70. Fischl B. FreeSurfer. *Neuroimage* 2012;**62**:774–81.

71. Lu D, Popuri K, Ding GW, Balachandar R, Beg MF. Multimodal and multiscale deep neural networks for the early diagnosis of Alzheimer's disease using structural MR and FDG-PET images. *Sci Rep* 2018;**8**:5697.

72. Young J, Modat M, Cardoso MJ, et al. Accurate multimodal probabilistic prediction of

317

conversion to Alzheimer's disease in patients with mild cognitive impairment. *Neuroimage Clin* 2013;2:735–45.

73. An L, Adeli E, Liu M, et al. A hierarchical feature and sample selection framework and its application for Alzheimer's disease diagnosis. *Sci Rep* 2017;7:45269.

74. Suk H-I, Lee S-W, Shen D, Initiative AsDN. Hierarchical feature representation and multimodal fusion with deep learning for AD/MCI diagnosis. *Neuromage* 2014;**101**:569–82.

75. Moradi E, Pepe A, Gaser C, Huttunen H, Tohka J, Initiative AsDN. Machine learning framework for early MRI-based Alzheimer's conversion prediction in MCI subjects. *Neuroimage* 2015;**104**:398–412.

76. Liu K, Chen K, Yao L, Guo X. Prediction of mild cognitive impairment conversion using a combination of independent component analysis and the Cox model. *Front Hum Neurosci* 2017;**11**:33.

77. Cheng B, Liu M, Zhang D, Munsell BC, Shen D. Domain transfer learning for MCI conversion prediction. *IEEE Trans Biomed Eng* 2015;**62**:1805–17.

78. Kaufmann T, van der Meer D, Doan NT, et al. Common brain disorders are associated with heritable patterns of apparent aging of the brain. *Nat Neurosci* 2019;**22**:1617–23.

79. Puntmann V. How-to guide on biomarkers: biomarker definitions, validation and applications with examples from cardiovascular disease. *Postgrad Med J* 2009;**85**:538–45.

80. Muller E, Shock JP, Bender A, et al. Outcome prediction with serial neuron-specific enolase and machine learning in anoxic-ischaemic disorders of consciousness. *Comput Biol Med* 2019;**107**:145–52.

81. Peacock WF IV, Van Meter TE, Mirshahi N, et al. Derivation of a three biomarker panel to improve diagnosis in patients with mild traumatic brain injury. *Front Neurol* 2017;8:641.

82. Tanioka S, Ishida F, Nakano F, et al. Machine learning analysis of matricellular proteins and clinical variables for early prediction of delayed cerebral ischemia after aneurysmal subarachnoid hemorrhage. *Mol Neurobiol* 2019;**56**:7128–35.

83. Olar A, Wani KM, Sulman EP, et al. Mitotic index is an independent predictor of recurrence-free survival in meningioma. *Brain Pathol* 2015;**25**:266–75.

84. Chang P, Malone H, Bowden S, et al. A multiparametric model for mapping cellularity in glioblastoma using radiographically localized biopsies. *Am Journal of Neuroradiol* 2017;**38**:890–8.

85. Orringer DA, Pandian B, Niknafs YS, et al. Rapid intraoperative histology of unprocessed surgical specimens via fibre-laser-based stimulated Raman scattering microscopy. *Nature Biomed Eng* 2017;**1**:0027.

86. Huang X, Liu H, Li X, et al. Revealing Alzheimer's disease genes spectrum in the whole-genome by machine learning. *BMC Neurol* 2018;**18**:5.

87. Zafeiris D, Rutella S, Ball GR. An artificial neural network integrated pipeline for biomarker discovery using Alzheimer's disease as a case study. *Comput Struct Biotechnol J* 2018;**16**:77–87.

88. Mika S, Ratsch G, Weston J, Scholkopf B, Mullers K-R. Fisher discriminant analysis with kernels. *Neural Networks for Signal Processing IX: Proceedings of the 1999 IEEE Signal Processing Society Workshop (Cat. No. 98TH8468)*. Madison, WI, 199941–8.

89. Crowgey EL, Marsh AG, Robinson KG, Yeager SK, Akins RE. Epigenetic machine learning: utilizing DNA methylation patterns to predict spastic cerebral palsy. *BMC Bioinformatics* 2018;**19**:225.

90. Bahado-Singh RO, Vishweswaraiah S, Aydas B, et al. Deep learning/artificial intelligence and blood-based DNA epigenomic prediction of cerebral palsy. *Int J Mol Sci* 2019;**20**:2075.

91. Aref-Eshghi E, Rodenhiser DI, Schenkel LC, et al. Genomic DNA methylation signatures enable concurrent diagnosis and clinical genetic variant classification in neurodevelopmental syndromes. *Am J Hum Genet* 2018;**102**:156–74.

92. Benghanem S, Paul M, Charpentier J, et al. Value of EEG reactivity for prediction of neurologic outcome after cardiac arrest: insights from the Parisian registry. *Resuscitation* 2019;**142**:168–74.

93. Ruijter BJ, Tjepkema-Cloostermans MC, Tromp SC, et al. Early EEG for outcome prediction of postanoxic coma: a prospective cohort study. *Ann Neurol* 2019;**86**:203–14.

94. Admiraal MM, Anne-Fleur van Rootselaar M, Hofmeijer J, et al. Electroencephalographic reactivity as predictor of neurological outcome in postanoxic coma: a multicenter prospective cohort study. *Ann Neurol* 2019;**86**:17–27.

95. Mayer SA, Claassen J, Lokin J, et al. Refractory status epilepticus: frequency, risk factors, and impact on outcome. *Arch Neurol* 2002;**59**:205–10.

96. Johnson EL, Martinez NC, Ritzl EK. EEG characteristics of successful burst suppression for

refractory status epilepticus. *Neurocrit Care* 2016;**25**:407–14.

97. Hirsch L, LaRoche S, Gaspard N, et al. American Clinical Neurophysiology Society's standardized critical care EEG terminology: 2012 version. *J Clin Neurophysiol* 2013;**30**:1–27.

98. Cruse D, Chennu S, Chatelle C, et al. Bedside detection of awareness in the vegetative state: a cohort study. *Lancet* 2011;**378**:2088–94.

99. Goldfine AM, Bardin JC, Noirhomme Q, et al. Reanalysis of "Bedside detection of awareness in the vegetative state: a cohort study." *Lancet* 2013;**381**:289–91.

100. Henriques J, Gabriel D, Grigoryeva L, et al. Protocol design challenges in the detection of awareness in aware subjects using EEG signals. *Clin EEG Neurosci* 2016;**47**:266–75.

101. Höller Y, Bergmann J, Thomschewski A, et al. Comparison of EEG-features and classification methods for motor imagery in patients with disorders of consciousness. *PloS One* 2013;**8**: e80479.

102. Claassen J, Doyle K, Matory A, et al. Detection of brain activation in unresponsive patients with acute brain injury. *N Engl J Med* 2019;**380**:2497–2505.

103. Edlow BL, Chatelle C, Spencer CA, et al. Early detection of consciousness in patients with acute severe traumatic brain injury. *Brain* 2017;**140**:2399–2414.

104. Pan J, Xie Q, He Y, et al. Detecting awareness in patients with disorders of consciousness using a hybrid brain–computer interface. *J Neural Eng* 2014;**11**:056007.

105. King J-R, Sitt JD, Faugeras F, et al. Information sharing in the brain indexes consciousness in noncommunicative patients. *Curr Biol* 2013;**23**:1914–19.

106. Geurts P, Ernst D, Wehenkel L. Extremely randomized trees. *Mach Learn* 2006;**63**:3–42.

107. Engemann DA, Raimondo F, King J-R, et al. Robust EEG-based cross-site and cross-protocol classification of states of consciousness. *Brain* 2018;**141**:3179–92.

108. Emami A, Kunii N, Matsuo T, et al. Seizure detection by convolutional neural network-based analysis of scalp electroencephalography plot images. *Neuroimage Clin* 2019;**22**:101684.

109. Schirrmeister RT, Springenberg JT, Fiederer LDJ, et al. Deep learning with convolutional neural networks for EEG decoding and visualization. *Hum Brain Mapp* 2017;**38**:5391–5420.

110. Acharya UR, Oh SL, Hagiwara Y, Tan JH, Adeli H. Deep convolutional neural network for the automated detection and diagnosis of seizure using EEG signals. *Comput Biol Med* 2018;**100**:270–8.

111. LeCun Y, Bengio Y, Hinton G. Deep learning. *Nature* 2015; **521**:436.

112. Varsavsky A, Mareels I, Cook M. *Epileptic Seizures and the EEG: Measurement, Models, Detection and Prediction*. Boca Raton: CRC Press, 2016.

113. Holzinger A. Interactive machine learning for health informatics: when do we need the human-in-the-loop? *Brain Inform* 2016;**3**:119–31.

114. Zou J, Schiebinger L. Design AI so that it's fair. *Nature* 2018;**559**:324–6.

115. Bouton CE, Shaikhouni A, Annetta NV, et al. Restoring cortical control of functional movement in a human with quadriplegia. *Nature* 2016;**533**:247.

116. Farina D, Vujaklija I, Sartori M, et al. Man/machine interface based on the discharge timings of spinal motor neurons after targeted muscle reinnervation. *Nat Biomed Eng* 2017;**1**:0025.

117. Beam AL, Kohane IS. Big data and machine learning in health care. *JAMA* 2018;**319**:1317–18.

Chapter 23

New Frontiers in Neuroprognostication: Biomarkers

Michael A. Pizzi and Katharina Busl

Introduction

The use of blood and cerebrospinal fluid (CSF) biomarkers for various neurological pathologies can augment the clinician's ability to prognosticate disease progression as well as functional and neurological outcomes. This chapter focuses on six common neurological pathologies seen in the neurological intensive care unit: secondary brain injury after cardiac arrest, intracranial hemorrhage (ICH), acute ischemic stroke, traumatic brain injury (TBI), aneurysmal subarachnoid hemorrhage (aSAH), and post-intensive care syndrome. Very few of the biomarkers have been clinically validated, but a number of biomarkers are promising in research studies and are also discussed. However, standardization of protocols and reference ranges has not been established for most biomarkers.

Cardiac Arrest

Cardiac arrest (CA) results in over 400,000 deaths in the United States annually. Approximately 25% of patients who suffer out-of-hospital cardiac arrest (OHCA) achieve return of spontaneous circulation (ROSC), and of those patients approximately 10% will survive to hospital discharge.[1] The most common reason for nonsurvival in patients who survive the original cardiac arrest is withdrawal of life support due to manifest or perceived poor neurological function or prognosis.[2] Self-fulfilling prophecy is a recognized challenge in this context, and biomarkers might aid in more accurate prognostication.

Neuron-Specific Enolase (NSE)

The most widely used serum biomarker to assist with neuroprognostication after cardiac arrest is neuron-specific enolase (NSE). NSE is a 78 kDa dimeric glycolytic enzyme with a half-life of approximately 24 hours.[3] Contrary to the name, NSE is also found in platelets and red blood cells, which can give false-positive results from hemolyzed blood samples.[4] Neuron-specific enolase is also a biomarker of neuroendocrine and small cell lung cancer.[5] The American Academy of Neurology (AAN) practice parameters, which were based on post-CA patients not treated with therapeutic hypothermia (TH), state that serum levels of NSE > 33 μg/L 1–3 days after CA were significant predictors of poor neurological outcome.[6] However, some post-CA patients with NSE levels > 33 μg/L in the first 72 hours after ROSC have been noted to have good neurological outcomes. In a cohort of post-CA patients treated with TH who survived to hospital discharge, 39% had a serum NSE concentration > 33 μg/L.[7] Furthermore, 10 of 12 patients with NSE > 33 μg/L who survived to hospital discharge had a favorable functional outcome defined as cerebral performance category (CPC) ≤ 2.[7] In another study investigating post-CA patients, approximately 11% of whom underwent TH, a level of NSE > 80 μg/L was needed in order to achieve 100% specificity for predicting persistent coma at 6 months.[8] Approximately one-third of post-CA patients treated with TH had a good functional outcome (CPC 1–2) with a serum concentration of NSE 40–80 μg/L; therefore, a serum NSE concentration of 78.9 μg/L was needed to yield a specificity of 100% to predict a poor functional outcome defined as CPC 3–5.[9] When both OHCA and in-hospital CA patients had NSE concentrations analyzed 3 days after ROSC, a serum NSE concentration > 90 μg/L had a 99% positive predictive value for a poor functional outcome defined as CPC 4–5.[10] Conversely, a serum NSE concentration < 17 μg/L had a negative predictive value of 92% excluding a CPC 4–5.

There is debate on the number and timing of obtaining blood samples for NSE concentrations post-CA. Available data suggest obtaining serial blood samples over multiple time points, in particular at 48 and 72 hours after CA.[3] In addition, when blood samples are obtained at 24, 48, and 72 hours after ROSC, the NSE measurements provided a better prediction ability compared to one NSE measurement at 48 hours after ROSC.[11]

When EEG findings were coupled with NSE levels in post-CA patients treated with TH, there was a correlation between absent EEG background reactivity and presence of epileptiform transients with elevated NSE in patients with poor neurological outcomes. However, this study also demonstrated that an elevated NSE > 33μg/L was seen in patients with good neurological recovery.[12] When NSE is combined with the clinical evaluation and EEG reactivity, neurological outcome prognostic utility increases. Post-CA patients were evaluated for pupillary, corneal, and oculocephalic reflexes after obtaining normothermia, off sedation and within 72 hours of CA. Reactivity of electroencephalogram (EEG) during hypothermia as well as NSE levels were also evaluated in these patients. Combining these data demonstrated the best prognostication for poor neurological outcome, defined as CPC 3–5, when there was incomplete return of brainstem reflexes or presence of myoclonus, absence of hypothermic reactivity on EEG, and serum NSE > 33 μg/L.[13] However, lack of EEG reactivity during hypothermia – as opposed to the biomarker – was found to be the most reliable predictor of poor neurological outcome, with a sensitivity of 74% and specificity of 99%.

S100 Protein

The S100 protein is a 21 kDa intracellular calcium-binding protein that is involved in neuronal differentiation, proliferation and apoptosis.[14] S100 has a half-life of approximately 2 hours, and peaks earlier in the blood than NSE.[15, 16] These characteristics of S100 made it a possible candidate biomarker; however, subsequent studies have not demonstrated S100 serum concentrations to be as good as NSE in predicting functional outcome after OHCA.[17] Furthermore, current guidelines do not recommend S100 as a biomarker for predicting functional outcome.[18]

In a review of studies evaluating biochemical markers as predictors of outcome after TH, the variability in testing parameters and outcome measures indicates insufficient data on the predictive accuracy of S100 and NSE.[19]

Neurofilament Light Chain (NFL)

Neurofilaments are components of the axonal cytoskeleton providing structural stability. Human neurofilament light chain (NFL) is a 70 kDa protein that assembles into heteropolymers. Recent development of single molecule array (SiMoA) assays have significantly increased the sensitivity of detecting NFL in serum samples.[20] Utilizing SiMoA analysis of serum samples of post-CA patients 24, 48, and 72 hours after CA demonstrated elevated NFL concentrations associated with poor functional outcomes (CPC 3–5) at 6 months post-CA.[21] Furthermore, NFL had greater sensitivity for poor functional outcome at 6 months than NSE, S100, and tau biomarkers, as well as somatosensory evoked potentials, computed tomography (CT), EEG, and both pupillary and corneal reflexes.

Micro-Ribonucleic Acid (miRNA)

Micro-ribonucleic acid (miRNA) are noncoding RNAs that regulate messenger RNA. Injured CNS cells and leukocytes have been shown to release miRNA exosomes and microvesicles into blood and saliva.[22] Post-CA patients treated with TTM (33°C and 36°C) had blood samples obtained 24 hours after ROSC, and miRNAs were characterized and quantified. Micro-RNA-124-3p levels significantly correlated with poor functional outcome (CPC 3–5) at 6 months post-CA.[23] There was no significant difference in miRNA124-3p levels between patients undergoing TTM of 33°C versus 36°C.

Proteomics

Serum proteomics have been utilized to investigate identification of novel biomarkers to aid in neuroprognostication.[24] Serum samples from post-CA patients were obtained within 6 hours of cardiac arrest and again at 24 hours. These serum samples were separated by 2D-gel electrophoresis followed by MALDI-TOF mass spectrometry. Two proteins were associated with poor functional outcome (CPC 3–5) at 3 months: muskelin and 14–3–3 (epsilon and zeta isoforms). Muskelin is highly expressed in metabolically active areas of the brain such as the hippocampus and cerebellum.[25] The 14–3–3 proteins are expressed in various tissues, but have the highest expression in the brain.[26] The 14–3–3 proteins account for approximately 1% of soluble proteins in the mammalian brain and have been shown to be involved in ion channel regulation, neuronal differentiation, and neurite outgrowth.[27]

Presepsin

Post-CA patients often have elevated inflammatory cytokines similar to that seen in septic patients. The hypothesis is that biomarkers of systemic inflammation in septic patients may also be potential biomarkers in post-CA patients. One such candidate inflammatory biomarker is presepsin, which is the soluble peptide product of CD14 proteolysis. A retrospective study of post-CA patients that underwent TTM of 33°C for 72 hours had blood samples obtained within 4 hours after ROSC, 12–36 hours after ROSC, and 60–84 hours after ROSC.[28] Serum presepsin concentration, at all time points analyzed, was an independent predictor of 28-day mortality and functional outcome. It should be noted that patients in this study underwent TTM for 72 hours instead of the standard 24 hours.

Intracerebral Hemorrhage

Intracerebral hemorrhage (ICH) accounts for approximately 10–15% of all strokes, but overall mortality is close to 50% at 3 months.[29] Functional outcome after ICH is also significant, since only approximately 15–25% of patients will be functionally independent at 12 months.[30]

Ferritin, CD163, and Hepcidin

Ferritin is an iron-carrying protein that has been shown to be a predictor of poor functional outcome in ICH. In a study of consecutive patients with ICH, blood samples were obtained on admission and days 3, 7, 14, and 21 after ictus. Controls were obtained from healthy sex- and age-matched volunteers.[31] Serum ferritin concentrations on days 1 and 7 were significantly higher in patients with poor neurological outcome (modified Rankin Scale [mRS] ≥ 3) versus good outcome. A similar study also demonstrated serum ferritin concentrations on days 1 and 7 after ictus were independently correlated with poor neurological outcome at 12 months after ICH. CD163 serum concentration on day 1 after ictus was independently correlated with poor neurological outcome (mRS 4–6) at both 3 months and 12 months after ICH.[32] Hepcidin is a peptide hormone that regulates iron hemostasis,[33] and has been associated with perihematomal edema volume after spontaneous ICH.[34] In the study by Garton and colleagues that investigated serum ferritin and CD163, as described above, hepcidin serum concentrations after ICH did not correlate

with poor functional outcome at either 3 months or 12 months after ICH.[32] However, in another study of hepcidin levels obtained 3 days after ICH, serum concentrations did correlate with poor functional outcome (mRS ≥ 3) at 3 months.[35]

Acute Ischemic Stroke

Various serum biomarkers associated with the blood–brain barrier (BBB) have been investigated after acute ischemic stroke in association with development of cerebral edema and hemorrhagic transformation of infarcted brain tissue.[36] This section will be limited to biomarkers that are associated with neuroprognostication, in particular regarding functional outcomes.

NFL

Blood samples were obtained from ischemic stroke patients upon arrival to emergency department, day 2, 3, 7, as well as 3 and 6 months post-stroke to analyze serum NFL concentrations. Functional outcome assessed by mRS at 3 months post-stroke correlated with serum NFL levels obtained on day 7 post-stroke. NFL levels on day 7 after ischemic stroke independently predicted functional outcome at 3 months post-stroke.[37]

S100

The S100B protein increases after acute ischemic stroke, and may help predict functional outcome when the serum concentration is > 140.5 ng/dL at 48 hours after stroke onset. This threshold level of S100B was associated with poor functional outcome (mRS ≥ 3) at 3 months post-stroke.[38]

Lipopolysaccharide-Binding Protein (LBP)

As mentioned above, the inflammatory cascade is upregulated after a variety of neurological insults. Identifying potential biomarkers associated with systemic inflammation has turned to candidate molecules that are upregulated after injection of lipopolysaccharide (LPS), which is endogenously located on the outer membrane of Gram-negative bacteria. One such molecule is lipopolysaccharide-binding protein (LBP), which was quantified within 24 hours of stroke onset. Serum levels of LBP predicted 3-and 12-month mortality, as well as poor functional outcome (mRS ≥ 3) at 3 months post-stroke.[39]

Traumatic Brain Injury (TBI)

Various biomarkers have been identified across the range from mild to severe TBI to assist with diagnosis and prognosis.[40] This section focuses on biomarkers in severe TBI that have been demonstrated to help predict functional outcome.

NSE and S100B

Neuron-specific enolase serum concentrations upon admission, 24, 48, 72, and 96 hours in severe TBI patients only predicted mortality at the 48 hour time point.[41] Poor functional outcomes.[42] have been correlated with serum NSE levels after severe TBI. However, when NSE is directly compared to S100B in TBI patients, serum S100B better predicted functional outcome (Glasgow Outcome Scale [GOS] at 3–6 months and 12 months) than did serum NSE concentrations. In particular, the predictive ability of S100B increased when blood samples were obtained between 12–30 hours after trauma.[43]

NFL

Neurofilament light chain has been shown to increase in the serum after TBI and correlates with poor functional outcome.[44] A prospective, single center study investigated severe TBI (GCS ≤ 8) patients who had serial serum NFL concentrations measured compared to controls, as well as a subset (44% of TBI patients) that had extraventricular drains (EVD) who also had cerebrospinal fluid (CSF) NFL levels measured.[45] Blood and CSF samples were obtained approximately daily from admission to day 12, with serum samples also obtained one year after TBI. Serum NFL concentrations obtained within 24 hours after TBI were significantly higher in patients with poor functional outcomes at 12 months (defined as GOS 1–3) as well as in nonsurvivors (follow-up was at 12 months after injury, yet all had died within 30 days of injury).

Glial Fibrillary Acidic Protein (GFAP)

Glial fibrillary acidic protein (GFAP) is an intermediate filament within astrocytes involved in cell migration, mitosis, and anchoring cell surface transporters.[46] In a meta-analysis of TBI studies evaluating the prognostic function of serum GFAP, 10 of the 15 studies only enrolled severe TBI with the other 4 including severe and moderate TBI, and 1 study including mild TBI. This analysis demonstrated serum GFAP levels drawn between 48 hours and 7 days after injury predicted poor functional outcome defined as GOS ≤ 3.[47]

Aneurysmal Subarachnoid Hemorrhage (aSAH)

Cleaved Receptor for Advanced Glycation End-Products (cRAGE)

Neuroinflammatory processes increase after aSAH and have been investigated as potential areas of biomarkers predicting functional outcomes, as well as possible mechanisms for therapeutic intervention. [48] The receptor for advanced glycation end-products (RAGE) is a group of cell surface receptors belonging to the immunoglobulin superfamily, which are expressed on neurons, microglia and astrocytes.[49] Upon binding ligands, such as S100B, RAGE activates inflammatory pathways. The soluble isoforms of RAGE are further subdivided into endogenous secretory and cleaved RAGE isoforms. Cleaved RAGE (cRAGE) has been shown to independently predict poor outcome after ischemic stroke.[50] Serum concentration of cRAGE was obtained from aSAH patients upon admission in one study. Serum concentrations of cRAGE were significantly higher in aSAH patients with poor functional outcome (GOS 1–3) at 6 months.[51]

Neuroglobulin

Neuroglobulin is a subtype of globin that is predominately expressed in the brain.[52] In a consecutive series of aSAH patients, neuroglobulin concentration was measured from blood samples obtained every 6 hours for the first 7 days.[53] Neuroglobulin concentration correlated with poor functional outcome (mRS > 3) at 12 months posthemorrhage. Furthermore, neuroglobulin levels were associated with poor neurocognitive function (Mini-Mental Status Exam [MMSE] < 24, clock drawing test < 10, and frontal assessment battery < 15) at 12 months post-hemorrhage.

Tumor Necrosis Factor-alpha (TNF-α) and TNF-α Receptor 1 (TNF-R1)

The inflammatory cytokine TNF-α increases after aSAH in the first 72 hours after the initial hemorrhage and is associated with cerebral vasospasm.[54] Serum concentrations of TNF-α were analyzed from serial blood samples during the first 2 weeks after SAH to determine levels correlated with cerebral vasospasm and functional outcome (mRS). Serum TNF-α levels on days 2–3 after SAH correlated with poor functional outcome (mRS > 2) at 3 months after aSAH.[55] Interestingly, TNF-α levels did not correlate with radiographic evidence of vasospasm (> 50% reduction in vessel diameter on angiography). Given the above findings implicating TNF-α as a biomarker of outcomes after aSAH, the main TNF-α receptor (TNF-R1) was also investigated as a potential biomarker. Serial blood samples from aSAH patients at time of cerebral angiogram, < 24 hours from admission, and < 72 hours after SAH onset were analyzed by ELISA for TNF-R1 concentrations.[56] Functional outcome was assessed by mRS at hospital discharge, 3 and 6 months. Elevated concentration of TNF-R1 was an independent predictor of poor outcome (mRS > 2) at 6 months after multivariate logistic regression.

Post-Intensive Care Syndrome

Worldwide, approximately 13–20 million people per year require ICU level of care.[57] A large number of patients afflicted with the above neurological disorders will commonly spend lengthy stays in the ICU. Some of these survivors develop cognitive, psychiatric, or physical disability, or a combination thereof, after the ICU stay, a phenomenon termed post-intensive care syndrome (PICS).[58] The exact pathophysiology of this syndrome is not yet entirely understood. A growing body of evidence has implicated acute and chronic inflammation, as evidenced by persistently upregulated inflammatory cytokines, to be associated with cognitive dysfunction.[59] In particular, interleukin-6 (IL-6) and IL-10 serum concentrations within 48 hours of hospital discharge were significantly higher in ICU survivors with cognitive dysfunction, which was assessed by MMSE (< 24 points) at a median follow-up of 48 months.[60]

The IMPROVE (Improving the Recovery and Outcome Every Day after the ICU) study is currently enrolling subjects to evaluate the impact of physical exercise and cognitive training on ICU patients.[61] As a secondary aim of this study, numerous acute phase reactants, glial activation, neurotrophic factors (CRP, S100B, GFAP, BDNF, VEGF, and IGF-1), and cytokines (IL-1, IL-6, IL-8, and TNF-α) will be measured in the intervention and control groups. This study may shed light on possible biomarkers associated with post-ICU cognitive dysfunction.

Conclusion

In summary, there are numerous biomarkers that are being investigated to augment the clinician's ability to prognosticate for various neurocritical care pathologies (Table 23.1). Caution is warranted, since most of these biomarkers have not been reproduced in various studies nor are there clearly defined reference ranges or cut-off values. The validation of these biomarkers for each of the pathologies discussed in this chapter requires continued research to accurately assess their prognostic utility.

References

1. Mozaffarian D, Benjamin EJ, Go AS, et al. Heart disease and stroke statistics – 2015 update: a report from the American Heart Association. *Circulation.* 2015;**131**:e29–322.

2. May TL, Ruthazer R, Riker RR, et al. Early withdrawal of life support after resuscitation from cardiac arrest is common and may result in additional deaths. *Resuscitation* 2019;**139**:308–13.

3. Stammet P. Blood biomarkers of hypoxic-ischemic brain injury after cardiac arrest. *Semin Neurol.* 2017;**37**:75–80.

4. Ramont L, Thoannes H, Volondat A, et al. Effects of hemolysis and storage condition on neuron-specific enolase (NSE) in cerebrospinal fluid and serum: implications in clinical practice. *Clin Chem Lab Med.* 2005;**43**:1215–17.

5. Kaiser E, Kuzmits R, Pregant P, Burghuber O, Worofka W. Clinical biochemistry of neuron specific enolase. *Clin Chim Acta.* 1989;**183**:13–31.

6. Wijdicks EF, Hijdra A, Young GB, Bassetti CL, Wiebe S ; QSSotAAo. Practice parameter: prediction of outcome in comatose survivors after cardiopulmonary resuscitation (an evidence-based review): report of the Quality Standards Subcommittee of the American Academy of Neurology. *Neurology.* 2006;**67**:203–10.

7. Fugate JE, Wijdicks EF, Mandrekar J, et al. Predictors of neurologic outcome in hypothermia after cardiac arrest. *Ann Neurol.* 2010;**68**:907–14.

8. Reisinger J, Höllinger K, Lang W, et al. Prediction of neurological outcome after cardiopulmonary resuscitation by serial determination of serum neuron-specific enolase. *Eur Heart J.* 2007;**28**:52–8.

9. Steffen IG, Hasper D, Ploner CJ, et al. Mild therapeutic hypothermia alters neuron specific enolase as an outcome predictor after resuscitation: 97 prospective hypothermia patients compared to 133 historical non-hypothermia patients. *Crit Care.* 2010;**14**:R69.

Table 23.1 Summary of biomarkers associated with functional outcomes of various neurocritical care pathologies

Clinical Condition	Biomarker	Timing of samples	Functional outcome
Cardiac arrest	Neuron-specific enolase	24, 48, 72 hours post-CA	Significantly greater poor outcome with NSE > 80 μg/L ((CPC 3–5 and CPC 4–5)
	Neurofilament light chain	24, 48, 72 hours post-CA	NFL serum concentration at 24 hours post-CA had 69% sensitivity and 98% specificity for poor outcome (CPC 3–5)
	Micro-RNA-124-3p	24 hours post-CA	Mean levels of miRNA-124-3p of 8408 copies/μL with poor outcome (CPC 3–5)
	Muskelin and 14–3–3	6 and 24 hours post-CA	Qualitatively increased in with poor outcome (CPC 3–5)
	Presepsin	4, 12–36, 60–84 hours post-CA	Significantly higher in patients with poor outcome (CPC 3–5)
Intracerebral hemorrhage	Ferritin	3, 7, 14, 21 days after initial hemorrhage	Significantly higher ferritin on days 3 and 7 with poor outcome (mRS ≥ 3)
	CD163	1 and 7 days after initial hemorrhage	Significantly higher on day 1 in patients with poor outcome (mRS 4–6)
	Hepcidin	1, 3, 5, 7 days after symptom onset	Significantly higher on day 3 patients in poor outcome (mRS 3)
Acute ischemic stroke	Neurofilament light chain	Upon arrival to ED, 2, 3, 7 days, and 3 and 6 months post-onset of symptoms	Levels on day 7 post-stroke independently predicted outcome (mRS)
	S100B	Admission and 48 hours after symptom onset	Significantly higher at 48 hours in patients with poor outcome (mRS ≥ 3)
	Lipopolysaccharide-binding protein	Within 24 hours of stroke symptoms onset	Higher levels in patients with poor outcome (mRS ≥ 3)
Traumatic brain injury	Neuron-specific enolase	Upon admission, 24, 48, 72, and 96 hours after admission	Level at 48 hours predicted in-hospital and 6-month mortality
	S100B	Upon admission, then twice daily for 3 days	Levels obtained 12–30 hours after TBI predicted unfavorable outcome (GOS 1–3)
	Neurofilament light chain	Upon admission, 1, 2, 3, 4, 6, 8–9, 10–12 days, and 12 months after injury	Level obtained within initial 24 hours predicted unfavorable outcome (GOS 1–3)
	Glial fibrillary acidic protein	48 hours to 7 days after injury	Significantly higher in patients with unfavorable outcome (GOS 1–3)
Aneurysmal subarachnoid Hemorrhage	Cleaved receptor for advanced glycation end-products	Upon arrival to ED	Levels predicted poor outcome at 6 months (GOS 1–3)
	Neuroglobulin	Every 6 hours from admission to day 7	Higher levels were associated with poor outcome at 12 months (mRS > 3)
	Tumor necrosis factor-α	Post-SAH days 01, 2–3, 4–5, 6–8, and 10–14	Levels on post-SAH days 2–3 associated with poor outcome at 3 months (mRS > 2)
	TNF-α receptor 1	Obtained at time of digital subtraction angiography, < 24 hours from admission and < 72 hours after SAH onset	Levels predicted poor outcome at 6 months (mRS > 2)
Post-intensive care syndrome	Interleukin-6 and -10	Obtained within 48 hours before hospital discharge	Patients with highest 25th percentile levels had worse cognitive outcome at a median follow-up of 48 months (MMSE)

Abbreviations: CA: cardiac arrest; CPC: cerebral performance category; ED: emergency department; GOS: Glasgow Outcome Scale; MMSE: Mini-Mental Status Exam; mRS: modified Rankin Scale; NSE: neuron-specific enolase; NFL: neurofilament light chain; SAH: subarachnoid hemorrhage; TBI: traumatic brain injury; TNF: tumor necrosis factor.

10. Streitberger KJ, Leithner C, Wattenberg M, et al. Neuron-specific enolase predicts poor outcome after cardiac arrest and targeted temperature management: a multicenter study on 1,053 patients. *Crit Care Med.* 2017;**45**:1145–51.

11. Wiberg S, Hassager C, Stammet P, et al. Single versus serial measurements of neuron-specific enolase and prediction of poor neurological outcome in persistently unconscious patients after out-of-hospital cardiac arrest – a TTM-trial substudy. *PLoS One.* 2017;**12**:e0168894.

12. Rossetti AO, Carrera E, Oddo M. Early EEG correlates of neuronal injury after brain anoxia. *Neurology.* 2012;**78**:796–802.

13. Oddo M, Rossetti AO. Early multimodal outcome prediction after cardiac arrest in patients treated with hypothermia. *Crit Care Med.* 2014;**42**:1340–7.

14. Donato R. Functional roles of S100 proteins, calcium-binding proteins of the EF-hand type. *Biochim Biophys Acta.* 1999;**1450**:191–231.

15. Böttiger BW, Möbes S, Glätzer R, et al. Astroglial protein S-100 is an early and sensitive marker of hypoxic brain damage and outcome after cardiac arrest in humans. *Circulation.* 2001;**103**:2694–8.

16. Shinozaki K, Oda S, Sadahiro T, et al. Serum S-100B is superior to neuron-specific enolase as an early prognostic biomarker for neurological outcome following cardiopulmonary resuscitation. *Resuscitation.* 2009;**80**:870–5.

17. Stammet P, Dankiewicz J, Nielsen N, et al. Protein S100 as outcome predictor after out-of-hospital cardiac arrest and targeted temperature management at 33 °C and 36 °C. *Crit Care.* 2017;**21**:153.

18. Sandroni C, Cariou A, Cavallaro F, et al. Prognostication in comatose survivors of cardiac arrest: an advisory statement from the European Resuscitation Council and the European Society of Intensive Care Medicine. *Resuscitation.* 2014;**85**:1779–89.

19. Samaniego EA, Persoon S, Wijman CA. Prognosis after cardiac arrest and hypothermia: a new paradigm. *Curr Neurol Neurosci Rep.* 2011;**11**:111–19.

20. Kuhle J, Barro C, Andreasson U, et al. Comparison of three analytical platforms for quantification of the neurofilament light chain in blood samples: ELISA, electrochemiluminescence immunoassay and Simoa. *Clin Chem Lab Med.* 2016;**54**:1655–61.

21. Moseby-Knappe M, Mattsson N, Nielsen N, et al. Serum neurofilament light chain for prognosis of outcome after cardiac arrest. *JAMA Neurol.* 2019;**76**:64–71.

22. Sun P, Liu DZ, Jickling GC, Sharp FR, Yin KJ. MicroRNA-based therapeutics in central nervous system injuries. *J Cereb Blood Flow Metab.* 2018;**38**:1125–48.

23. Devaux Y, Dankiewicz J, Salgado-Somoza A, et al. Association of circulating microRNA-124-3p levels with outcomes after out-of-hospital cardiac arrest: a substudy of a randomized clinical trial. *JAMA Cardiol.* 2016;**1**:305–13.

24. Boyd JG, Smithson LJ, Howes D, Muscedere J, Kawaja MD ; Group CCCTB. Serum proteomics as a strategy to identify novel biomarkers of neurologic recovery after cardiac arrest: a feasibility study. *Intensive Care Med Exp.* 2016;**4**:9.

25. Tagnaouti N, Loebrich S, Heisler F, et al. Neuronal expression of muskelin in the rodent central nervous system. *BMC Neurosci.* 2007;**8**:28.

26. Foote M, Zhou Y. 14–3–3 proteins in neurological disorders. *Int J Biochem Mol Biol.* 2012;**3**:152–64.

27. Berg D, Holzmann C, Riess O. 14–3–3 proteins in the nervous system. *Nat Rev Neurosci.* 2003;**4**:752–762.

28. Qi Z, Zhang Q, Liu B, Shao F, Li C. Presepsin as a biomarker for evaluating prognosis and early innate immune response of out-of-hospital cardiac arrest patients after return of spontaneous circulation. *Crit Care Med.* 2019;**47**:e538–e546.

29. van Asch CJ, Luitse MJ, Rinkel GJ, et al. Incidence, case fatality, and functional outcome of intracerebral haemorrhage over time, according to age, sex, and ethnic origin: a systematic review and meta-analysis. *Lancet Neurol.* 2010;**9**:167–76.

30. Pinho J, Costa AS, Araújo JM, Amorim JM, Ferreira C. Intracerebral hemorrhage outcome: A comprehensive update. *J Neurol Sci.* 2019;**398**:54–66.

31. Yang G, Hu R, Zhang C, et al. A combination of serum iron, ferritin and transferrin predicts outcome in patients with intracerebral hemorrhage. *Sci Rep.* 2016;**6**:21970.

32. Garton ALA, Gupta VP, Christophe BR, Connolly ES. Biomarkers of functional outcome in intracerebral hemorrhage: interplay between clinical metrics, CD163, and ferritin. *J Stroke Cerebrovasc Dis.* 2017;**26**:1712–20.

33. Zhao N, Zhang AS, Enns CA. Iron regulation by hepcidin. *J Clin Invest.* 2013;**123**:2337–43.

34. Mehdiratta M, Kumar S, Hackney D, Schlaug G, Selim M. Association between serum ferritin level and perihematoma edema volume in patients with spontaneous intracerebral hemorrhage. *Stroke.* 2008;**39**:1165–70.

35. Xiong XY, Chen J, Zhu WY, et al. Serum hepcidin concentrations correlate with serum iron level and outcome in patients with intracerebral hemorrhage. *Neurol Sci.* 2015;**36**:1843–9.

36. Li W, Pan R, Qi Z, Liu KJ. Current progress in searching for clinically useful biomarkers of

blood-brain barrier damage following cerebral ischemia. *Brain Circ.* 2018;**4**:145–52.

37. Tiedt S, Duering M, Barro C, et al. Serum neurofilament light: A biomarker of neuroaxonal injury after ischemic stroke. *Neurology.* 2018;**91**: e1338–e1347.

38. Branco JP, Oliveira S, Sargento-Freitas J, et al. S100β protein as a predictor of poststroke functional outcome: a prospective study. *J Stroke Cerebrovasc Dis.* 2018;**27**:1890–6.

39. Klimiec E, Pasinska P, Kowalska K, et al. The association between plasma endotoxin, endotoxin pathway proteins and outcome after ischemic stroke. *Atherosclerosis.* 2018;**269**:138–43.

40. Gan ZS, Stein SC, Swanson R, et al. Blood biomarkers for traumatic brain injury: a quantitative assessment of diagnostic and prognostic accuracy. *Front Neurol.* 2019;**10**:446.

41. Rodríguez-Rodríguez A, Egea-Guerrero JJ, Gordillo-Escobar E, et al. S100B and Neuron-Specific Enolase as mortality predictors in patients with severe traumatic brain injury. *Neurol Res.* 2016;**38**:130–7.

42. Cheng F, Yuan Q, Yang J, Wang W, Liu H. The prognostic value of serum neuron-specific enolase in traumatic brain injury: systematic review and meta-analysis. *PLoS One.* 2014;**9**: e106680.

43. Thelin EP, Jeppsson E, Frostell A, et al. Utility of neuron-specific enolase in traumatic brain injury; relations to S100B levels, outcome, and extracranial injury severity. *Crit Care.* 2016;**20**:285.

44. Al Nimer F, Thelin E, Nyström H, et al. Comparative assessment of the prognostic value of biomarkers in traumatic brain injury reveals an independent role for serum levels of neurofilament light. *PLoS One.* 2015;**10**:e0132177.

45. Shahim P, Gren M, Liman V, et al. Serum neurofilament light protein predicts clinical outcome in traumatic brain injury. *Sci Rep.* 2016;**6**:36791.

46. Hol EM, Pekny M. Glial fibrillary acidic protein (GFAP) and the astrocyte intermediate filament system in diseases of the central nervous system. *Curr Opin Cell Biol.* 2015;**32**:121–30.

47. Shemilt M, Boutin A, Lauzier F, et al. Prognostic value of glial fibrillary acidic protein in patients with moderate and severe traumatic brain injury: a systematic review and meta-analysis. *Crit Care Med.* 2019;**47**:e522–e529.

48. de Oliveira Manoel AL, Macdonald RL. Neuroinflammation as a target for intervention in subarachnoid hemorrhage. *Front Neurol.* 2018;**9**:292.

49. Choi BR, Cho WH, Kim J, et al. Increased expression of the receptor for advanced glycation

end products in neurons and astrocytes in a triple transgenic mouse model of Alzheimer's disease. *Exp Mol Med.* 2014;**46**:e75.

50. Tang SC, Yeh SJ, Tsai LK, et al. Cleaved but not endogenous secretory RAGE is associated with outcome in acute ischemic stroke. *Neurology.* 2016;**86**:270–6.

51. Yang DB, Dong XQ, Du Q, et al. Clinical relevance of cleaved RAGE plasma levels as a biomarker of disease severity and functional outcome in aneurysmal subarachnoid hemorrhage. *Clin Chim Acta.* 2018;**486**:335–40.

52. Burmester T, Weich B, Reinhardt S, Hankeln T. A vertebrate globin expressed in the brain. *Nature.* 2000;**407**:520–3.

53. Ding CY, Kang DZ, Wang ZL, et al. Serum Ngb (neuroglobin) is associated with brain metabolism and functional outcome of aneurysmal subarachnoid hemorrhage. *Stroke.* 2019;**50**:1887–90.

54. Miller BA, Turan N, Chau M, Pradilla G. Inflammation, vasospasm, and brain injury after subarachnoid hemorrhage. *Biomed Res Int.* 2014;**2014**:384342.

55. Chou SH, Feske SK, Atherton J, et al. Early elevation of serum tumor necrosis factor-α is associated with poor outcome in subarachnoid hemorrhage. *J Investig Med.* 2012;**60**:1054–8.

56. Fragata I, Bustamante A, Penalba A, et al. Venous and arterial TNF-R1 predicts outcome and complications in acute subarachnoid hemorrhage. *Neurocrit Care.* 2019;**31**:107–15.

57. Adhikari NK, Fowler RA, Bhagwanjee S, Rubenfeld GD. Critical care and the global burden of critical illness in adults. *Lancet.* 2010;**376**:1339–46.

58. Inoue S, Hatakeyama J, Kondo Y, et al. Post-intensive care syndrome: its pathophysiology, prevention, and future directions. *Acute Med Surg.* 2019;**6**:233–46.

59. van den Boogaard M, Kox M, Quinn KL, et al. Biomarkers associated with delirium in critically ill patients and their relation with long-term subjective cognitive dysfunction; indications for different pathways governing delirium in inflamed and noninflamed patients. *Crit Care.* 2011;**15**:R297.

60. Maciel M, Benedet SR, Lunardelli EB, et al. Predicting long-term cognitive dysfunction in survivors of critical illness with plasma inflammatory markers: a retrospective cohort study. *Mol Neurobiol.* 2019;**56**:763–7.

61. Wang S, Hammes J, Khan S, et al. Improving Recovery and Outcomes Every Day after the ICU (IMPROVE): study protocol for a randomized controlled trial. *Trials.* 2018;**19**:196.

Chapter 24

New Frontiers in Neuroprognostication: Point-of-Care Ultrasonography

Collin Herman, Jonathan Gomez, and Aarti Sarwal

Background

Clinical examination is central to prognostication in acute brain injury but it has its limitations, especially in presence of confounders like sedation, recent cardiac arrest or lack of access to full exam due to concomitant injuries.[1–3] Lack of robust clinical prognostication tools has allowed the possibility of scenarios where clinicians may withdraw care prematurely due to a presumed poor prognosis based on a poor neurological exam.[4] Conversely, clinicians may defer prognostication in a confounded neurological exam and maintain patients on advanced life support for days before the degree of neurological injury becomes manifest.[5] In some of these scenarios, cerebral hemodynamic evaluation using transcranial Doppler (TCD) may provide a noninvasive surrogate to assess cerebral perfusion and augment available information to aid in prognostication.

Introduced in 1982 as a noninvasive means of assessing cerebral blood flow by measuring velocities in intracranial vasculature, TCD has become a mainstay for evaluation of cerebrovascular hemodynamics in stroke and subarachnoid hemorrhage. [6] TCD is a noninvasive tool for point-of-care assessment without any risk of radiation that is amenable to serial bedside evaluations. This portability and convenience of use has enabled novel explorations in understanding changes in cerebrovascular physiology in various diseases that cause acute brain injury and has opened an opportunity for integrating this modality into neuroprognostication.

In this chapter, we describe a case-based review to highlight use of TCD to help in prognostication from different perspectives (Table 24.1).

- Predict and manage an impending neurological insult
- Identify patients with significantly impaired perfusion where progression to irreversible injury is imminent

Table 24.1 Contribution of TCD as an imaging adjunct in various pathologies

Benefit of TCD in various pathologies	
Indication	**Contribution of TCD**
SAH	Detection of vasospasm or cerebral auto-regulatory dysfunction to guide clinical monitoring and treatment goals
ICP	Serial monitoring of ICP in patients where placement of invasive monitoring devices is contraindicated such as in the setting of coagulopathy, active anticoagulation therapy, or thrombocytopenia
Brain death	Ancillary test for determination of need of formal diagnostic assessment for cerebral circulatory arrest
Cardiovascular disease	Risk stratification for stroke and/or cognitive decline in cardiothoracic procedures, ECMO, and carotid disease
Cardiac arrest	Prognostication of survival by detection of unfavorable CBF characteristics and guide ECMO goals in critically ill patients
TBI	Assessment of CPP, ICP, and CBF for goal-oriented management to mitigate mortality
Ischemic stroke	Detection of patency of vessels post-thrombectomy/thrombolysis vs. re-occlusion, risk stratification of stroke reoccurrence, and goal-oriented management of BP in recanalized patients

Abbreviations: BP: blood pressure; CBF: cerebral blood flow; CPP: cerebral perfusion pressure; ECMO: extracorporeal membrane oxygenation; ICP: increased intracranial pressure; SAH: subarachnoid hemorrhage; TCD: transcranial Doppler.

- Provide surrogate of intact cerebral perfusion where additional clinical time and neurodiagnostics can be justified in a resource intensive environment

Epidemiology

Neurological disease accounts for significant morbidity and mortality in the United States (US). Stroke is also the fifth most common cause of death in the US, accounting for 1 out of every 20 deaths nationally.[7] The majority of mortality from stroke continues to be related to withdrawal of care, highlighting the importance of having objective neuroprognostication tools. In addition to stroke, other neurological conditions, for example, traumatic brain injury, hypoxic-ischemic brain injury, and brain tumors, result in significant hospitalizations and intensive care unit (ICU) admissions each year. Traumatic brain injury (TBI) affects 2.87 million people annually and nearly 57,000 of those die of TBI-related factors.[8] About 350,000 out-of-hospital and 750,000 in-hospital resuscitations are attempted for cardiac arrests each year with a survival rate of 5–9% and 20%, respectively. [9] Only 3–7% of survivors are estimated to recover to their pre-arrest functional status.[10] Any tools that can improve our prognostication algorithms in these neurological conditions could have a huge public health impact.

Public Health Impact

Approximately 795,000 people in the US have a stroke each year.[11] Most stroke patients require hospitalization, with an estimated $34 billion of direct and indirect annual costs associated with stroke.[11] This figure accounts for healthcare services, medications, long-term care in post-acute facilities, and productivity loss from disabled patients. Stroke is also a major cause of disability with over half of stroke survivors age 65 years or older suffering impaired mobility. Given the enormous financial cost of caring for patients with neurological disease and societal costs of disabled patients, it is crucial that we focus our care paradigms involving diagnostic testing, treatments, and level of care for each of these patients aimed at preventing further neurological morbidity. More than half of the total annual costs associated with stroke come from direct patient care.[11] Any interventions that can predict neurological decline in a high-risk patient and target early therapies especially in the critical care setting can have a significant financial impact. It is estimated that the incidence of stroke will continue to rise, with the majority of this expected increase occurring in the ever-growing elderly population (≥ 75 years old).[12] The annual direct medical costs from stroke are projected to triple by 2030. [13] Appropriate neuroprognostication to target level of care, early goal directed therapies, patient selection for resource intensive interventions, integrating quick and inexpensive testing like TCD can help optimize the ICU length-of-stay and total hospital length-of-stay, possibly mitigating this financial burden to some extent.

Neuroprognostication in Acute Settings

Predicting and Preventing Vasospasm in Subarachnoid Hemorrhage

Cerebral vasospasm is a well-known complication of aneurysmal subarachnoid hemorrhage (SAH), though it also occurs less commonly with traumatic SAH and ruptured vascular malformations. Cerebral vasospasm has a high incidence following aneurysmal SAH and is a significant contributor to morbidity and mortality by way of delayed cerebral ischemia.[14–16] TCD can be used to diagnose vasospasm by detecting characteristic changes of increased velocities on insonation. TCD has high sensitivity 90% (95% confidence interval [CI]: 77%–96%), specificity 71% (95% CI: 51%–84%), positive predictive value 57% (95% CI: 38%–71%), and negative predictive value 92% (95% CI: 83%–96%) in the diagnosis of vasospasm. [6, 17–21] Daily TCD screening during the window of vasospasm days 4–10 may help target patients who needs more frequent neuromonitoring. Much research has been devoted to cutoffs on TCD to predict clinical decline. Low or very high middle cerebral artery (MCA) flow velocities (< 120 or >2 00 cm/s) reliably predict the absence or presence of clinically significant vasospasm. Presence of sonographic vasospasm itself even without clinical symptoms is associated with poor outcome.[22] TCD evaluated derangement of autoregulation in SAH may also foretell vasospasm, which further causes worsening of autoregulatory response. Presence of cerebral autoregulatory dysfunction in the first few days after the event (days 1–6) has been shown to have a negative prognostic value.[23, 24] Combining such TCD parameters can guide patient selection for intensive clinical monitoring and treatment goals like

Case Study 24.1 An 82-year-old male was admitted with diffuse SAH secondary to ruptured left anterior communicating artery aneurysm. He was intubated in the emergency room due to low Glasgow Coma Scale (GCS) score with admission to the ICU and started on nimodipine prophylaxis. Patient underwent daily TCD examinations for surveillance of vasospasm. On hospital day 6, the left MCA mean velocity (MV) increased from 101 cm/s to 179 cm/s (Figure 24.1). No clinical decline was detected off sedation while patient remained intubated. Patient was taken for emergent cerebral angiography where he was found to have severe left MCA vasospasm and treated with intra-arterial verapamil. A follow-up magnetic resonance imaging (MRI) demonstrated left MCA territory infarction. Patient progressed to malignant cerebral edema and eventually transitioned to comfort care given poor prognosis.

Pearl: Our case highlights use of TCD monitoring in predicting vasospasm in absence of clinical decline.

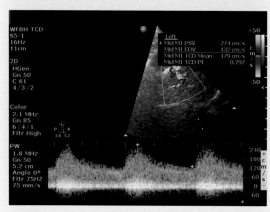

Figure 24.1 Left middle cerebral artery (MCA) velocity 179 cm/s with turbulent waveforms is consistent with moderate-severe vasospasm.

permissive hypertension prior to a neurological decline (Case Study 24.1).

Predicting or Ruling Out Increased Intracranial Pressure and Brain Death

Elevation in intracranial pressure (ICP) is a potentially lethal side effect of acute brain injury from various etiologies. The Monro–Kellie doctrine states that the volume within the cranial cavity, composed of blood, brain parenchyma, and cerebral spinal fluid (CSF), remains constant. Thus, a change of volume in any of these components will result in compensatory changes of the others, altering intracranial pressure.[25] Reliable ICP monitoring is of paramount importance with respect to neuroprognostication in many critically ill patients, and TCD is one of the few non-invasive options available to measure serial changes in ICP. Patients with elevated ICP may have contraindications to placement of an invasive ICP monitor such as anticoagulation or

thrombocytopenia. TCD may be an appealing option in such scenarios. TCD waveforms represent surrogates of cerebral perfusion pressure (CPP) and can represent response to ICP lowering therapies. TCD waveforms show predictable change in waveforms as cerebral blood flow is impaired in patients progressing with malignant cerebral edema. With gradual increase in ICP, the waveforms progress from resistive morphology with low diastolic flow, to obliterated diastolic flow, to reversal of diastole when ICP exceeds patient's diastolic blood pressure. If cerebral edema continues to progress despite therapy, these waveforms progress to systolic spikes and then complete absence of flow consistent with cerebral circulatory arrest. Insonation of patients revealing any of the resistive or oscillating waveforms can reflect upon patient's high ICP and serve as a poor prognostic sign unless the underlying injury is amenable to therapy.

A subset of critically ill patients may not be able to get traditional neuroimaging like computed tomography (CT) or MRI to assist in neuroprognostication. Such patients may be on high ventilator settings, high-dose vasopressors, on continuous dialysis that makes transport for CT or MRI challenging, or on extracorporeal membrane oxygenation (ECMO) for a cardiac arrest. They may have confounders like sedation, paralysis, and organ failure that impair ability to perform and use clinical neurological assessment and instrumentation challenges prohibiting convenient transport for neuroimaging. Surveillance TCDs can be key markers of physiological cerebral perfusion pressure to show whether or not a patient has malignant cerebral edema or CPP-impairing brain pathology (see Figure 24.2). It is important to note that parenchymal brain injury without mass effect cannot be ruled out with normal TCDs.[26] Side-to-side comparison of cerebral artery waveforms can be additionally helpful in ruling out compartmentalized caused of cerebral edema.

Transcranial Doppler is a useful ancillary test for determination of death by neurological criteria.[27] TCD provides a visual confirmation for impending cerebral circulatory arrest (CCA) when clinical scenario and underlying brain injury are consistent with irreversible malignant cerebral edema. Serial evaluations showing obliteration of the diastolic flow progressing to diastolic flow reversal despite maximal therapeutic interventions can be a negative prognostication sign and very accurate in indicating CCA. [28] Presence of small systolic spikes of < 50 cm/s amplitude and < 200 ms duration in intracranial vessels can be another sign of progression to CCA. A point-of-care study may trigger need for initiating clinical exam with apnea test and a follow up confirmatory full TCD study for brain death. While a full diagnostic study assessing anterior and posterior circulation would be necessary for declaration of brain death evaluation, a limited point-of-care evaluation can be very helpful to clinicians in distinguish brain death from mimics where TCD will show physiological waveforms (Case Study 24.2).

Predicting Stroke in Cardiovascular Disease and Cardiothoracic Procedures

Neurological complications occur in about 20% of patients undergoing cardiothoracic interventions and most occur in the perioperative period.[29]

Case Study 24.2 A 44-year-old female with a history of multiple myeloma presented to the emergency room after being found down at home by her family. She was found to have underlying cerebral venous sinus thrombosis requiring therapeutic anticoagulation and precluding the placement of an invasive ICP monitor. She underwent daily TCD examinations that showed a progressive change in waveforms to resistive and then reversed diastolic flow, consistent with increased ICP (Figure 24.2). This triggered aggressive medical management via osmotic therapy. Her cerebral perfusion was monitored using daily diagnostic TCD studies with limited point-of-care examinations as needed to guide further medical management. She experienced significant improvement in her waveforms and responded to venous thrombectomy with anticoagulation. She was eventually discharged to a skilled nursing facility.

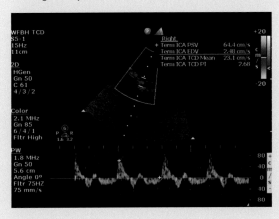

Figure 24.2 Intracranial internal carotid artery waveforms show an oscillating pattern with reversal of cerebral flow during diastole. If persistent, this pattern is consistent with grim prognosis and likely progression to brain death.

These complications may range from focal neurological deficits, confusion and memory deficits, and stroke with an incidence of 2–8%.[30] Patients who experience postoperative strokes exhibit an increased mortality.[31] There has been an emerging interest in the prevention of neurological injury in these patients by way of preoperative selection and intraoperative monitoring for patients deemed highest risk for intraoperative stroke. TCD has found a role in cerebrovascular monitoring both during preoperative evaluation as well as during cardiothoracic surgery. [32] TCD can detect hemodynamically significant stenosis in intracranial vessels, which predisposes patients to perioperative stroke. Positive emboli monitoring during some procedures has been directly linked to postoperative stroke.[33] Intraoperatively, patients may experience cardioembolic phenomena or sequelae of hypoperfusion during bypass transitions. [29,33] TCD can directly assess cerebral perfusion patterns and their responses, allowing for dynamic intraoperative monitoring of embolic signals.[34] The role of emboli phenomena in predicting stroke risk has been seen in infective endocarditis, myocardial infarction and other cardiovascular pathologies. [35]

Patients who undergo ECMO also have a high risk of neurological complications. [26,36] In children who did not suffer clinically apparent neurological injury, cerebral blood flow velocities were lower than normal while on ECMO and increased after decannulation.[37,38] However, children who developed cerebral hemorrhage had higher than normal cerebral blood flow velocities noted for days prior to clinical recognition of bleeding. Cerebral blood flow velocity measurement may represent a portable, noninvasive way to predict cerebral complications of ECMO and warrants further study.[38]

While current guidelines rely largely on degree of carotid stenosis to direct management, there is growing interest in further stratifying stroke risk in patients with asymptomatic carotid lesions to ensure optimal treatment. The identification of microemboli despite maximal medical therapy in these patients can help triage appropriate management of their lesion prior to a neurological event.[39]

Under physiological conditions, hypercapnia induces cerebral arterial dilation and increases cerebral blood flow that can be measured by TCD.[40] Cerebral vasomotor reactivity may be quantified by change in TCD-measured MCA mean flow velocities by inhaling 5% CO_2 in air as well as by hyperventilation.[41] In the presence of a flow-limiting stenotic lesion, compensatory intracranial vasodilation may be limited in response to hypercapnia. Studies have suggested that impaired vasoreactivity confers an increased risk for ischemic stroke ipsilateral to the stenotic lesion.[42–44] This can be of tremendous significance in patients with either symptomatic or asymptomatic carotid stenosis when the optimal management strategy is unclear. In such situations, TCD assessment of vasoreactivity helps assess risk of stroke and can guide the decision between surgical and medical management of the stenosed vessel. One study has demonstrated that impaired cerebral vasoreactivity in the setting of carotid stenosis was associated with a more rapid cognitive decline in patients with Alzheimer's dementia than in those with normal vasoreactivity.[45] Further investigation is warranted to determine whether vasoreactivity assessment may play a neuroprognostic role in this patient population (Case Study 24.3).

Prognostication after Cardiac Arrest

Survival rates are approximately 5–9% for out-of-hospital and 20% for in-hospital cardiac arrests.[9] Only 3–7% of survivors recover to their pre-arrest

---

Case Study 24.3 A 65-year-old patient with a history of lacunar stroke with no residual deficits but known left middle cerebral artery stenosis on dual antiplatelets agents needing coronary artery bypass surgery for coronary artery disease was evaluated using TCD. TCD confirmed hemodynamic significant stenosis preoperatively. Intraoperatively, the patient was monitored using continuous TCD to assess for drops in velocities during different stages of cardiopulmonary bypass. The anesthesia team targeted the patient's systemic blood pressure, carbon dioxide levels in blood, and flow metrics on the bypass pump to maintain perfusion across the left middle cerebral artery as reflected by TCD. Patient had an uneventful course and was extubated postoperatively without any neurological deficits.

functional status.[10] This is largely due to hypoxic-ischemic injury occurring during cardiac arrest itself as well as secondary injury occurring in the days following arrest. Multiple studies have demonstrated that TCD-derived values may predict functional outcome and survival in this patient population.[46–48]

Transcranial Doppler studies done during cardiac arrest showed that favorable outcomes were associated with higher MV and end diastolic velocities (EDV) suggesting that a lower cerebral vascular resistance (CVR) may yield a survival benefit in these patients.[49,50] Post-arrest patients who survive tend to have higher flow velocities, lower resistivity indices and no correlation between TCD velocities and systemic blood pressure suggesting preserved cerebral autoregulation.[46,47] In post-arrest patients who are too unstable to transport for conventional neuroimaging, such as in a those on ECMO, TCD has been shown to be a reliable modality to assess for certain neuropathology such as elevated ICP. Reversal of diastolic flow during post-arrest resuscitation has been shown to be associated with death or severe neurological deficits.[46,48] Normal mean flow velocity in the rewarming phase was associated with survival with favorable prognosis.[51] Using serial TCD examinations, patients with severely disabling or fatal outcome can be identified within the first 24 hours. TCD also has a role in individualization of hemodynamic and ventilation goals to ensure adequate cerebral perfusion and blood flow.[9] Specifically, TCD can help direct ECMO hemodynamic parameters to ensure adequate cerebral perfusion and promote favorable neurological outcome in such patients (Case Study 24.4).[52]

Case Study 24.4 A 33-year-old female suffered a witnessed out-of-hospital ventricular fibrillation arrest and was resuscitated to return of spontaneous circulation. She was admitted to the ICU for cardiogenic shock requiring veno-arterial ECMO. Deep sedation and paralysis while on ECMO impaired reliable neurological assessments. Patient also required hemodialysis. Patient's family and critical care providers requested neurological prognostication prior to the initiation of dialysis to ensure that patient was not kept alive in presence of malignant cerebral edema that would predict severe neurological injury in line with known advance directives. Patient was deemed too unstable for transport to obtain CT brain or other neuroimaging. TCD showed significant positive flow correlating to her mean arterial pressures and inconsistent with malignant cerebral edema (see Figure 24.3). This discovery encouraged continuation of aggressive resuscitative efforts directed at the management of underlying cardiac pathology. Patient continued to improve and was weaned off ECMO one week later. She eventually recovered kidney function and was discharged to an acute rehabilitation center.

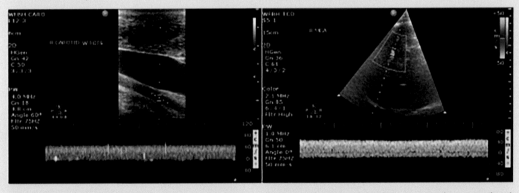

Figure 24.3 Right MCA waveforms in a patient on veno-arterial ECMO that shows a steady non-pulsatile waveform with a mean flow velocity of 40 cm/s consistent with physiological perfusion. Right carotid insonation in the patient showed microembolic signals that may be caused by air or thrombi. Prognostic significance of microembolic signals in ECMO is currently being investigated. ECMO: extracorporeal membrane oxygenation; MCA: middle cerebral artery

Traumatic Brain Injury

Neurological outcomes in TBI are contingent on the severity of initial injury as well as the degree of secondary cerebral injury from hypoxia, hypotension and ischemia.[53] TCD offers a noninvasive modality to measure real-time cerebral flow velocities to help assess CPP and cerebral blood flow (CBF).[24,54] Management strategies in TBI targeting optimal CBF, ICPs and CPPs have been shown to reduce mortality.[55,56]

In mild to moderate TBI, TCD-measured diastolic flow and pulsatility index (PI) may complement brain imaging as a screening tool to identify patients at risk of further neurological deterioration. [53] Cerebral hypoperfusion, measured through TCD as low-flow velocity in middle cerebral artery during first 72 hours of TBI, has been correlated with poor outcome at 6 months following TBI. [57,58] TCD evidence of vasospasm and hyperemia in the first 7 days after TBI also predicts a worse outcome at 6 months.[59] The highest mean flow velocity recorded, independent of vasospasm or hyperemia, has also shown to be also predictive of outcome.[59] Multiple studies have demonstrated the association between elevated PIs and poor neurological outcome in patients with TBI.[53,54,60]

Current guidelines in management of TBI, regardless of severity, do not include monitoring with TCD, but TCD can be used for CPP directed care as suggested by the guidelines to mitigate secondary ischemic injury (Case Study 24.5).

Outcomes after Ischemic Stroke

In patients with acute ICA thrombosis, TCD evidence of arterial occlusion together with stroke severity at 24 hours and CT lesion size have proven to be independent predictors of outcome at 30 days.[61] It is universally recognized that clinical course of stroke may present either spontaneous improvements or worsening in relation to dynamic changes in CBF. Thus, the detection of such hemodynamic changes with the use of TCD may have an important prognostic role.[62] This role has obviously changed with thrombectomy becoming standard of care for large vessel obstructions. In patients who are not thrombectomy candidates or unable to be recanalized, recanalization detected by TCD within 6 hours of symptom onset is related to clinical outcomes at 48 hours (odds ratio [OR]: 4.31, 95% CI: 2.67–6.97) and functional status at 3 months (OR: 6.75, 95% CI: 3.47–13.12). [63] Mortality is higher in MCA occlusion versus patent MCA on admission in patients when MCA occlusion persists hours after tissue plasminogen activator (tPA) bolus.[64] Early re-occlusion can be measured by TCD and predicts a significantly worse outcome at 3 months and a higher in-hospital mortality compared to sustained recanalization.[64] The presence of microembolic signals on TCD during the acute phase of stroke showed a correlation with early stroke recurrence.[39]

Transcranial Doppler may also play a prognostic role in post-recanalization management of cerebral

---

Case Study 24.5 A 36-year-old male presented with severe TBI manifested by low GCS score without evidence of polytrauma. Nonconstrasted CT scan of his head showed a traumatic right convexity SAH. TCD performed 3 hours following admission showed PCA pulsatility indices of 1.78 and 1.87 (see Figure 24.4). Given concern for increased ICP, an ICP monitor was placed and confirmed the presence of such. Patient was managed aggressively with hyperosmotic therapy but experienced minimal improvement in exam over the hospital stay. He was ultimately discharged to a skilled nursing facility.

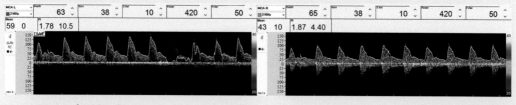

Figure 24.4 Left MCA showing resistive waveforms with a mean flow velocity of 59 cm/s but PI of 1.78 (normal 0.6–1.2). Right MCA shows a resistive waveform as well with mean flow velocity of 43 cm/s but PI 1.87. MCA: middle cerebral artery; PI: pulsatility index.

perfusion. Current stroke guidelines call for a blood pressure (BP) goal of < 180/105 mmHg in patients post-tPA therapy to prevent hemorrhage and to limit reperfusion injury.[65] Emerging literature suggests that in patients after thrombectomy achieving a Thrombolysis in Cerebral Infarction (TICI) score of 2B or 3 reperfusion, further blood pressure reduction to systolic BP < 140 mmHg in the first 24 hours may be beneficial despite engagement of collaterals in patients at higher blood pressure.[66–68] While induced hypertension can augment cerebral perfusion prior to recanalization, reperfusion injury after recanalization can cause cerebral edema and hemorrhage. A patient's underlying autoregulatory status may also play a role in this since long standing large vessel occlusions may cause loss of autoregulation and perfusion through collateralization. TCD is able to quickly and noninvasively assess the status of intracranial collateral circulation.[69] TCD markers of asymmetry in large vessels may portend ongoing ischemic and perfusion dependent symptoms.

In addition to the prognostic role that TCD can play in the acute setting of perfusion-dependent strokes and in predicting stroke risk in the outpatient setting, there is interest in the potential utility of TCD with respect to predicting functional recovery post-stroke. One small study has previously suggested that increased cerebral blood flow in the contralateral MCA is associated with improved aphasia recovery following ischemic stroke (Case Study 24.6).[70]

Gaps in Current Knowledge

Currently, many guidelines recommend the use of diagnostic studies such as MRI, EEG, and somatosensory evoked potentials (SSEP) in neuroprognosticating various conditions.[1,71] None of the algorithms has incorporated cerebral hemodynamic assessments like that which is offered by noninvasive TCD. While numerous studies have demonstrated that TCD is useful in the neuroprognostication of multiple disease states, there is still much to be established regarding the specific role TCD should play before it is included in these paradigms. For instance, while normal physiological waveforms can rule out the diagnosis of malignant cerebral edema at the time of assessment, it is unclear what the optimal frequency of serial examinations should be to detect sonographic changes prior to significant progression of the disease process itself. While it is known that TCD can help guide ECMO settings to ensure adequate cerebral perfusion, specific physiological ranges have yet to be established. Finally, certain waveforms that were once thought to represent poor prognosis (i.e. oscillatory waveform preceding CCA) may actually be reversible with aggressive therapy based on anecdotal reports. [72] The point at which these sonographic waveforms become truly irreversible and representative of a poor prognosis needs further evaluation in large clinical studies.

Ongoing Research

With growing concerns over the enormous expense of healthcare today, there is great interest in novel means of diagnosing, treating, and prognosticating disease in a cost-effective manner. Transcranial Doppler is actively being investigated in many conditions as a novel prognostic tool to identify high-risk patients and add to clinical prognostication.

Case Study 24.6 A 67-year-old male presented to the emergency department with dysarthria and a left hemiparesis concerning for acute stroke. CT angiogram revealed a complete right internal carotid artery occlusion that was recanalized emergently with mechanical thrombectomy and complete revascularization. He was admitted to the ICU for antihypertensive management to achieve a systolic blood pressure goal < 140 mmHg. Given persistence of symptoms in the hours post-reperfusion, an MRI brain was performed and showed no restricted diffusion. TCD showed relative hypoperfusion of the right middle cerebral artery compared to the left (see Figure 24.5A and 24.5B). Assuming patient had collateralization dependent perfusion with loss of autoregulation of right-side systolic blood pressure was augmented to 160 mm Hg resulting in clinical improvement. A follow-up TCD study showed improvement in right MCA perfusion (see Figure 24.5C and 24.5D). He was eventually discharged with more gradual normalization of blood pressures with a National Institutes of Health Stroke Scale (NIHSS) score of 0.

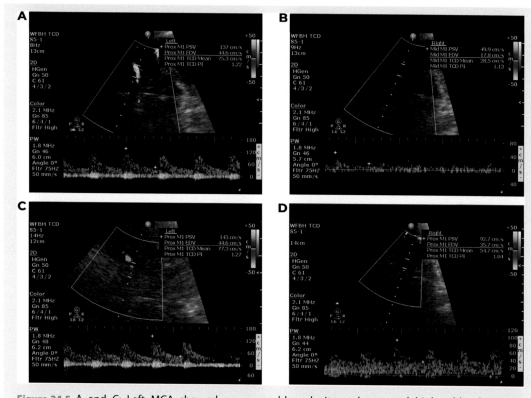

Figure 24.5 A and C: Left MCA showed a comparable velocity at lower and higher blood pressure suggesting preserved autoregulation. B and D: Right MCA showed hypoperfusion with low velocities that improved with induced hypertension. MCA: middle cerebral artery.

References

1. Sandroni, C, A Cariou, F Cavallaro, et al. Prognostication in comatose survivors of cardiac arrest: an advisory statement from the European Resuscitation Council and the European Society of Intensive Care Medicine. *Resuscitation* 2014;**85** (12):1779–89.

2. Samaniego, EA, M Mlynash, AF Caulfield, I Eyngorn, CA Wijman. Sedation confounds outcome prediction in cardiac arrest survivors treated with hypothermia. *Neurocrit Care* 2011;**15**(1):113–119.

3. Greer, DM, J Yang, PD Scripko, et al. Clinical examination for prognostication in comatose cardiac arrest patients. *Resuscitation* 2013;**84**(11):1546–51.

4. Geocadin, RG, CW Callaway, EL Fink, et al. Standards for studies of neurological prognostication in comatose survivors of cardiac arrest: a scientific statement from the American Heart Association. *Circulation* 2019;**140**(9): e517–e542.

5. Lorusso, R. Extracorporeal life support and neurologic complications: still a long way to go. *J Thorac Dis* 2017;**9**(10):e954–e956.

6. Aaslid, R, TM Markwalder, H Nornes. Noninvasive transcranial Doppler ultrasound recording of flow velocity in basal cerebral arteries. *J Neurosurg* 1982;**57**(6):769–74.

7. Yang, Q, X Tong, L Schieb, et al. Vital signs: recent trends in stroke death rates – United States, 2000–2015. *MMWR Morbid Mortal Wkly Rep* 2017;**66** (35):933–9.

8. Centers for Disease Control and Prevention. Surveillance report of traumatic brain injury-related emergency department visits, hospitalizations, and deaths – United States, 2014. US Department of Health and Human Services, 2019. Available at: www.cdc.gov/traumaticbraininjury/pdf/TBI-Surveillance-Report-FINAL_508.pdf.

9. Sinha, N, S Parnia. Monitoring the brain after cardiac arrest: a new era. *Curr Neurol Neurosci Rep* 2017;**17**(8):62.

10. Lim, C, MP Alexander, G LaFleche, DM Schnyer, M Verfaellie. The neurological and cognitive sequelae of cardiac arrest. *Neurology* 2004;**63**(10):1774–8.

11. Benjamin, EJ, MJ Blaha, SE Chiuve, et al. Heart disease and stroke statistics-2017 update: a report from the American Heart Association. *Circulation* 2017;**135**(10):e146–e603.

12. Howard, G, DC Goff. Population shifts and the future of stroke: forecasts of the future burden of stroke. *Ann N Y Acad Sci* 2012;**1268**:14–20.

13. Ovbiagele, B, LB Goldstein, RT Higashida, et al. Forecasting the future of stroke in the United States: a policy statement from the American Heart Association and American Stroke Association. *Stroke* 2013;**44**(8):2361–75.

14. Macdonald, RL, TA Schweizer. Spontaneous subarachnoid haemorrhage. *Lancet* 2017;**389** (10069):655–66.

15. Findlay, JM, J Nisar, T Darsaut. Cerebral vasospasm: a review. *Can J Neurol Sci* 2016 **43** (1):15–32.

16 Munoz-Sanchez, MA, F Murillo-Cabezas, JJ Egea-Guerrero, et al. [Emergency transcranial doppler ultrasound: predictive value for the development of symptomatic vasospasm in spontaneous subarachnoid hemorrhage in patients in good neurological condition]. *Med Intensiva* 2012;**36** (9):611–18.

17. Mascia, L, L Fedorko, K terBrugge, et al. The accuracy of transcranial Doppler to detect vasospasm in patients with aneurysmal subarachnoid hemorrhage. *Intensive Care Med* 2003;**29**(7):1088–94.

18. Rigamonti, A, A Ackery, AJ Baker. Transcranial Doppler monitoring in subarachnoid hemorrhage: a critical tool in critical care. *Can J Anaesth* 2008;**55** (2):112–23.

19. Lau, VI, RT Arntfield. Point-of-care transcranial Doppler by intensivists. *Crit Ultrasound J* 2017;**9** (1):21.

20. Connolly, ES Jr, AA Rabinstein, JR Carhuapoma, et al. Guidelines for the management of aneurysmal subarachnoid hemorrhage: a guideline for healthcare professionals from the American Heart Association/American Stroke Association. *Stroke* 2012;**43**(6):1711–37.

21. Kumar, G, RB Shahripour, MR Harrigan. Vasospasm on transcranial Doppler is predictive of delayed cerebral ischemia in aneurysmal subarachnoid hemorrhage: a systematic review and meta-analysis. *J Neuro*surg 2016;124(5):1257–64.

22. Schmidt, B, M Gunawardene, D Krieg, et al. A prospective randomized single-center study on the risk of asymptomatic cerebral lesions comparing irrigated radiofrequency current ablation with the cryoballoon and the laser balloon. *J Cardiovasc Electrophysiol* 2013;**24**(8):869–74.

23. Lang, EW, RR Diehl, HM Mehdorn. Cerebral autoregulation testing after aneurysmal subarachnoid hemorrhage: the phase relationship between arterial blood pressure and cerebral blood flow velocity. *Crit Care Med* 2001;**29**(1):158–63.

24. D'Andrea, A, M Conte, R Scarafile, et al. Transcranial Doppler ultrasound: physical principles and principal applications in neurocritical care unit. *J Cardiovasc Echogr* 2016;**26** (2):28–41.

25. Pinto, VL, P Tadi, A Adeyinka. *Increased Intracranial Pressure*. StatPearls. Treasure Island (FL): StatPearls Publishing, 2020.

26. Marinoni, M, G Cianchi, S Trapani, et al. Retrospective analysis of transcranial doppler patterns in veno-arterial extracorporeal membrane oxygenation patients: feasibility of cerebral circulatory arrest diagnosis. *Asaio J* 2018;**64** (2):175–82.

27. Ducrocq, X, W Hassler, K Moritake, et al. Consensus opinion on diagnosis of cerebral circulatory arrest using Doppler-sonography: task force group on cerebral death of the Neurosonology Research Group of the World Federation of Neurology. *J Neurol Sci* 1998;**159** (2):145–50.

28. Chang, JJ, G Tsivgoulis, AH Katsanos, MD Malkoff, AV Alexandrov. Diagnostic accuracy of transcranial Doppler for brain death confirmation: systematic review and meta-analysis. *Am J Neuroradiol* 2016;**37** (3):408–14.

29. Xu, B, Q Qiao, M Chen, et al. Relationship between neurological complications, cerebrovascular and cerebral perfusion following off-pump coronary artery bypass grafting. *Neurol Res* 2015;**37**(5):421–6.

30. van Dijk, D, M Spoor, R Hijman, et al. Cognitive and cardiac outcomes 5 years after off-pump vs on-pump coronary artery bypass graft surgery. *JAMA* 2007;**297**(7):701–8.

31. Palmerini, T, C Savini, M Di Eusanio. Risks of stroke after coronary artery bypass graft – recent insights and perspectives. *Interv Cardiol* 2014;**9** (2):77–83.

32. Thudium, M, I Heinze, RK Ellerkmann, T Hilbert. Cerebral function and perfusion during cardiopulmonary bypass: a plea for a multimodal monitoring approach. *Heart Surg Forum* 2018;**21** (1):E028–E035.

33. Bismuth, J, Z Garami, JE Anaya-Ayala, et al. Transcranial Doppler findings during thoracic

endovascular aortic repair. *J Vasc Surg* 2011;**54**(2):364–9.

34. Russell, D, R Brucher. Embolus detection and differentiation using multifrequency transcranial Doppler. *Stroke* 2006;**37**(2):340–1; author reply 341–2.

35. Dittrich, R, EB Ringelstein. Occurrence and clinical impact of microembolic signals (MES) in patients with chronic cardiac diseases and atheroaortic plaques–a systematic review. *Curr Vasc Pharmacol* 2008;**6**(4):329–34.

36. Melmed, KR, KH Schlick, B Rinsky, et al. Assessing cerebrovascular hemodynamics using transcranial Doppler in patients with mechanical circulatory support devices. *J Neuroimaging* 2020;**30**(3):297–302.

37. Salna, M, H Ikegami, JZ Willey, et al. Transcranial Doppler is an effective method in assessing cerebral blood flow patterns during peripheral venoarterial extracorporeal membrane oxygenation. *J Card Surg* 2019;**34**(6):447–52.

38. O'Brien, NF, MW Hall. Extracorporeal membrane oxygenation and cerebral blood flow velocity in children. *Pediatr Crit Care Med* 2013;**14**(3):e126–34.

39. Bazan, R, GJ Luvizutto, GP Braga, et al. Relationship of spontaneous microembolic signals to risk stratification, recurrence, severity, and mortality of ischemic stroke: a prospective study. *Ultrasound J* 2020;**12**(1):6.

40. Dahl, A, KF Lindegaard, D Russell, et al. A comparison of transcranial Doppler and cerebral blood flow studies to assess cerebral vasoreactivity. *Stroke* 1992;**23**(1):15–19.

41. Wolf, ME. Functional TCD: regulation of cerebral hemodynamics – cerebral autoregulation, vasomotor reactivity, and neurovascular coupling. *Front Neurol Neurosci* 2015;**36**:40–56.

42. Silvestrini, M, F Vernieri, P Pasqualetti, et al. Impaired cerebral vasoreactivity and risk of stroke in patients with asymptomatic carotid artery stenosis. *JAMA* 2000;**283**(16):2122–7.

43. Yonas, H, HA Smith, SR Durham, SL Pentheny, DW Johnson. Increased stroke risk predicted by compromised cerebral blood flow reactivity. *J Neurosurg* 1993;**79**(4):483–9.

44. Gur, AY, I Bova, NM Bornstein. Is impaired cerebral vasomotor reactivity a predictive factor of stroke in asymptomatic patients? *Stroke* 1996;**27**(12):2188–90.

45. Silvestrini, M, G Viticchi, L Falsetti, et al. The role of carotid atherosclerosis in Alzheimer's disease progression. *J Alzheimers Dis* 2011;**25**(4):719–26.

46. Wessels, T, JU Harrer, C Jacke, U Janssens, C Klotzsch. The prognostic value of early transcranial Doppler ultrasound following cardiopulmonary resuscitation. *Ultrasound Med Biol* 2006;**32**(12):1845–51.

47. Rafi, S, JM Tadie, A Gacouin, et al. Doppler sonography of cerebral blood flow for early prognostication after out-of-hospital cardiac arrest: DOTAC study. *Resuscitation* 2019;**141**: 188–94.

48. Lemiale, V, O Huet, B Vigue, et al. Changes in cerebral blood flow and oxygen extraction during post-resuscitation syndrome. *Resuscitation* 2008;**76**(1):17–24.

49. Blumenstein, J, J Kempfert, T Walther, et al. Cerebral flow pattern monitoring by transcranial Doppler during cardiopulmonary resuscitation. *Anaesth Intensive Care* 2010;**38**(2):376–80.

50. Lewis, LM, CR Gomez, BE Ruoff, et al. Transcranial Doppler determination of cerebral perfusion in patients undergoing CPR: methodology and preliminary findings. *Ann Emerg Med* 1990;**19**(10):1148–51.

51. Lin, JJ, SH Hsia, HS Wang, MC Chiang, KL Lin. Transcranial Doppler ultrasound in therapeutic hypothermia for children after resuscitation. *Resuscitation* 2015;**89**: 182–7.

52. Baghshomali, S, P Reynolds, A Sarwal. Transcranial doppler to assess cerebral blood flow in patients on extra corporeal membrane oxygenation (P4.236). *Neurology* 2014;**82**(10 Supplement):236.

53. Bouzat, P, M Oddo, JF Payen. Transcranial Doppler after traumatic brain injury: is there a role? *Curr Opin Crit Care* 2014;**20**(2):153–160.

54. Czosnyka, M, P Smielewski, P Kirkpatrick, DK Menon, JD Pickard. Monitoring of cerebral autoregulation in head-injured patients. *Stroke* 1996;**27**(10):1829–34.

55. Coles, JP. Regional ischemia after head injury. *Curr Opin Crit Care* 2004;**10**(2):120–5.

56. Rosner, MJ, S Daughton. Cerebral perfusion pressure management in head injury. *J Trauma* 1990;**30**(8):933–40.

57. Jaggi, JL, WD Obrist, TA Gennarelli, TW Langfitt. Relationship of early cerebral blood flow and metabolism to outcome in acute head injury. *J Neurosurg* 1990;**72**(2):176–82.

58. van Santbrink, H, JW Schouten, EW Steyerberg, CJ Avezaat, AI Maas. Serial transcranial Doppler measurements in traumatic brain injury with special focus on the early posttraumatic period. *Acta Neurochir (Wien)* 2002;**144**(11):1141–9.

59. Zurynski, YA, NW Dorsch, MR Fearnside. Incidence and effects of increased cerebral blood flow velocity after severe head injury: a transcranial Doppler ultrasound study II. Effect of vasospasm and hyperemia on outcome. *J Neurol Sci* 1995;**134** (1-2):41–6.

60. Jaffres, P, J Brun, P Declety, et al. Transcranial Doppler to detect on admission patients at risk for neurological deterioration following mild and moderate brain trauma. *Intensive Care Med* 2005;**31**(6):785–90.

61. Camerlingo, M L Casto, B Censori, MC, et al. Prognostic use of ultrasonography in acute non-hemorrhagic carotid stroke. *Ital J Neurol Sci* 1996;**17**(3):215–18.

62. D'Andrea, A, M Conte, R Scarafile, et al. Transcranial Doppler ultrasound: physical principles and principal applications in neurocritical care unit. *J Cardiovasc Echogr* 2016;**26**(2):28–41.

63. Stolz, E, F Cioli, J Allendoerfer, et al. Can early neurosonology predict outcome in acute stroke?: a metaanalysis of prognostic clinical effect sizes related to the vascular status. *Stroke* 2008;**39** (12):3255–61.

64. Alexandrov, AV, JC Grotta. Arterial reocclusion in stroke patients treated with intravenous tissue plasminogen activator. *Neurology* 2002;**59** (6):862–7.

65. Powers, WJ, AA Rabinstein, T Ackerson, et al. Guidelines for the early management of patients with acute ischemic stroke: 2019 update to the 2018 Guidelines for the Early Management of Acute

Ischemic Stroke: a guideline for healthcare professionals from the American Heart Association/American Stroke Association. *Stroke* 2019;**50**(12):e344–e418.

66. Nogueira, RG, AP Jadhav, DC Haussen, et al. Thrombectomy 6 to 24 hours after stroke with a mismatch between deficit and infarct. *N Engl J Med* 2018;**378**(1):11–21.

67. Goyal, M, AM Demchuk, BK Menon, et al. Randomized assessment of rapid endovascular treatment of ischemic stroke. *N Engl J Med* 2015;**372**(11):1019–30.

68. Hong, L, X Cheng, L Lin, et al. The blood pressure paradox in acute ischemic stroke. *Ann Neurol* 2019;**85**(3):331–9.

69. Gomez, J, S Wolfe, A Sarwal. Sonographic demonstration of a perfusion-dependent stroke with negative MRI and a flow-limiting stenosis. *Neurocrit Care* 2019;**32**(3):883–8.

70. Silvestrini, M, E Troisi, M Matteis, C Razzano, C Caltagirone. Correlations of flow velocity changes during mental activity and recovery from aphasia in ischemic stroke. *Neurology* 1998;**50** (1):191–5.

71. Carney, N, AM Totten, C O'Reilly, et al. Guidelines for the Management of Severe Traumatic Brain Injury, Fourth Edition. *Neurosurgery* 2017;**80** (1):6–15.

72. Kumar, G, AV Alexandrov. Vasospasm surveillance with transcranial doppler sonography in subarachnoid hemorrhage. *J Ultrasound Med* 2015;**34**(8):1345–50.

Index

Printed in the United States
by Baker & Taylor Publisher Services